Grant's Dissector

Edition 18

Grant's Dissector

Edition 18

Alan J. Detton, PhD
Associate Professor
Department of Pathology and Cell Biology at CUIMC
Columbia University Vagelos College of Physicians & Surgeons
New York, New York

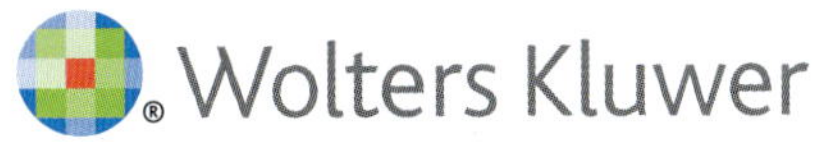

Philadelphia • Baltimore • New York • London
Buenos Aires • Hong Kong • Sydney • Tokyo

Acquisitions Editor: Crystal Taylor
Development Editor: Greg Nicholl (freelance); Amy Millholen
Editorial Coordinator: Marisa Solorzano-Taylor
Editorial Assistant: Parisa Saranj
Marketing Manager: Danielle Klahr
Production Project Manager: Bridgett Dougherty
Design Coordinator: Stephen Druding
Art Director: Jennifer Clements
Artists: Imagineeringart.com, Inc.; Dragonfly Media Group
Manufacturing Coordinator: Margie Orzech
Prepress Vendor: Absolute Service, Inc.

Eighteenth Edition

By A. J. Detton: Seventeenth Edition, 2021; Sixteenth Edition, 2017
By P. W. Tank: Fifteenth Edition, 2013; Fourteenth Edition, 2009; Thirteenth Edition, 2005
By E. K. Sauerland: Twelfth Edition, 1999; Eleventh Edition, 1994; Tenth Edition, 1991; Ninth Edition, 1984; Eighth Edition, 1978; Seventh Edition, 1974
By J. C. B. Grant: Sixth Edition, 1967; Fifth Edition, 1959
By J. C. B. Grant and H. A. Cates: Fourth Edition, 1953; Third Edition, 1948; Second Edition, 1945; First Edition, 1940

Seventeenth edition translations:
Chinese, Simplified (Beijing Science & Technology Publishing Co., Ltd.) (BSTP)
Spanish (Wolters Kluwer)

10 9 8 7 6 5 4 3 2

Printed in Mexico

Library of Congress Cataloging-in-Publication Data

Names: Detton, Alan J., author.
Title: Grant's dissector / Alan J. Detton.
Other titles: Dissector
Description: Edition 18. | Philadelphia : Wolters Kluwer, [2025] | Includes bibliographical references and index.
Identifiers: LCCN 2023043815 (print) | LCCN 2023043816 (ebook) | ISBN 9781975193669 | ISBN 9781975193683 (epub) | ISBN 9781975193690
Subjects: MESH: Dissection | Laboratory Manual | BISAC: MEDICAL / Anatomy
Classification: LCC QM34 (print) | LCC QM34 (ebook) | NLM QS 130 | DDC 611--dc23/eng/20231122
LC record available at https://lccn.loc.gov/2023043815
LC ebook record available at https://lccn.loc.gov/2023043816

shop.lww.com

QUADM0824

To the incredible women who have taught me so much and continue to bring inspiration to my life. Thank you for your examples of strength and determination through new beginnings, and for showing me how compassion, love, and character can always be present no matter the situation. I am so fortunate to have you in my life and love you all more than I can express.

I also wish to express my sincere gratitude and appreciation to the donors who have given all to the advancement of education and research without whom this work would not be possible.

Reviewers

Language and Inclusivity Consultant

Yasmin Carter, PhD
Associate Professor
Division of Translational Anatomy, Department of Radiology
UMass Chan Medical School
Worcester, Massachusetts

Clinical Reviewer

Alan M. Engler, MD
Clinical Assistant Professor
Department of Anatomy and Structural Biology
Albert Einstein College of Medicine
Bronx, New York

Faculty Reviewers

Abduelmenem Alashkham, PhD, MSc (Distinction), MBBCh
Anatomy, School of Biomedical Sciences
University of Edinburgh
Edinburgh, Scotland, United Kingdom

Steven W. Kubalak, PhD
Medical University of South Carolina
Charleston, South Carolina

Robert Terreberry, PhD
Jerry M. Wallace School of Osteopathic Medicine
Campbell University
Buies Creek, North Carolina

Brent J. Thompson, PhD
DeBusk College of Osteopathic Medicine
Lincoln Memorial University-Knoxville
Knoxville, Tennessee

Daniel B. Topping, MD
College of Medicine
University of Florida
Gainesville, Florida

Christopher T. York
Wake Forest University School of Medicine
Winston-Salem, North Carolina

Robert W. Zajdel, PhD
Upstate Medical University
State University of New York
Syracuse, New York

Jiepei Zhu, MD, PhD
Morehouse School of Medicine
Atlanta, Georgia

Preface

Grant's Dissector is intended to provide dissection instructions and enough anatomical detail to help students observe and recognize important relationships revealed through human dissection. The eighteenth edition of *Grant's Dissector* aims to continue the strong tradition of previous editions as a regional dissection instruction manual with an emphasis on streamlining the content for today's gross anatomy courses. As curricula are constantly changing, the modifications described here are intended to increase the adaptability of *Grant's Dissector* to a variety of dissection needs while maintaining an appropriate level of depth.

UNIT ORGANIZATION

The organizational flow in the eighteenth edition has been maintained for consistency throughout every chapter. The chapters are subdivided into units, which begin with a clearly labeled title and short summary of the region of interest followed by three key aspects to each dissection: an overview, the instructions, and a follow-up.

Dissection Overview

Clinical Correlations

The summary lists of clinical correlations are meant to provide a quick point of reference for students interested in the application of anatomical knowledge in the clinical setting, a key component to clinical gross anatomy instruction. The list of clinical correlates is found throughout the text at the start of each chapter and has been updated to include figure references from *Grant's Atlas of Anatomy*. For the first time, figures have been included within select clinical correlates to highlight anatomical variants or relationships key to comprehension of the anatomy related to a clinical condition or procedure.

Diversity and Inclusion

A conscious effort was made in this text to address inclusive language as well as highlighting the difference between sex and gender. Sex and gender are recognized as nonbinary distinctions, and acknowledgment is made that not all individuals may feel represented in the figures and descriptions in this text. It is hoped that the efforts to portray female representative anatomy first throughout this text, most notably in the chapter on pelvis and perineum, alongside references for female and male structures are seen as progress toward a more inclusive teaching and learning environment for all.

Skeletal and Surface Anatomy

The dissection overview introduces what is to be accomplished during the dissection session and includes step-by-step instructions to guide students through the relevant skeletal anatomy subdivided topically, followed by applicable surface anatomy. Commencing a dissection with the relevant skeletal features is meant to reinforce their anatomical relevance and lay a foundation for the surface anatomy that is then palpable on the cadaver. Similar to a clinical exam, a proper understanding of the skeletal and surface landmarks plays a key role in comprehension of the underlying anatomy during a dissection.

Dissection Instructions

Figure References

All dissection overview and dissection instruction sequences begin with a figure reference for the anatomical terms included in the subsequent instructions. The streamlined method of figure reference is meant to facilitate student comprehension of the association of multiple structures, minimize the amount of back-and-forth figure referencing, and provide a much higher association of all bolded terms to the presented figure.

Subcutaneous Tissue and Body Habitus

Definitions for *skin removal* versus *skin reflection*, as well as *full-* and *partial-skinning* techniques are provided in the Introduction Chapter. Additionally, each dissection sequence related to skinning includes updates to the colors used in the figures for required versus optional cut lines for improved clarity. The introduction figure representing the subcutaneous tissue has been updated to include a more detailed representation of the fat and fascial layers deep to the skin. Additionally, a more inclusive dialogue has been added to address varying amounts of subcutaneous tissue as related to body habitus.

Dissection Follow-up

Cadaver Care

Each dissection sequence ends with a Dissection Follow-up and includes a numbered list of tasks for the students to perform in the lab following the dissection and reminds students of proper care and cadaver maintenance throughout the entire dissection protocol. The numbered tasks highlight the important features of the dissection and encourage the synthesis of information through review of the material. The Dissection Follow-up also serves as a reminder of the text in the Introduction Chapter on cadaver care which includes a description of the students' "first patient" and the responsibility to properly care for the donor's remains.

Muscle Summary Tables

The 33 muscle summary tables introduced in the sixteenth edition in the Dissection Follow-up have been maintained and improved for accuracy in the eighteenth edition. The muscle summary tables provide succinct information related to muscles names, attachments, actions, and innervations of the key muscles identified during each dissection unit. The muscle tables provide a key review opportunity for students while simultaneously making the dissections steps in the instructions more task oriented and approachable.

KEY FEATURES

Expansion of Representative Skin Tones

A significant effort has been undertaken in this eighteenth edition to represent a broad and inclusive range of representative skin tones in patient populations. Figures include a range of skin tone variations throughout each chapter of the text.

New Illustrations

Significant effort has been made to update the style of many older illustrations in this volume of work including but not limited to those of the vertebral column, spinal cord, breast, diaphragm, and orbit. Cross-sectional images including the pelvis, abdomen, and neck have been updated to depict similar colors associated with fascial layers as seen in *Grant's Atlas of Anatomy*. New figures have been added for an alternative method of abdominal dissection with removal of the small intestine in isolation, as well as for clarification of the sequences pertaining to the pharynx, and head reflection or bisection. Additionally, figures for the external genitalia have been created or updated, including new figures of the female pelvis and perineum, as well as the cross-sectional anatomy of the clitoris.

ADDITIONAL RESOURCES

References to companion atlas and video material in the eighteenth edition of *Grant's Dissector* are now consistently listed next to the correlating section headings. In the printed text, two primary resources have been highlighted for supplemental instruction: *Grant's Atlas of Anatomy* (Atlas) and *Grant's Dissection Videos* (Video).

References to Atlas Illustrations

The student is encouraged to rely on *Grant's Dissector* for dissection instruction and to use *Grant's Atlas of Anatomy* for additional portrayal of anatomical structures. To facilitate figure searching, atlas references now refer to specific figure numbers rather than page numbers as seen in previous editions.

- Agur AMR, Dalley AF. *Grant's Atlas of Anatomy*. 16th ed. Wolters Kluwer; 2025.

References to Dissection Videos

The time stamp references (identified as "VIDEO" in the text) correlate to the companion series of high-definition videos, *Grant's Dissection Videos*, paralleling the instructions for each region of the body. Each dissection instruction protocol of the videos was performed, filmed, and edited by the author, Dr. Alan J. Detton. The dissections were performed on a single female and single male cadaver to replicate the dissection experience encountered by students within the laboratory environment.

Acknowledgments

Working on the eighteenth edition of *Grant's Dissector* has taught me perhaps more than ever the powerful and unique educational value that dissection offers. It is an incredible privilege to be able to appreciate first-hand the texture and feel of the tissues of the human body and to witness that despite the beauty of anatomical variation, each of us are far more similar than we are different. As I have progressed in my career while writing each edition of this text, I have felt a growing bond to those who also dedicate their time, passion, and energy to providing clarity in this unique educational modality.

I wish to express my continued and expanded gratitude for the significant contributions of the authors involved in the development of previous editions of *Grant's Dissector*. I look back on conversations with Patrick Tank with extreme fondness and hope that my vision for this work has aligned with the potential he would have also seen as efforts are made to make a more inclusive dissection companion.

I have been fortunate to have so many incredible colleagues and mentors along my somewhat unique career path. I acknowledge I cannot reference you all by name but know that I value our conversations at annual meetings, committees, and social settings and that I look forward to continued interactions with each of you.

To my incredible colleagues Anne Agur and Arthur (Art) Dalley, you continue to impress me with your dedication to creating educational resources of the highest quality. You have taught me so much about being an educator in all senses of the word, and I feel so honored to continue to have increased interactions with you in personal and professional capacities. I would like to express my thanks to Yasmin Carter who has helped this work progress in both subtle and direct ways. Yasmin, your passion for inclusion and raising awareness of the beautiful range of all people is truly inspirational. To have worked with you on elements in this text has been a privilege, and I look forward to increased collaborative efforts in the future. I wish to also express my appreciation for the advice, support, and guidance I received from Bob Acland while creating the dissection videos. Each time I reflect on how to demonstrate something, or portray a technique to be filmed, I reflect on his timeless advice that "the words must come first."

As always, I am so appreciative for the entire Wolters Kluwer team. Working with you at national and international events has been such a remarkable opportunity for which I am truly appreciative. Crystal Taylor, I value your support so much and hope to continue brainstorming new ideas and projects. Greg Nicholl, I am so glad you were brought in on this project once again and hope you remain involved moving forward. I put you through a lot in this edition, yet you continued to be supportive as you negotiated and delivered so much more than I could have hoped for. I would also like to thank Jennifer Clements and the entire art and editorial teams for the support of changing and incorporating so many figures and updates to a single edition. This has truly been a team effort and your work is recognized and greatly appreciated.

Alan J. Detton

Contents

CHAPTER 7
Neck and Head 265

List of Clinical Correlations

List of Tables

Figure Credits

CHAPTER 1

FIGURE 1.1B Modified from Gest TR. *Lippincott Atlas of Anatomy.* 2nd ed. Wolters Kluwer; 2020.

FIGURE B1.1 Modified from Agur AMR, Dalley AF. *Moore's Essential Clinical Anatomy.* 7th ed. Wolters Kluwer; 2024.

CHAPTER 2

FIGURE 2.9 Modified from Agur AMR, Dalley AF. *Grant's Atlas of Anatomy.* 16th ed. Wolters Kluwer; 2025.

FIGURE 2.14 Modified from Agur AMR, Dalley AF. *Grant's Atlas of Anatomy.* 16th ed. Wolters Kluwer; 2025.

FIGURE 2.15 Modified from Agur AMR, Dalley AF. *Grant's Atlas of Anatomy.* 16th ed. Wolters Kluwer; 2025.

FIGURE 2.23 Modified from Agur AMR, Dalley AF. *Grant's Atlas of Anatomy.* 16th ed. Wolters Kluwer; 2025.

FIGURE 2.26 Modified from Agur AMR, Dalley AF. *Grant's Atlas of Anatomy.* 16th ed. Wolters Kluwer; 2025.

FIGURE 2.27 Modified from Agur AMR, Dalley AF. *Grant's Atlas of Anatomy.* 16th ed. Wolters Kluwer; 2025.

FIGURE 2.28 Modified from Agur AMR, Dalley AF. *Grant's Atlas of Anatomy.* 16th ed. Wolters Kluwer; 2025.

FIGURE 2.29 Modified from Agur AMR, Dalley AF. *Grant's Atlas of Anatomy.* 16th ed. Wolters Kluwer; 2025.

FIGURE 2.32 Modified from Agur AMR, Dalley AF. *Grant's Atlas of Anatomy.* 16th ed. Wolters Kluwer; 2025.

FIGURE 2.40 Modified from Agur AMR, Dalley AF. *Grant's Atlas of Anatomy.* 16th ed. Wolters Kluwer; 2025.

FIGURE 2.41 Modified from Agur AMR, Dalley AF. *Grant's Atlas of Anatomy.* 16th ed. Wolters Kluwer; 2025.

FIGURE 2.42 Modified from Agur AMR, Dalley AF. *Grant's Atlas of Anatomy.* 16th ed. Wolters Kluwer; 2025.

FIGURE 2.43 Modified from Agur AMR, Dalley AF. *Grant's Atlas of Anatomy.* 16th ed. Wolters Kluwer; 2025.

FIGURE 2.46 Modified from Agur AMR, Dalley AF. *Grant's Atlas of Anatomy.* 16th ed. Wolters Kluwer; 2025.

FIGURE 2.47A Modified from Agur AMR, Dalley AF. *Grant's Atlas of Anatomy.* 16th ed. Wolters Kluwer; 2025.

FIGURE 2.48 Modified from Agur AMR, Dalley AF. *Grant's Atlas of Anatomy.* 16th ed. Wolters Kluwer; 2025.

CHAPTER 3

FIGURE 3.7 Modified from Agur AMR, Dalley AF. *Grant's Atlas of Anatomy.* 16th ed. Wolters Kluwer; 2025.

FIGURE 3.9 Modified from Agur AMR, Dalley AF. *Moore's Essential Clinical Anatomy.* 7th ed. Wolters Kluwer; 2024.

FIGURE 3.11 Modified from Gest TR. *Lippincott Atlas of Anatomy.* 2nd ed. Wolters Kluwer; 2020.

FIGURE 3.12 Modified from Gest TR. *Lippincott Atlas of Anatomy.* 2nd ed. Wolters Kluwer; 2020.

FIGURE 3.13 Modified from Agur AMR, Dalley AF. *Moore's Essential Clinical Anatomy.* 7th ed. Wolters Kluwer; 2024.

FIGURE 3.15 Modified from Gest TR. *Lippincott Atlas of Anatomy.* 2nd ed. Wolters Kluwer; 2020.

FIGURE 3.16 Modified from Gest TR. *Lippincott Atlas of Anatomy.* 2nd ed. Wolters Kluwer; 2020.

FIGURE 3.17B Modified from Agur AMR, Dalley AF. *Grant's Atlas of Anatomy.* 16th ed. Wolters Kluwer; 2025.

FIGURE 3.18 Modified from Gest TR. *Lippincott Atlas of Anatomy.* 2nd ed. Wolters Kluwer; 2020.

FIGURE 3.19 Modified from Gest TR. *Lippincott Atlas of Anatomy.* 2nd ed. Wolters Kluwer; 2020.

FIGURE 3.22 Modified from Gest TR. *Lippincott Atlas of Anatomy.* 2nd ed. Wolters Kluwer; 2020.

FIGURE 3.24 Modified from Agur AMR, Dalley AF. *Grant's Atlas of Anatomy.* 16th ed. Wolters Kluwer; 2025.

FIGURE 3.25 Modified from Agur AMR, Dalley AF. *Moore's Essential Clinical Anatomy.* 7th ed. Wolters Kluwer; 2024.

FIGURE 3.26 Modified from Agur AMR, Dalley AF. *Moore's Essential Clinical Anatomy.* 7th ed. Wolters Kluwer; 2024.

FIGURE 3.27 Modified from Gest TR. *Lippincott Atlas of Anatomy.* 2nd ed. Wolters Kluwer; 2020.

FIGURE 3.28 Modified from Gest TR. *Lippincott Atlas of Anatomy.* 2nd ed. Wolters Kluwer; 2020.

CHAPTER 4

FIGURE 4.16 Modified from Gest TR. *Lippincott Atlas of Anatomy.* 2nd ed. Wolters Kluwer; 2020.

FIGURE 4.17 Modified from Gest TR. *Lippincott Atlas of Anatomy.* 2nd ed. Wolters Kluwer; 2020.

FIGURE 4.18 Modified from Gest TR. *Lippincott Atlas of Anatomy.* 2nd ed. Wolters Kluwer; 2020.

FIGURE 4.19 Modified from Agur AMR, Dalley AF. *Grant's Atlas of Anatomy.* 16th ed. Wolters Kluwer; 2025.

FIGURE 4.21 Modified from Agur AMR, Dalley AF. *Grant's Atlas of Anatomy.* 16th ed. Wolters Kluwer; 2025.

FIGURE 4.27 Modified from Agur AMR, Dalley AF. *Grant's Atlas of Anatomy.* 16th ed. Wolters Kluwer; 2025.

FIGURE 4.28 Modified from Gest TR. *Lippincott Atlas of Anatomy.* 2nd ed. Wolters Kluwer; 2020.

FIGURE 4.29 Modified from Gest TR. *Lippincott Atlas of Anatomy.* 2nd ed. Wolters Kluwer; 2020.

FIGURE 4.31 Modified from Gest TR. *Lippincott Atlas of Anatomy.* 2nd ed. Wolters Kluwer; 2020.

FIGURE 4.32 Modified from Gest TR. *Lippincott Atlas of Anatomy.* 2nd ed. Wolters Kluwer; 2020.

FIGURE 4.47 Modified from Agur AMR, Dalley AF. *Grant's Atlas of Anatomy.* 16th ed. Wolters Kluwer; 2025.

FIGURE B4.2 Dalley AF, Agur AMR. *Moore's Clinically Oriented Anatomy*. 9th ed. Wolters Kluwer; 2023.

CHAPTER 5

FIGURE 5.2 Modified from Gest TR. *Lippincott Atlas of Anatomy*. 2nd ed. Wolters Kluwer; 2020.

FIGURE 5.8 Modified from Gest TR. *Lippincott Atlas of Anatomy*. 2nd ed. Wolters Kluwer; 2020.

FIGURE 5.11 Modified from Agur AMR, Dalley AF. *Moore's Essential Clinical Anatomy*. 7th ed. Wolters Kluwer; 2024.

FIGURE 5.13 Modified from Agur AMR, Dalley AF. *Grant's Atlas of Anatomy*. 16th ed. Wolters Kluwer; 2025.

FIGURE 5.18 Modified from Gest TR. *Lippincott Atlas of Anatomy*. 2nd ed. Wolters Kluwer; 2020.

FIGURE 5.20 Modified from Gest TR. *Lippincott Atlas of Anatomy*. 2nd ed. Wolters Kluwer; 2020.

FIGURE 5.35 Modified from Dalley AF, Agur AMR. *Moore's Clinically Oriented Anatomy*. 9th ed. Wolters Kluwer; 2023.

FIGURE 5.40 Modified from Gest TR. *Lippincott Atlas of Anatomy*. 2nd ed. Wolters Kluwer; 2020.

FIGURE 5.41 Modified from Gest TR. *Lippincott Atlas of Anatomy*. 2nd ed. Wolters Kluwer; 2020.

CHAPTER 6

FIGURE 6.19 Modified from Gest TR. *Lippincott Atlas of Anatomy*. 2nd ed. Wolters Kluwer; 2020.

FIGURE 6.22 Modified from Gest TR. *Lippincott Atlas of Anatomy*. 2nd ed. Wolters Kluwer; 2020.

FIGURE 6.30 Modified from Gest TR. *Lippincott Atlas of Anatomy*. 2nd ed. Wolters Kluwer; 2020.

FIGURE 6.31 Modified from Gest TR. *Lippincott Atlas of Anatomy*. 2nd ed. Wolters Kluwer; 2020.

FIGURE 6.32 Modified from Gest TR. *Lippincott Atlas of Anatomy*. 2nd ed. Wolters Kluwer; 2020.

FIGURE 6.33 Modified from Gest TR. *Lippincott Atlas of Anatomy*. 2nd ed. Wolters Kluwer; 2020.

CHAPTER 7

FIGURE 7.12 Modified from Gest TR. *Lippincott Atlas of Anatomy*. 2nd ed. Wolters Kluwer; 2020.

FIGURE 7.14 Modified from Gest TR. *Lippincott Atlas of Anatomy*. 2nd ed. Wolters Kluwer; 2020.

FIGURE 7.16 Modified from Agur AMR, Dalley AF. *Grant's Atlas of Anatomy*. 16th ed. Wolters Kluwer; 2025.

FIGURE 7.17 Modified from Agur AMR, Dalley AF. *Grant's Atlas of Anatomy*. 16th ed. Wolters Kluwer; 2025.

FIGURE 7.21 Modified from Gest TR. *Lippincott Atlas of Anatomy*. 2nd ed. Wolters Kluwer; 2020.

FIGURE 7.25 Modified from Gest TR. *Lippincott Atlas of Anatomy*. 2nd ed. Wolters Kluwer; 2020.

FIGURE 7.38 Modified from Agur AMR, Dalley AF. *Grant's Atlas of Anatomy*. 16th ed. Wolters Kluwer; 2025.

FIGURE 7.69 Modified from Agur AMR, Dalley AF. *Grant's Atlas of Anatomy*. 16th ed. Wolters Kluwer; 2025.

Introduction

YOUR FIRST PATIENT

The opportunity to dissect a human body is a once in a lifetime experience. It is not possible to fully appreciate the motivation of an individual to become a full body donor, but most of us will try to imagine the circumstances leading to that decision. The value of the gift that has been given to you cannot be measured and can only be repaid by proper care and use of the cadaver. The cadaver must be treated with the same respect and dignity reserved for the living patient. It is recommended that prior to commencing dissection, a moment be taken to consider the life of your donor, the incredible gift your donor has provided for your education, and the proper amount of care and respect you wish to honor your donor with during the dissections.

CADAVER CARE

Upon entering the laboratory, you will find that the cadaver has been embalmed with a strong fixative. The whole body has been kept moist by wrappings, submersion under preservative fluid, or a body bag. Desiccation of the cadaver will make the specimen much more difficult to work with and study because once a part has been allowed to become dry, it can never be fully restored. Therefore, expose only those parts of the body that you are currently working on and moisten any exposed regions periodically throughout the dissection. At the end of each dissection session, moisten the wrappings and cadaver with wetting solution and properly cover the cadaver following the protocols of your laboratory.

DISSECTION INSTRUMENTS

It is generally true that large dissection equipment (hammers, chisels, saws, etc.) will be provided for you, but personal dissection instruments may need to be purchased. The well-equipped dissector should have the following instruments (FIGURE I.1):

- **Probe**—an excellent blunt dissection tool to be used for investigation of a new region along with your fingers. A probe is designed to tear connective tissue and allow the user to feel the nerves and vessels before they

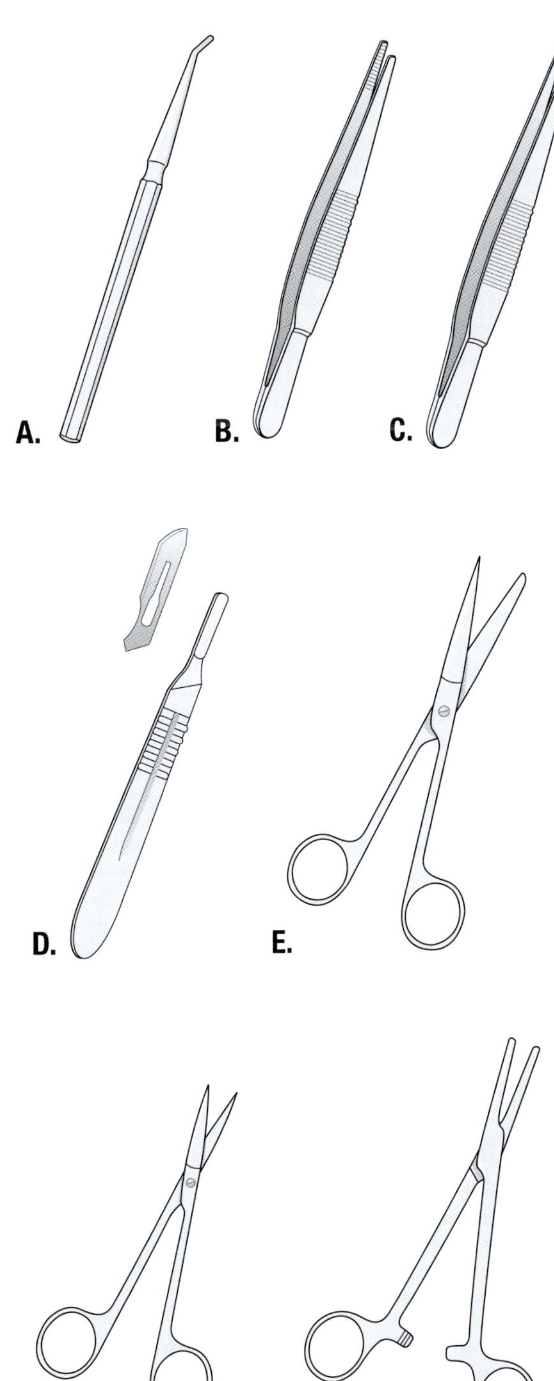

FIGURE I.1 ● Dissection instruments. **A.** Probe. **B.** Forceps. **C.** Tissue (rat-toothed) forceps. **D.** Scalpel handle and blade. **E.** Large blunt-ended scissors. **F.** Small sharp-ended scissors. **G.** Hemostat.

are damaged. With practice, the probe can become a primary dissection instrument to isolate and clean delicate structures.

- **Forceps**—used to lift and hold vessels, nerves, and other structures while blunt dissecting with a probe. Two pairs of forceps are needed. One pair should have tips that are blunt and rounded, and the gripping surfaces should be corrugated. The second pair should have teeth (also known as tissue forceps or rat-toothed forceps) for gripping tissue.
- **Scalpel**—primarily used as a skinning tool. Scalpels are not recommended for general dissection because they cut small structures without allowing you to feel them. The scalpel handle should be made of metal (not plastic). The blade should be about 3.5 to 4 cm long. The cutting edge must have some convexity near the point. The scalpel should be held in a grip similar to holding a pencil, and a sharp blade must be used at all times for most effective implementation. Therefore, a sufficient supply of blades will be needed. To avoid injury, seek assistance the first time you place and remove a scalpel blade.
- **Scissors**—useful in cutting, blunt dissection, and transection. Two pairs of scissors are recommended: a large, heavy pair of dissecting scissors (about 15 cm in length) and a small pair of scissors with two sharp points for the dissection of delicate structures.
- **Hemostat**—a powerful grasping tool that is helpful in skin removal. The advantage of hemostats is the ability to lock the grip on the slippery surfaces such as skin to facilitate reflection or removal of tissue. However, the hemostat has two disadvantages: First, it crushes delicate structures. Second, it cannot be repositioned quickly like forceps can, thereby slowing progress. Hemostats and scissors should be held with the thumb and 4th finger in the finger loops for the most control and precision.

GLOSSARY OF DISSECTION TERMS

This dissection manual repeatedly uses dissection terms. Before beginning to dissect, learn the meaning of the following:

- **Dissect**—to cut apart. In the context of this dissection manual, the meaning of dissect is to tear apart or separate. The recommended dissection approach throughout this manual is blunt dissection. The scalpel should only be used for skin incisions or as a tool of last resort for crude cuts to dissect extremely tough connective tissues.
- **Blunt dissection**—to separate structures with your fingers, a probe, or scissors by tearing (not cutting) connective tissues.
- **Scissors technique**—a method of blunt dissection in which the tips of a closed pair of scissors are inserted into connective tissue and then opened, tearing the connective tissue with the back edge of the tips. The scissors technique is an effective way to dissect vessels and nerves as illustrated in FIGURE I.2.

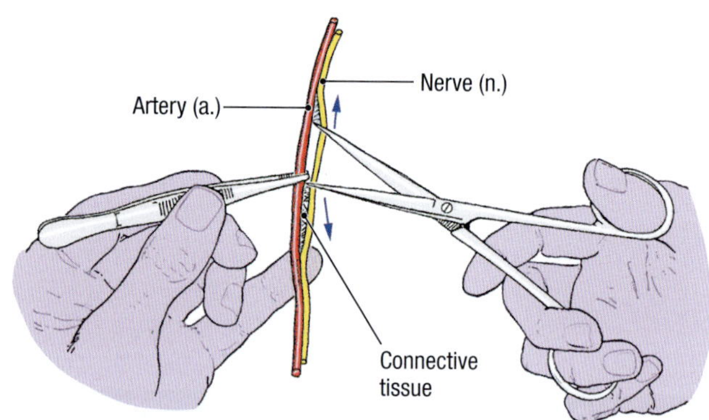

FIGURE I.2 ● Scissors technique for separating structures with blunt dissection.

- **Sharp dissection**—to dissect by use of a scalpel or the cutting edge of the scissors. The scalpel or scissors should only be used in conjunction with forceps.
- **Clean**—to remove fat and connective tissue, by means of blunt dissection (preferred) or sharp dissection, to expose the surface of an anatomical structure for study. Tissue from the surface of a structure can be removed by sharp dissection by cutting through the fascia and connective tissue after it has been separated from the desired structure with blunt dissection.
  - **Clean the surface of a muscle**—to remove all fat and connective tissue so the muscle fascicles become obvious and the direction of force can be understood.
  - **Clean the border of a muscle**—to define the border of a muscle with blunt dissection by breaking the loose connective tissue that binds the muscle to surrounding structures.
  - **Clean a nerve**—to use a probe (or scissors technique) to strip the connective tissue around the nerve for purposes of observing its relationships and branches.
  - **Clean a vessel**—to use a probe (or scissors technique) to strip the fat and connective tissue off the surface of a vessel, or its branches, to illustrate its relationships.
- **Define**—to use blunt dissection to enhance a structure to better illustrate its relationships. Defining a structure usually involves bluntly dissecting the loose connective tissue away from it.
- **Retract**—to pull a structure to one side to visualize another structure that lies more deeply. Retraction is a temporary displacement and is not intended to harm the retracted structure.
- **Transect**—to cut a structure in two in the transverse plane, as in transection of a muscle belly or tendon.
- **Reflect**—to fold back from a cut edge, as in folding back a transected muscle to view what is beneath it. The reflected tissue should remain attached to the specimen.
- **Strip a vein**—to remove a vein and its tributaries from the dissection field so that the artery and related structures can be seen more clearly. Veins are stripped either by blunt dissection using a probe or carefully with scissors using a combination of blunt and sharp dissection techniques.

ANATOMICAL POSITION

Anatomists describe the position and relation of structures of the body relative to the *anatomical position* as illustrated in FIGURE I.3. In anatomical position, an able-bodied person would stand erect with the face and feet directed forward and arms by the sides with palms facing forward. During dissection, structures are described as though the body was in the anatomical position, even though the cadaver is lying on a dissection table either **supine** (face up) or **prone** (face down). When encountering a structure during dissection, be aware of its position, its relationship to other structures, its size and shape, its function, its blood supply, and its nerve supply. Learn to give an accurate account of each important structure in an orderly and logical fashion by describing it to your lab partners. Always base your descriptions of structures and relationships on anatomical position.

ANATOMICAL PLANES

With the body in anatomical position, anatomists describe three directional planes that intersect the body as points of reference for either structure location or movement (FIGURE I.3). With the exception of the **median (midsagittal) plane**, the anatomical planes may be found at any level parallel to the original point of reference. A clear understanding of anatomical planes will assist your understanding of cross-sectional anatomy and diagnostic imaging. The cross-sectional images seen in this dissection guide represent axial views of various body regions as viewed from inferior to superior.

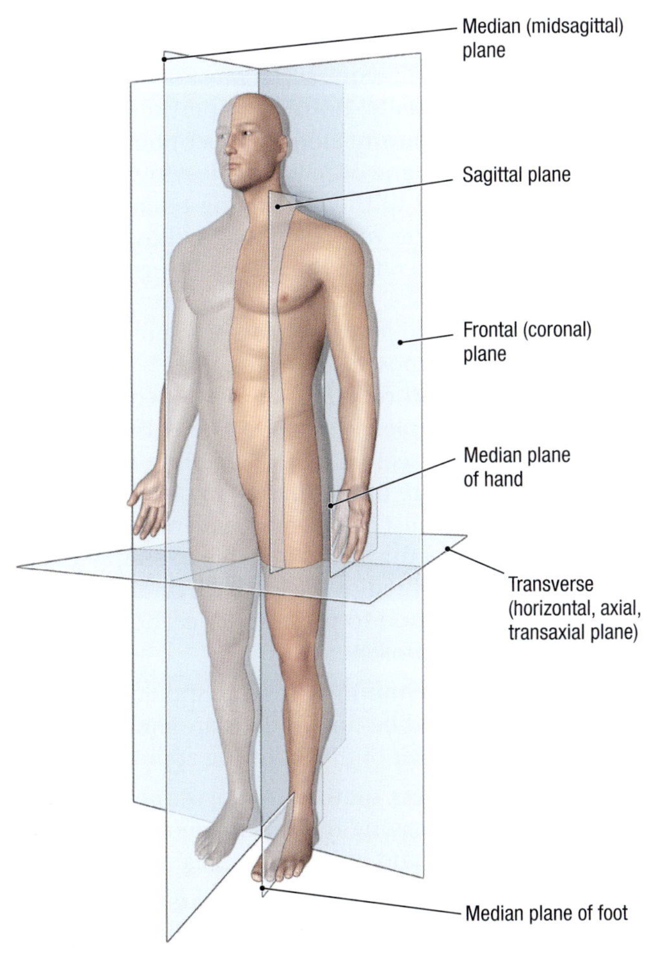

FIGURE I.3 ● Anatomical position and anatomical planes. Anterolateral view.

- **Sagittal planes** course vertically through the body and divide the body into right and left halves. Often, sagittal planes are given a specific point of reference to assist physicians in identification of structures correlating to that point, such as a midclavicular, a sagittal plane passing midway through the clavicle.
  - **Median plane (midsagittal plane)** is the sagittal plane that lies in the midline of the body cutting vertically through the axis to divide the body into "equal" right and left halves. **Medial** is a term used to describe structures closer to the median plane, and **lateral** is a term used to describe structures further from the median plane.
- **Frontal (coronal) planes** course vertically through the body at a right angle to the median plane and divide the body into **anterior/ventral** (the portion of the body in front of the plane) and **posterior/dorsal** (the portion of the body behind the plane) parts.
- **Transverse (horizontal, axial, transaxial) planes** course horizontally through the body at right angles to both the frontal and sagittal planes and divide the body into **superior** (the portion of the body above the plane) and **inferior** (the portion of the body below the plane) parts.

It is important to note that the hands and feet have their own unique median planes to reference movement of the digits. The median plane of the hand runs through the 3rd metacarpal and digit, whereas the median plane of the foot runs through the 2nd metatarsal and digit.

ANATOMICAL VARIATION

All bodies have the same basic architectural plan, but just as no two bodies are identical on the outside, it should be no surprise that no two bodies are identical on the inside. Minor variations, such as variation in size, color, and pathway of a vessel, commonly occur in all regions of the body and should be expected. At the onset of dissection, the focus should be on learning normal (average) anatomy rather than variants unless specifically instructed to do otherwise. Take time during each dissection period to view several dissections on neighboring cadavers so that you can learn to appreciate anatomical variations and be better prepared for identification examinations.

Before beginning to dissect, consult your textbook for additional **terms of relationship and comparison**, **terms of laterality**, and **terms of movement**. These terms form an important part of the language of anatomy, and it is not possible to understand anatomical descriptions without understanding and using these terms.

DAILY DISSECTION ROUTINE

To get the most out of dissection, it is recommended that you establish a routine approach to each day's dissection, such as the following:

- **Prepare before the lab.** Read the dissection assignment in this book and become familiar with the new vocabulary, the structures to be dissected, and the dissection approach. When actively dissecting, you must deliberately search for structures, and a small amount of advance preparation will make the exercise go more quickly and be much more productive.
- **Watch the corresponding *Grant's Dissection Videos*** either before or during lab to gain a better visual perspective of the techniques and steps to be used in the dissection. Throughout the text, you will see the term VIDEO beneath the corresponding dissection heading with the associated video and sequence numbers listed to facilitate your search of the appropriate dissection demonstration footage.
- ***Grant's Atlas of Anatomy*** is the recommended atlas to use in the dissection lab, although alternative atlases may be similarly implemented. Corresponding page numbers have been provided to the 16th edition of *Grant's Atlas of Anatomy* to help you quickly find illustrations that support the dissection protocol as outlined.
- **Palpate bony landmarks** as indicated in the skeletal and surface anatomy sequences and use them in the search for soft tissue structures.
- **Cleaning an area** refers to removing fat, connective tissue, and smaller veins to make the details of the more emphasized structures more obvious.
- **Review the completed dissection** at the end of the dissection period and again at the start of the next dissection period. To help you do this, review exercises are included at strategic points in each chapter.
- **Complete each dissection before proceeding to the next** because most dissections will be an extension of the previous dissection.

LAB SAFETY

Follow your laboratories guidelines, which may include the following:

- **Scrubs, white coats, or aprons** should be worn while in the laboratory. For sanitary reasons, this outer layer of clothing should not be worn outside of the dissection laboratory, and scrubs should immediately be changed upon exiting the lab.
- **Do not wear sandals or open-toed shoes in the laboratory** because a dropped scalpel, dissection instrument, or other piece of lab equipment can result in serious injury.
- **Nitrile or latex gloves** must be worn to prevent contact with human tissue and fixatives.
- **Always wear eye protection** such as goggles or glasses when using a bone saw to protect your eyes from potential projectiles.

REMOVING SKIN

Removal of the skin is a key component of the dissection protocol and often sets the tone of the entire dissection. Prior to commencing a new region of study, the decision to either **reflect** or **remove** the skin must be made. As part of your consideration for which set of instructions to follow, it should be noted that the skin is impermeable to water; hence, an advantage of leaving a portion of the skin and subcutaneous tissue connected to the cadaveric specimen is increased "working time" by preventing desiccation. In all skinning methods, care must be taken to accurately remove the skin without damaging the underlying structures. For each sequence of dissection instructions related to skin incisions, the following approaches may be applied:

- **Skin reflection** will require that most of the sequential cuts be made initially; however, a portion of skin will be left uncut, typically along the periphery of the region, to have a plane of reflection leaving a section of the skin attached to the underlying tissue. The plane of connected tissue will be used as a "hinge" to move the section of skin out of the way while performing the dissection sequence and then allow it to be replaced back to anatomical position to assist in preventing desiccation of the exposed structures.
- **Skin removal** will require that all the sequential cuts be made to completely remove the entire region of skin from the dissection field. Removing the skin will allow full exposure of the underlying structures; however, more care must be taken to prevent desiccation of the exposed structures. It is possible to simply overlay the entire piece of removed skin back on the body in a full removal method to prevent desiccation similar to the reflection approach.

In addition to determining if the skin should be removed or reflected, it should be noted that skin removal may be completed using either of the following approaches:

- A **partial-thickness method** removes the dermis and epidermis only, leaving the subcutaneous tissue intact to better identify and isolate superficial veins and cutaneous nerves coursing within the fat as demonstrated in FIGURE I.4A. A partial-thickness technique offers the advantage of increased visibility of some structures;

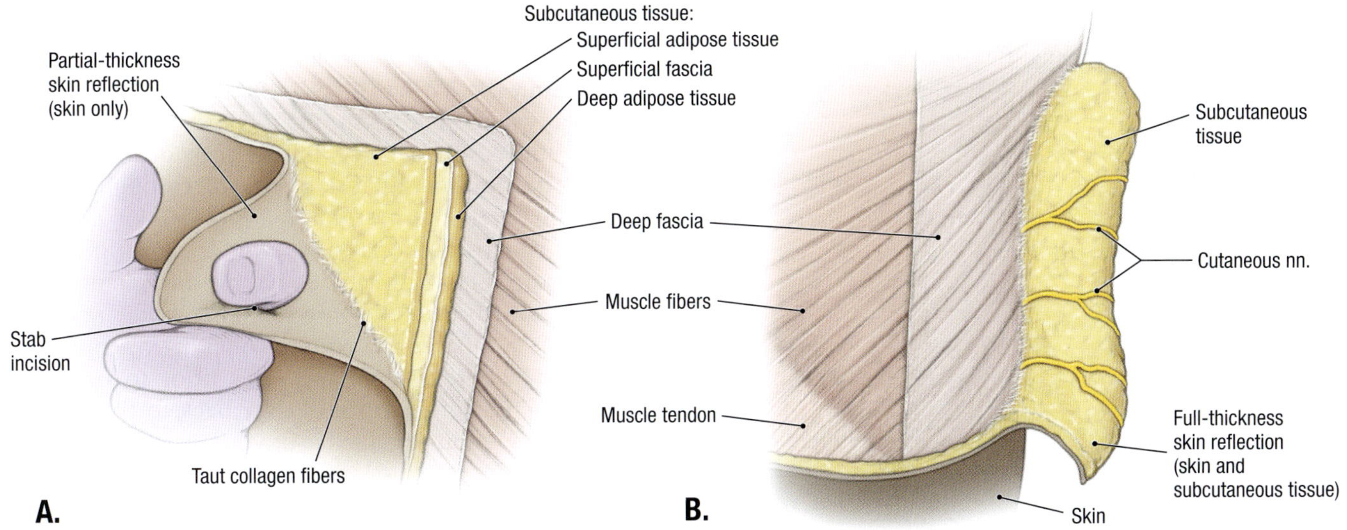

FIGURE I.4 ● **A.** Buttonhole technique in partial-thickness skin reflection. **B.** Full-thickness skin reflection.

however, it does require more time, a potentially limiting consideration for some dissection courses.

- A **full-thickness method** describes removal of the dermis, epidermis, and underlying subcutaneous tissue together in a deeper block simultaneously as demonstrated in FIGURE I.4B. For shorter courses with less space in the lab, full removal of skin may be preferred as the working space remains "cleaner" with less oil, fat, and fluids from the embalming process on the dissection table, which may continue to release from the subcutaneous tissue during your dissection.

Often, a mixed approach to partial- and full-thickness removal is optimal to offer an accelerated pace in some body regions while allowing for more care and caution in others. For the provided dissection instructions in this text, all sections related to skin removal are assumed to be partial thickness, and all those described as skin reflection are assumed as full thickness.

A variable amount of subcutaneous tissue lies immediately deep to the skin. It is important to note that varying amounts of subcutaneous tissue are common and to be expected in individuals with larger body habitus. Pay attention to the comments made for donors with a larger body habitus, and keep in mind the respect you would demonstrate to a living individual or patient and appreciate that often larger muscle tone may accompany increased amounts of subcutaneous tissue.

The subcutaneous tissue contains fat, fascia, cutaneous nerves, and superficial blood vessels. Subcutaneous tissue throughout the body maintains a general pattern from superficial to deep of skin, superficial adipose tissue, superficial fascia, deep adipose tissue, and deep fascia. The superficial adipose tissue and superficial fascia correlate to autonomic patterns of innervation, while the deep adipose tissue and investing fascia, parallel somatic patterns of distribution with the musculofascial system.

Variations of layer thickness within the subcutaneous tissue occur throughout the body. For example, in the abdominal region, the superficial adipose tissue is named *Camper's fascia*, while the superficial fascial layer is termed *Scarpa's fascia*. Deep to the Scarpa's fascia, a relatively thin layer of deep adipose tissue separates it from the underlying deep or investing fascia surrounding the muscles in the region. In the neck and face, the superficial fat may be nearly absent as the superficial fascia layer is intimately connected to the muscles of facial expression, a layer often referred to as the superficial musculoaponeurotic system (SMAS), of particular concern for plastic and reconstructive surgeries.

The thickness of skin also varies from region to region. For example, the skin is relatively thin on the dorsum of the hand and considerably thicker over palm of the hand. Generally, skin incisions should not extend into the subcutaneous tissue; therefore, a general understanding of regional skin thickness is important.

To begin skinning, make incision lines of the appropriate depth, either full or partial, along the recommended incision lines as instructed in this manual. Following the initial incision, use toothed forceps or hemostats to grasp the skin at the intersection of two incision lines. Once a skin flap has been raised, place traction on the skin as it is being removed and direct the scalpel blade toward the deep surface of the skin to cut the underlying taut collagen fibers. Avoid directing the scalpel toward the body because the blade will readily cut through and destroy underlying subcutaneous tissue, muscle, and neurovascular structures. To steady your scalpel hand, rest it against the cadaver and hold the scalpel as you would hold a pencil and make short (5 to 10 cm) sweeping motions as demonstrated in FIGURE I.5. To prevent accidents, do not work too close to your lab partners and always hold the skin with dissection instruments and **not your fingers** when making new incisions with a scalpel.

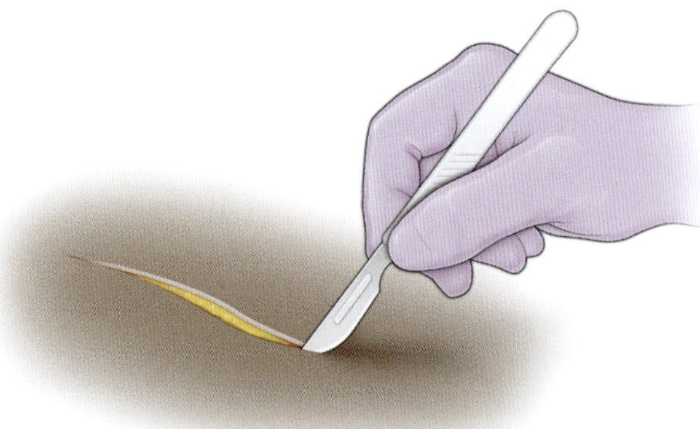

FIGURE I.5 ● Scalpel dissection technique with hand resting on body surface for stability.

FIGURES

Throughout the various dissection chapters, you will see many illustrative figures meant to assist you in your dissection efforts. In each region, the provided figures will guide you from the initial skin removal through the various tissue layers to the underlying organs or joints. As many of the instructional steps will be similar in nature, a standardized labeling scheme has been implemented in the figures with the following line and abbreviation features. Take a moment to review **TABLE I.1** of commonly used figure abbreviations and lines prior to beginning your dissection protocols and refer back to this table as needed throughout the course of your dissection.

TABLE I.1 Commonly Used Figure Abbreviations and Lines

Anatomical Structure or Reference	*Abbreviation or Figure Element*
Artery and arteries	a. and aa.
Vein and veins	v. and vv.
Nerve and nerves	n. and nn.
Muscle and muscles	m. and mm.
Cranial nerve	CN (followed by roman numeral)
Point of reference line(s)	....
Incision line(s) and sequence	1 .... 2 :
Optional incision or reflection line(s)	----------------------
Previously made incision line(s)	______________________
Boundary or border line(s)	
Directional movement line(s)	——————→

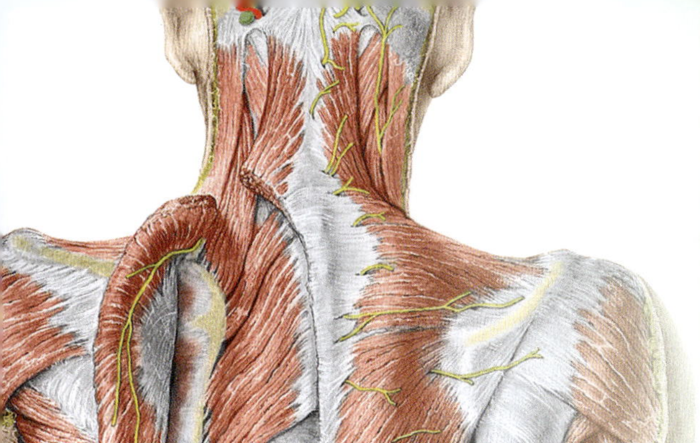

CHAPTER 1
Back

REFERENCES

ATLAS = *Grant's Atlas of Anatomy*, 16th ed., figure number	VIDEO = *Grant's Dissection Videos*, video sequence number

The back is the posterior aspect of the trunk extending from the base of the skull to the superior aspect of the gluteal region. The back plays important roles in posture, upper limb stability and movement, and protection of visceral and neurovascular structures. The bones of the vertebral column along with the spinal cord and meninges will be studied with the back.

The vertebral column consists of 33 vertebrae: 7 cervical (C), 12 thoracic (T), 5 lumbar (L), 5 sacral (S), and 4 coccygeal (Co). The vertebrae are numbered within each region from superior to inferior. The upper 24 vertebrae (cervical, thoracic, and lumbar) allow flexibility and movement of the vertebral column. The lower vertebrae (sacral and coccygeal) are fused to provide rigid support of the pelvic girdle and to transmit forces to and from the lower limb.

CLINICAL CORRELATIONS

During your dissection protocol, you may encounter anatomical variations, clinical conditions, disease processes, or medical devices in your cadaveric donor. The following select clinical correlations will be described in more detail throughout this chapter.

Back

1.1. Excessive Vertebral Curvature (Kyphosis, Lordosis, and Scoliosis), see **Thoracic Vertebrae** sequence. ATLAS 1.1A, 1.2, 1.6
1.2. Herniated Disc, see **Cervical and Lumbar Vertebrae** sequence. ATLAS 1.14, 1.16
1.3. Triangles of Back, see **Latissimus Dorsi** sequence. ATLAS 1.26, 2.33
1.4. Back Pain, Sprains, and Strains, see **Erector Spinae** sequence. ATLAS 1.14, 1.29, 1.30
1.5. Lumbar Puncture and Epidural Anesthesia, see **Laminectomy** sequence. ATLAS 1.40, 1.41

SKIN OF BACK AND SUPERFICIAL SUBOCCIPITAL REGION

Dissection Overview

The skin of the back, underlying subcutaneous tissue, and deep muscles of the back receive innervation segmentally from the posterior (dorsal) primary rami. Posterior primary rami are unnamed and referred to by their corresponding vertebral levels except for the suboccipital nerve (C1), the greater occipital nerve (C2), and the cluneal nerves in the gluteal region.

The order of dissection will be as follows: Skeletal anatomy of the vertebral column and the surface anatomy of the back will be studied. The skin will be either reflected or removed from the back, posterior surface of the neck, and posterior surface of the proximal upper limb. The subcutaneous tissue will either be removed or reflected in a full- or partial-thickness approach. Superficial neurovascular structures in the occipital region will be studied.

Skeletal Anatomy

Refer to an articulated skeleton or individual bones and identify the following skeletal features.

Posterior Skull and Scapula

ATLAS 1.23, 1.36, 2.3

1. Refer to FIGURE 1.1.
2. On the **occipital bone**, identify the **external occipital protuberance**.
3. Identify the **superior nuchal line** arching laterally from the external occipital protuberance and observe that it runs parallel to the more inferiorly located **inferior nuchal line**.
4. On the **temporal bone**, identify the large **mastoid process** inferolaterally, posterior to the **external acoustic meatus**.
5. Observe that the **scapula** is triangular with the **superior angle**, acromion process, and **inferior angle** forming the points of the triangle, and the **medial (vertebral) border** and **lateral (axillary) border** forming the lower two sides of the triangle.
6. Identify the **spine of the scapula**, the large ridge along the posterior surface of the scapula.
7. Follow the spine of the scapula laterally and identify the **acromion process**, the most lateral portion of the bone.

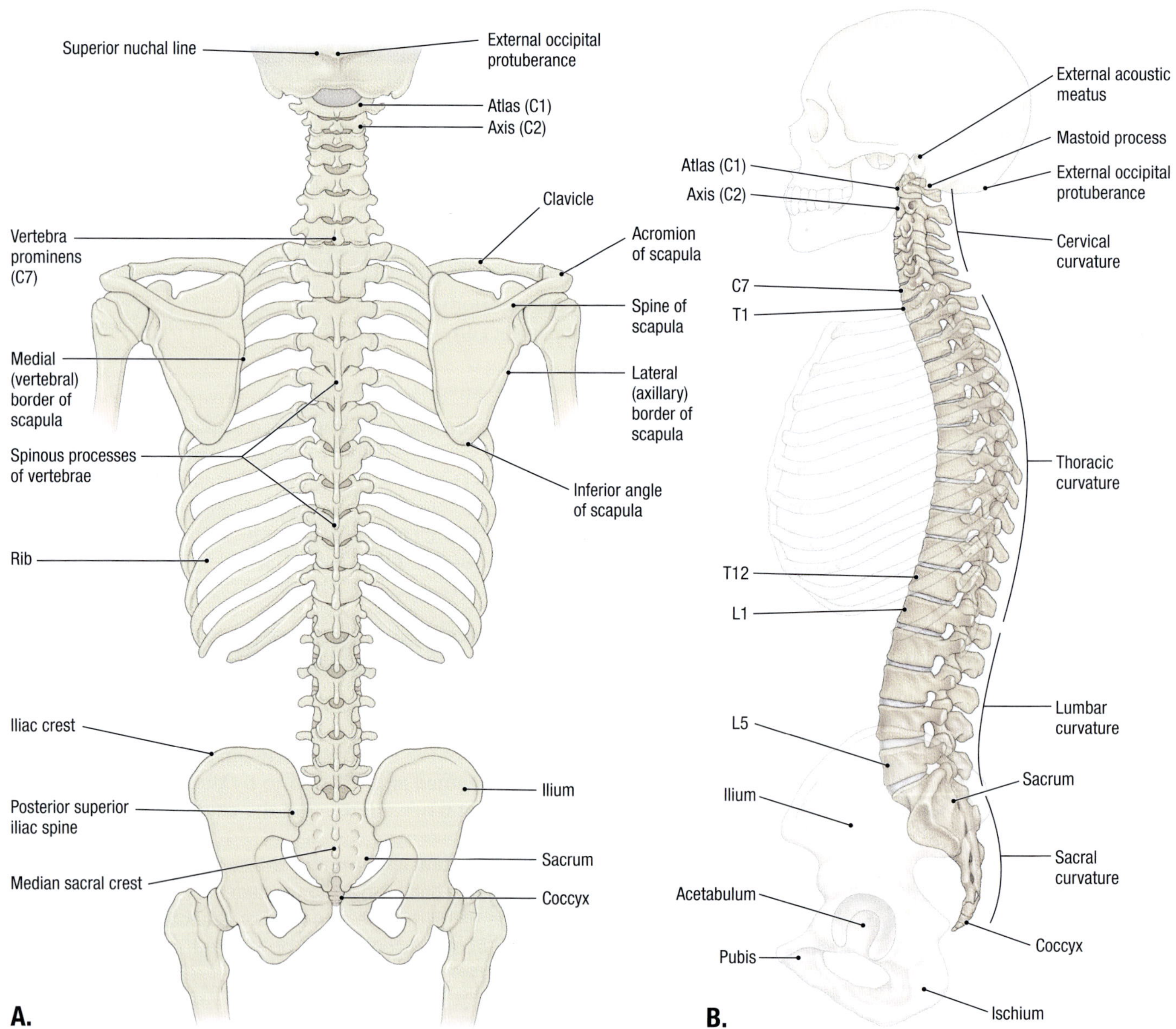

FIGURE 1.1 ● Skeleton of back. **A.** Posterior view. **B.** Lateral view.

Thoracic Vertebrae

ATLAS 1.12

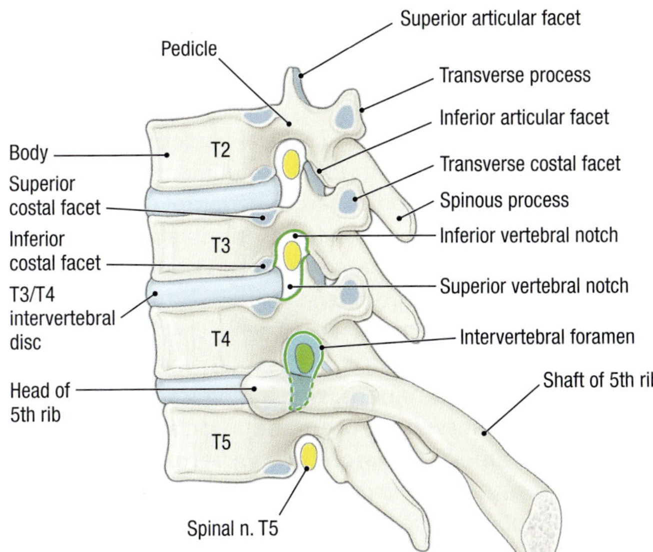

FIGURE 1.2 ■ Thoracic vertebrae. Lateral view.

1. Refer to FIGURE 1.2.
2. On a **thoracic vertebra**, identify the large bony mass of the **vertebral body** anteriorly.
3. Observe that articulation with ribs is a unique characteristic of thoracic vertebrae. On an articulated skeleton, verify that the head of ribs 1, 10, 11, and 12 articulate with the body of one vertebra while the remaining ribs articulate with the **demifacets**, the **superior** and **inferior costal facets**, of two adjacent vertebrae and the associated **intervertebral (IV) disc**.
4. Identify the pedicles, the short bony processes arching posteriorly from the vertebral body bilaterally.
5. Identify the **superior vertebral notch** on the superior aspect of a pedicle and the **inferior vertebral notch** along the inferior aspect of a pedicle.
6. Identify an inferior vertebral notch of one vertebra and the superior vertebral notch of the vertebra immediately inferior and observe how together they form an **IV foramen**. *Note that a spinal nerve passes through the IV foramen from the vertebral canal where it arose from the spinal cord.*
7. Identify the **transverse processes** and associated **transverse costal facets**.
8. Observe that the tubercle of a rib articulates with the transverse costal facet of the thoracic vertebra of the same number (i.e., the tubercle of rib 5 articulates with the transverse costal facet of vertebra T5).
9. Identify the **superior** and **inferior articular processes** with their associated **facets (surfaces)**. Observe that in the thoracic region, the articular facets are orientated in the coronal plane, allowing for some rotation and lateral flexion while limiting flexion and extension anteriorly and posteriorly.
10. Identify the spinous process of a thoracic vertebra and observe that it is relatively long and slender, is directed inferiorly and posteriorly, and at lower thoracic levels overlaps the adjacent spinous process of the inferiorly located vertebra.
11. From a superior view, identify the **vertebral arch** formed by the posterior aspect of the vertebral body, pedicles, transverse processes, **laminae**, and spinous process to encircle the **vertebral foramen**.
12. On an articulated skeleton, observe that when individual vertebrae are stacked to form the **vertebral column** that the vertebral foramina align to form the **vertebral canal** to protect the spinal cord from the base of the skull to the sacrum.
13. Verify from a lateral perspective that the vertebral column has natural curves, with the **thoracic** and **sacral curvatures** being concave anteriorly in a kyphotic orientation, and the **cervical** and **lumbar curvatures** concave posteriorly in a lordotic orientation (see **Clinical Correlation 1.1**). *Note that primary curvature relates to the alignment of the vertebral column during development which is maintained in the thoracic and sacral regions, while secondary curvature develops in the cervical and lumbar regions in response to an infant learning to hold up their head or walk, respectively.*

CLINICAL CORRELATION 1.1

Excessive Vertebral Curvature (Kyphosis, Lordosis, and Scoliosis)

ATLAS 1.1A, 1.2, 1.6

Congenital abnormalities, degenerative diseases, or other pathologic processes such as osteoporosis can lead to excessive vertebral curvature. Kyphosis is an exaggeration of thoracic curvature in the sagittal plane, often caused by degeneration of the anterior aspect of the vertebral bodies. Lordosis is an exaggeration of the lumbar curvature in the sagittal plane, often due to rotation of the hips caused by weakened trunk muscles. Scoliosis is an abnormal amount of lateral curvature of the vertebral column in the coronal plane, often accompanied by rotation of the vertebrae and ribs due to muscular weakness or developmental anomalies.

Cervical and Lumbar Vertebrae

ATLAS 1.7, 1.13

1. Refer to FIGURE 1.3.
2. On a set of disarticulated **cervical vertebrae**, observe that they differ from thoracic vertebrae as they have smaller vertebral bodies, larger vertebral foramina, and lack transverse costal facets for rib attachment.
3. Identify the spinous process of a cervical vertebra and observe that they are often "split" or **bifid**.
4. Identify the C7 vertebra and observe that it has the most prominent spinous process in the cervical region, the **vertebra prominens**, which is typically not bifid.
5. Identify a transverse process and associated **transverse foramen (foramen transversarium)**. *Note that the transverse foramina of the cervical vertebrae, with the exception of the C7 foramina, allow for passage of the vertebral arteries bilaterally.*
6. Identify the **superior** and **inferior articular processes** of a cervical vertebra with the associated **superior** and **inferior articular facets**, respectively. Observe that in the cervical region, the articular facets are orientated approximately in the horizontal plane, allowing for increased rotational movement while maintaining large degrees of flexion and extension.
7. Refer to a set of disarticulated **lumbar vertebrae** and observe that they differ from thoracic vertebrae as they have larger vertebral bodies, more prominent processes, and lack costal facets for rib attachment.
8. Identify the **superior** and **inferior articular processes** of a lumbar vertebra and the associated **superior** and **inferior articular facets**. Observe that in the lumbar region, the articular facets are orientated in a sagittal plane, allowing for increased flexion and extension anteriorly and posteriorly with limited rotation or lateral flexion.
9. Identify the spinous process of a lumbar vertebra and observe that it is broad, blunt, and does not overlap adjacent vertebrae.
10. On an articulated skeleton, observe that IV discs become progressively larger from the cervical to the lumbar regions due to the increased weight and support required at the base of the vertebral column (see **Clinical Correlation 1.2**).

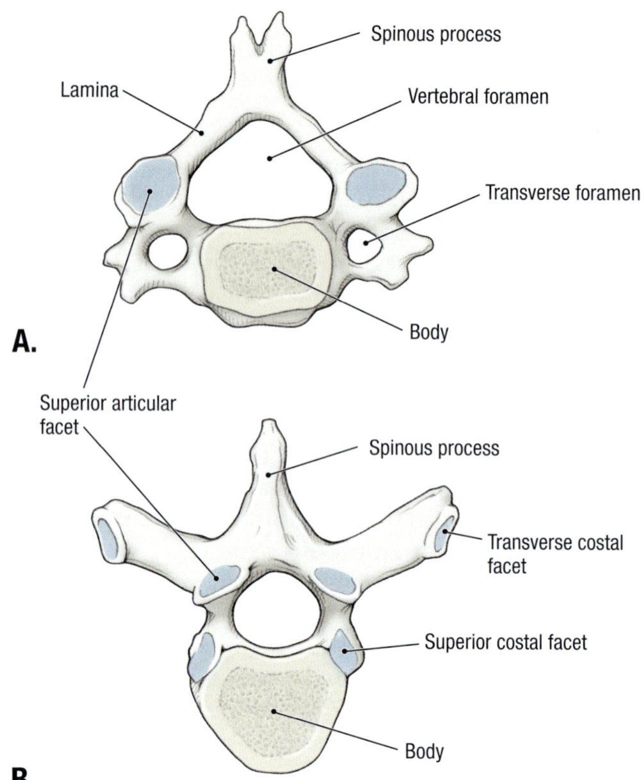

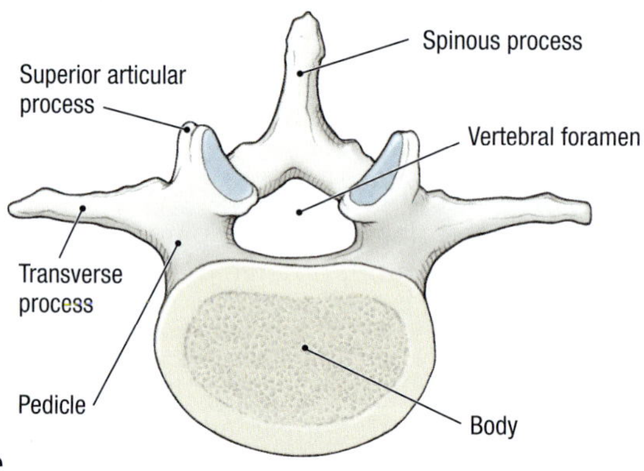

FIGURE 1.3 ● **A.** Cervical (C4) vertebra. **B.** Thoracic (T6) vertebra. **C.** Lumbar (L4) vertebra. Superior views.

CLINICAL CORRELATION 1.2

Herniated Disc

ATLAS 1.14, 1.16

Intervertebral discs are composed of an outer anulus fibrosus, a series of concentric rings of tough fibrocartilage, and an inner nucleus pulposus, a gelatinous mass assisting in shock absorption. Herniation occurs when the inner nucleus pulposus extrudes through the outer anulus fibrosus, most commonly at the L4/L5 or L5/S1 vertebral levels. Herniation of the nucleus pulposus typically occurs posterolaterally into the vertebral canal or an IV foramen to either side of the posterior longitudinal ligament. Herniation may lead to spinal cord or spinal nerve compression resulting in sensory and/or motor deficits, and possible pain in the region supplied by the compressed nervous structure. Herniation may occur following a traumatic injury or evolve over time as seen with bone degeneration or poor posture.

Sacrum and Ilium

ATLAS 1.18, 1.19, 1.20

1. Refer to FIGURE 1.4.
2. Identify the **sacrum** and observe that it is formed by five fused sacral vertebrae.
3. On the posterior surface of the sacrum, identify the **median sacral crest**, the fused rudimentary spinous processes of the upper three or four sacral vertebrae.
4. On the lateral aspect of the sacrum, identify the **ala**, the fused rudimentary transverse processes of the sacral vertebrae, and the **auricular surface**, which articulates with the ilium.
5. Identify the **anterior** and **posterior sacral foramina**, which allow the anterior and posterior rami of sacral spinal nerves to exit from the vertebral canal anteriorly and posteriorly as the sacrum articulates on its lateral surfaces with the hip bones.
6. On the posterior inferior aspect of the sacrum, identify the **sacral hiatus**, the inferior opening at the termination of the vertebral canal.
7. Inferior to the sacrum identify the **coccyx**, a small triangular bone formed by a single coccygeal vertebra, or the fusion of two to four rudimentary coccygeal vertebrae.
8. Observe that the coccygeal vertebrae lack the features of typical vertebrae apart from the vertebral bodies.
9. Refer back to FIGURE 1.1.
10. Identify the **hip bone** (os coxae or innominate bone) and observe that in the adult it is formed by the fusion of three separate bones: **ilium**, the superior most bone; **ischium**, the inferior most bone; and **pubis**, the bone directed anteriorly toward the opposite hip bone at the midline.
11. Identify the **acetabulum**, the socket of the hip joint. *Note that during development, the three bones of the hip meet in the acetabulum as the triradiate cartilage, one of the last points of skeletal fusion as the cartilage is replaced by bone.*
12. Identify the **iliac crest**, the large bony ridge extending along the superior aspect of the ilium from the **anterior superior iliac spine (ASIS)** to the **posterior superior iliac spine (PSIS)**.

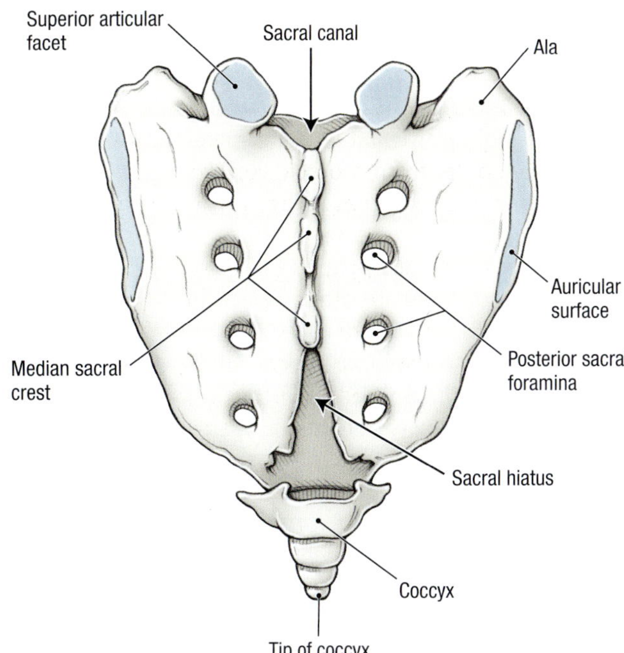

FIGURE 1.4 ● Sacrum and coccyx. Posterior view.

Surface Anatomy

The surface anatomy of the back may be studied on a living subject or on a cadaver. On the cadaver, fixation of tissue during embalming may make it difficult to distinguish bone from well-preserved soft tissues in some specimens.

Back

ATLAS 1.23, 1.25

1. Refer to FIGURE 1.5.
2. With the cadaver in the prone position, palpate the external occipital protuberance on the posterior aspect of the head.
3. Palpate the mastoid process at the base of the skull posterior to the external ear, along with the superior attachment of the sternocleidomastoid, a large muscle in the anterior lateral aspect of the neck.
4. Move inferiorly along the posterior midline and make attempts to palpate the cervical spinous processes. *Note that depending on body type and varying amounts of spinal curvature that cervical spinous processes may be difficult to palpate with the exception of the spinous process of the vertebra prominens (C7) at the base of the neck.*
5. Beginning at the vertebra prominens, palpate laterally to identify the superior border of the **trapezius** and follow it inferolaterally toward its attachment to the acromion process of the scapula and **lateral (acromial) end of the clavicle**.
6. Palpate from the acromion process posteriorly and medially along the spine of the scapula toward the medial (vertebral) border of the scapula, approximately at the T3 vertebral level.
7. Follow the medial border of the scapula inferiorly toward the inferior angle of the scapula, approximately at the T7 vertebral level.
8. In the thoracic midline, palpate the spinous processes of the thoracic vertebrae.

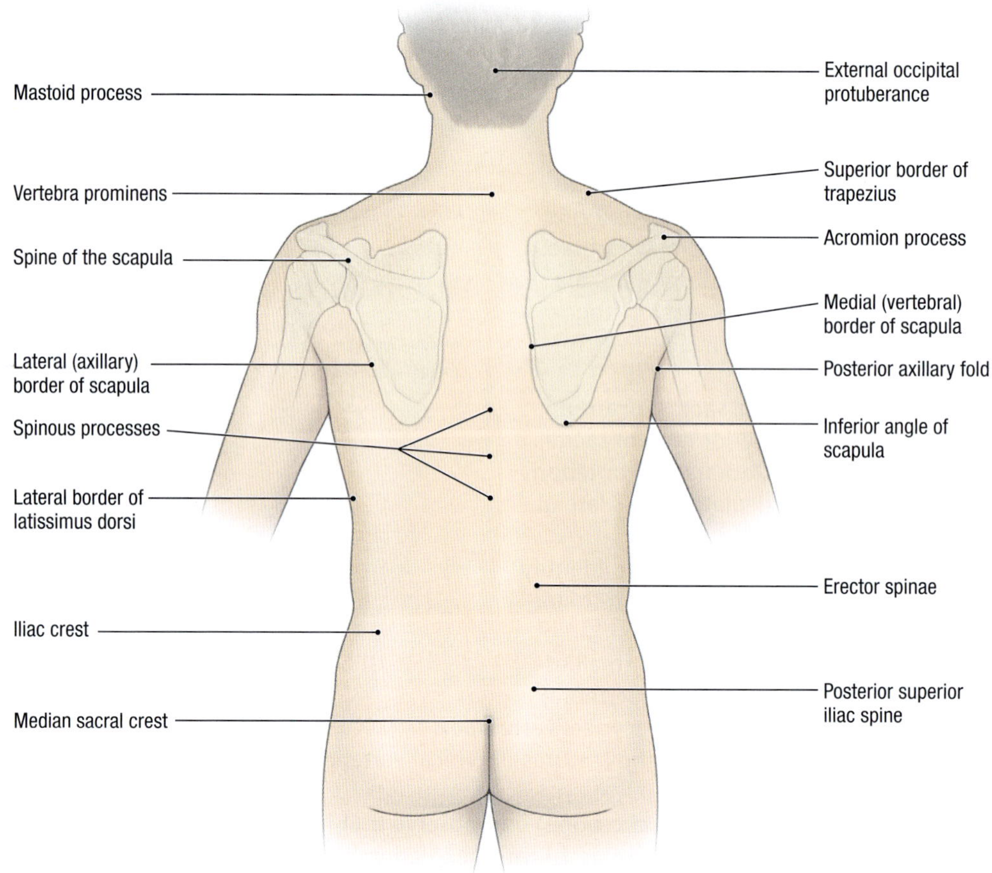

FIGURE 1.5 ● Surface anatomy of back. Posterior view.

9. Progress inferiorly to the lumbar region and palpate the **erector spinae**, the mass of postural muscles located bilaterally to either side of the vertebral column.
10. Palpate along the lateral margin of the erector spinae inferiorly and identify the iliac crest at the L4 vertebral level.
11. Follow the iliac crest posteriorly and medially and identify the **PSIS**, approximately at the S2 vertebral level along the **median sacral crest** of the sacrum.
12. Palpate from the iliac crest superiorly along the lateral aspect of the trunk and identify the lateral border of the **latissimus dorsi**.
13. Follow the lateral border of the latissimus dorsi superiorly to the axilla and observe that it forms the **posterior axillary fold**.

Dissection Instructions

Dissection Note: Prior to commencing with skin incisions, decide to perform either a full- or partial-thickness approach and to either reflect or remove the skin from the dissection field. See **Removing Skin** in the **Introduction Chapter** for descriptions.

Skin Incisions of Back

VIDEO 1.1.1

1. Refer to FIGURE 1.6.
2. With the cadaver in the prone position, use a scalpel to make a skin incision in the midline from the external occipital protuberance (X) to the median sacral crest of the sacrum (S). *Note that the skin is approximately 6 mm thick in this region, and thus, only the edge of the scalpel blade needs to penetrate the surface of the skin.*
3. To verify the thickness of the skin, make an initial small incision along the midline and use forceps or hemostats to pull the sides apart to observe the cut edge of skin. In an appropriately deep skin incision, you should see underlying adipose tissue but no muscle tissue.
4. Make an incision from the inferior aspect of the median sacral crest (S) arching superiorly and laterally to the midaxillary line (T) approximating the curve of the iliac crests.

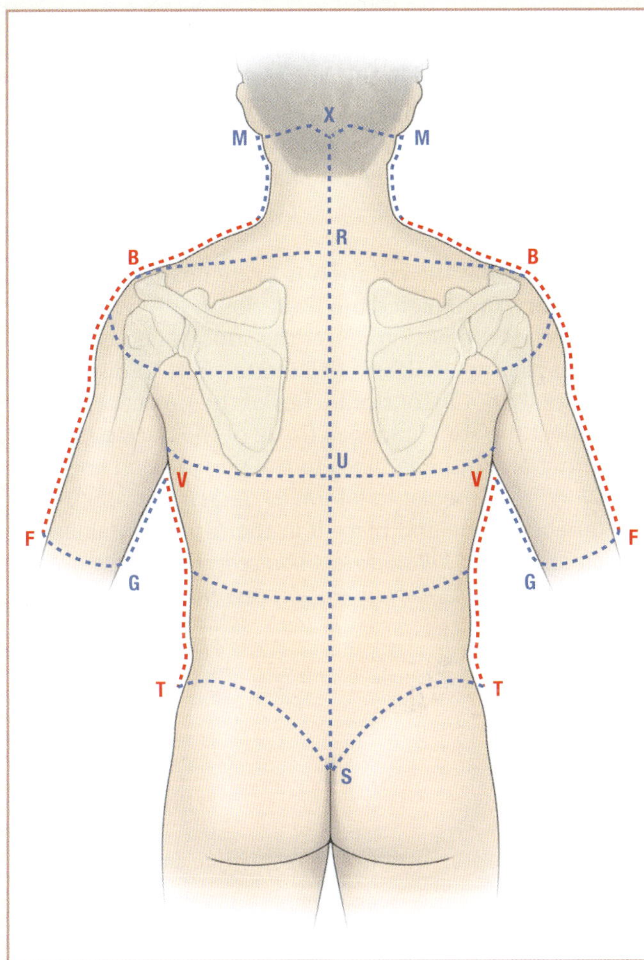

FIGURE 1.6 ● Skin incisions of back. Posterior view.

5. Make a shallow transverse skin incision from the external occipital protuberance (X) to the mastoid process (M) laterally.
6. Make a transverse skin incision superior to the scapula from the midline (R) to the acromion process (B).
7. At the level of the inferior angle of the scapula, make a transverse skin incision from the midline (U) to the midaxillary line (V).
8. To facilitate skinning, make several parallel transverse incisions about 8 cm above and below the horizontal incisions described in steps 6 and 7.
9. Make a vertical incision on the inner aspect of the upper limb from the axilla to a point halfway down the arm (G).
10. Beginning on the medial aspect of the arm (G), make a shallow incision around the posterior surface of the arm toward the lateral aspect of the limb (F).

Dissection Note: If reflecting the skin, skip steps 11 through 13.

11. Make a superficial skin incision down the lateral surface of the neck beginning at the mastoid process (M) along the superior border of the trapezius to its attachment at the acromion process (B).
12. Continue the incision along the lateral aspect of the shoulder from the acromion process (B) to the midpoint of the arm laterally (F), connecting it with the horizontal incision made approximately halfway down the arm.
13. Make a vertical skin incision along the lateral surface of the trunk along the midaxillary line from the axilla superiorly (V) to the hip inferiorly (T).
14. Beginning in the middle of the back, reflect the skin from medial to lateral using either a pair of locking forceps or the buttonhole technique. At any point, the portions of skin may be cut into smaller segments to facilitate removal. *Note that even if a full-thickness reflection is desired, it may prove beneficial to begin with a partial-thickness approach until an appropriate depth of reflection is verified based on visualization of the underlying deep fascia covering the muscles.*
15. In the occipital region, stay as superficial as possible to avoid damaging the underlying neurovascular structures in either a full- or partial-thickness approach.
16. In the posterior neck, reflect or remove the subcutaneous tissue only as far laterally as the superior border of the trapezius as nerves coursing superficially in the region are in danger of being cut.
17. If reflecting the skin, utilize the uncut sections of skin laterally as hinge points to leave the skin attached along the peripheral aspect of the back. *Note that leaving the skin attached peripherally is a good technique to prevent desiccation of underlying structures by returning the reflected skin to its original orientation between dissection protocols.*
18. If removing the skin, once the lateral incision points are reached, detach the skin and place it in the tissue container.

Superficial Suboccipital Region

ATLAS 1.26; VIDEO 1.1.2

1. Refer to FIGURE 1.7.
2. In the subcutaneous tissue at the base of the skull, locate the **occipital artery** and the **greater occipital nerve**, the posterior (dorsal) ramus of spinal nerve C2. *Note that the superficial veins in the region may serve as guides to identify the location of the occipital artery but care need not be taken to preserve them.*

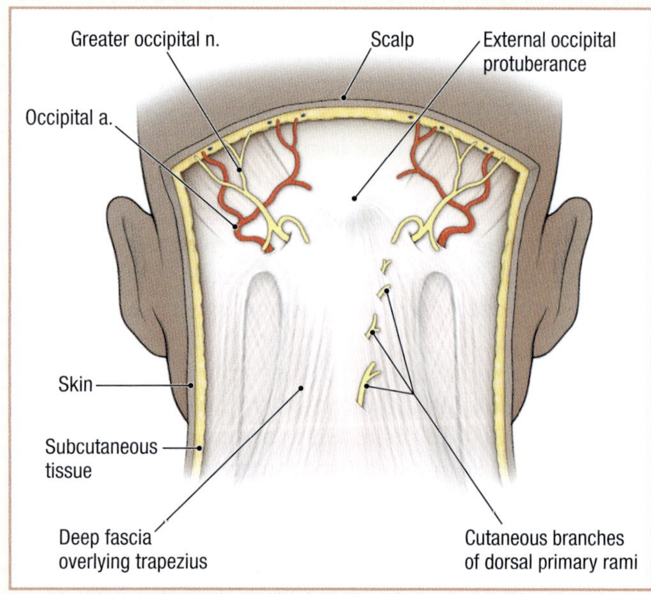

FIGURE 1.7 ● Superficial dissection of occipital region. Posterior view.

3. Use blunt dissection to isolate the greater occipital nerve and observe that it pierces the trapezius about 3 cm inferolateral to the external occipital protuberance and may cross the occipital artery along its path to the skin on the posterior aspect of the head. *Note that the deep fascia in this area is very dense and tough and it may be difficult to find or isolate the greater occipital nerve.*
4. Observe that the **cutaneous branches of the dorsal primary rami** pierce the trapezius in the posterior aspect of the neck to enter the subcutaneous tissue. To save time, make no deliberate effort to display posterior cutaneous branches of the posterior rami.
5. Reflect the subcutaneous tissue of the back by cutting it along similar lines to the skin incision lines. Work from medial to lateral to detach the subcutaneous tissue and place it in the tissue container. *Note that if a full-thickness skin reflection or removal has been implemented, this process has already been performed.*

Dissection Follow-up

1. Review the key anatomical landmarks for the surface anatomy of the back.
2. Review the anatomical features of the cervical, thoracic, and lumbar vertebrae noting the respective similarities and differences.
3. Review the pattern of innervation of posterior rami of the back and suboccipital region.
4. Study a dermatome chart and become familiar with the concept of segmental innervation.
5. If a full- or partial-thickness skin reflection was performed, replace the reflected portions of skin back to anatomical position.

SUPERFICIAL MUSCLES OF BACK

Dissection Overview

The back contains three groups of muscles separated by layers of deep fasciae: superficial, intermediate, and deep. The muscles in all three groups attach to the vertebral column which forms the axis of the trunk, supports the weight of the body, transmits forces generated by movement, and provides a protective bony covering for the spinal cord and nerve roots.

The superficial muscles of the back are the trapezius, latissimus dorsi, rhomboid major, rhomboid minor, and levator scapulae. Unlike the skin of the back and the deep muscle layer, the superficial muscles of the back are innervated by anterior (ventral) primary rami and serve to affect movement and stability of the upper limb through attachment to the scapula.

The order of dissection will be as follows: The trapezius will be identified, cleaned, and reflected. The latissimus dorsi will be identified, cleaned, and reflected. The rhomboid major and rhomboid minor will be identified, cleaned, and reflected. The levator scapulae will be identified and cleaned.

Dissection Instructions

Dissection Note: If available, place a block under the shoulder to facilitate dissection of the superficial muscles of the back by relieving tension in the region. Perform the following dissection instructions bilaterally. *Note that this may not be advisable in some donors as increased pressure on the anterior thoracic wall risks fracturing the ribs.*

Trapezius

ATLAS 1.25, 1.26; VIDEO 1.2.1

1. Refer to FIGURE 1.8.
2. Identify the **trapezius,** a large diamond-shaped superficial muscle of the back consisting of three parts: descending (superior), transverse (middle), and ascending (inferior).
3. Clearly define the inferolateral border of the trapezius and remove any remaining superficial fascia from its superficial surface, but do not disturb its superolateral border at this time.
4. Review the attachments and actions of the trapezius (see **TABLE 1.1**).
5. Prepare the trapezius for reflection by using blunt dissection to lift the muscle away from the underlying tissue medial to the inferior angle of the scapula. *Note that it is important to use caution while breaking the fascial connections deep to the trapezius as the muscle can easily be torn with excessive force.*
6. Make a shallow vertical incision along the medial attachment of the trapezius to detach it from the spinous processes in the thoracic region and the **nuchal ligament** in the cervical region, continuing superiorly until you reach the external occipital protuberance (**Cut 1**).
7. Make a short transverse cut with a scalpel (2.5 cm) across the superior end of the trapezius to detach it from the superior nuchal line while sparing the greater occipital nerve and the occipital artery (**Cut 2**). Do not extend the transverse cut beyond the superolateral border of the trapezius.
8. Use sharp dissection to cut the trapezius as close as possible from its lateral attachments on the superior aspect of the spine and acromion of the scapula (**Cut 3**).
9. Leave the trapezius attached to the clavicle and cervical fascia and carefully reflect the muscle superolaterally.
10. On the deep surface of the reflected trapezius, identify the plexus of nerves formed by the **spinal accessory nerve (CN XI)** providing motor innervation, and branches of the **anterior rami of spinal nerves C3** and **C4** providing proprioception. *Note that at this point in the dissection, it may not be possible to distinguish which portion of the plexus arises from which source.*
11. Identify branches of the **transverse cervical artery** with its associated veins on the deep surface of the trapezius accompanying the plexus of nerves.
12. Remove the transverse cervical veins to clear the dissection field.
13. Observe that superiorly the spinal accessory nerve passes through the lateral (posterior) triangle of the neck. Do not make attempts to follow the nerve into the lateral triangle at this time as it will be dissected further in the neck dissections.

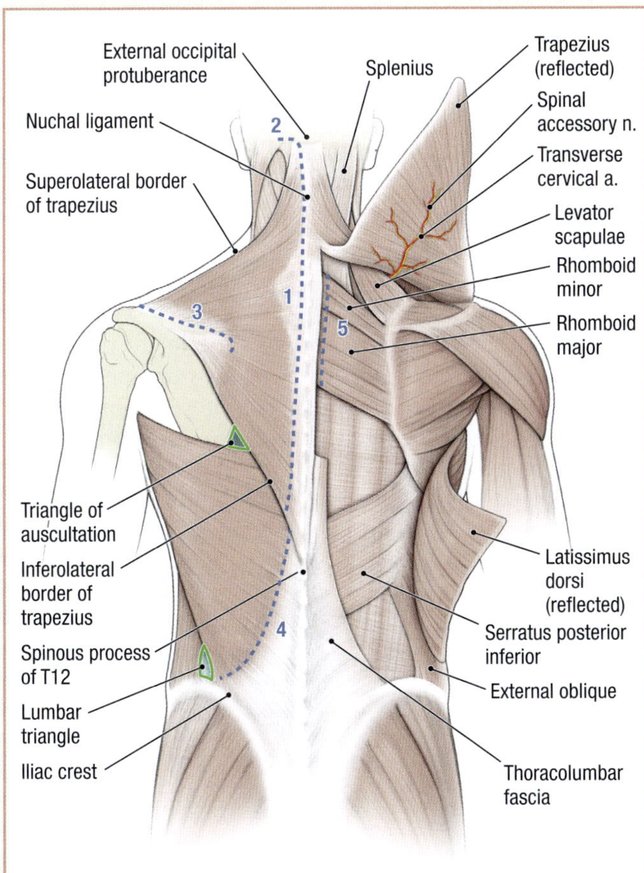

FIGURE 1.8 ● Superficial muscles of back. Posterior view.

Latissimus Dorsi

ATLAS 1.25, 1.26; VIDEO 1.2.2

1. Refer to FIGURE 1.8.
2. Identify the **latissimus dorsi**, the broad flat muscle of the back inferior to the trapezius, and clean its superficial surface and borders.
3. Review the attachments and actions of the latissimus dorsi (see **TABLE 1.1**).
4. To reflect the medial aspect of the latissimus dorsi, use blunt dissection deep to the superior border of the muscle (medial to the inferior angle of the scapula) and break the plane of loose connective tissue that lies between it and the deeper muscles.

5. Elevate the latissimus dorsi enough to insert scissors and cut through its medial attachment along the curve of the thoracolumbar fascia (**Cut 4**), not along the lumbar spinous processes.
6. Reflect the latissimus dorsi laterally and observe that it often has a strong fascial connection to the inferior angle of the scapula on its deep surface.
7. Continue reflecting the latissimus dorsi laterally, making an effort to not disturb its attachment to the ribs or the possible attachment to the inferior angle of the scapula (see **Clinical Correlation 1.3**). *Note that the serratus posterior inferior, an intermediate layer of back muscle, is often inadvertently reflected with the latissimus dorsi.*

CLINICAL CORRELATION 1.3

Triangles of Back

ATLAS 1.26, 2.33

The triangle of auscultation is bound by the trapezius superiorly, latissimus dorsi inferiorly, and rhomboid major and scapula laterally. The triangle of auscultation is approximately at intercostal space 6 and is particularly well suited for auscultation (listening to sounds produced by thoracic organs, particularly the lungs) as it has little overlying muscles.

The lumbar triangle is bound by the latissimus dorsi medially, external oblique laterally, and iliac crest inferiorly. The floor of the lumbar triangle is bound by the internal abdominal oblique. Due to the gap in muscle tissue on rare occasions, the lumbar triangle is the site of lumbar hernias.

8. The latissimus dorsi receives the **thoracodorsal nerve** and **artery** on its anterior surface near the posterior axillary fold. You may elect to further reflect the latissimus dorsi laterally and isolate its associated nerve and artery from the posterior view, but this will be more readily visible with the dissection of the axilla and is not necessary at this time.

Rhomboid Major and Rhomboid Minor

ATLAS 1.26, 1.27; VIDEO 1.2.3

1. Refer to FIGURE 1.8.
2. Medial to the scapula, identify the more inferiorly located **rhomboid major** and the more superiorly located **rhomboid minor**. Clean the superficial surface and borders of the rhomboid muscles.
3. Review the attachments and actions of the rhomboid major and minor (see **TABLE 1.1**).
4. Use blunt dissection to separate the rhomboid muscles from one another using the lateral attachments along the scapula as a guide. Observe that the rhomboid minor typically attaches at the level of the spine of the scapula, whereas the rhomboid major attaches inferior to the spine along the medial (vertebral) border of the scapula.
5. To reflect the rhomboid muscles, use blunt dissection deep to the inferior border of the rhomboid major and separate it from the deeper muscles.
6. Working from inferior to superior, use sharp dissection to detach the rhomboid major from its medial attachments on the spinous processes, and the rhomboid minor from its medial attachments on the spinous processes and inferior aspect of the nuchal ligament (**Cut 5**).
7. Reflect the rhomboid major and minor laterally. *Note that the serratus posterior superior, an intermediate layer of back muscle, is often inadvertently reflected with the rhomboid muscles.*
8. On the deep surface of the two rhomboid muscles near their lateral attachments on the medial border of the scapula, use blunt dissection to find the **dorsal scapular nerve** and **dorsal scapular vessels**. *Note that the dorsal scapular artery may branch directly from the subclavian artery, or from the transverse cervical artery, in which case it is also known as the deep branch of the transverse cervical artery.*

Levator Scapulae

ATLAS 1.26, 1.27; VIDEO 1.2.4

1. Refer to FIGURE 1.8.
2. Identify the **levator scapulae** superior to the rhomboid minor. *Note that at this stage of the dissection, the levator scapulae can be seen only near its inferior attachment to the superior angle of the scapula.*
3. Clean the inferior surfaces and borders of the levator scapulae, but do not dissect its superior attachments to the transverse processes of the upper four cervical vertebrae at this time.
4. Observe that the dorsal scapular nerve and artery supply the levator scapulae prior to reaching the rhomboid muscles and that they pass anterior (deep) to the inferior end of the muscle.
5. Review the attachments and actions of the levator scapulae (see **TABLE 1.1**).

Dissection Follow-up

1. Review the attachments, actions, and innervations of the superficial muscles of the back in **TABLE 1.1**.
2. Review the movements that occur between the scapula and the thoracic wall.
3. Review the boundaries of the triangle of auscultation and lumbar triangle and the clinical significance of each.
4. Replace the superficial muscles of the back and any portion of reflected skin back to their correct anatomical positions.
5. Use an illustration to observe the origin of the transverse cervical artery and the origin of the dorsal scapular artery.

TABLE 1.1 Superficial Muscles of Back

Muscle	*Medial Attachments*	*Lateral Attachments*	*Actions*	*Innervation*
Trapezius	Superior nuchal line, external occipital protuberance, ligamentum nuchae, SP C7–T12	Lateral one-third of the clavicle and acromion and spine of scapula	Rotates scapula to tilt the glenoid cavity superiorly, elevates (superior part), retracts (middle part), and depresses (inferior part) scapula	Motor: spinal accessory n. (CN XI) Proprioception: C3–C4
Latissimus dorsi	SP T7–T12, thoracolumbar fascia, iliac crest, ribs 10–12, inferior angle of scapula[a]	Floor of intertubercular sulcus of humerus	Extends, adducts, and medially rotates humerus	Thoracodorsal n. (middle subscapular n.)
Levator scapulae	TP C1–C4	Superior part of medial border of scapula	Elevates and rotates the scapula to tilt the glenoid cavity inferiorly	Dorsal scapular n.
Rhomboid major	SP T2–T5	Medial border of scapula to inferior spine	Retracts and rotates the scapula to tilt the glenoid cavity inferiorly	
Rhomboid minor	Ligamentum nuchae, SP C7–T1	Medial border of scapula at spine		

Abbreviations: C, cervical vertebrae; CN, cranial nerve; n., nerve; SP, spinous process; T, thoracic vertebrae; TP, transverse process.
[a]Intermediate attachment.

INTERMEDIATE AND DEEP MUSCLES OF BACK

Dissection Overview

The intermediate muscles of the back are the serratus posterior superior and the serratus posterior inferior, thin muscles attaching to the spinous processes and ribs. The intermediate muscles of the back act as accessory muscles of respiration and are innervated by intercostal nerve branches.

The deep muscles of the back include the splenius capitis, splenius cervicis, erector spinae, and transversospinales. The deep muscles of the back stabilize the vertebral column and act to cause extension, rotation, and lateral flexion and are innervated by posterior rami of spinal nerves. The deep muscles of the back are surrounding by the thick investing fascia of the thoracolumbar fascia, which plays a key role in transferring loads from the trunk and extremities while assisting in stabilization of the lumbosacral area.

The order of dissection will be as follows: The serratus posterior superior and inferior will be identified, cleaned, and reflected. The splenius capitis and splenius cervicis will be identified, cleaned, and reflected. The erector spinae will be identified and cleaned, and the semispinalis capitis will be identified, cleaned, and reflected. The semispinalis cervicis and multifidus muscles will be identified and cleaned.

Dissection Instructions

Dissection Note: Perform the following dissection instructions bilaterally.

Serratus Posterior Superior

ATLAS 1.27; VIDEO 1.3.1

1. Refer to FIGURE 1.9.
2. Identify the **serratus posterior superior** deep to the rhomboid muscles. *Note that if you do not see the serratus posterior superior, it may be attached to the deep surface of the reflected rhomboid muscles.*
3. Clean the surface and borders of the serratus posterior superior.
4. Review the attachments and actions of the serratus posterior superior (see **TABLE 1.2**).
5. Use a probe or blunt instrument to gently elevate the serratus posterior superior from the underlying erector spinae muscles.
6. Use sharp dissection to cut the medial attachments of the serratus posterior superior along the nuchal

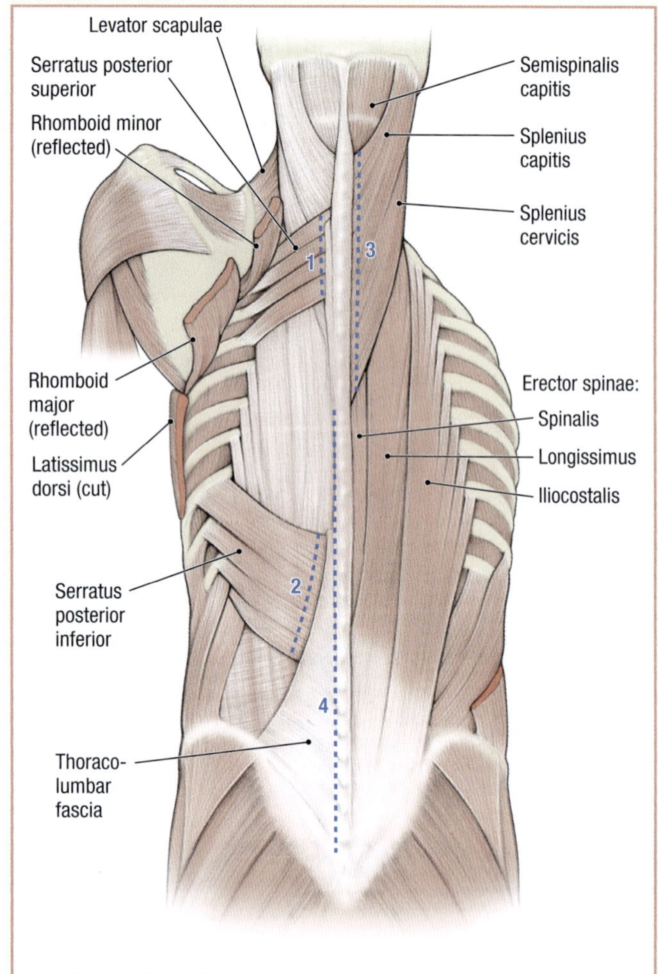

FIGURE 1.9 ● Intermediate (*left*) and superficial (*right*) layers of deep back muscles. Posterior view.

ligament and the spinous processes of vertebrae C7–T3 (**Cut 1**).

7. Reflect the serratus posterior superior laterally leaving its attachments intact along the superior borders of ribs 2 to 5 lateral to their angles.

Serratus Posterior Inferior

ATLAS 1.27; VIDEO 1.3.2

1. Refer to FIGURE 1.9.
2. Identify the **serratus posterior inferior** deep to the latissimus dorsi. *Note that if you do not see the serratus posterior inferior, it may be attached to the deep surface of the reflected latissimus dorsi.*
3. Continue reflecting the latissimus dorsi laterally by detaching the muscle from its attachments to the ribs and possible attachment to the inferior angle of the scapula to achieve greater visibility of the serratus posterior inferior.
4. Clean the surface and borders of the serratus posterior inferior.
5. Review the attachments and actions of the serratus posterior inferior (see **TABLE 1.2**).
6. Use a probe or blunt instrument to gently elevate the serratus posterior inferior from the underlying erector spinae muscles.
7. Use sharp dissection to cut the medial attachments of the serratus posterior inferior along the spinous processes of vertebrae T11–L2 (**Cut 2**).
8. Reflect the serratus posterior inferior laterally, leaving its attachments intact lateral to the angles of the ribs.

Splenius

ATLAS 1.28, 1.33E; VIDEO 1.3.3

1. Refer to FIGURE 1.9.
2. Identify the two portions of the **splenius**: **splenius capitis** attaching to the skull, and **splenius cervicis** to the cervical vertebrae. *Note that the two parts of the splenius are not easily distinguished from each other at this stage of the dissection.*
3. Clean the surface of the splenius deep to the serratus posterior superior. Observe that the fibers of the splenius course obliquely across the neck from inferior to superior.
4. Review the attachments and actions of the splenius capitis and cervicis (see **TABLE 1.2**).
5. Use sharp dissection to detach the inferior attachments of the splenius from the nuchal ligament and spinous processes of vertebrae C7–T6 (**Cut 3**).
6. Reflect the splenius laterally leaving the superior attachments undisturbed.

Erector Spinae

ATLAS 1.28, 1.33; VIDEO 1.3.4

1. Refer to FIGURE 1.9.
2. To either side of the midline, identify the location of the **erector spinae**, the large collective mass of muscles deep to the investing fascia of the region, the **thoracolumbar fascia.**
3. Use scissors to carefully incise the posterior surface of the thoracolumbar fascia from the midthoracic level superiorly to the sacrum inferiorly (**Cut 4**). Observe that the thoracolumbar fascia is thin at thoracic levels and thick at lumbar and sacral levels.
4. Use blunt dissection to separate and reflect the thoracolumbar fascia from the posterior surface of the erector spinae. *Note that the thoracolumbar fascia surrounds the deep muscles of the back both anteriorly and posteriorly, creating a dense connective tissue sheath around the erector spinae and transversospinales groups of muscles.*

5. Observe that the erector spinae are split into three longitudinal columns: **spinalis** medially, **longissimus** centrally, and **iliocostalis** laterally.
6. Observe that the columns of the erector spinae fuse inferiorly at the level of the sacrum and ilium as the **common erector spinae tendon** (see **Clinical Correlation 1.4**).

CLINICAL CORRELATION 1.4

Back Pain, Sprains, and Strains

ATLAS 1.14, 1.29, 1.30

Back pain is one of the most common health problems experienced by adults and may relate to a variety of structures in the back including skeletal, joints, IV discs, meninges, muscles, or nerves. Back strains involve tears in the muscle tissue, commonly in the postural muscles of the erector spinae, whereas back sprains are injuries to the ligamentous tissue without dislocation or fracture. Pain may stem from local injuries to the muscles, bones, joints, or discs, leading to spasms and loss of blood supply or guarding of the patient with acute or chronic injuries and illness. Compression or injury to nerves or nerve roots may refer pain to corresponding myotomes or dermatomes supplied by the affected nerve. Back pain may also be referred to the back from retroperitoneal organs within the abdominal cavity.

7. Beginning at the midthoracic level, use blunt dissection to separate the three columns of the erector spinae as far inferiorly as the common erector spinae tendon.
8. Review the attachments and actions of the erector spinae (see **TABLE 1.2**).

Semispinalis Capitis

ATLAS 1.29, 1.35; VIDEO 1.3.5

1. Refer to FIGURE 1.10.
2. Identify and clean the **semispinalis capitis**, the most superficial member of the transversospinales group of muscles, deep to the splenius capitis and cervicis.
3. Observe that the fibers of the semispinalis capitis course vertically, parallel to the vertebral column.
4. Review the attachments and actions of the semispinalis capitis (see **TABLE 1.2**).
5. Find the greater occipital nerve where it penetrates the semispinalis capitis and use blunt dissection to follow it deeply by widening the point of passage of the nerve through the muscle.
6. Detach the semispinalis capitis close to the occipital bone while preserving the greater occipital nerve (**Cut 1**).

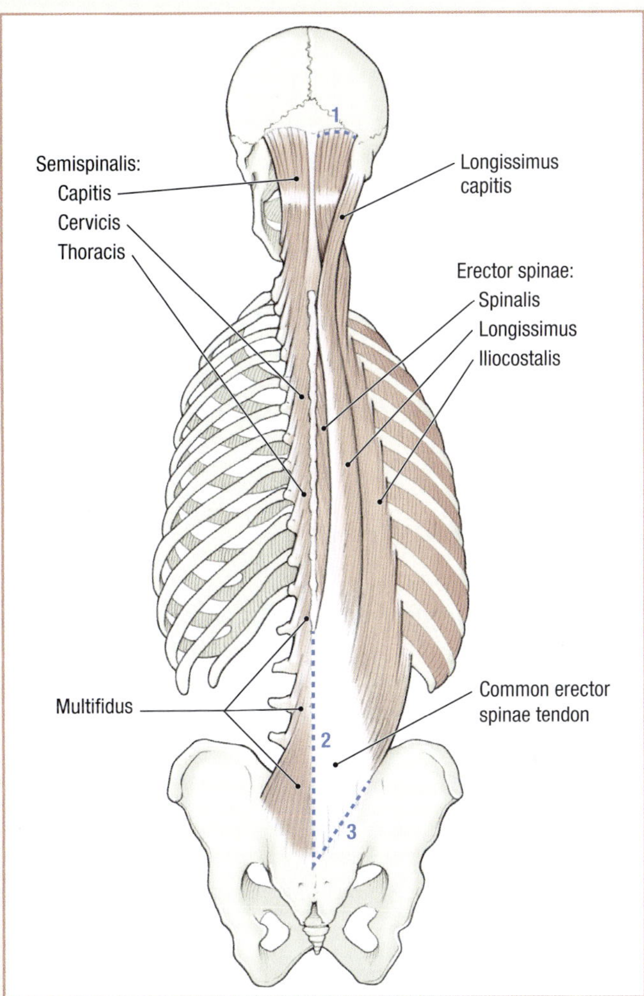

FIGURE 1.10 ■ Deep muscles of back isolated with erector spinae (*right*) and transversospinales (*left*). Posterior view.

7. Reflect the semispinalis capitis inferiorly while continuing to preserve the greater occipital nerve. *Note that it may be necessary to split the muscle superiorly around the nerve to facilitate reflection.*

Semispinalis Cervicis

ATLAS 1.29, 1.35; VIDEO 1.3.6

1. Refer to FIGURE 1.10.
2. Deep to the semispinalis capitis, identify the **semispinalis cervicis.**
3. Verify that the superior attachment of the semispinalis cervicis is the spinous process of the axis (C2). *Note that the semispinalis additionally has a thoracic component, semispinalis thoracis, but do not make an attempt to dissect it.*
4. Clean the superior extent of the semispinalis cervicis.
5. Review the attachments and actions of the semispinalis cervicis (see **TABLE 1.2**).

Multifidus

ATLAS 1.29, 1.31; VIDEO 1.3.7

1. Refer to FIGURE 1.10.
2. On one side of the body only, make a vertical incision through the common erector spinae tendon along the lumbar spinous processes to the median sacral crest inferiorly at approximately the S2 vertebral level (**Cut 2**).
3. From the inferior extent of the vertical incision, make a superolateral incision through the common erector spinae tendon from the median sacral crest to the iliac crest (**Cut 3**) to create a "V"-shaped incision.
4. Detach the common erector spinae tendon from its inferior attachments on the lumbar and sacral spinous processes and reflect it superolaterally.
5. Deep to the reflected common erector spinae tendon, identify and clean the **multifidus**.
6. Observe that the multifidus is very wide and thick over the sacrum and that it narrows in the lumbar region. *Note that the multifidus has components in the lumbar, thoracic, and cervical regions and terminates superiorly at vertebral level C2. Do not follow it superiorly beyond the lumbar region.*
7. Review the attachments and actions of the multifidus (see **TABLE 1.2**).

Dissection Follow-up

1. Refer to **TABLE 1.2**.
2. Review the locations and actions of the intermediate group of back muscles.
3. Review the locations and actions of the deep back muscles (splenius, erector spinae, and transversospinales).
4. Review the pattern of motor innervation to the deep group of back muscles.
5. Replace the intermediate and deep muscles of the back and any portion of reflected tissue back to their correct anatomical positions.

TABLE 1.2 Intermediate and Deep Muscles of Back

Muscle	*Medial Attachments*	*Lateral Attachments*	*Actions*	*Innervation*
INTERMEDIATE LAYER				
Serratus posterior superior	SP C7–T3	Superior borders of ribs 2–5, lateral to their angles	Elevates ribs 2–5	Anterior rami T2–T5
Serratus posterior inferior	SP T11–L2	Inferior border of ribs 9–12, lateral to their angles	Depresses ribs 9–12	Anterior rami T9–T12
DEEP LAYER				
Splenius capitis	Ligamentum nuchae, SP C7–T4	Mastoid process, lateral one-third of superior nuchal line	Unilateral—laterally flexes and rotates head or neck to same side Bilateral—extends head and neck	Posterior rami of middle cervical nerves
Splenius cervicis	SP T3–T6	TP C1–C3		
Spinalis	Median sacral crest, posterior surface sacrum, SP L and lower T, medial part iliac crest	SP of T and C	Unilateral—laterally flexes VT to same side Bilateral—extends VT and head, stabilizes VT	Posterior rami of lower cervical nerves
Longissimus		Between tubercles and angles of ribs, TP of T and C, and mastoid process		
Iliocostalis		Angles of lower ribs and TP of C		
Semispinalis capitis	TP C7–T6/T7, AP C4–C6	Between superior and inferior nuchal lines of occipital bone medially	Unilateral—extends and laterally rotates head to opposite side Bilateral—extends head	Posterior rami of spinal nerves
Semispinalis cervicis	TP T1–T5/T6	SP C2–C5	Unilateral—extends and laterally rotates neck to opposite side Bilateral—extends neck	
Multifidus	Sacrum, ilium, TP T1–L5, and AP C4–C7	SP L5–C2	Extends and rotates VT to opposite side	

Abbreviations: AP, articular process; C, cervical vertebrae; L, lumbar vertebrae; SP, spinous process; T, thoracic vertebrae; TP, transverse process; VT, vertebral column.

SUBOCCIPITAL REGION

Dissection Overview

The suboccipital region is located at the base of the skull in the posterior neck and classified as the most superior aspect of the back. Three small muscles lie within the suboccipital region bilaterally creating boundaries of the suboccipital triangle: rectus capitis posterior major, obliquus capitis superior, and obliquus capitis inferior. A fourth muscle is located medial to the suboccipital triangle near the midline, the rectus capitis posterior minor. All four suboccipital muscles are innervated by the suboccipital nerve (C1).

The order of dissection will be as follows: The bones of the suboccipital triangle will be reviewed. The muscles of the suboccipital triangle will be identified. The contents of the suboccipital triangle will be studied.

Skeletal Anatomy

Refer to an articulated skeleton and identify the following skeletal features.

Suboccipital Region

ATLAS 1.9, 1.10

1. Refer to FIGURES 1.1 and 1.11.
2. On the posterior aspect of the skull, identify the external occipital protuberance and the bilaterally located superior and inferior nuchal lines.
3. Observe the relationship of the areas of muscle attachment between the nuchal lines and their proximity to the base of the skull and **foramen magnum**.
4. Observe that the **atlas** (C1) does not have a body and that the **axis** (C2) has the **dens**, the body of C1 that fused to C2 during development.
5. Identify the **posterior arch** of the atlas, and the **posterior tubercle** approximately at the midpoint of the posterior arch. Observe that unlike other vertebrae, the atlas does not have a spinous process.
6. On the superior aspect of the posterior arch, identify the **groove for the vertebral artery** and observe its relationship to the **transverse foramen** on the **transverse process**.
7. Identify the bifid spinous process of the axis.

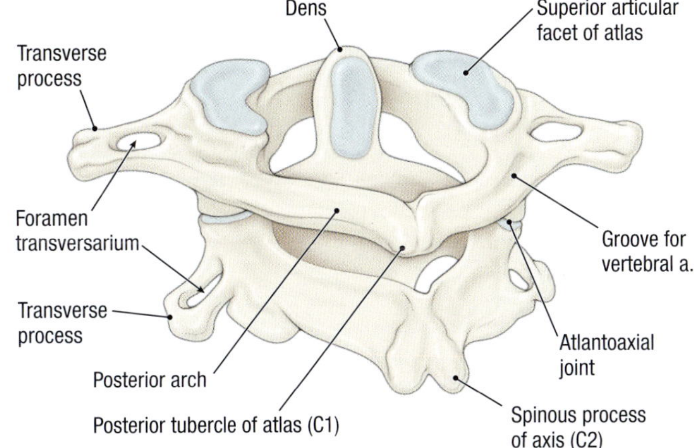

FIGURE 1.11 ■ Atlas (C1) and axis (C2). Posterolateral view.

Dissection Instructions

Suboccipital Muscles

ATLAS 1.35, 1.36; VIDEO 1.4.1

Dissection Note: The spinous process of C2 and the external occipital protuberance will be key landmarks for this dissection and should be used as points of reference for the suboccipital region.

1. Refer to FIGURE 1.12.
2. Identify the **spinous process of the axis** using the superior extent of the semispinalis cervicis as a reference point.
3. Using the spinous process of the axis as a landmark, identify and clean the **obliquus capitis inferior**, the inferior boundary of the suboccipital triangle.
4. Beginning superficially, use blunt dissection to follow the greater occipital nerve inferior to the inferior border of the obliquus capitis inferior. *Note that the greater occipital nerve (posterior ramus of C2) emerges between vertebrae C1 and C2.*
5. Using the spinous process of the axis as a landmark, identify and clean the **rectus capitis posterior major**, the medial boundary of the suboccipital triangle.
6. Medial to the rectus capitis posterior major, identify and clean the **rectus capitis posterior minor**.
7. Beginning at the occipital bone, identify and clean the **obliquus capitis superior**, the lateral boundary of the suboccipital triangle.
8. Review the attachments and actions of the suboccipital muscles (see **TABLE 1.3**).

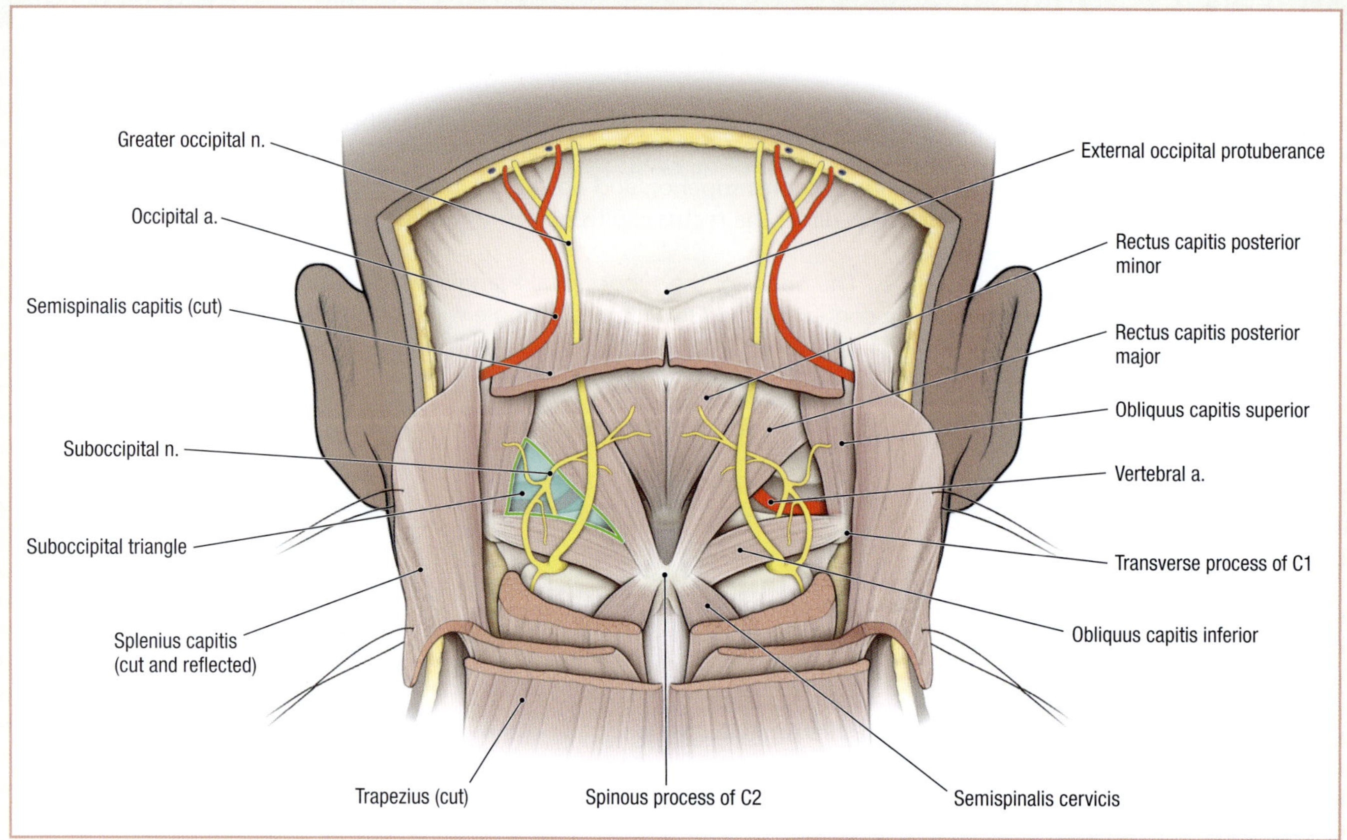

FIGURE 1.12 ● Suboccipital region. Posterior view.

Contents of Suboccipital Triangle

ATLAS 1.35B; VIDEO 1.4.2

1. Refer to FIGURE 1.12.
2. On one side, remove any veins found within the suboccipital region.
3. Follow the suboccipital nerve (posterior ramus of C1) to where it emerges between the occipital bone and the atlas (C1 vertebra). *Note that the suboccipital nerve supplies motor innervation to all the muscles of the suboccipital region and is the only posterior ramus of a cervical spinal nerve with no cutaneous distribution.*
4. Deep within the suboccipital triangle, identify and clean the **vertebral artery** superior to the posterior arch of C1. Do not follow the vertebral artery superiorly or inferiorly at this point in the dissection as this will be done with dissection of the neck.
5. To increase visibility of the path of the vertebral artery, detach the obliquus capitis superior and rectus capitis posterior major from their attachments on the inferior nuchal line and reflect them laterally and inferiorly, respectively.

Dissection Follow-up

1. Review the locations and actions of the suboccipital muscles in **TABLE 1.3**.
2. Review the path of the vertebral artery from the thorax to the posterior aspect of the brain and identify possible points of constriction of the vessel.
3. Return any reflected muscles and portions of skin back to their correct anatomical positions.
4. Review the skeletal anatomy of C1 and C2.
5. Review the movements allowed between the skull and C1 (atlantooccipital joint) and between C1 and C2 (atlantoaxial joint).

TABLE 1.3 Muscles of Suboccipital Region

Muscle	Medial Attachments	Lateral Attachments	Actions	Innervation
Rectus capitis posterior major	SP of C2 (axis)	Lateral inferior nuchal line of occipital bone	Extends head and rotates face to same side	Suboccipital n. (Posterior ramus C1)
Rectus capitis posterior minor	Posterior tubercle of C1 (atlas)	Medial inferior nuchal line of occipital bone	Extends head	
Obliquus capitis superior	TP of C1 (atlas) (inferior attachment)	Between lateral aspect of superior and inferior nuchal lines of occipital bone (superior attachment)	Extends head	
Obliquus capitis inferior	SP of C2 (axis)	TP of C1 (atlas)	Rotates face to same side	

Abbreviations: C, cervical vertebrae; n., nerve; SP, spinous process; TP, transverse process.

VERTEBRAL CANAL, SPINAL CORD, AND MENINGES

Dissection Overview

The vertebral canal extends from foramen magnum at the base of the skull through the stacked vertebral foramina of the cervical, thoracic, and lumbar vertebrae to terminate at the sacral hiatus. The vertebral canal encloses and protects the spinal cord, origin of spinal nerves, spinal meninges, and associated blood vessels.

The spinal cord begins at the inferior extent of the brainstem within the skull at the level of the foramen magnum and terminates in the adult at the level between the first and second lumbar vertebrae. Thirty-one pairs of spinal nerves (8 cervical, 12 thoracic, 5 lumbar, 5 sacral, and 1 coccygeal) arise from the spinal cord and emerge between adjacent vertebrae via the IV foramina. In the cervical region, the spinal nerves emerge superior to the corresponding vertebrae, leaving the C8 spinal nerve inferior to the C7 vertebral body. In the thoracic, lumbar, and sacral regions, the spinal nerves emerge inferior to the corresponding vertebral levels. Two prominent enlargements are visible along the length of the spinal cord correlating to an increased amount of neural tissue: the cervical enlargement, spinal cord segments C4–T1 which supply the upper limb, and the lumbar enlargement, spinal cord segments L2–S3 which supply the lower limb, as shown in FIGURE 1.13.

The order of dissection will be as follows: The erector spinae and transversospinales will be removed to expose the laminae of the vertebrae. A laminectomy will be performed to expose the spinal meninges from midthoracic to sacral levels. The spinal meninges will be examined, cut, and reflected to expose the spinal cord. The spinal cord and related structures will be studied.

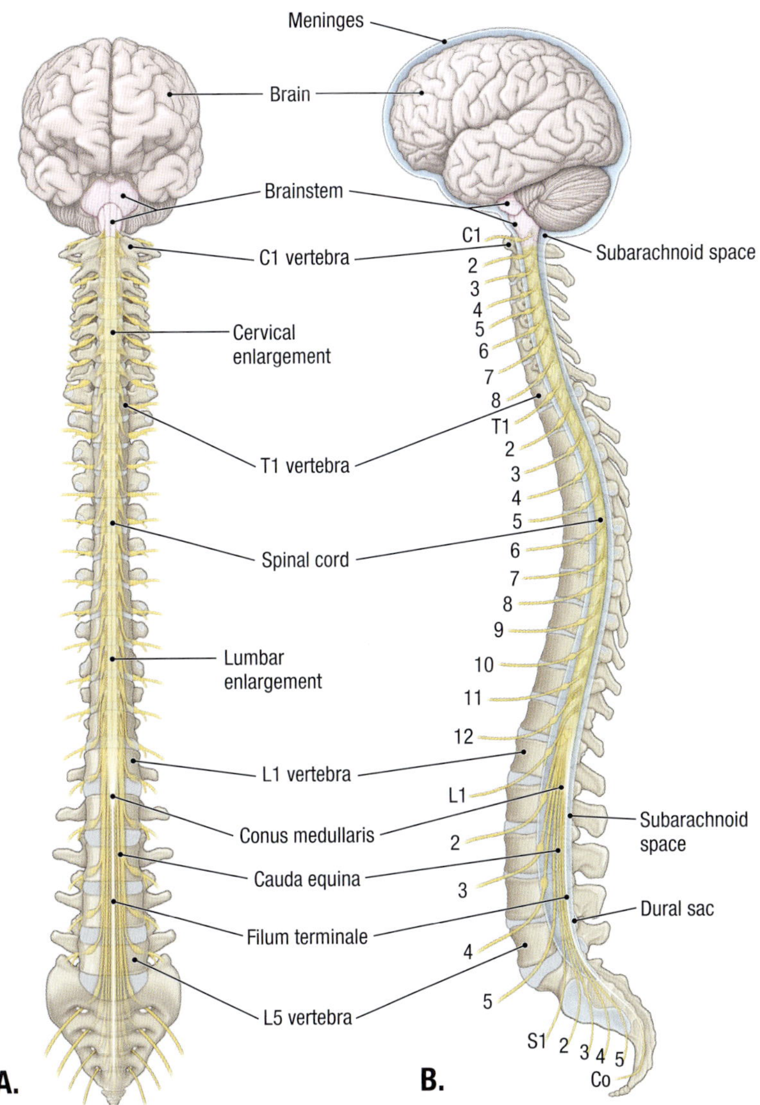

FIGURE 1.13 Spinal cord within vertebral canal. **A.** Anterior view. **B.** Lateral view.

Dissection Instructions

Laminectomy

ATLAS 1.37, 1.39; VIDEO 1.5.1

Dissection Note: A laminectomy is the surgical excision of one or more spinous processes and their supporting laminae to provide access to, or relieve pressure on, the spinal cord or nerve roots. Perform the following dissection instructions bilaterally and wear eye protection for all steps that require the use of a chisel, bone saw, or bone cutters.

1. Refer to FIGURE 1.14.
2. Make a horizontal cut with a scalpel at the level of T4 through the erector spinae.
3. Elevate the superior edge of the cut erector spinae and reflect the entire group of muscles inferiorly as far as S3. As you progress inferiorly, detach the muscles from the vertebral column with a scalpel to cleanly expose the underlying laminae.
4. Use scraping motions with a chisel to clean remaining muscle fragments off the laminae.
5. Use a chisel, power saw, or bone nibblers to cut the laminae of vertebrae T6 on both sides of the spinous processes. Make this cut at the lateral end of the laminae to gain wide exposure to the vertebral canal and ensure you are in the correct location prior to continuing. The cutting instrument should be angled at 45° to the vertical to maximize exposure of the vertebral canal.
6. Extend the laminectomy cut in the thoracic region to the T12 vertebral level. Be careful to not cut through the transverse processes and thus enter the thoracic cavity.
7. Use a scalpel to cut the **interspinous ligament** between vertebrae T6 and T7 and between vertebrae T12 and L1. Preserve the interspinous ligaments between T7 and T12 vertebral levels to keep the intervening spines together upon removal.
8. Use a chisel to pry the spinous processes and their laminae out as a unit paying attention to not damage the underlying structures. If done properly, the dura mater will remain in the vertebral canal with the spinal cord and remain undamaged.
9. On the posterior surface of the removed skeletal and ligamentous specimen, identify the **supraspinous ligament** overlying adjacent spinous processes. *Note that the supraspinous ligament extends from the sacrum to the C7 vertebral level where it blends with the ligamentum nuchae to continue to the external occipital protuberance.*
10. Identify the **interspinous ligaments** connecting adjacent spinous processes.
11. On the internal aspect of the removed portion of vertebral canal, identify the **ligamentum flavum** connecting adjacent laminae.
12. Use a chisel or bone nibblers to widen the created canal and remove any sharp edges of bone remaining after the initial cuts.
13. Continue the laminectomy procedure inferiorly in the lumbar region using direct observation of the exposed vertebral canal to help you make the cuts correctly. The laminae of lower lumbar levels may be quite deep due to the lordotic curvature of the region.
14. Make a "V-shaped" cut in the posterior surface of the sacrum with the inferior point of the wedge terminating at vertebral level S3. Exercise caution as the sacrum and sacral canal curve sharply posteriorly (superficially) due to the kyphotic curvature of the region.
15. Use a chisel to pry the spinous processes and their laminae out as a unit, paying attention to not damage the underlying structures, and place the removed spinous specimen in the tissue container.
16. When finished with the laminectomy, you should see the posterior surface of the dura mater from vertebral levels T6–S2 (see **Clinical Correlation 1.5**).

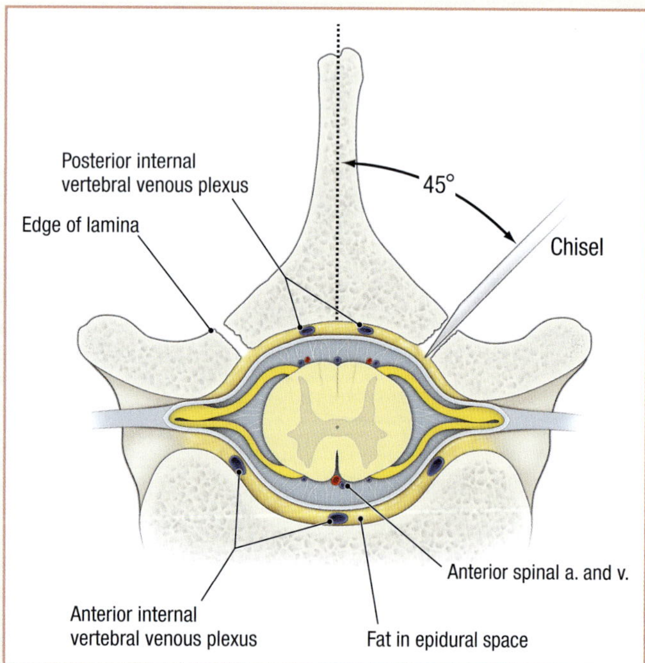

FIGURE 1.14 ● Laminectomy cuts into vertebral canal. Inferior view.

CLINICAL CORRELATION 1.5

Lumbar Puncture and Epidural Anesthesia

ATLAS 1.40, 1.41

Lumbar puncture, spinal anesthesia, and epidural anesthesia are performed in the lumbar region between L3 and L4 or L4 and L5 spinous process with the patient leaning forward or lying on their side. In the adult, the spinal cord typically terminates as the conus medullaris at the L1/L2 IV disc with the roots and rootlets of the cauda equina extending inferiorly, making lower lumbar levels comparatively safe locations for needle insertion (FIGURE B1.1). During a lumbar puncture (spinal tap), the inserted needle pierces the dura and arachnoid mater to reach the subarachnoid space to sample cerebrospinal fluid (CSF). In an epidural, an anesthetic agent is injected into the epidural space to block pain in a prolonged procedure such as child birth, whereas for spinal anesthesia, the anesthetic agent is introduced directly to the subarachnoid space to block sensation during lower limb arthroplasties, C-sections, or other procedures when the duration can be predicted.

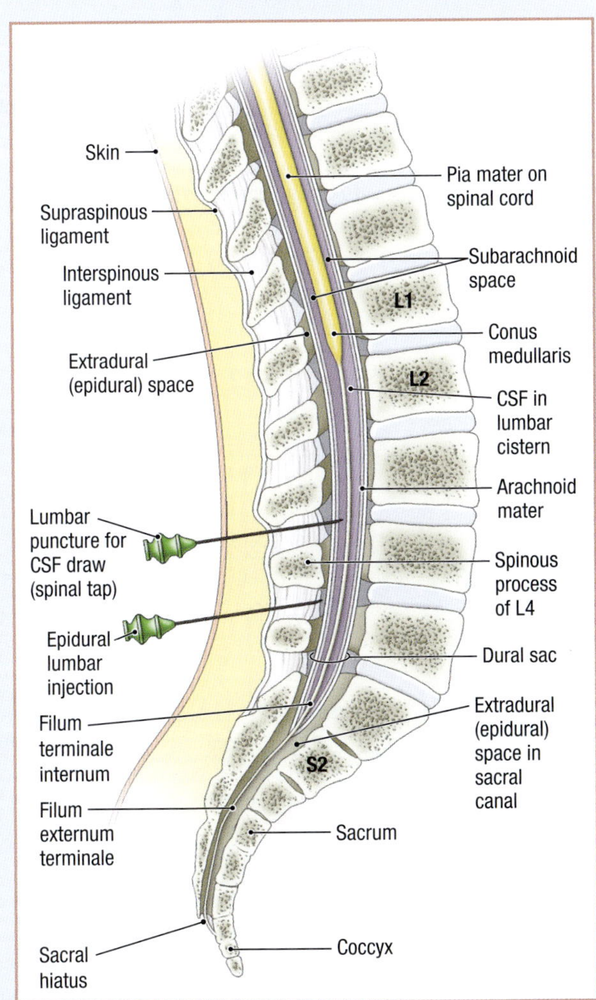

FIGURE B1.1 ■ Spinal cord and dural sac in vertebral canal. Midsagittal view.

Spinal Meninges

ATLAS 1.38, 1.39, 1.40; VIDEO 1.5.2

1. Within the **epidural (extradural) space** identify **epidural fat** and veins of the **internal vertebral venous plexus**. *Note that although the veins may be difficult to identify due to the embalming process, they are important as they may serve as a route for the spread of infection or metastasis of cancer from breast tissue in the thoracic region, or from pelvic tissue to the vertebrae, vertebral canal, and cranial cavity.*
2. Use blunt dissection to remove the epidural fat and veins from the epidural space.
3. Identify the **dural sac**, a longitudinal sheath within the vertebral canal formed by the **dura mater**, the most superficial meningeal layer. Observe that the dural sac surrounds and protects the spinal cord and ends inferiorly at vertebral level S2.
4. In the thoracic region, lift a fold of **dura mater** with forceps and use scissors to cut a small opening in its posterior midline.
5. Extend the cut inferiorly from the thoracic region to vertebral level S2 making efforts to avoid damaging the underlying arachnoid mater by retracting the dura mater laterally as you progress inferiorly. *If pins are available, use them to hold the cut edges of dura mater laterally to expose the underlying structures.*
6. Deep to the dura mater, identify the delicate and thin **arachnoid mater**, the middle meningeal layer.
7. Incise the arachnoid mater in the posterior midline and observe the **subarachnoid space**. *Note that the subarachnoid space contains CSF in the living person but not in the cadaver as it drains during the embalming process.*
8. Refer to FIGURE 1.15.
9. Retract the arachnoid mater laterally and identify the **spinal cord**. Observe that the spinal cord is completely invested by the **pia mater**, the deepest meningeal layer. *Note that the pia mater is the thinnest of the meningeal layers, lies directly on the surface of the spinal cord, and cannot be dissected.*
10. On the surface of the spinal cord, identify the **posterior spinal arteries and veins** coursing parallel to the **posterior median sulcus**, the centrally located groove.
11. On the spinal cord at lower thoracic vertebral levels, identify the **lumbar enlargement** (spinal cord segments L2–S3) providing innervation to the lower limb.
12. Inferior to the lumbar enlargement, identify the **conus medullaris (medullary cone)** demarcating the end of the spinal cord between vertebral levels L1 and L2.
13. Identify the collection of anterior and posterior nerve roots surrounding the conus medullaris in the lower vertebral canal forming the **cauda equina**, the collection of nervous tissue resembling a horse's tail within the dural sac.
14. Centrally within the cauda equina, identify the **filum terminale internum**, a delicate collection of pia

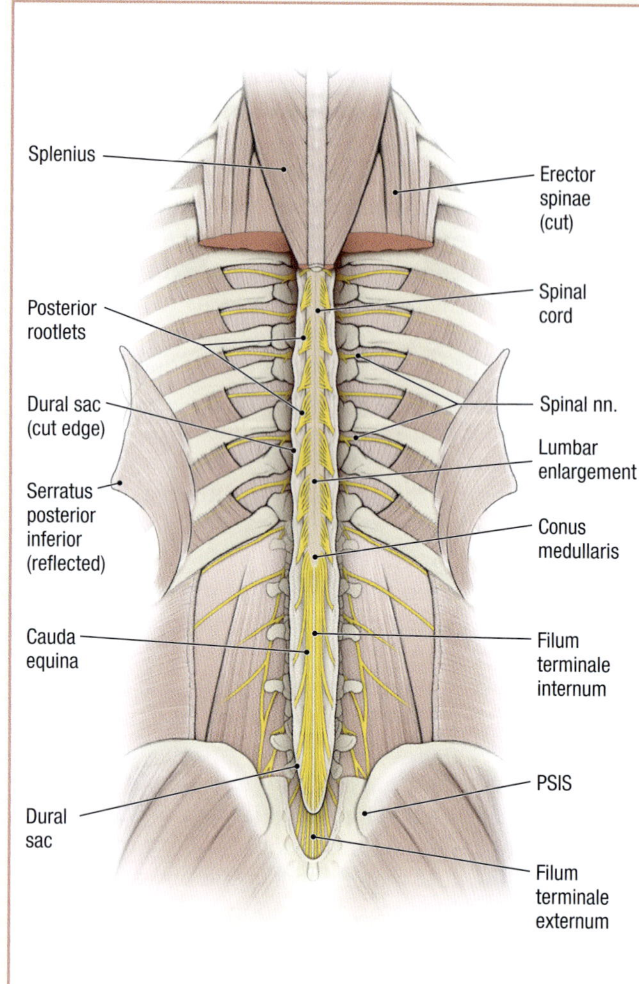

FIGURE 1.15 ■ Exposure of lower vertebral canal, spinal cord, and cauda equina. Posterior view.

mater extending inferiorly from the tip of the conus medullaris.

15. Observe that inferiorly, the filum terminale internum becomes encircled by the lower end of the dural sac and continues as the **filum terminale externum (coccygeal ligament)** below vertebral level S2 within the sacral canal. *Note that the filum terminale externum passes through the sacral hiatus and ends by attaching to the coccyx.*
16. Refer to FIGURE 1.16.
17. Identify the **denticulate ligaments**, extensions of pia mater attaching to the inner surface of the arachnoid lined dural sac on each side of the spinal cord.
18. Observe that the **posterior (dorsal) roots** are on the posterior side of the denticulate ligaments, whereas the **anterior (ventral) roots** are on the anterior side of the denticulate ligaments.
19. Use a probe to follow the posterior and anterior roots to the point where they pierce the dura mater laterally to enter the IV foramina.
20. Follow the posterior roots medially to observe that they are formed by the merging of **posterior rootlets** arising from the spinal cord.
21. Observe that the anterior roots are formed by **anterior rootlets,** although visibility may be somewhat restricted due to the orientation of the spinal cord.
22. Make an effort to observe the small **blood vessels** coursing along the anterior and posterior roots. Depending on the vertebral level, the small blood vessels may be branches of posterior intercostal, lumbar, or vertebral arteries. The arteries pass into the vertebral canal via the IV foramen and supply blood to the spinal cord.
23. In the thoracic region, insert a probe into an IV foramen posterior to the posterior roots.

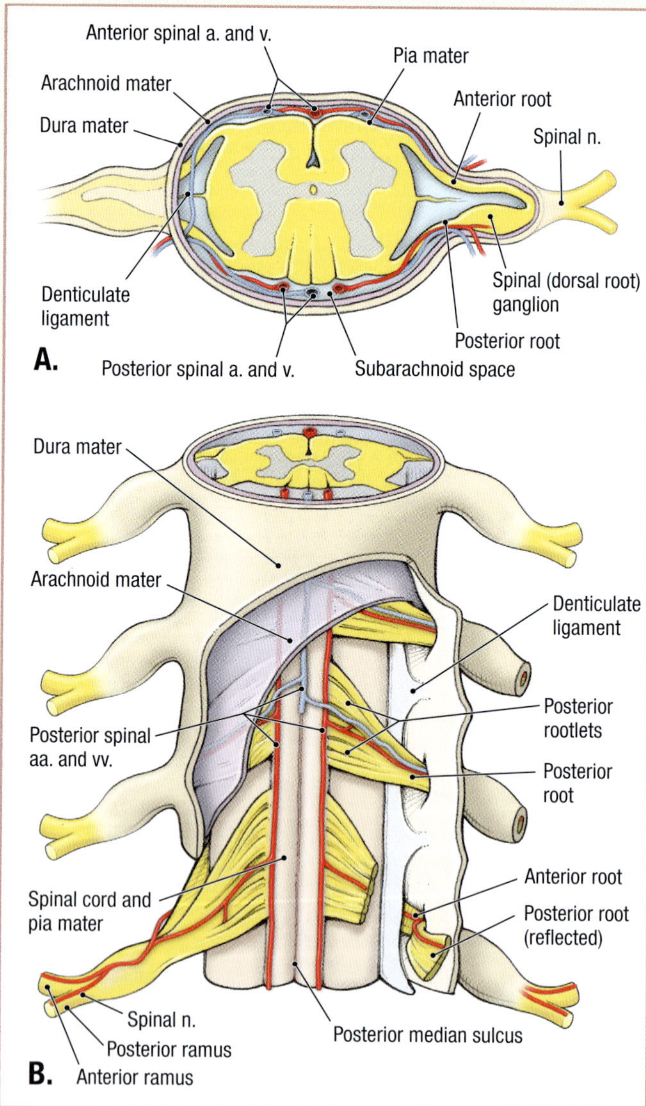

FIGURE 1.16 ■ **A.** Axial section of spinal cord. Superior view. **B.** Relationship of meninges to the spinal cord, spinal nerves, roots, and rootlets. Posterior view.

24. Use bone cutters to remove the posterior wall of the IV foramen and expose the **spinal (dorsal root) ganglion**. *Note that the spinal ganglion is the location of the sensory cell bodies of the spinal nerves.*
25. Lateral to the spinal ganglion, identify the **spinal nerve,** the point where the posterior and anterior roots merge.
26. Follow the spinal nerve laterally a short distance to the point where it divides into a **posterior ramus** and an **anterior ramus**. *Note that the posterior ramus will supply the deep muscles of the back and the overlying skin, whereas the anterior ramus will be responsible for the anterolateral trunk and limbs.*

Dissection Follow-up

1. Review the formation and branches of a typical spinal nerve.
2. Review the pattern of motor innervation to the deep back muscles as compared to the superficial muscles of the back.
3. Review the coverings and parts of the spinal cord and study an illustration that shows the blood supply to the spinal cord.
4. Consult a dermatome chart and relate this pattern of cutaneous innervation to the spinal cord segments.

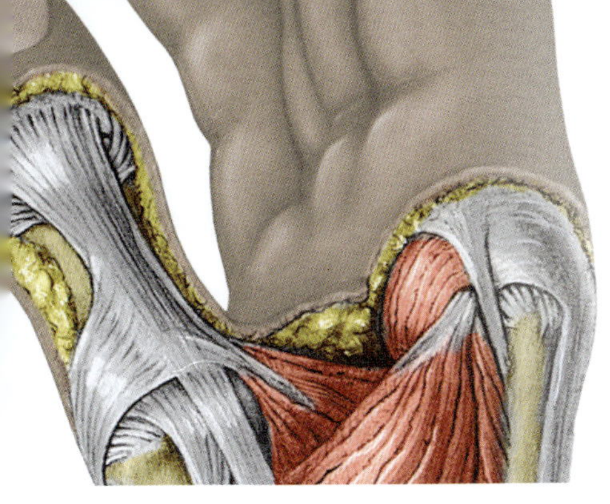

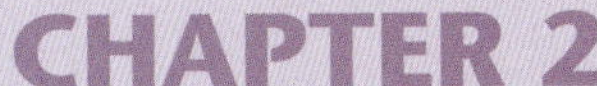

CHAPTER 2
Upper Limb

REFERENCES

ATLAS = *Grant's Atlas of Anatomy*, 16th ed., figure number

VIDEO = *Grant's Dissection Videos*, video sequence number

The upper limb extends from the shoulder to the tips of the fingers and is divided into four regions: shoulder (pectoral girdle), arm (brachium), forearm (antebrachium), and hand (manus). The upper limb is structured for mobility so we can place our hands, fundamentally grasping organs, in a variety of orientations within a large area of space. Some of the muscles that control the upper limb are intrinsic, those which originate and terminate within the upper limb, and some are extrinsic, those which either originate or terminate outside the upper limb.

Dissection of the upper limb will commence with dissection of the scapular region with the body in a prone position. By starting with the scapular region, the ongoing study of the superficial muscles of the back will continue into the upper limb and minimizes the number of full body rotations required. Once the scapular dissection has been completed, the body will be turned to a supine position and dissection of the upper limb will continue from an anterior approach.

CLINICAL CORRELATIONS

During your dissection protocol, you may encounter anatomical variations, clinical conditions, disease processes, or medical devices in your cadaveric donor. The following select clinical correlations will be described in more detail throughout this chapter.

Upper Limb

2.1. Rotator Cuff Injury, see **Rotator Cuff** sequence. ATLAS 2.37
2.2. Breast Quadrants, Cancer, and Implants, see **Breast** sequence. ATLAS 3.5, 3.6
2.3. Long Thoracic, Thoracodorsal, and Axillary Nerve Injuries, see **Brachial Plexus** sequence. ATLAS 2.4A, 2.30A, 2.32, 2.46
2.4. Brachial Artery Variants and Damage, see **Neurovasculature of Arm** sequence. ATLAS 2.11, 2.30B, 2.54F
2.5. Median and Ulnar Nerve Injuries, see **Neurovasculature of Anterior Forearm** sequence. ATLAS 2.5, 2.6, 2.53
2.6. Carpal Tunnel Syndrome, see **Carpal Tunnel** sequence. ATLAS 2.69, 2.71
2.7. Recurrent Branch of Median Nerve Injury, see **Thenar Eminence** sequence. ATLAS 2.73, 2.78
2.8. Radial Nerve Injury, see **Superficial Layer of Posterior Forearm** sequence. ATLAS 2.7, 2.88
2.9. Shoulder Injuries, see **Glenohumeral Joint** sequence. ATLAS 2.50, 2.51

SKIN AND SUPERFICIAL MUSCLES OF BACK

If the upper limb is your first dissection unit, place the cadaver in a prone position and follow the dissection protocols outlined in Chapter 1 for **Skin Incisions of Back**, **Superficial Suboccipital Region**, and **Superficial Muscles of Back**.

SHOULDER AND POSTERIOR ARM

Dissection Overview

There are six shoulder (scapulohumeral) muscles attached between the scapula and the humerus: deltoid, supraspinatus, infraspinatus, teres major, teres minor, and subscapularis. The triceps brachii, located within the posterior compartment of the arm, passes between the attachment sites of the two teres muscles to create spaces, or windows, through which neurovascular structures may be found. The anconeus, the other muscle in the posterior compartment of the arm, will be studied with the posterior forearm. Further examination of the fascia, contents, and organization of the arm will be studied when the anterior compartment of the arm is dissected.

The order of dissection will be as follows: The skeletal anatomy of the shoulder will be studied. The deltoid will be studied, detached from the spine of the scapula, and the course of its nerve and artery will be explored. The four muscles arising from the posterior surface of the scapula (supraspinatus, infraspinatus, teres major, and teres minor) will be studied, and their nerves and blood vessels will be demonstrated. The boundaries and contents of the quadrangular and triangular spaces will be identified. The posterior arm will be cleaned and studied.

Skeletal Anatomy

Refer to an articulated skeleton or disarticulated scapula and humerus to identify the following skeletal features.

Posterior Scapula

ATLAS 2.1B, 2.3E, 2.3F

1. Refer to FIGURE 2.1.
2. On the posterior aspect of the scapula, identify the **spine of the scapula** and observe that it separates the **supraspinous fossa** from the **infraspinous fossa** and terminates laterally as the **acromion process**.
3. Along the superior border of the scapula, identify the **suprascapular notch** along the anterior aspect of the supraspinous fossa.
4. On the lateral aspect of the scapula, inferior to the acromion, identify the **glenoid cavity** forming the "socket" of the glenohumeral joint.
5. Superior and inferior to the depression of the glenoid cavity, identify the **supraglenoid** and **infraglenoid tubercles**, respectively. *Note that the roughened regions of the tubercles serve as attachment sites for muscles of the upper limb.*

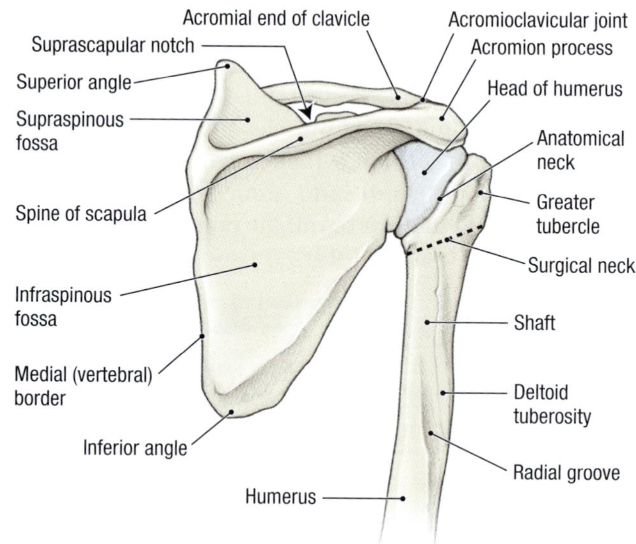

FIGURE 2.1 ● Skeleton of right shoulder. Posterior view.

Proximal Posterior Humerus

ATLAS 2.3E, 2.38D

1. On the proximal aspect of the humerus medially, identify the smooth surface of the **head of the humerus**, the "ball" of the glenohumeral joint.
2. Inferolateral to the head of the humerus, locate the **anatomical neck** coursing obliquely through the thick epiphysis of the bone.
3. Inferior to the greater and lesser tubercles, where the bone begins to narrow, identify the **surgical neck of the humerus**.
4. Identify the **shaft** of the humerus and the **deltoid tuberosity** along its lateral aspect.
5. On the posterior surface of the shaft, identify the **radial groove** coursing obliquely.

Surface Anatomy

The surface anatomy of the shoulder may be studied on a living subject or on a cadaver. On the cadaver, note that fixation of tissue during embalming may make it difficult to distinguish bone from well-preserved soft tissues in some specimens.

Posterior Shoulder

ATLAS 1.23, 2.1B, 2.33

1. Refer to FIGURE 2.2.
2. Place the cadaver in the prone (face down) position.
3. Palpate the **spine of the scapula** coursing horizontally along an oblique line on the posterior surface of the scapula and observe that it subdivides the scapular region into a portion superior (supraspinous) and inferior (infraspinous) to it.
4. Progress medially from the spine of the scapula toward the **medial (vertebral) border of the scapula**. *Note that the medial aspect of the spine of the scapula is approximately at the T3 vertebral level.*
5. Follow the medial border of the scapula inferiorly toward the **inferior angle of the scapula** (at vertebral level T7).
6. Progress laterally from the inferior angle along the path of the latissimus dorsi and identify the **posterior axillary fold**. *Note that the lateral (axillary) border of the scapula is not readily palpable because the latissimus dorsi, teres major, and teres minor lie along the lateral aspect of the scapula.*
7. Return to the spine of the scapula and palpate laterally to the **acromion process of the scapula**. Observe that the acromion process is a palpable landmark of the shoulder and that it articulates anteriorly with the **lateral (acromial) end of the clavicle** at the **acromioclavicular (AC) joint**.

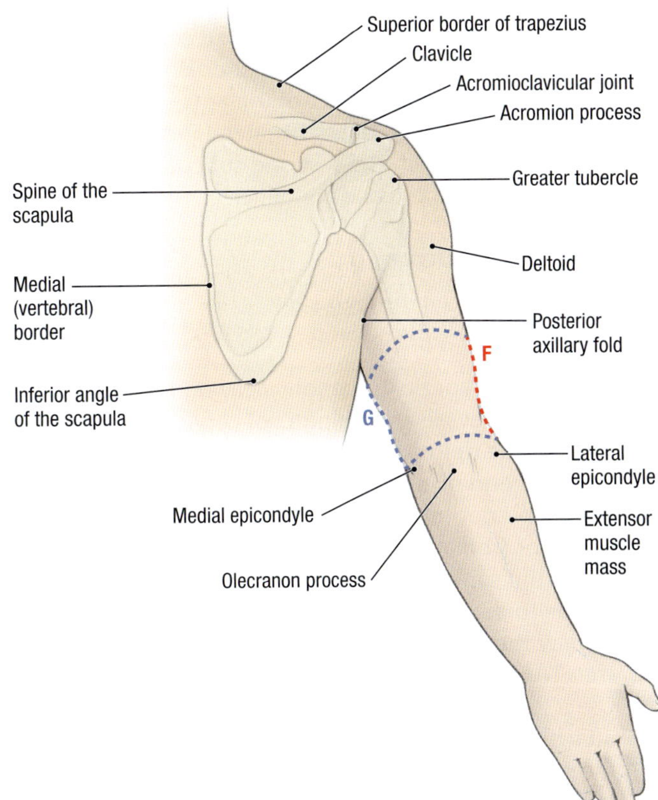

FIGURE 2.2 ● Surface anatomy of shoulder. Posterior view.

8. Palpate the triangular-shaped **deltoid** along the posterior aspect of the shoulder and observe that it attaches inferior to the spine, the acromion of the scapula, and the lateral aspect of the clavicle.
9. Palpate inferiorly along the lateral aspect of the deltoid to where it attaches to the **deltoid tuberosity of the humerus**.
10. Using the deltoid as a landmark, palpate the muscles within the **anterior** and **posterior compartments of the arm**.

Dissection Instructions

Skin Incisions of Posterior Arm

VIDEO 2.1.1

Dissection Note: Prior to commencing with skin incisions, decide to perform either a full- or partial-thickness approach and to either reflect or remove the skin from the dissection field. See **Removing Skin** in the **Introduction Chapter** for descriptions.

1. Refer to FIGURE 2.2.
2. With the cadaver in the prone position, abduct the upper limb to 45° or as far as possible. If a block is available, place it under the chest and shoulder to facilitate dissection of the region.
3. Use a scalpel to make a vertical skin incision along the medial aspect of the arm from the midpoint of the arm (G) to a point superior to the medial epicondyle of the humerus.
4. Beginning near the medial epicondyle where the vertical incision stopped, make a shallow incision around the posterior surface of the elbow toward the lateral aspect of the limb parallel to the cut along the posterior aspect of the arm (G to F).

Dissection Note: If reflecting the skin, skip step 5.

5. Make a vertical incision along the lateral aspect of the arm from the midpoint of the arm (F) to a point superior to the lateral epicondyle connecting with the horizontal incision.
6. Reflect the skin of the posterior arm from medial to lateral using either a pair of locking forceps or the buttonhole technique.
7. Perform either a full- or partial-thickness reflection of the skin and subcutaneous tissue to expose the underlying deep fascia of the posterior compartment of the arm.

8. If reflecting the skin, utilize the uncut sections of skin laterally as hinge points to leave the skin attached along the peripheral aspect of the arm.
9. If removing the skin, once the lateral incision points are reached, detach the skin and subcutaneous tissue and place it in the tissue container.

Posterior Shoulder

ATLAS 2.42, 2.46, 2.47; VIDEO 2.1.2

1. Refer to FIGURE 2.3.
2. Reflect the trapezius superiorly, leaving it attached along the clavicle and "hinge" of cervical fascia.
3. Identify the **deltoid** forming the contours of the shoulder and observe that it is composed of three parts: anterior (clavicular), middle (acromial), and posterior (spinal).
4. Clean the surface and borders of the posterior part of the deltoid.
5. Review the attachments and actions of the deltoid (see **TABLE 2.1**).
6. Use a scalpel to detach the deltoid from its posterior attachments along the inferior aspect of the spine of the scapula and acromion process. Leave the deltoid attached anteriorly along the clavicle and inferiorly where it attaches to the humerus at the deltoid tuberosity.
7. Reflect the posterior part of the deltoid laterally, taking care not to tear the vessel and nerve branches on its deep surface.
8. Identify the **axillary nerve** and the **posterior circumflex humeral artery** and **vein** on the deep surface of the deltoid near the surgical neck of the humerus. *Note that the axillary nerve innervates the deltoid and the teres minor.*
9. Clean the axillary nerve and posterior circumflex humeral vessels using blunt dissection and trace them around the posterior aspect of the surgical neck of the humerus deeply into the **quadrangular space**.
10. Observe that the quadrangular space is bound superiorly by the teres minor, inferiorly by the teres major, and medially by the long head of the triceps brachii. The lateral border of the quadrangular space is the surgical neck of the humerus, which may not visible at this time.
11. Identify and clean the proximal end of the **long head of the triceps brachii**. Observe that the long head passes posterior to the teres major and anterior to the teres minor to insert at the infraglenoid tubercle of the scapula. *Note that the triceps brachii will be further dissected with the posterior compartment of the arm.*

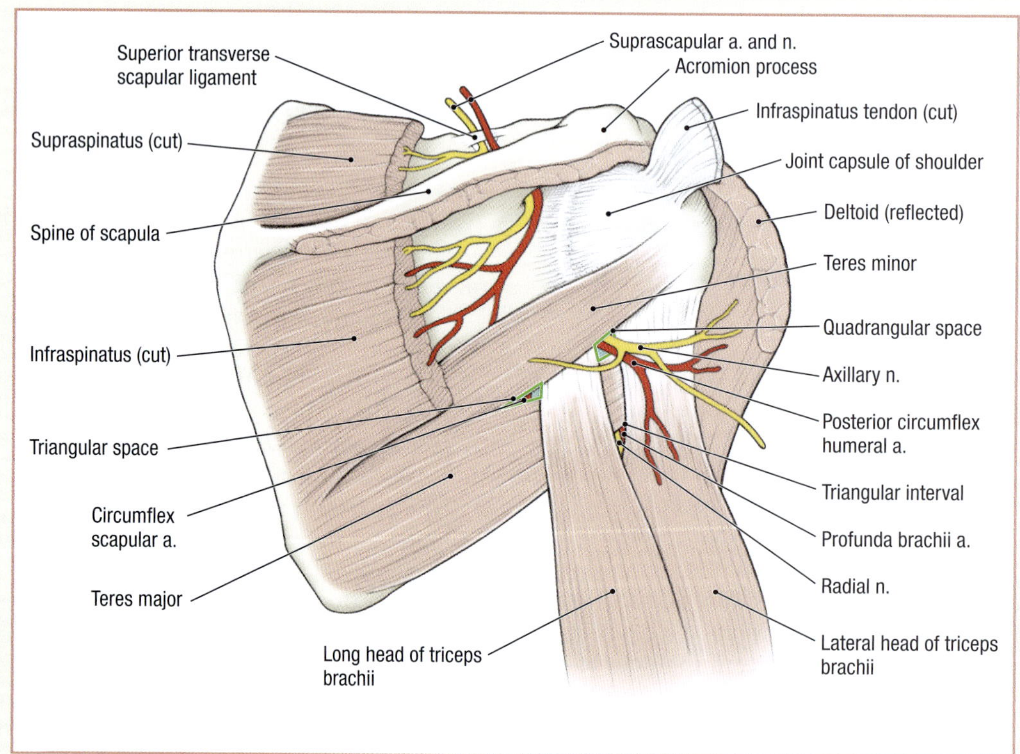

FIGURE 2.3 ● Neurovasculature of shoulder. Posterior view.

12. Clean and define the borders of the **teres major**. If the teres major is partially covered by the latissimus dorsi, simply loosen the connective tissue surrounding the latissimus dorsi to gently pull it laterally.
13. Review the attachments and actions of the teres major (see **TABLE 2.1**).

Rotator Cuff

ATLAS 2.37, 2.46; VIDEO 2.1.3

1. Refer to FIGURE 2.3.
2. The four muscles of the **rotator cuff** are the supraspinatus, infraspinatus, teres minor, and subscapularis. *Note that the subscapularis will be dissected with the axilla.*
3. Inferior to the spine of the scapula, identify and clean the **infraspinatus** within the infraspinous fossa of the scapula. *Note that the infraspinatus is often covered by tough connective tissue, which may need to be removed with sharp dissection.*
4. Inferolateral to the infraspinatus, identify and clean the **teres minor** along the lateral border of the scapula. Make an effort to clearly define its superior and inferior borders but not its medial and lateral attachments.
5. Review the attachments and actions of the infraspinatus and teres minor (see **TABLE 2.1**).
6. Identify the **triangular space** medial to the quadrangular space and observe that it is bound superiorly by the teres minor, inferiorly by the teres major, and laterally by the long head of the triceps brachii.
7. Identify the **circumflex scapular artery** and **vein** within the triangular space. Make no deliberate effort to follow the vessels deep to the muscles at this time.
8. Superior to the spine of the scapula, identify and clean the **supraspinatus** within the supraspinous fossa (see **Clinical Correlation 2.1**).
9. Review the attachments and actions of the supraspinatus (see **TABLE 2.1**).
10. Use a scalpel to transect the supraspinatus about 5 cm lateral to the superior angle of the scapula and medial to the suprascapular notch. If a disarticulated scapula is available, hold it over the scapula of the cadaver to help you locate the proper level of the cut.
11. Use blunt dissection to loosen and reflect the lateral portion of the supraspinatus from the supraspinous fossa.

CLINICAL CORRELATION 2.1

Rotator Cuff Injury

ATLAS 2.37

The muscles of the rotator cuff collectively act to maintain glenohumeral stability by keeping the head of the humerus in the glenoid fossa. Repetitive use of the glenohumeral joint may lead to inflammation of the capsule, the bursae, or nearby tendons resulting in shoulder pain. Trauma or calcification of the joint structures may lead to a tear through the tendinous attachment of one of the rotator cuff muscles. The most torn of which is the supraspinatus tendon where it courses superior to the glenohumeral joint to assist shoulder abduction. The supraspinatus is also particularly susceptible to injury as its tendon is in a largely avascular region of the joint.

Suprascapular Artery and Nerve

ATLAS 2.46, 2.47; VIDEO 2.1.4

1. Refer to FIGURE 2.3.
2. Identify the **suprascapular artery** and **nerve** in the supraspinous fossa.
3. Follow the artery and nerve anteriorly to demonstrate their relationship with the **superior transverse scapular ligament**. Observe that the suprascapular artery passes superior to the superior transverse scapular ligament and that the suprascapular nerve passes inferior to it. *Note that this relationship can be remembered by use of a mnemonic: **A**rmy (**a**rtery) goes over the bridge; **N**avy (**n**erve) goes under the bridge, with the "bridge" being the superior transverse scapular ligament.*
4. Transect the infraspinatus about 5 cm lateral to the medial border of the scapula.
5. Use blunt dissection to loosen and reflect the lateral portion of the infraspinatus from the infraspinous fossa.
6. Follow the **suprascapular artery** and **nerve** laterally around the spine of the scapula deep to the acromion process to the infraspinous fossa where they supply the infraspinatus.
7. Observe that the suprascapular artery sends branches to the circumflex scapular and dorsal scapular arteries to contribute to the collateral circulation of the scapular anastomoses.

Posterior Compartment of Arm

ATLAS 2.42, 2.45, 2.46; VIDEO 2.1.5

1. Refer to FIGURE 2.4.
2. With the cadaver in the prone position, rotate the upper limb medially to gain better access to the posterior compartment of the arm.
3. Use sharp dissection to open the posterior compartment of the arm by making a longitudinal incision through the brachial fascia from the teres minor superiorly to the olecranon of the ulna inferiorly.
4. Use blunt dissection to spread and reflect the cut edges of the brachial fascia.

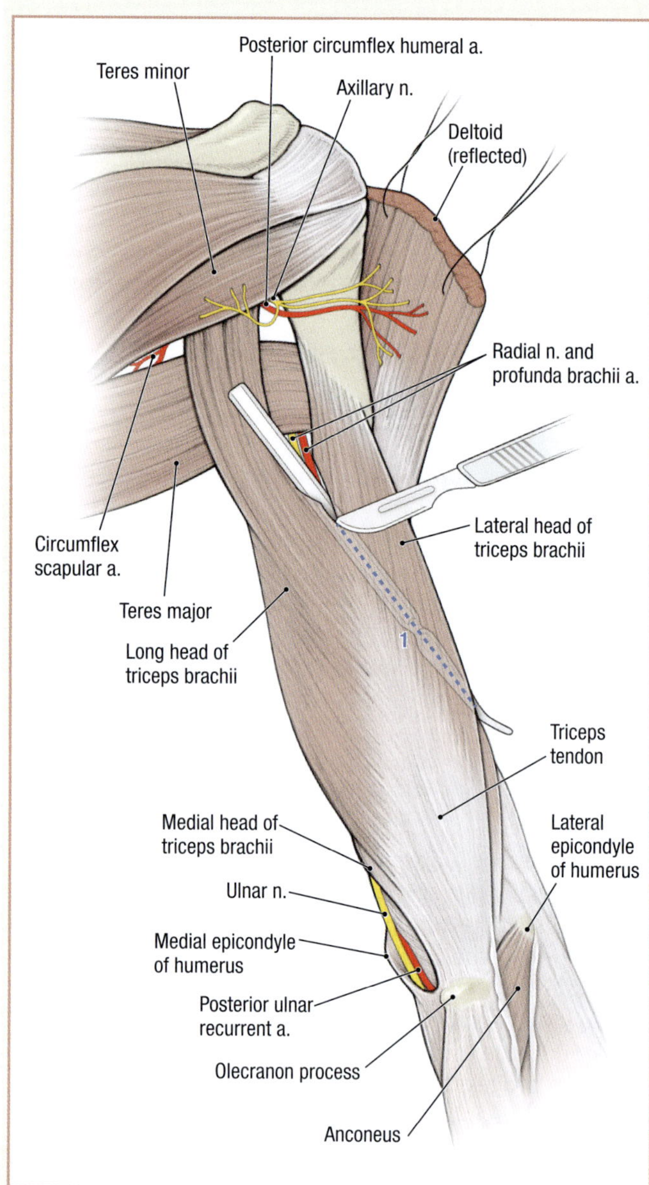

FIGURE 2.4 ● Shoulder and posterior compartment of arm. Posterior view.

5. On the periphery of the arm, use sharp dissection to detach the brachial fascia from the medial and lateral intermuscular septa and place it in the tissue container.
6. Identify the **triceps brachii** and observe the arrangement of its three muscular heads: the **long head**, more superficial and posterior to the other heads; the **lateral head**, lateral to the radial groove; and the **medial head**, medial to the radial groove.
7. Review the attachments and actions of the triceps brachii (see **TABLE 2.1**).
8. Use blunt dissection to separate the long head of the triceps brachii from the lateral head, inferior to where the teres major crosses the anterior surface of the long head.
9. Identify the **triangular interval** inferior to the quadrangular space and observe that it is bound medially by the long head of the triceps brachii, laterally by the lateral head of the triceps brachii, and superiorly by the inferior border of the teres major.
10. Widen the triangular interval and identify the **radial nerve** and the **profunda brachii artery (deep artery of the arm** or **deep brachial artery)** within the space.
11. Push a probe from superior to inferior along the course of the radial nerve between the lateral head of the triceps brachii and the humerus.
12. On one side of the body only, use a scalpel to transect the lateral head of the triceps brachii where it merges with the long head over the probe.
13. Spread apart the heads of the triceps and use blunt dissection to clean the radial nerve and the deep artery of the arm within the radial groove of the humerus. Do not follow the radial nerve or deep artery of the arm distally at this time as this will be performed with dissection of the cubital fossa.

Dissection Follow-up

1. Review the innervations and attachments of the scapulohumeral muscles in **TABLE 2.1**.
2. List the action of each muscle of the rotator cuff individually as well as the combined action of the rotator cuff group of muscles.
3. Review the origin, course, and distribution of the transverse cervical, dorsal scapular, and suprascapular arteries and their roles in the scapular anastomoses.
4. Review the relationship of the suprascapular artery and nerve to the superior transverse scapular ligament.
5. Review the boundaries and contents of the triangular and quadrangular spaces, and the triangular interval.
6. Replace the muscles of the scapular region and posterior arm in their correct anatomical positions.

TABLE 2.1 Scapulohumeral Muscles

Muscle	*Proximal Attachments*	*Distal Attachments*	*Actions*	*Innervation*
Deltoid	Spine of the scapula, acromion of the scapula, lateral one-third of the clavicle	Deltoid tuberosity of the humerus	Abducts, flexes, extends, and medially and laterally rotates the humerus	Axillary n.
Supraspinatus	Supraspinous fossa of the scapula	Superior facet of the greater tubercle of the humerus	Abducts the humerus	Suprascapular n.
Infraspinatus	Infraspinous fossa of the scapula	Middle facet of the greater tubercle of the humerus	Laterally rotates the humerus	Suprascapular n.
Teres major	Inferior angle of the scapula	Medial lip of the intertubercular sulcus of the humerus	Adducts and medially rotates the humerus	Lower subscapular n.
Teres minor	Lateral border of the scapula	Inferior facet of the greater tubercle of the humerus	Laterally rotates the humerus	Axillary n.
Subscapularis	Subscapular fossa	Lesser tubercle of the humerus	Medially rotates the humerus	Upper and lower subscapular nn.

Abbreviations: n., nerve; nn., nerves.

PECTORAL REGION AND SUBCUTANEOUS TISSUE OF UPPER LIMB

Dissection Overview

The pectoral region covers portions of the anterior and lateral thoracic walls. The breast, a major content of the pectoral region, commonly extends from the lateral border of the sternum to the midaxillary line and from ribs 2 to 6, although the amount of breast tissue is quite variable. The breast is positioned anterior to the pectoral fascia and separated from the underlying muscle and fascia by the retromammary space. The breast contains mammary glands, which are modified sweat glands compartmentalized into lobules. The lobules are separated by suspensory ligaments that attach the underlying fascia to the skin.

The subcutaneous tissue of the upper limb contains fat, superficial fascia, lymphatics, superficial veins, and cutaneous nerves. In the living body, the superficial veins may be visible through the skin and are frequently used for venipuncture. In the cadaver, the superficial veins are not conspicuous.

The order of dissection will be as follows: The skeletal anatomy of the pectoral region will be studied. The skin will be either reflected or removed from the pectoral region and upper limb. The breast will be dissected in female cadaveric specimens. The subcutaneous tissue will either be removed or reflected in a full- or partial-thickness approach. Select superficial veins and cutaneous nerves will be dissected.

Skeletal Anatomy

Refer to an articulated skeleton or individual bones and identify the following skeletal features.

Scapula and Clavicle

ATLAS 2.2, 2.3

1. Refer to FIGURE 2.5.
2. On a clavicle, identify the **medial (sternal) end** and the **lateral (acromial) end**.
3. Observe that the medial end of the clavicle articulates with the **manubrium of the sternum** to create the **sternoclavicular (SC) joint** medially.
4. Observe that the lateral end of the clavicle articulates with the **acromion of the scapula** to create the **AC joint** laterally.
5. On the anterior aspect of the scapula, identify the **subscapular fossa** bound medially and laterally by the **medial (vertebral)** and **lateral (axillary) borders**, respectively.
6. Identify the **coracoid process**, the "beak-like" prominence extending anteriorly from the scapula lateral to the **suprascapular notch** and medial to the **glenoid fossa**.

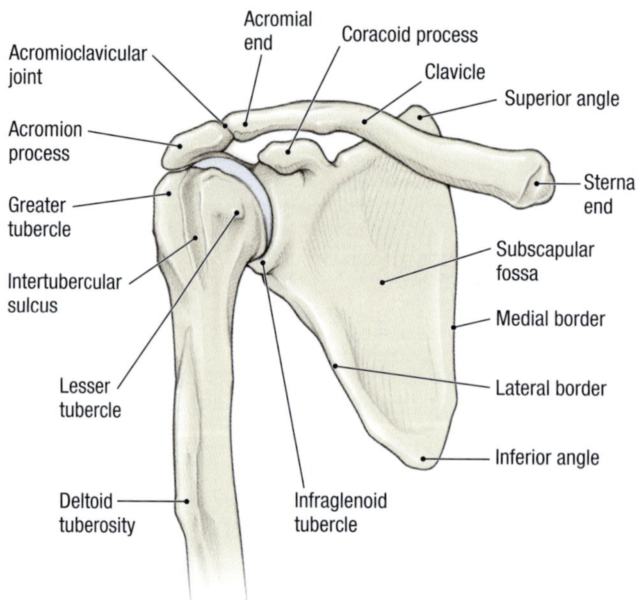

FIGURE 2.5 ● Skeleton of right shoulder. Anterior view.

Proximal Anterior Humerus

ATLAS 2.3D, 2.38A

1. Identify the **head of the humerus** on the proximal medial aspect of the bone and observe that it articulates with the glenoid fossa of the scapula to create the glenohumeral (shoulder) joint.
2. Identify the large bony prominence of the **greater tubercle** on the proximal aspect of the humerus laterally.
3. Identify the **lesser tubercle** on the proximal aspect of the humerus anteriorly and note its separation from the greater tubercle by the **intertubercular sulcus (bicipital groove)**.
4. Identify the **deltoid tuberosity** along the midshaft of the humerus laterally.

Surface Anatomy

The surface anatomy of the upper limb and pectoral region may be studied on a living subject or on a cadaver. On the cadaver, note that fixation of tissue during embalming may make it difficult to distinguish bone from well-preserved soft tissues in some specimens.

Pectoral Region

ATLAS 2.18, 3.1, 3.3

1. Refer to FIGURE 2.6.
2. Place the cadaver in the supine position.
3. Beginning at the midline of the neck, palpate the **jugular notch** between the sternal ends of the **clavicles** where they articulate with the manubrium of the sternum at the SC joints.
4. On the anterior chest wall, identify and palpate the **sternal angle** (manubriosternal joint) at the level of the **2nd costal cartilage**.
5. Palpate inferiorly along the sternum toward the **xiphisternal junction** at the level of the 6th costal cartilage.
6. Palpate laterally from the xiphisternal junction along the curved **costal margin** toward the midaxillary line.
7. Identify the **nipple** and the surrounding tissue of the **areola**. Observe that the nipple is located superficial to the 4th intercostal space, although this relationship is variable due to the amount of glandular and subcutaneous tissue of the breast.
8. In the female, return to the midline and identify the **intermammary cleft** overlying the body of the sternum between the right and left **breasts**.
9. Palpate from the nipple superolaterally toward the axilla and attempt to identify the location of the **axillary process (tail) of the breast**. *Note that in cadavers with advanced age, it may be difficult to identify the tail of the breast due to atrophy of the mamillary tissue.*

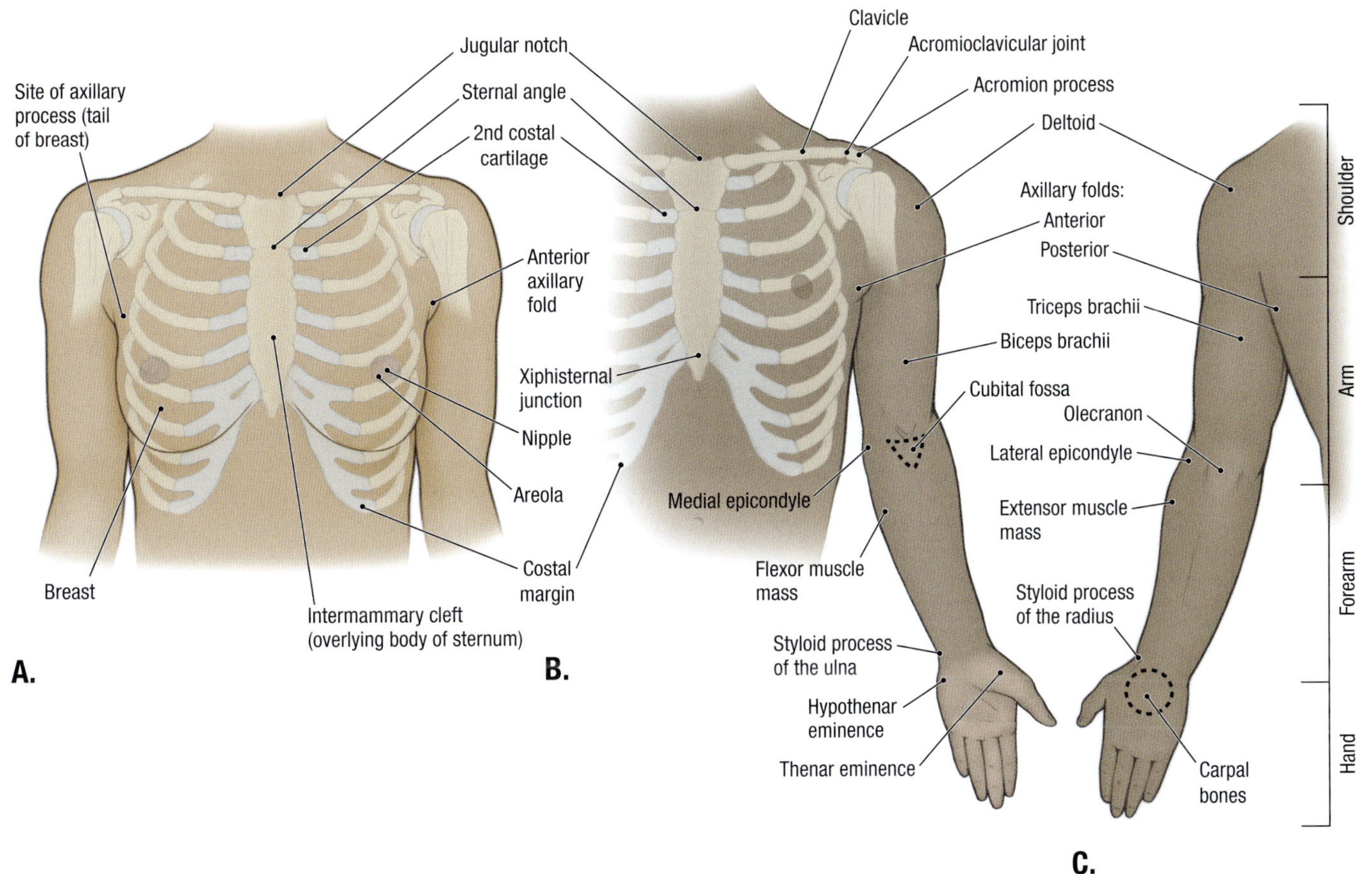

FIGURE 2.6 ● **A.** Surface anatomy of female pectoral region and breast. Anterior view. **B.** Surface anatomy of male pectoral region and upper limb. Anterior view. **C.** Surface anatomy of upper limb. Posterior view.

Upper Limb

ATLAS 2.1, 2.14, 2.20

1. Refer to FIGURE 2.6.
2. Palpate laterally along the clavicle toward the **acromion process** and identify the location of the **AC joint**.
3. Palpate the large muscle mass of the **deltoid** along the lateral shoulder and observe that it attaches inferior to the lateral one-third of the clavicle and acromion process.
4. In the axilla (armpit), palpate the free edges of both the **anterior** and **posterior axillary folds**.
5. On the anterior aspect of the arm, palpate the **biceps brachii** and follow it inferiorly toward the **cubital fossa** anterior to the elbow.
6. On the medial aspect of the cubital fossa, palpate the **medial epicondyle** and the associated **flexor muscle mass** in the anterior forearm.
7. On the lateral aspect of the cubital fossa, palpate the **lateral epicondyle** and the **extensor muscle mass** in the posterior forearm.
8. At the wrist, palpate the **styloid process of the radius** laterally and the **styloid process of the ulna** medially and posteriorly just proximal to the **carpal bones**.
9. In the palm, palpate the **thenar eminence** at the base of the thumb and the **hypothenar eminence** on the medial aspect of the hand.

Dissection Instructions

Dissection Note: Prior to commencing with skin incisions, decide to perform either a full- or partial-thickness approach and to either reflect or remove the skin from the dissection field. See **Removing Skin** in the **Introduction Chapter** for descriptions.

Perform the following dissection sequence bilaterally in the male and unilaterally in the female because the breast will be dissected differently on the contralateral side.

Skin Incisions of Pectoral Region

ATLAS 2.15, 2.17; VIDEO 2.2.1 (MALE), 2.3.1 (FEMALE)

1. Refer to FIGURE 2.7.
2. Make a midline skin incision from the jugular notch (A) to the xiphisternal junction (C).
3. Elevate a small portion of skin and verify that the skin on the thorax is thinner than the skin on the back, and thus, care must be taken to avoid damaging superficial structures in the region.
4. Make a skin incision from the jugular notch (A) along the clavicle laterally to the acromion process (B).
5. Make an incision from the xiphisternal junction (C) along the costal margin inferolaterally to the midaxillary line (V).
6. Make a transverse skin incision from the middle of the body of the sternum to the midaxillary line passing around the nipple. The nipple may be kept attached to the subcutaneous tissue and left intact as it is often a good superficial landmark for the 4th intercostal space.
7. Make a transverse skin incision from the xiphisternal junction (C) to the midaxillary line.
8. Make a transverse skin incision halfway between the incision line along the clavicle and the incision encircling the nipple.
9. Make an incision beginning on the medial surface of the arm (G) extending superiorly to the axilla.
10. Make an incision from the midpoint of the arm medially (G) around the anterior surface of the arm toward the lateral surface of the arm (F).

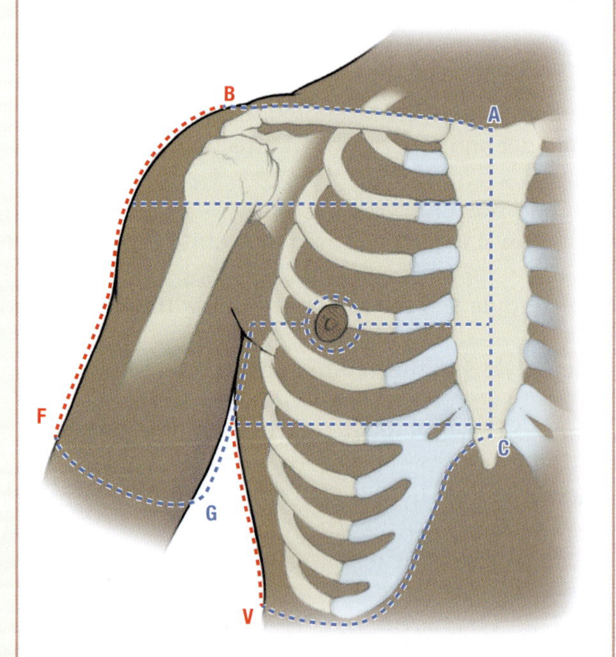

FIGURE 2.7 ■ Skin incisions of pectoral region. Anterior view.

Dissection Note: If reflecting the skin, skip steps 11 and 12.

11. Continue the incision from the acromion (B) down the lateral side of the arm to a point approximately halfway down the arm (F). *Note that if the back has previously been dissected, this cut has already been made.*
12. Make a vertical incision along the midaxillary line from the inferior extent of the ribs (V) to the axilla. *Note that if the back has previously been dissected, this cut has already been made.*
13. Beginning in the middle of the thorax, reflect the skin from medial to lateral using either a pair of locking forceps or the buttonhole technique. At any point, the portions of skin may be cut into smaller segments to facilitate removal. *Note that even if a full-thickness reflection is desired, it may prove beneficial to begin with a partial-thickness approach until an appropriate depth of reflection is verified based on visualization of the underlying deep fascia covering the muscles of the region.*
14. If removing the skin, detach the skin along the midaxillary line and lateral aspect of the arm and place it in the tissue container.
15. If reflecting the skin, make an effort to "tuck" the skin from the back underneath the cadaver to provide stability for the portions of skin now being reflected from the thorax and arm. Utilize the uncut sections of skin laterally as hinge points to leave the skin attached along the peripheral aspect of the back.

Breast

ATLAS 3.4, 3.5, 3.7; VIDEO 2.3.2

Dissection Note: Due to the advanced age of some cadavers, expect the lobes of the gland to be replaced by fat, and note that it may be difficult to dissect and identify all structures listed. Perform the following dissection sequence on the contralateral side from where the skin was removed.

1. Refer to FIGURE 2.8.
2. Identify the **areola** and the **nipple**.

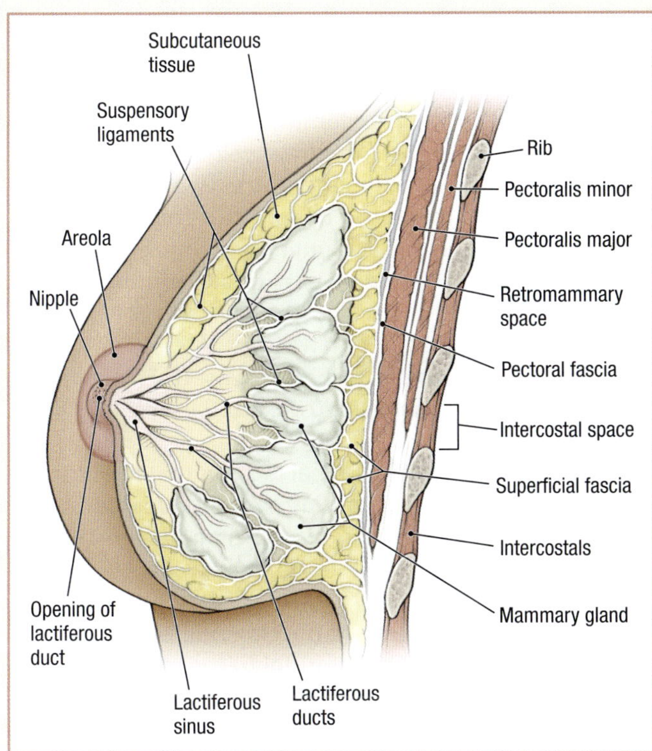

FIGURE 2.8 ■ Sagittal section of right breast. Medial view.

3. Make a parasagittal (superior to inferior) cut through the nipple to divide the breast into medial and lateral halves.
4. Take a moment to examine the cut surface of the breast tissue, and then use sharp dissection to remove the medial aspect of the breast from the dissection field, being careful not to cut through the underlying deep fascia and place it in the tissue container.
5. On the cut edge of the breast, use a probe to dissect through the fat within 3 cm deep to the nipple and find and clean 1 of the 15 to 20 **lactiferous ducts** converging on the nipple.
6. Identify a **lactiferous sinus**, which is an expanded part of the lactiferous duct.
7. Trace one lactiferous duct to the nipple and attempt to identify its opening.
8. Use the handle of a forceps or a blunt instrument to gently remove the fat from several compartments between the **suspensory ligaments**, the regions that once contained lobes of functional glandular tissue.
9. Insert your fingers deep to the breast and open the **retromammary space** immediately superficial to the pectoral fascia (see **Clinical Correlation 2.2**). *Note that healthy breast tissue can readily be separated from the underlying pectoral fascia.*

CLINICAL CORRELATION 2.2

Breast Quadrants, Cancer, and Implants

ATLAS 3.5, 3.6

For descriptive purposes, clinicians divide the breast into four quadrants centered on the nipple. The superolateral (upper outer) quadrant contains the "axillary tail" of breast tissue, which often extends into the axilla and is a common site for breast cancers to develop. As breast tumors enlarge, increased tension places traction on the suspensory ligaments resulting in dimpling of the skin overlying the tumor or an "orange peel" appearance. In advanced stages of breast cancer, the tumor may invade the pectoralis major, pectoral fascia, and skin, which may be detected by palpation in a physical examination.

In cases of breast cancer or as a preventive option for those at high risk of cancer, a mastectomy may be performed to surgically remove breast tissue and associated lymphatics in the pectoral and axillary regions. Breast implants may be inserted to change the appearance, shape, and size of the breast following a mastectomy (reconstructive) or for cosmetic (aesthetic) augmentation. Breast implants may be "above the muscle" (retromammary or subglandular) or "below the muscle" (subpectoral or submuscular) in reference to the pectoralis major.

10. Use sharp dissection to carefully remove the remaining breast tissue from the anterior surface of the pectoralis major.
11. Remove the contralateral breast tissue from the dissection field and follow the instructions for removal of the remaining subcutaneous tissue.

Superficial Pectoral Region

ATLAS 2.17, 2.19, 2.32; VIDEO 2.2.2

Dissection Note: Dissection of the subcutaneous tissue of the anterior thoracic wall will be performed on all cadavers.

1. Refer to FIGURE 2.9.
2. Identify the **platysma**, a thin but broad muscle of facial expression, which extends inferiorly through the neck into the subcutaneous tissue of the superior thorax.
3. Isolate the platysma from the surrounding superficial fat and reflect the muscle superiorly out of the dissection field superior to the clavicles.
4. Identify an **anterior cutaneous nerve** emerging from an intercostal space lateral to the borders of the sternum.

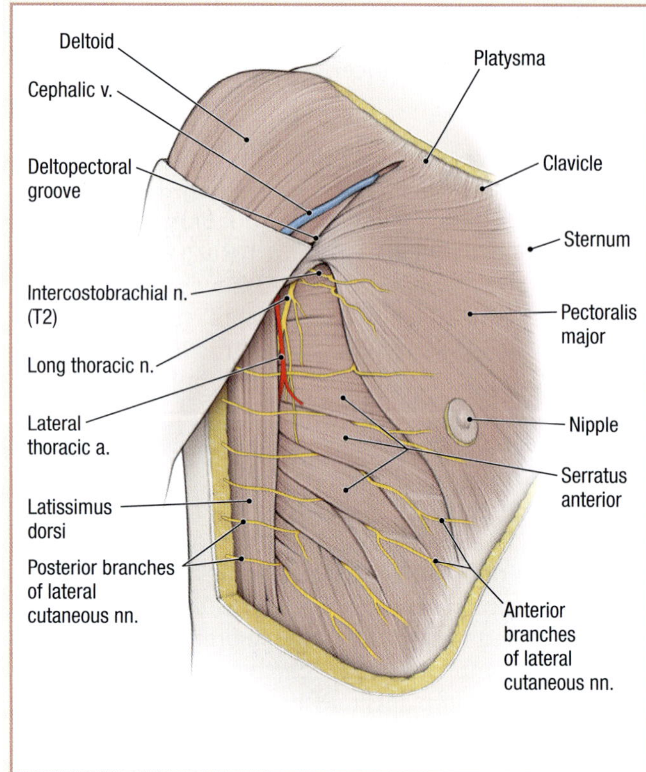

FIGURE 2.9 ● Distribution of lateral cutaneous nerves of trunk and pectoral region. Anterior view.

5. If using a partial-thickness skin removal, remove the remaining subcutaneous tissue of the pectoral region proceeding from medial to lateral.
6. Palpate an intercostal space near the midaxillary line and identify a **lateral cutaneous branch of the intercostal nerve** where it leaves the intercostal space to enter the subcutaneous tissue, and make attempts to trace its **anterior and posterior branches** for a short distance.
7. Emerging from the 2nd intercostal space, identify the **intercostobrachial nerve**, a somewhat larger lateral cutaneous nerve that supplies the skin of the armpit.
8. Medial to the deltoid, identify and clean a short portion of the **cephalic vein** where it courses in the **deltopectoral groove**, the depression between the deltoid and pectoralis major.
9. Follow the cephalic vein superiorly and observe that near the clavicle it penetrates the **clavipectoral fascia** within the **deltopectoral triangle** to join the axillary vein. *Note that the apex of the deltopectoral triangle narrows to form the deltopectoral groove.*
10. Detach the subcutaneous tissue along the midaxillary line sparing any identified cutaneous nerves and place it in the tissue container.

Skin Incisions of Arm and Forearm

ATLAS 2.14; VIDEO 2.2.3

Dissection Note: Prior to commencing with skin incisions, note that the superficial veins and cutaneous nerves are easily damaged in the upper limb if skin incisions are made too deeply. It is thus recommended that along the periphery and anterior surface of the limb, a partial-thickness skinning technique be implemented.

1. Refer to FIGURE 2.10.
2. Make an incision encircling the wrist (E). *Note that the skin is very thin (2 mm) around the wrist—do not cut too deeply.*
3. Make a shallow longitudinal incision on the anterior surface of the upper limb from the midpoint of the arm (G) to the incision encircling the wrist (E), paying particular attention to remain shallow at the cubital fossa.
4. Make an incision around the circumference of the upper limb at a level just distal to the elbow.
5. Beginning from the midline incision, reflect the skin of the upper limb laterally using either a pair of locking forceps or the buttonhole technique. At any point, the portions of skin may be cut into smaller segments to facilitate removal.
6. Remove the skin from the arm and forearm and place it in the tissue container.
7. Because reflecting the skin with portions still attached will block views of the underlying anatomy, it is recommended to keep the removed portions of skin in large pieces, which may be used later to wrap the limb post dissection to prevent desiccation.

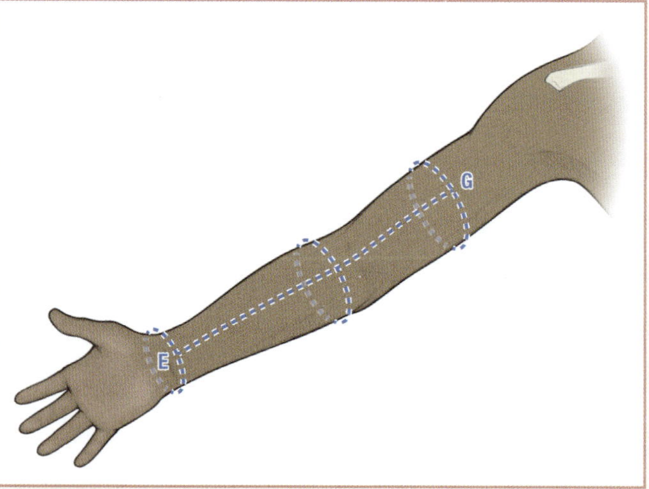

FIGURE 2.10 ● Skin incisions of upper limb. Anterior view.

Superficial Arm and Forearm

ATLAS 2.8, 2.13, 2.14; VIDEO 2.2.4, 2.2.5

1. Refer to FIGURE 2.11.
2. With the body lying supine, rotate the upper limb or flex the elbow to increase visibility of structures and use blunt dissection with a probe, forceps, or dissecting scissors to demonstrate the superficial veins of the arm and forearm.
3. Beginning near the wrist in the posterior forearm, identify the basilic and cephalic veins, but do not follow them distally as the superficial veins of the dorsum of the hand will be studied when the hand is dissected.
4. Use blunt dissection to follow the cephalic and basilic veins proximally freeing them from the surrounding fat and connective tissue. *Note that it may be useful to abduct the upper limb to 45° if possible and to have your dissection partner hold it in the abducted position.*
5. Demonstrate that the cephalic and basilic veins are joined across the cubital fossa by the **median cubital vein.** *Note that the venous pattern in this region can be quite variable and should be observed on other cadavers as an example of anatomical variation.*
6. Follow the cephalic vein proximally into the pectoral region where it courses in the deltopectoral groove.
7. Follow the basilic vein proximally and observe that superior to the medial epicondyle, it pierces the deep fascia to join the deep veins. Do not follow it into the axilla at this time.
8. Use a probe to elevate the superficial veins and observe that several **perforating veins** penetrate the deep fascia to connect the superficial and deep veins of the upper limb.
9. Identify the **lateral cutaneous nerve of the forearm** within the subcutaneous tissue anterior to the lateral epicondyle of the humerus lateral to the distal tendon of the biceps brachii.
10. Clean the lateral cutaneous nerve of the forearm and observe its close relationship to the cephalic and median cubital veins near the cubital fossa.
11. On the medial side of the biceps brachii tendon, identify and clean the **medial cutaneous nerve of the forearm**, noting its close relationship to the basilic vein.
12. Near the wrist, identify and clean the **superficial branch of the radial nerve** near the styloid process of the radius for 2 or 3 cm making an effort to not disrupt the nearby structures in the anatomical snuffbox.
13. On the medial aspect of the wrist posteriorly, identify and clean the **dorsal branch of the ulnar nerve** near the styloid process of the ulna for 2 or 3 cm.
14. Remove all remaining subcutaneous tissue from the arm and forearm, preserving the dissected superficial veins, nerves, and deep fascia overlying the muscles. Place the removed subcutaneous tissue in the tissue container.
15. Examine the deep (investing) fascia of the upper limb and observe that it extends from the shoulder to the wrist. *Note that the deep fascia continues into the hand all the way to the fingertips with palmar fascia on the anterior (ventral) surface of the hand, and dorsal fascia of the hand on the posterior (dorsal) surface of the hand.*
16. Identify the **brachial fascia** in the arm surrounding the anterior and posterior compartments.
17. Identify the **antebrachial fascia** in the forearm surrounding the anterior and posterior compartments.

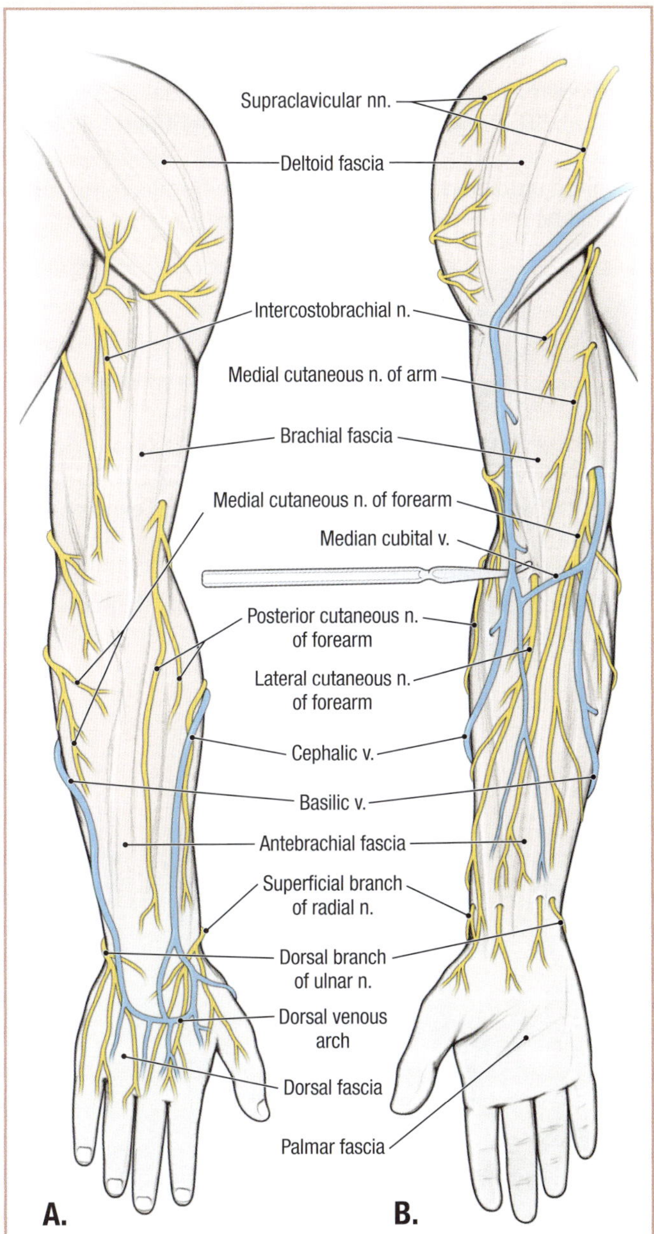

FIGURE 2.11 Superficial veins and cutaneous nerves of upper limb. **A.** Posterior view. **B.** Anterior view.

Dissection Follow-up

1. Review the location and parts of the breast.
2. Familiarize yourself with the vascular supply and lymphatic drainage of the breast.
3. Trace the course of the superficial veins of the upper limb from distal to proximal noting important access sites for venipuncture.
4. Review the path of the cutaneous nerves of the upper limb.
5. Review and name the various components of the deep fascia of the upper limb.
6. Replace the removed portions of skin back to anatomical position.

PECTORAL REGION

Dissection Overview

There are four muscles in the pectoral region: pectoralis major, pectoralis minor, subclavius, and serratus anterior. The muscles of the pectoral region, also classified as anterior axioappendicular muscles, attach between the axial and appendicular skeletons and provide movement and stability to the upper limb. The serratus anterior will be identified following reflection of the pectoralis major but will be dissected with the axilla.

The order of dissection will be as follows: The pectoralis major will be studied and reflected. The pectoralis minor and clavipectoral fascia will be studied, and the muscle reflected. The subclavius will be identified, and the branches of the thoracoacromial artery will be dissected.

Dissection Instructions

Pectoralis Major

ATLAS 2.17, 2.23; VIDEO 2.4.1

1. Refer to FIGURE 2.12.
2. Clean the superficial surface of the **pectoralis major** and clearly define its borders. *Note that the deep fascia on the superficial and deep surfaces of the pectoralis major, the pectoral fascia, is continuous with the axillary fascia forming the base of the axilla.*
3. Observe that the pectoralis major has two heads which meet at the SC joint: the **clavicular** attaching along the clavicle, and the **sternocostal** attaching along the body of the sternum and costal cartilage.
4. Review the attachments and actions of the pectoralis major (see **TABLE 2.2**).

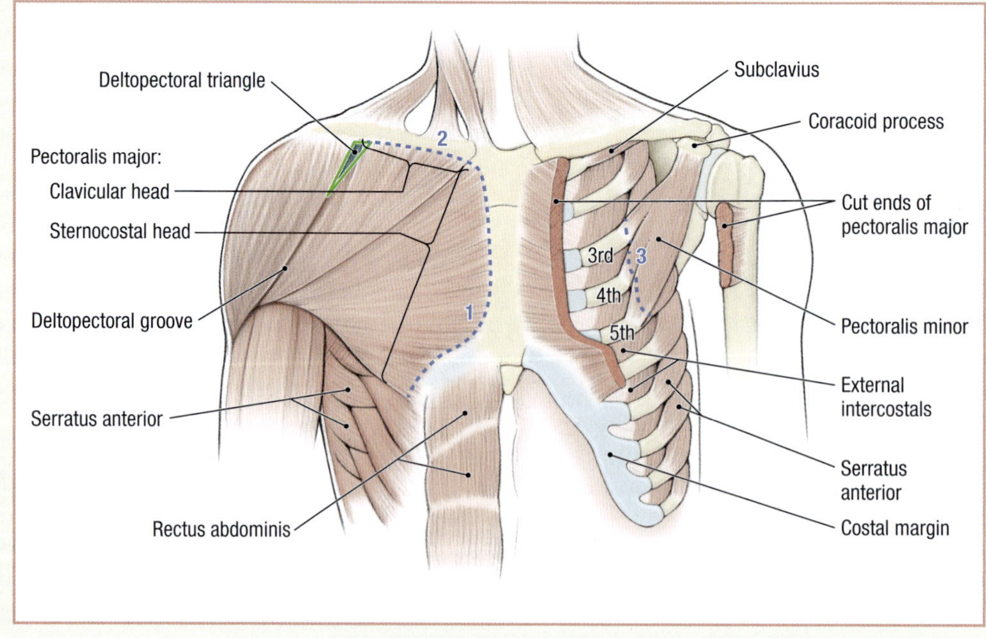

FIGURE 2.12 ■ Superficial (*right*) and deep (*left*) dissections of pectoral region. Anterior view.

5. Clean the anterior and middle surfaces of the deltoid if not already done, taking care to preserve the cephalic vein.
6. To prepare the pectoralis major for reflection, relax the sternocostal head by flexing and adducting the arm or by placing a dissection block under the ipsilateral shoulder.
7. Use blunt dissection deep to the inferior border of the pectoralis major and its surrounding pectoral fascia to create a space between it and the underlying pectoralis minor and its surrounding clavipectoral fascia.
8. Beginning at the inferior border of the pectoralis major, detach the sternocostal head from its attachment to the costal cartilages and sternum (**Cut 1**).
9. Working from inferior to superior, insert your fingers deep to the clavicular head to palpate the location of the nerves and vessels inserting on the deep surface of the muscle.
10. Use sharp dissection to detach the clavicular head as close to the clavicle as possible (**Cut 2**).
11. Gently elevate the pectoralis major superolaterally, leaving it attached to the humerus while preserving the nerves and vessels that enter its deep surface. Do not yet fully reflect the muscle or the neurovascular structures will be torn.
12. Identify the **clavipectoral fascia** immediately deep to the pectoralis major. *Note that superiorly the clavipectoral fascia attaches to the clavicle and lies both superficial and deep to the subclavius and pectoralis minor, while inferiorly, it attaches to the axillary fascia.*
13. On the deep surface of the clavicular head, identify the **lateral pectoral nerve** and the **pectoral branch of the thoracoacromial artery**. *Note that the medial and lateral pectoral nerves are named according to the cord of the brachial plexus from which they arise and not their relative anatomical locations to the midline.*

Pectoralis Minor and Thoracoacromial Artery

ATLAS 2.23, 2.27, 2.29; VIDEO 2.4.2

1. Refer to FIGURE 2.12.
2. Identify the **pectoralis minor**.
3. Observe that the cephalic vein passes from superficial to deep on the medial side of the pectoralis minor through the costocoracoid membrane part of the clavipectoral fascia.
4. Locate the **medial pectoral nerve** where it pierces the pectoralis minor and follow it to where it enters the deep surface of the pectoralis major.

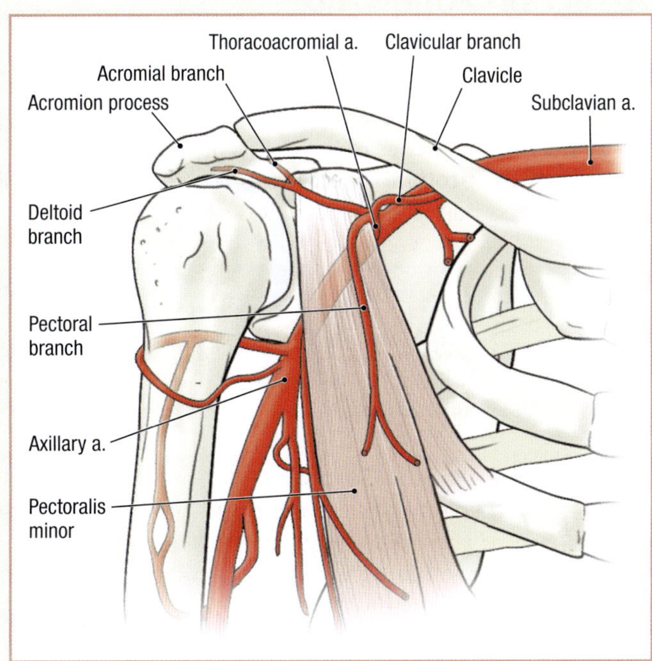

FIGURE 2.13 Arterial supply of pectoral region isolated. Anterior view.

5. Clean the surface of the pectoralis minor and clearly define its borders sparing the medial pectoral nerve.
6. Scrape any remaining portions of pectoralis major from the clavicle.
7. Deep to the clavicle, identify and clean the visible portions of the **subclavius**.
8. Review the attachments and actions of the pectoralis minor and subclavius (see **TABLE 2.2**).
9. Use sharp dissection to detach the pectoralis minor from its inferior attachments on ribs 3 to 5 (**Cut 3**).
10. Reflect the pectoralis minor superiorly, leaving it attached to the coracoid process of the scapula.
11. Refer to FIGURE 2.13.
12. Medial to the reflected pectoralis minor, identify branches of the **thoracoacromial artery** and the **lateral pectoral nerve**. *Note that these neurovascular structures also pass through the costocoracoid membrane.*
13. Identify and clean the branches of the thoracoacromial artery beginning with the **pectoral branch**, typically the largest of the branches which descends between the pectoralis major and pectoralis minor.
14. The **deltoid branch** courses laterally in the deltopectoral groove between the deltoid and pectoralis major and accompanies the cephalic vein.
15. The **acromial branch** courses superior to the coracoid process toward the acromion.
16. The **clavicular branch** courses medially to supply the subclavius and the SC joint.

Dissection Follow-up

1. Review the attachments, actions, and innervations of the pectoralis major, pectoralis minor, and subclavius in **TABLE 2.2**.
2. Review the relationship of the clavipectoral and pectoral fascial layers to the muscles, vessels, and nerves of this region and its role in supporting the base of the axilla.
3. Identify the branches of the thoracoacromial artery and the structures supplied by each.
4. Replace the pectoral muscles into their correct anatomical positions.

TABLE 2.2 Muscles of Pectoral Region

Muscle	*Medial Attachments*	*Lateral Attachments*	*Actions*	*Innervation*
Pectoralis major	Medial half of clavicle, sternum, costal cartilages 1–7	Lateral lip of the intertubercular sulcus	Medially rotates, flexes, and adducts the humerus	Medial and lateral pectoral nn.
Pectoralis minor	Ribs 3–5	Coracoid process of the scapula	Anteriorly tilts and depresses the scapula	Medial pectoral n.
Subclavius	Rib 1	Clavicle	Depresses the clavicle and stabilizes the SC joint	Nerve to subclavius

Abbreviations: n., nerve; nn., nerves; SC, sternoclavicular.

AXILLA

Dissection Overview

The axilla ("armpit") is the region between the pectoral muscles, scapula, arm, and thoracic wall. Due to its central location, the axilla is a key region of passage for vessels and nerves coursing between the root of the neck, the thorax, and the upper limb. The axilla contains the axillary sheath, brachial plexus, axillary vessels, lymph nodes and lymphatic vessels, muscular attachments, and a considerable amount of fat and connective tissue as shown in FIGURE 2.14.

The brachial plexus is a network of nerves originating from spinal cord levels C5–T1, which descend posterior to the clavicle through the apex of the axilla, to then pass inferolaterally toward the base of the axilla. Only the infraclavicular part of the brachial plexus (cords and branches) will be dissected at this time. The supraclavicular part (roots, trunks, and divisions) will be dissected with the root of the neck.

The order of dissection will be as follows: The axillary vein and its tributaries will be identified and removed. The branches of the axillary artery will be dissected. The cords and branches of the brachial plexus will be studied.

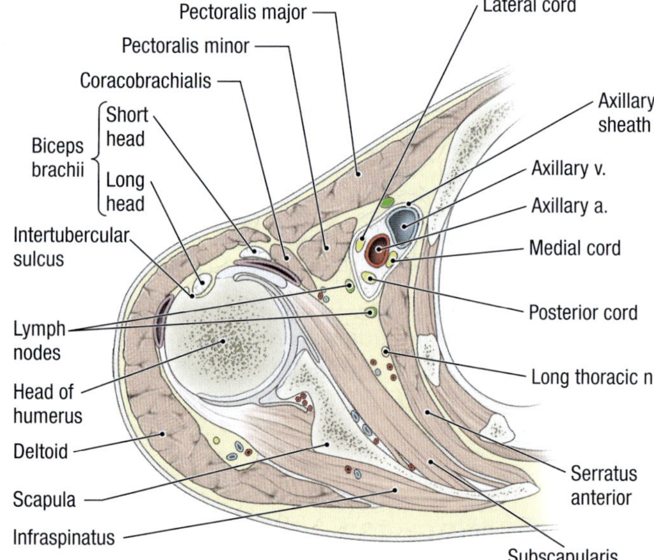

FIGURE 2.14 ● Axial section of right shoulder and axilla. Inferior view.

Dissection Instructions

Axilla

ATLAS 2.25, 2.26; VIDEO 2.5.1

1. Refer to FIGURE 2.15.
2. Review the walls and boundaries of the axilla beginning superiorly near the clavicle.
3. The **apex of the axilla** (cervicoaxillary canal) is bound by the clavicle anteriorly, the superior border of the scapula posteriorly, and the 1st rib medially.
4. The **base of the axilla** is formed by the skin and subcutaneous tissue of the armpit.
5. The **anterior wall of the axilla** is defined by the anterior axillary fold containing the pectoralis major, part of the pectoralis minor, and the clavipectoral fascia.

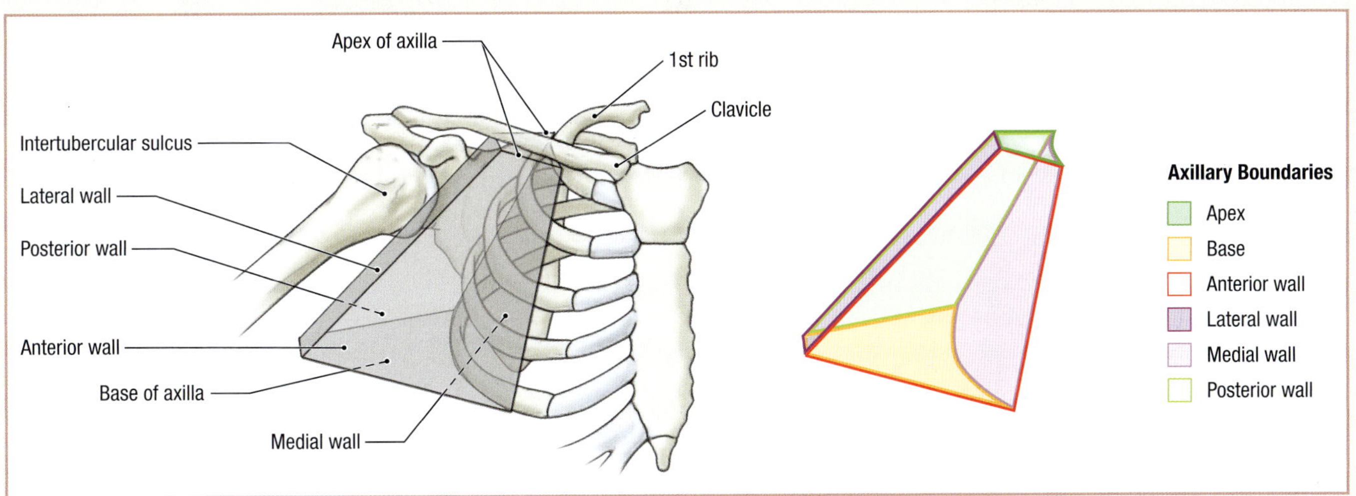

FIGURE 2.15 ■ Walls and boundaries of axilla. Anterior view.

6. The **posterior wall of the axilla** is defined by the posterior axillary fold containing the teres major and latissimus dorsi inferiorly, and the subscapularis covering the anterior surface of the scapula.
7. The **medial wall of the axilla** is the upper portion of the lateral thoracic wall and the serratus anterior.
8. The **lateral wall of the axilla** is the intertubercular sulcus of the humerus.
9. Reflect the pectoralis major laterally and the pectoralis minor superiorly.
10. Abduct the upper limb to approximately 45°.
11. Observe that the axilla contains a large amount of axillary fat to protect the contents of the region while allowing for mobility of the upper limb.
12. Within the axillary fat, identify the **axillary sheath,** a thin layer of connective tissue surrounding the axillary vessels and components of the brachial plexus extending from the lateral border of the 1st rib to the inferior border of the teres major.
13. Use blunt dissection to open the anterior surface of the axillary sheath.
14. Identify the **axillary vein** and observe that it is formed near the lateral border of the teres major by the joining of the brachial and basilic veins.
15. Follow the axillary vein medially toward the lateral border of the 1st rib where it is joined by the cephalic vein to form the subclavian vein. To increase visibility of the arteries and nerves in the axilla, the axillary vein must be removed.
16. Use sharp dissection to cut the axillary vein near the lateral border of the 1st rib lateral to the point of drainage of the cephalic vein and reflect it laterally.
17. While reflecting the axillary vein laterally, use blunt dissection to separate it from the structures that lie posterior to it (axillary artery and brachial plexus), and scissors to cut the small tributary veins draining into it along its length.
18. Use sharp dissection to cut the axillary vein near the inferior border of the teres major and remove it from the dissection field.
19. Remove any lymph nodes in the region associated with the veins.

Axillary Artery

ATLAS 2.27, 2.29, 2.30; VIDEO 2.5.2

Dissection Note: The branching pattern of the axillary artery may vary from that which is commonly illustrated. If the pattern is different in your specimen, understand that the branches are named according to their region of distribution rather than by their point of origin. As the dissection proceeds, remove all veins accompanying the arteries within the axilla while preserving the structures of the brachial plexus.

1. Refer to FIGURE 2.16.
2. Identify the **axillary artery** within the axilla. The axillary artery begins at the lateral border of the 1st rib as the continuation of the subclavian artery and ends at the inferior border of the teres major where it becomes the brachial artery.
3. Using the pectoralis minor as a landmark, identify the three parts of the axillary artery: the **first part** between the lateral border of the 1st rib and the medial border of the pectoralis minor, the **second part** posterior to the pectoralis minor, and the **third part** between the lateral border of the pectoralis minor and the inferior border of the teres major.
4. Observe that typically the first part of the axillary artery has one branch, the second part has two branches, and the third part has three branches.
5. Identify and clean the **superior thoracic artery,** which arises near the apex of the axilla to supply blood to the 1st and 2nd intercostal spaces.

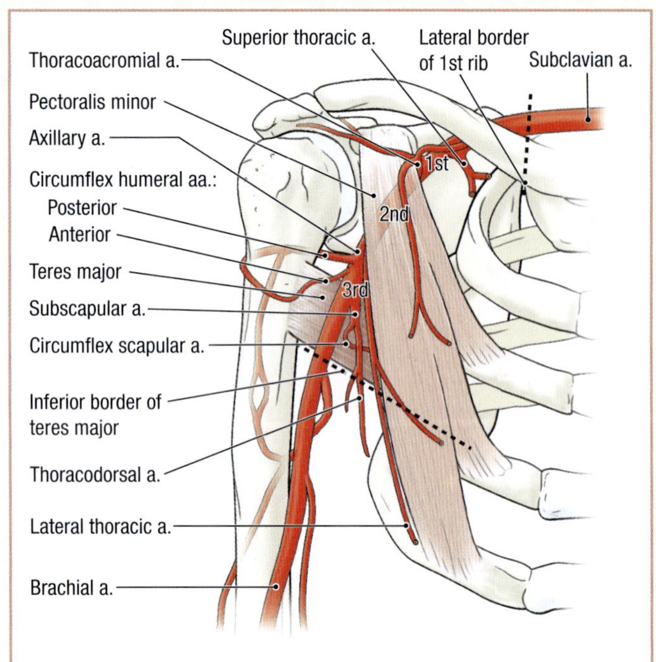

FIGURE 2.16 Three parts and branches of axillary artery isolated. Anterior view.

6. Identify the **thoracoacromial artery** near the medial border of the pectoralis minor and review its branches previously dissected: pectoral, acromial, deltoid, and clavicular.
7. Identify and clean the **lateral thoracic artery**, which typically branches off the axillary artery near the lateral border of the pectoralis minor, although it may arise from the subscapular or thoracoacromial arteries, to supply pectoral muscles, serratus anterior, axillary lymph nodes, and the lateral thoracic wall. *Note that the lateral thoracic artery also supplies the lateral portion of the breast and is often referred to as the lateral mammary artery.*
8. Identify and clean the **subscapular artery**, the largest branch of the axillary artery.
9. Identify the terminal branches of the subscapular artery, the **circumflex scapular artery** supplying muscles on the posterior surface of the scapula, and the **thoracodorsal artery** supplying the latissimus dorsi. *Note that the subscapular artery also gives rise to several unnamed muscular branches and may be the origin of the lateral thoracic artery.*
10. Identify and clean the **anterior** and **posterior circumflex humeral arteries,** which arise from the lateral surface of the axillary artery distal to the origin of the subscapular artery. *Note that the circumflex humeral arteries supply the deltoid, anastomose around the surgical neck of the humerus, and may arise from a short common trunk.*
11. Observe that the posterior circumflex humeral artery is typically the larger of the two circumflex humeral arteries.
12. Follow the posterior circumflex humeral artery posterior to the surgical neck of the humerus and observe its proximity to the axillary nerve as these structures pass through the quadrangular space.
13. Follow the **anterior circumflex humeral artery** for a short distance and observe that this vessel courses around the anterior surface of the humerus at the surgical neck deep to the tendon of the long head of the biceps brachii.

Brachial Plexus

ATLAS 2.28, 2.29, 2.31; VIDEO 2.5.3

Dissection Note: The branching pattern of the nerves of the brachial plexus varies somewhat between individuals. Use the peripheral relationships of the nerves including their region of distribution or point of exit from the axilla for positive identification. Minimal force is required to separate the cords and terminal branches of the brachial plexus, and much of the dissection can be done gently with blunt dissection.

1. Refer to FIGURE 2.17.
2. Follow the pectoralis minor deep into the axilla and identify the location of the coracoid process.
3. Observe that the coracoid process serves as the attachment for three muscles: pectoralis minor, coracobrachialis, and short head of the biceps brachii.
4. Using the pectoralis minor as a landmark, identify the second part of the axillary artery and the three **cords of the brachial plexus** (lateral, medial, and posterior), named according to their relationship to the axillary artery.

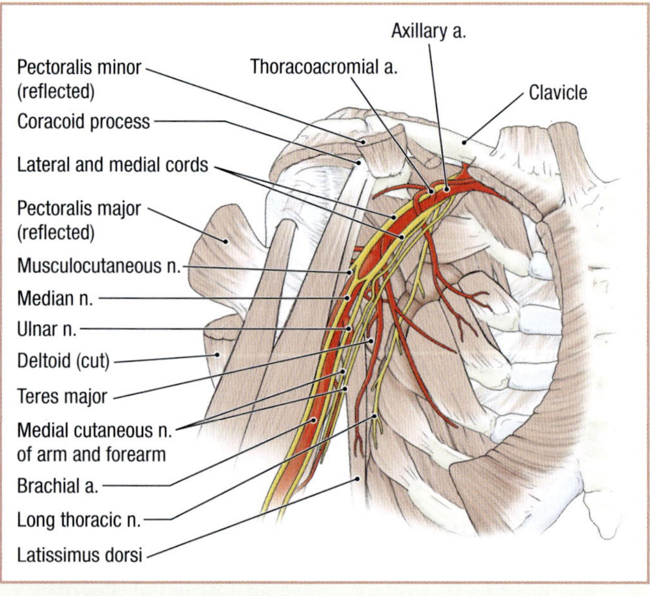

FIGURE 2.17 Infraclavicular (axillary) portion of brachial plexus. Anterior view.

5. Identify the **musculocutaneous nerve** where it pierces the coracobrachialis. *Note that the musculocutaneous nerve is the most lateral terminal branch of the brachial plexus.*
6. Use blunt dissection to follow the musculocutaneous nerve proximally to the **lateral cord of the brachial plexus.**
7. Observe that the lateral cord gives rise to the **lateral root of the median nerve**. Follow the lateral root distally and identify the **median nerve**.
8. Trace the **medial root of the median nerve** proximally to the **medial cord** near the medial aspect of the axillary artery.
9. Identify the **ulnar nerve** arising from the medial cord.
10. Use the cadaver or an illustration to observe that the three **terminal branches** you have just identified (musculocutaneous, median, and ulnar nerves) form a rough letter "M" anterior to the third part of the axillary artery.
11. Trace the medial pectoral nerve to the medial cord for which it is named.
12. Trace the lateral pectoral nerve to the lateral cord for which it is named, observing that it often arises distal to the medial pectoral nerve.
13. Identify the **medial cutaneous nerve of the arm** and **medial cutaneous nerve of the forearm** originating from the medial cord proximal to the ulnar nerve. Use blunt dissection to trace these nerves a short distance into the arm.
14. Refer to FIGURE 2.18.
15. Gently retract the axillary artery, the lateral cord, and the medial cord superiorly and identify the **posterior cord** of the brachial plexus.
16. Identify and clean the **axillary nerve** arising from the posterior cord.
17. Follow the axillary nerve to verify that it passes through the quadrangular space with the posterior circumflex humeral artery to reach the deltoid and teres minor.
18. Identify and clean the **radial nerve** arising from the posterior cord.
19. Follow the radial nerve laterally and observe that it leaves the axilla by passing anterior to the latissimus dorsi and teres major and that it courses toward the triceps brachii in the posterior compartment of the arm.
20. Observe that the radial nerve is larger than the axillary nerve and that it courses within the radial groove near the midshaft of the humerus. *Note that the radial nerve is the only motor and sensory nerve to the posterior compartments of the upper limb.*

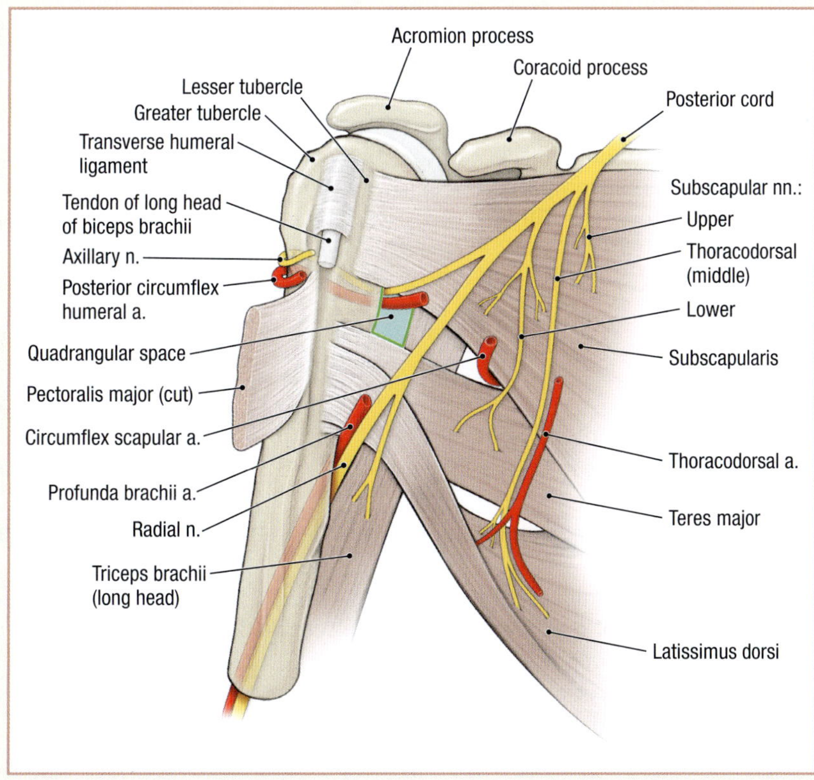

FIGURE 2.18 ■ Posterior cord of brachial plexus and posterior wall of axilla. Anterior view.

21. Beginning centrally, identify and isolate the **thoracodorsal nerve** arising off the posterior cord and trace it inferiorly to the latissimus dorsi.
22. Distal to the branch point of the thoracodorsal nerve, identify and isolate the **lower subscapular nerve** and follow it a short distance toward the subscapularis and teres major.
23. Proximal to the thoracodorsal nerve, identify the **upper subscapular nerve**, the first of three branches from the posterior cord and often the most difficult to identify. Trace the upper subscapular nerve distally to the subscapularis.
24. Observe that the posterior cord gives rise to the upper and lower subscapular nerves and the thoracodorsal nerve prior to terminating as the axillary and radial nerves.
25. Identify the three muscles forming the posterior wall of the axilla: latissimus dorsi, teres major, and subscapularis.
26. Observe that the subscapularis covers the anterior surface of the scapula and recall that it is a member of the rotator cuff group of muscles.
27. Review the attachments and actions of the subscapularis (see **TABLE 2.3**).
28. Identify the **serratus anterior** and recall that it forms the medial wall of the axilla.
29. Slide your hand into the axilla and verify that the serratus anterior attaches to the medial border of the scapula. Observe that with your palm against the serratus anterior, the dorsum of your hand is against the subscapularis.
30. On the superficial surface of the serratus anterior, identify and clean the **long thoracic nerve** coursing vertically and observe that it sends multiple branches to the serratus anterior, which often accompany branches of the lateral thoracic artery (see **Clinical Correlation 2.3**).

CLINICAL CORRELATION 2.3

Long Thoracic, Thoracodorsal, and Axillary Nerve Injuries

ATLAS 2.4A, 2.30A, 2.32, 2.46

The long thoracic nerve is vulnerable to surgical injury during mastectomy, or trauma to the lateral thoracic wall leading to impaired function of the serratus anterior. When a patient with paralysis of the serratus anterior is asked to push with both hands against a wall, the medial border of the scapula protrudes on the affected side, a condition known as "winged scapula."

The thoracodorsal nerve is vulnerable to compression injuries and surgical trauma during mastectomy and/or axillary dissection (removal of the lymph nodes). Injury of the thoracodorsal nerve affects the latissimus dorsi, resulting in a weakened ability to extend, adduct, and medially rotate the arm.

The axillary nerve courses around the surgical neck of the humerus and may be injured in proximal humeral fractures or inferior dislocations of the shoulder joint. Injury of the axillary nerve affects the deltoid and teres minor, resulting in a weakened ability to abduct and laterally rotate the arm.

31. Follow the long thoracic nerve superiorly toward the apex of the axilla as far as possible. *Note that the long thoracic nerve does not arise from the cords of the brachial plexus like the other nerves in the region; rather, it arises from the roots of the brachial plexus (C5–C7).*
32. Clean the surface of the serratus anterior, paying attention not to disrupt the long thoracic nerve.
33. Review the actions and innervations of the serratus anterior (see **TABLE 2.3**).

Dissection Follow-up

1. Review the boundaries and major contents of the axilla.
2. Review the relationship of the three parts of the axillary artery to the pectoralis minor and name the arterial branches of each part.
3. Review the subdivisions of the brachial plexus focusing on the orientation of the infraclavicular portion within the axilla.
4. Review the target structures of each terminal branch of the brachial plexus.
5. Review the movements of the groups of muscles acting on the scapula in **TABLE 2.3**.
6. Replace the pectoralis major and pectoralis minor into their correct anatomical positions.
7. Examine other cadavers to gain an appreciation of variations in the branching pattern of arteries and nerves.
8. Familiarize yourself with the lymphatic drainage of the axilla.

TABLE 2.3 Muscles of Axilla

Muscle	*Medial Attachments*	*Lateral Attachments*	*Actions*	*Innervation*
MEDIAL WALL				
Serratus anterior	Anterior surface of the medial border of the scapula	Ribs 1–9 lateral parts	Rotates the glenoid cavity superiorly and protracts the scapula	Long thoracic n.
POSTERIOR WALL				
Subscapularis	Subscapular fossa	Lesser tubercle of the humerus	Medially rotates the humerus	Upper and lower subscapular nn.
Latissimus dorsi	Thoracolumbar fascia, iliac crest	Intertubercular groove (floor)	Extends, adducts, and medially rotates the humerus	Thoracodorsal n.
Teres major	Inferior angle of the scapula	Medial lip of the intertubercular sulcus	Adducts and medially rotates the humerus	Lower subscapular n.

Abbreviations: n., nerve; nn., nerves.

ANTERIOR ARM AND CUBITAL FOSSA

Dissection Overview

The brachial fascia (deep fascia of the arm) is a sleeve of tough connective tissue investing the compartments of the arm. Brachial fascia is continuous at its proximal end with the pectoral, axillary, and deep fascia covering the deltoid and latissimus dorsi. Distally, the brachial fascia is continuous with the antebrachial fascia (deep fascia of the forearm). The brachial fascia is connected to the medial and lateral sides of the humerus by intermuscular septa creating an anterior (flexor) compartment and a posterior (extensor) compartment as shown in FIGURE 2.19. The anterior compartment contains three muscles (biceps brachii, brachialis, and coracobrachialis), whereas the posterior compartment predominately contains the triceps brachii along with the small anconeus distally.

The cubital fossa is the depression on the anterior surface of the elbow. The cubital fossa is a clinically important region as it contains the brachial artery and accompanying veins, the median nerve, and the superficial veins commonly used for venipuncture.

The order of dissection will be as follows: The skeletal anatomy of the arm and elbow will be studied. The fascia of the anterior compartment of the arm will be reflected, and its contents studied. Nerves and blood vessels will be traced from the axilla through the arm to the cubital fossa.

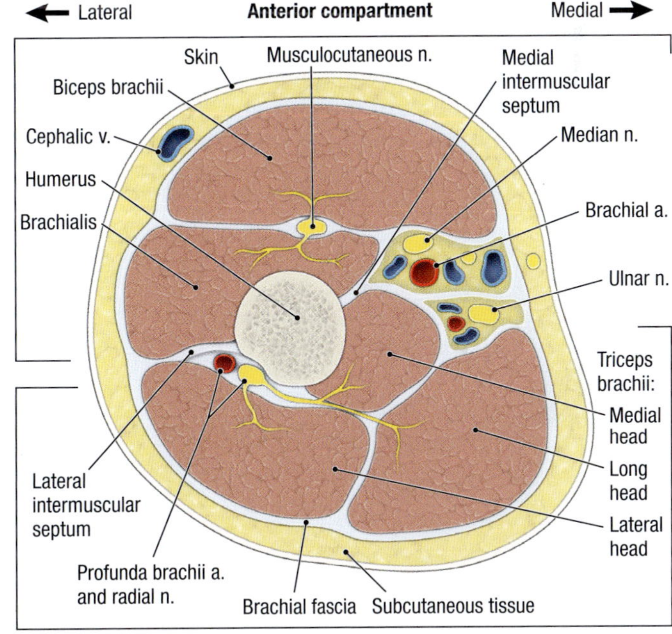

FIGURE 2.19 ● Axial section of right arm. Inferior view.

Skeletal Anatomy

Refer to an articulated skeleton or isolated humerus, radius, and ulna and identify the following skeletal features.

Distal Anterior Humerus

ATLAS 2.3C, 2.38A

1. Refer to FIGURE 2.20.
2. On the distal end of the humerus, identify the **medial epicondyle** medially and the **lateral epicondyle** laterally.
3. Between the epicondyles, identify the depression of the **olecranon fossa** posteriorly and the **coronoid fossa** anteriorly.
4. Inferior to the epicondyles, identify the **trochlea** medially and the **capitulum** laterally.

Proximal Radius and Ulna

ATLAS 2.3C, 2.57

1. Refer to FIGURE 2.20.
2. On the proximal end of the radius, identify the **head of the radius**.
3. Inferior to the head of the radius, identify the narrowed **neck of the radius**.
4. Distal to the neck of the radius, identify the **radial tuberosity**, the attachment site of the biceps brachii.
5. Place the head of the radius in the **radial notch** of the ulna and observe that the rotational movements of pronation and supination occur at the **proximal radioulnar joint**.
6. On the proximal end of the ulna, identify the **trochlear notch** between the **olecranon process** and the **coronoid process**.
7. Articulate the ulna with the humerus and observe that flexion is limited by contact of the coronoid process in the coronoid fossa and that extension is limited by contact of the olecranon process in the olecranon fossa.
8. On an articulated skeleton, examine the **elbow joint** and confirm that it is composed of the articulation between the trochlear notch of the ulna and trochlea of the humerus (humeroulnar), and the head of the radius and capitulum of the humerus (humeroradial), which together account for the hinge action (flexion/extension) of the elbow joint.

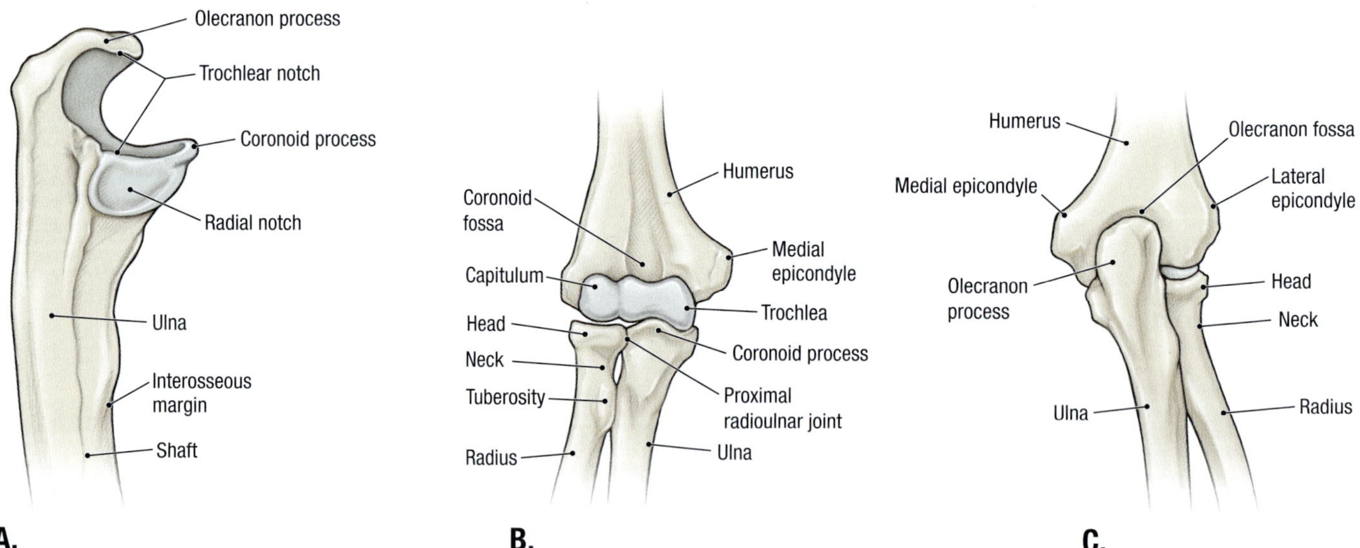

FIGURE 2.20 ■ **A.** Proximal ulna. Lateral view. **B.** Skeleton of right elbow. Anterior view. **C.** Skeleton of right elbow. Posterior view.

Dissection Instructions

Anterior Compartment of Arm

ATLAS 2.41, 2.42; VIDEO 2.6.1

1. Refer to FIGURE 2.21.
2. With the cadaver in the supine position, make a longitudinal incision in the anterior surface of the brachial fascia from the level of the pectoralis major to the elbow.
3. Use blunt dissection to separate the brachial fascia from the underlying muscles.
4. From the longitudinal incision, work your fingers laterally to identify the **lateral intermuscular septum**, and medially to identify the **medial intermuscular septum**. Detach the brachial fascia from the intermuscular septa and place it in the tissue container.

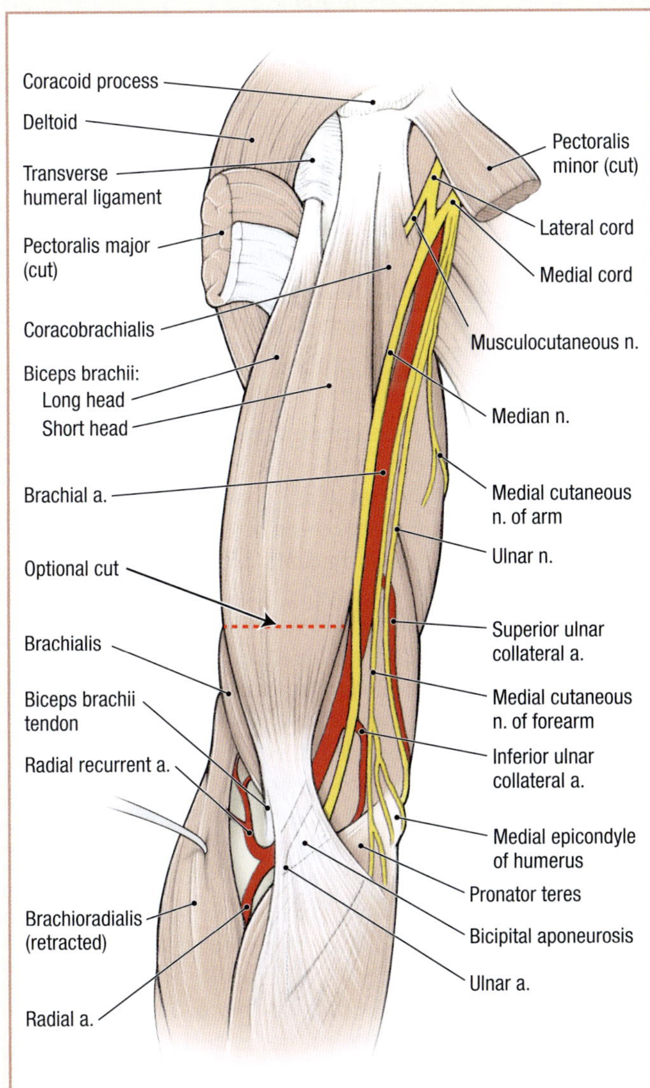

FIGURE 2.21 ■ Anterior compartment of right arm. Anterior view.

5. Use blunt dissection to separate the three muscles in the anterior compartment of the arm: coracobrachialis, brachialis, and biceps brachii.
6. Use blunt dissection to separate the two muscular bellies of the **biceps brachii** and identify the more medially located **short head of the biceps brachii**. Clean the surface of the short head of the biceps brachii and confirm its attachment to the coracoid process of the scapula.
7. Identify and clean the more laterally located **long head of the biceps brachii**. Superiorly, the tendon of the long head of the biceps brachii courses in the intertubercular sulcus of the humerus deep to the **transverse humeral ligament**, passes through the glenohumeral joint, and attaches to the **supraglenoid tubercle**. Do not follow the tendon of the long head to its attachment on the scapula or deep to the transverse humeral ligament at this time.
8. Clean the surface of the biceps brachii inferiorly and identify the **biceps brachii tendon** passing into the cubital fossa.
9. Identify the **bicipital aponeurosis**, an extension of the biceps brachii tendon that broadens medially and attaches to the antebrachial fascia. *Note that the bicipital aponeurosis separates the superficially located median cubital vein from the underlying brachial artery and median nerve making this a safe place for venipuncture.*
10. Review the attachments and actions of the biceps brachii (see **TABLE 2.4**).
11. Clean the surface of the **coracobrachialis**, paying attention to not disrupt the course of the musculocutaneous nerve. Confirm that the proximal attachment of the coracobrachialis is the coracoid process of the scapula and that its distal attachment is on the medial side of the shaft of the humerus.
12. Review the attachments and actions of the coracobrachialis (see **TABLE 2.4**).
13. Flex the elbow about 45° and gently pull the biceps brachii medially or laterally to observe the more deeply located **brachialis**.
14. On one side of the cadaver, you may choose to transect the biceps brachii about 5 cm proximal to the elbow, taking care to not cut the musculocutaneous nerve.
15. If the optional cut was made, reflect the two portions of the biceps brachii superiorly and inferiorly, respectively, to increase visibility of the underlying musculocutaneous nerve and brachialis.
16. Follow the brachialis distally into the cubital fossa and confirm that it attaches to the ulna.
17. Review the attachments and actions of the brachialis (see **TABLE 2.4**).

Neurovasculature of Arm

ATLAS 2.4C, 2.43A; VIDEO 2.6.2

1. Refer to FIGURE 2.21.
2. Identify the **musculocutaneous nerve** where it pierces the coracobrachialis and recall that it innervates the three muscles of the anterior compartment of the arm.
3. Find the musculocutaneous nerve where it emerges from the coracobrachialis and follow it through the plane of loose connective tissue between the biceps brachii and brachialis. Observe that after the musculocutaneous nerve gives off its muscular branches, it continues distally as the **lateral cutaneous nerve of the forearm.**
4. Follow the lateral cutaneous nerve of the forearm to the cubital fossa where it emerges lateral to the biceps brachii tendon.
5. Review the relationship of the lateral cutaneous nerve of the forearm to the cephalic vein.
6. On the medial aspect of the arm, identify the **medial cutaneous nerve of the forearm** and follow it from the medial cord of the brachial plexus to the level of the cubital fossa.
7. Use blunt dissection to follow the **median nerve** distally from the axilla where it arises from the medial and lateral cords of the brachial plexus, to where it enters the cubital fossa medial to the biceps brachii tendon. *Note that the median nerve courses medial to the biceps brachii within the medial intermuscular septum.*
8. Use blunt dissection to follow the **ulnar nerve** from the medial cord of the brachial plexus to a location posterior to the medial epicondyle of the humerus. *Note that the ulnar nerve courses in the medial intermuscular septum in the proximal arm and then comes to lie on the posterior surface of the medial intermuscular septum in the distal one-third of the arm.*
9. Follow the ulnar nerve posteriorly at the elbow and observe that it is in contact with the posterior surface of the medial epicondyle of the humerus. *Note that at this location, the nerve is commonly referred to as the "funny bone" and induces the tingling sensation commonly felt with impact to the elbow.*
10. Refer to FIGURE 2.22.
11. Identify the **brachial artery**, the continuation of the axillary artery. The brachial artery begins at the inferior border of the teres major and ends at the level of the elbow by branching into the ulnar and radial arteries.
12. Remove the surrounding brachial fascia covering the brachial artery and verify that it courses with the median nerve within the medial intermuscular septum. Observe that the median nerve is the only large structure to course along the anterior surface of the brachial artery.

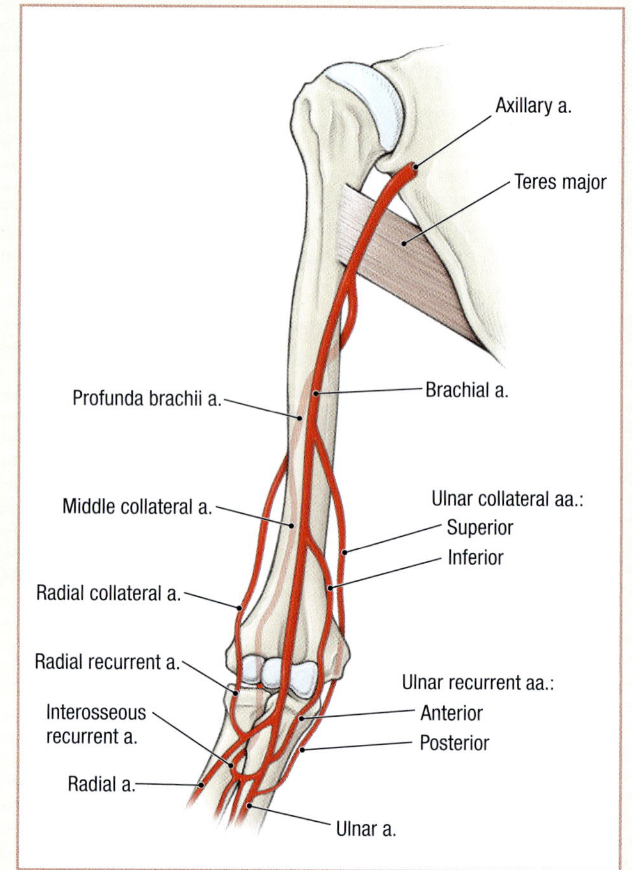

FIGURE 2.22 ● Brachial artery and collateral circulation of elbow. Anterior view.

13. The deep veins of the upper limb are named according to the corresponding artery that they follow and typically occur in pairs known as **venae comitantes.** *Note that the two-to-one relationship of deep veins per artery will be seen throughout the limbs and is a good way to differentiate the appearance of vessels and nerves.*
14. Observe that the **brachial veins** join the basilic vein near the axilla to form the axillary vein.
15. Remove the brachial veins and their tributaries to clear the dissection field while preserving the branches of the brachial artery.
16. The brachial artery has three named branches in the arm arising medially: deep artery of the arm, superior ulnar collateral artery, and inferior ulnar collateral artery. *Note that several unnamed muscular branches also arise along the length of the brachial artery.*
17. In the proximal arm, find the **profunda brachii artery** where it arises from the brachial artery.
18. Follow the profunda brachii artery around the posterior surface of the humerus and confirm that it accompanies the radial nerve in the radial groove between the superior attachments of the medial and lateral heads of the triceps brachii (see **Clinical Correlation 2.4**).

CLINICAL CORRELATION 2.4

Brachial Artery Variants and Damage

ATLAS 2.11, 2.30B, 2.54F

When taking a blood pressure reading, the brachial artery is purposely compressed where it lies close to the shaft of the humerus medial to the biceps brachii. Midshaft fractures of the humerus may sever the profunda brachii artery of the arm as it wraps around the shaft, whereas more distal fractures may damage the brachial artery itself where it courses anteriorly. The profunda brachii artery can provide some collateral circulation to the rest of the arm particularly if a reduction of flow to the main artery occurs gradually.

Occasionally, the brachial artery bifurcates in the arm rather than in the cubital fossa, a "high bifurcation"; thus, the ulnar artery may course superficial to the superficial layer of flexor muscles and be mistaken for a vein. Injection of drugs and medications into the artery, if mistaken for a vein, can have catastrophic consequences.

19. Identify and clean the **superior ulnar collateral artery** where it arises from the brachial artery about halfway down the arm. Observe that the superior ulnar collateral artery courses distally with the ulnar nerve to pass posterior to the medial epicondyle of the humerus. *Note that the superior ulnar collateral artery may arise from the profunda brachii artery.*
20. Identify and clean the **inferior ulnar collateral artery** where it arises from the brachial artery about 3 cm above the medial epicondyle of the humerus. Observe that the inferior ulnar collateral artery passes anterior to the medial epicondyle, deep to the brachialis.

Cubital Fossa

ATLAS 2.53, 2.54; VIDEO 2.6.3

1. Refer to FIGURE 2.23.
2. Observe that the triangular-shaped **cubital fossa** is bound laterally by the brachioradialis and medially by the pronator teres.
3. Identify the location of the superior boundary of the cubital fossa, an imaginary line connecting the medial and lateral epicondyles of the humerus.
4. Observe that the superficial boundary (roof of the cubital fossa) is the antebrachial fascia and bicipital aponeurosis and that the deep boundary (floor of the cubital fossa) is the brachialis and supinator.
5. Review the positions of the cephalic, basilic, and median cubital veins anterior to the cubital fossa. To gain access to deeper structures, it may be necessary

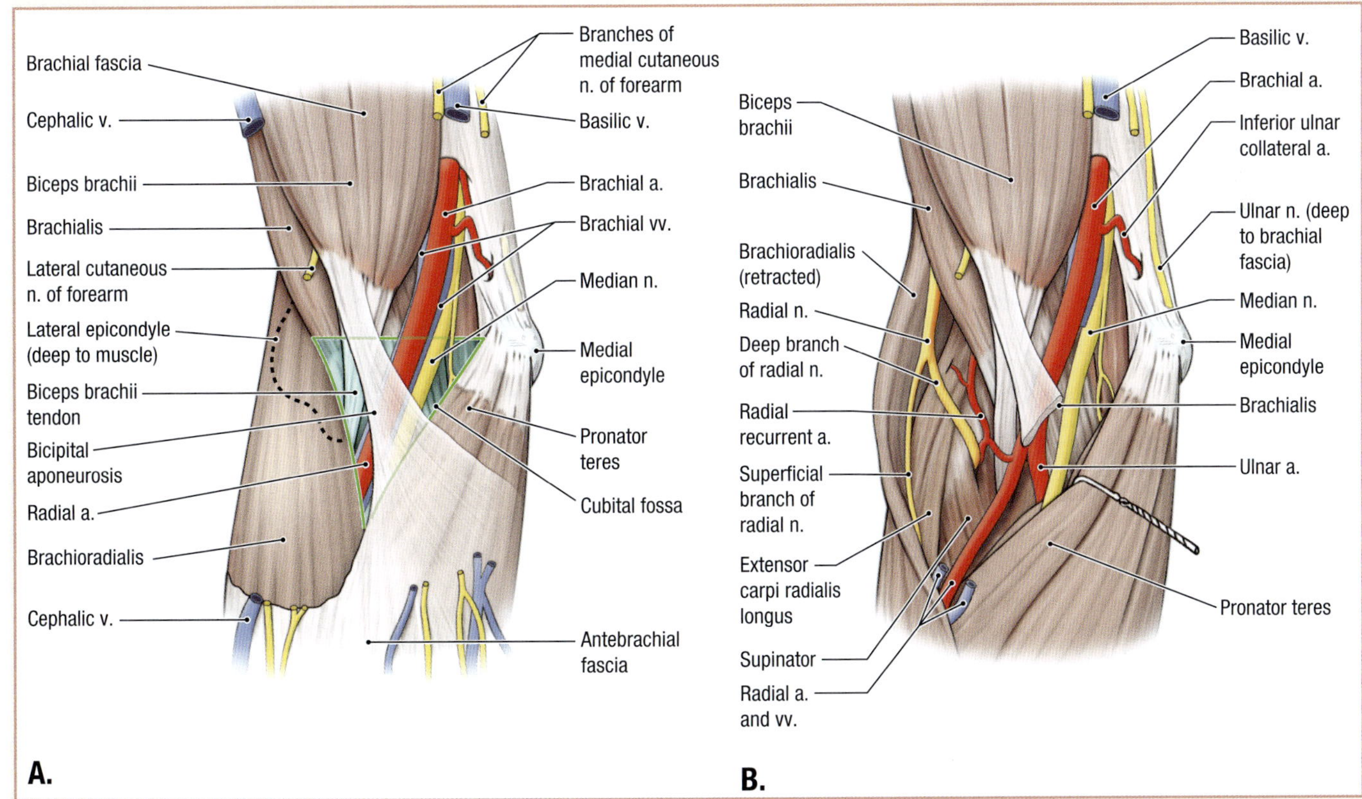

FIGURE 2.23 ● **A.** Superficial dissection of cubital fossa with representative superficial fascia, veins, and cutaneous nerves. **B.** Deep dissection of cubital fossa. Anterior views.

to cut the perforating veins that connect the deep veins to the superficial veins and retract the vessels either medially or laterally as a group.

6. Identify and clean the tendon of the biceps brachii in the cubital fossa.
7. Insert a probe deep to the bicipital aponeurosis near the biceps brachii tendon and gently slide it distally. Use scissors to cut the bicipital aponeurosis as far distally as possible to allow for lateral reflection of the portion still attached to the biceps tendon. Do not cut the brachial artery lying deep to the bicipital aponeurosis.
8. Follow the median nerve and brachial artery from the arm into the cubital fossa removing any fat, veins, or lymphatics that may obstruct your view of these structures.
9. On the lateral aspect of the forearm, identify and clean the proximal end of the **brachioradialis**.
10. Use blunt dissection to open the connective tissue plane between the brachioradialis and the brachialis in the arm to observe that the brachioradialis originates in the posterior compartment of the arm.
11. Deep to the brachioradialis, identify the radial nerve in the superolateral aspect of the cubital fossa lateral to the brachialis.
12. Observe that the radial nerve passes anterior to the elbow joint near the lateral epicondyle and that it is accompanied by the **radial recurrent artery** at this location.
13. Observe the relative positions of three important structures in the cubital fossa from lateral to medial: biceps brachii **t**endon, brachial **a**rtery, and median **n**erve. *Note that the sequence of structures in the cubital fossa may be remembered by the simple mnemonic TAN (tendon, artery, nerve).*
14. Deep to the contents of the cubital fossa, identify and clean the **brachialis** forming the medial aspect of the floor of the cubital fossa. *Note that the supinator also forms part of the floor of the cubital fossa but will be dissected with the posterior compartment of the forearm.*

Dissection Follow-up

1. Review the attachments, innervations, and actions of the muscles in the anterior and posterior compartments of the arm in **TABLE 2.4**.
2. Review the origin, course, termination, and branches of the brachial artery.
3. Trace the paths of the musculocutaneous, median, ulnar, and radial nerves from the brachial plexus to the elbow, reviewing the key relationships of each.
4. Review the position of the neurovascular structures within the fascia and intermuscular septa.
5. Describe the pattern of compartment innervation of the arm.
6. Replace the muscles of the anterior compartment of the arm in their correct anatomical positions.

TABLE 2.4 Muscles of Arm

Muscle	Proximal Attachments	Distal Attachments	Actions	Innervation
ANTERIOR COMPARTMENT OF ARM				
Coracobrachialis	Coracoid process of the scapula	Medial side of shaft of the humerus	Adducts and flexes the humerus	Musculocutaneous n.
Biceps brachii	Long head—supraglenoid tubercle of the scapula; short head—coracoid process of the scapula	Radial tuberosity and antebrachial fascia	Supinates and flexes the forearm	
Brachialis	Anterior aspect of the humerus	Tuberosity of the ulna	Flexes the forearm	
POSTERIOR COMPARTMENT OF ARM				
Triceps brachii	Long head—infraglenoid tubercle of the scapula; medial and lateral heads—posterior surface of the humerus	Olecranon process of the ulna	Extends the forearm	Radial n.
Anconeus	Lateral epicondyle of the humerus	Lateral surface of the olecranon and posterior surface of the proximal ulna	Assists the triceps in extension of the elbow	

Abbreviation: n., nerve.

ANTERIOR COMPARTMENT OF FOREARM

Dissection Overview

The antebrachial fascia (deep fascia of the forearm) is a sleeve of tough connective tissue investing the forearm, which also serves as a site of some muscle attachments. Antebrachial fascia is continuous at its proximal end with brachial fascia and distally with the palmar and dorsal fascia of the hand. Medial and lateral intermuscular septa project deeply from the antebrachial fascia to the radius and ulna.

The intermuscular septa, interosseous membrane, radius, and ulna combine to divide the forearm into anterior and posterior compartments as shown in FIGURE 2.24. The anterior compartment of the forearm contains the forearm flexors and pronators, which receive motor innervation from the median and ulnar nerves. The anterior forearm compartment muscles are arranged in three layers or groups: superficial (first layer), intermediate (second layer), and deep (third layer).

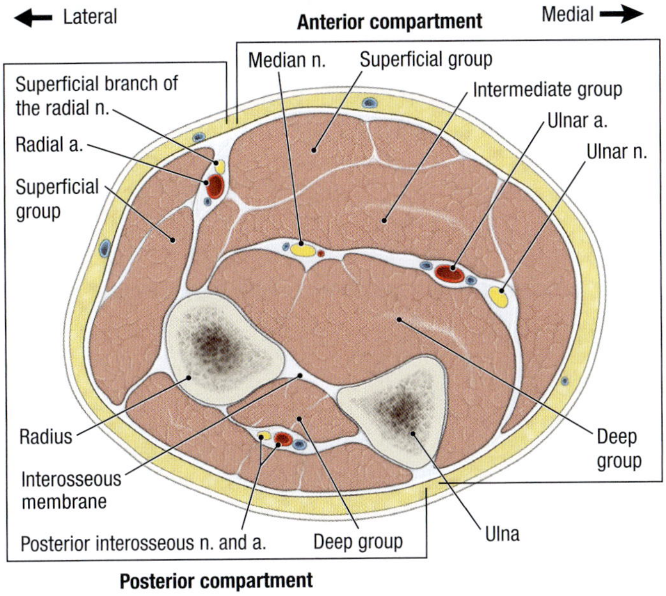

FIGURE 2.24 ● Axial section of right forearm. Inferior view.

The order of dissection will be as follows: The skeletal anatomy of the forearm will be studied. The structures in the subcutaneous tissue of the forearm will be reviewed. The subcutaneous tissue and antebrachial fascia will be removed. At the level of the wrist, the relative positions of tendons, vessels, and nerves will be studied. The superficial and intermediate layers of flexor muscles will be studied and reflected on one side. Vessels and nerves that lie between the intermediate and deep layers of flexor muscles will be studied. The deep layer of flexor muscles will be dissected.

Skeletal Anatomy

Refer to a skeleton or isolated humerus, radius, and ulna to identify the following skeletal features.

Distal Humerus

ATLAS 2.38, 2.57

1. Refer to FIGURE 2.25.
2. On the distal humerus, identify the **medial supraepicondylar ridge** superior to the medial epicondyle as well as the **lateral supraepicondylar ridge** superior to the lateral epicondyle.
3. Review the location of the capitulum, trochlea, coronoid fossa, and olecranon fossa.

Radius and Ulna

ATLAS 2.57, 2.65, 2.85

1. Refer to FIGURE 2.25.
2. Review the location of the **head**, **neck**, and **radial tuberosity** of the radius.
3. Review the location of the **olecranon process**, **trochlear notch**, and **coronoid process of the ulna**.
4. Identify the **anterior oblique line** on the anterior surface of the radius.
5. Along the medial edge of the radius, identify the **interosseous border**, the thin region of the bone serving as an attachment site of the **interosseous membrane**.
6. At the distal end of the radius, identify the **ulnar notch** and the inferiorly oriented **styloid process**.

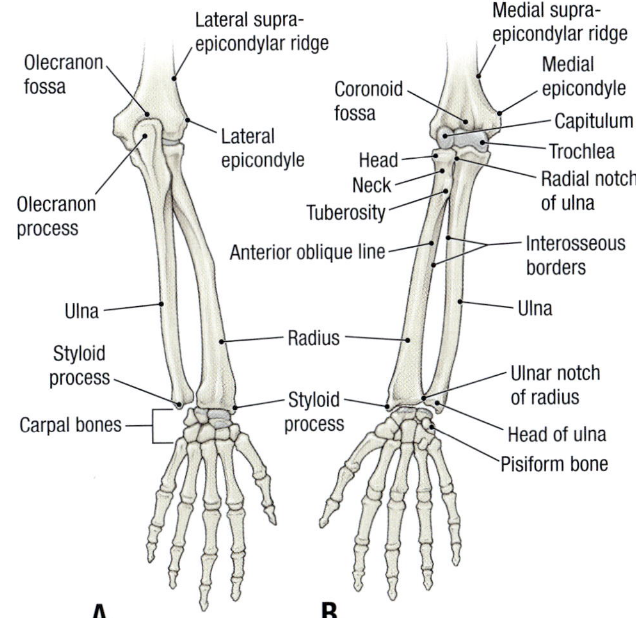

FIGURE 2.25 ● Skeleton of right forearm. **A.** Posterior view. **B.** Anterior view.

7. Articulate the radius and ulna and observe that the **head of the ulna** fits into the depression of the ulnar notch of the radius to create the **distal radioulnar joint**.
8. Observe that the interosseous border of each bone is oriented at the corresponding ridge of the other bone.
9. Pronate and supinate the forearm of the skeleton and notice the rotational movements that occur at the proximal and distal radioulnar joints. In the position of supination (anatomical position), observe that the radius and ulna are parallel, whereas in the position of pronation, the radius crosses anterior to the ulna.
10. On the palmar surface of the articulated hand, identify the **pisiform bone**.

Dissection Instructions

Superficial Layer of Anterior Forearm

ATLAS 2.67; VIDEO 2.7.1

1. Refer to FIGURE 2.26.
2. With the cadaver in the supine position, abduct the upper limb and actively supinate the forearm either using string to hold it in this position or have your dissection partner assist in orienting the upper limb throughout the dissection.
3. Remove the remnants of any remaining subcutaneous tissue of the forearm, taking care to preserve the cephalic and basilic veins while removing any other small veins in the region.
4. Incise the anterior surface of the antebrachial fascia from the cubital fossa to the wrist.
5. Use blunt dissection to spread apart and separate the antebrachial fascia from the muscles that lie deep to it.
6. Detach the antebrachial fascia from its attachments to the radius and ulna along the intermuscular septa peripherally and place it in the tissue container. *Note that the fascia on the medial aspect of the forearm is connected to the underlying tissue and sharp dissection may be needed to fully remove the antebrachial fascia.*
7. Beginning on the medial aspect of the elbow, identify the four muscles in the superficial layer of the anterior forearm: pronator teres, flexor carpi radialis, palmaris longus, and flexor carpi ulnaris.
8. Identify the **common flexor tendon** attached to the medial epicondyle of the humerus and observe that it forms part of the proximal attachment of the muscles of the superficial layer.
9. Use blunt dissection to separate the tendons of the superficial layer of anterior forearm muscles and observe that they cannot be easily separated proximally due to the common tendon.
10. Identify and clean the proximal surface of the **pronator teres** and use blunt dissection to trace it toward its attachment to the middle of the radius on its lateral surface.
11. Identify the two heads of the pronator teres: the **superficial (humeral) head** and the **deep (ulnar) head**. Observe that the median nerve passes between the two heads of the pronator teres.
12. Clean the surface of the **flexor carpi radialis** and follow its tendon toward its distal attachment.
13. In the middle of the forearm, identify the thin **palmaris longus tendon**. Follow and clean the palmaris longus distally toward its attachment to the palmar aponeurosis in the hand. *Note that this muscle and tendon are absent in some individuals.*
14. On the medial aspect of the forearm, identify and clean the **flexor carpi ulnaris** and follow its tendon toward its distal attachment.
15. Review the attachments and actions of the muscles in the superficial layer of the anterior forearm (see **TABLE 2.5**).
16. On the anterior surface of the wrist, identify and clean the **radial artery** deep and lateral to the tendon of the flexor carpi radialis. *Note that the pulse of the radial artery can be felt at this location on the anterior distal surface of the radius in living individuals as well as between the abductor pollicis longus and flexor carpi radialis tendons.*
17. Identify the **median nerve** deep and lateral to the **palmaris longus tendon**. *Note that the median nerve is superficial at the wrist and can be easily injured.*
18. Identify and clean the **ulnar artery** and **ulnar nerve** deep and lateral to the tendon of the flexor carpi ulnaris. *Note that the pulse of the ulnar artery can be felt lateral to the flexor carpi ulnaris and pisiform bone.*

Intermediate Layer of Anterior Forearm

ATLAS 2.68; VIDEO 2.7.2

Dissection Note: Perform the following dissection sequence on only one side of the cadaver. Maintain the superficial relationships on the contralateral side. On the side where the deep dissection cuts are not made, simply use blunt dissection to retract the muscles and tendons to expose the underlying structures.

1. Refer to FIGURE 2.26.
2. Deep to the superficial layer tendons, identify the distal portion of the **flexor digitorum superficialis**, the muscle of the intermediate layer. *Note that to see the intermediate muscle fully, several muscles of the superficial layer must be transected and reflected on one limb.*
3. Use sharp dissection to cut the tendon of the palmaris longus proximal to the wrist (**Cut 1**) and reflect the tendon and muscle belly superiorly.
4. Use sharp dissection to cut the tendon of the flexor carpi radialis proximal to the wrist (**Cut 2**) and reflect the tendon and muscle belly superiorly.

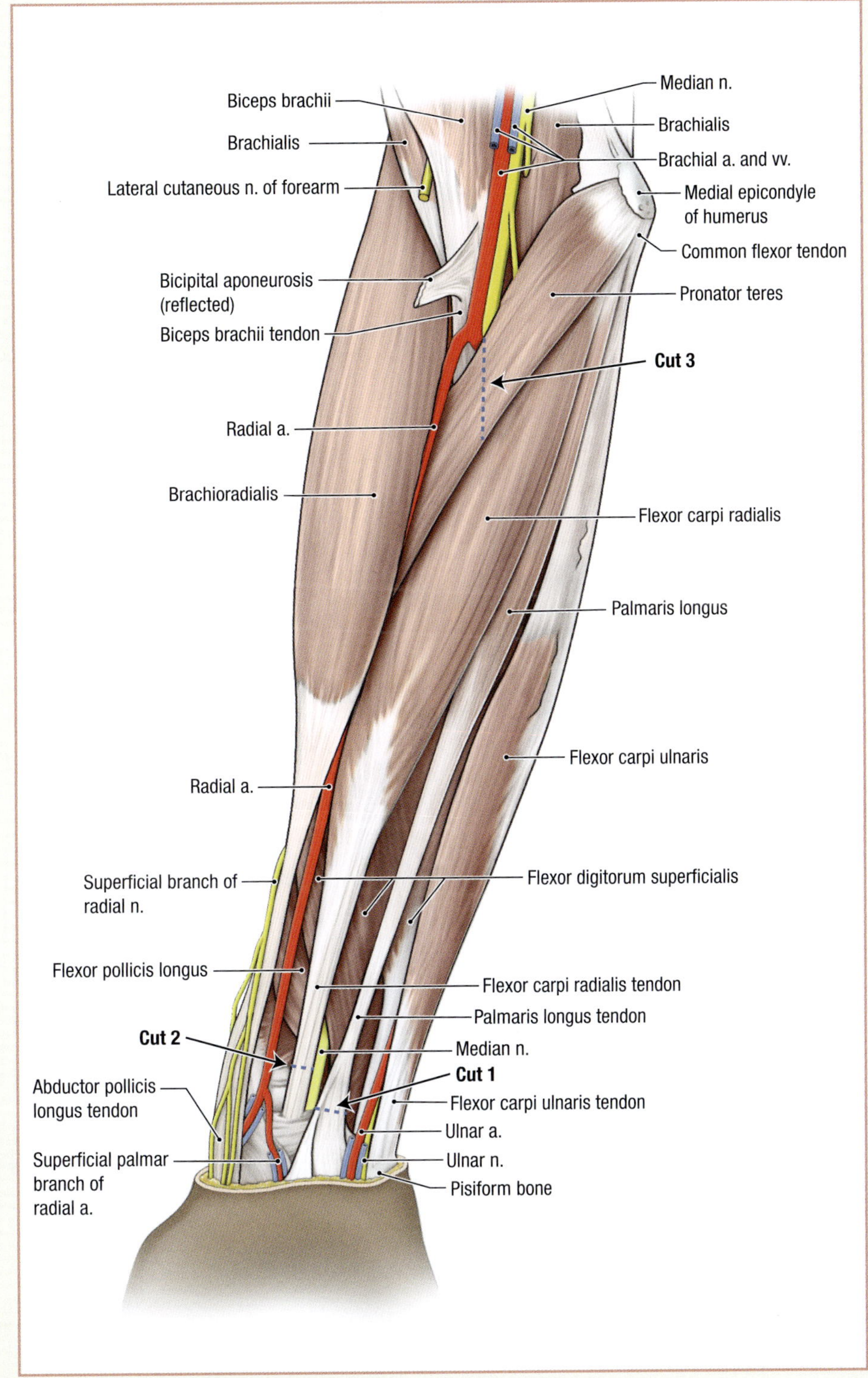

FIGURE 2.26 ■ Superficial layer of anterior compartment of right forearm. Anterior view.

5. Insert a probe between the two heads of the pronator teres along the anterior surface of the median nerve.
6. Use a scalpel to transect the humeral head of the pronator teres anterior to the probe sparing the median nerve (**Cut 3**) and reflect the cut portion of muscle medially.
7. Refer to FIGURE 2.27.
8. Identify the proximal portion of the flexor digitorum superficialis and observe that its proximal attachments create a tendinous arch spanning over the path of the ulnar artery and median nerve.
9. Observe that distally, the flexor digitorum superficialis gives rise to four individual tendons which

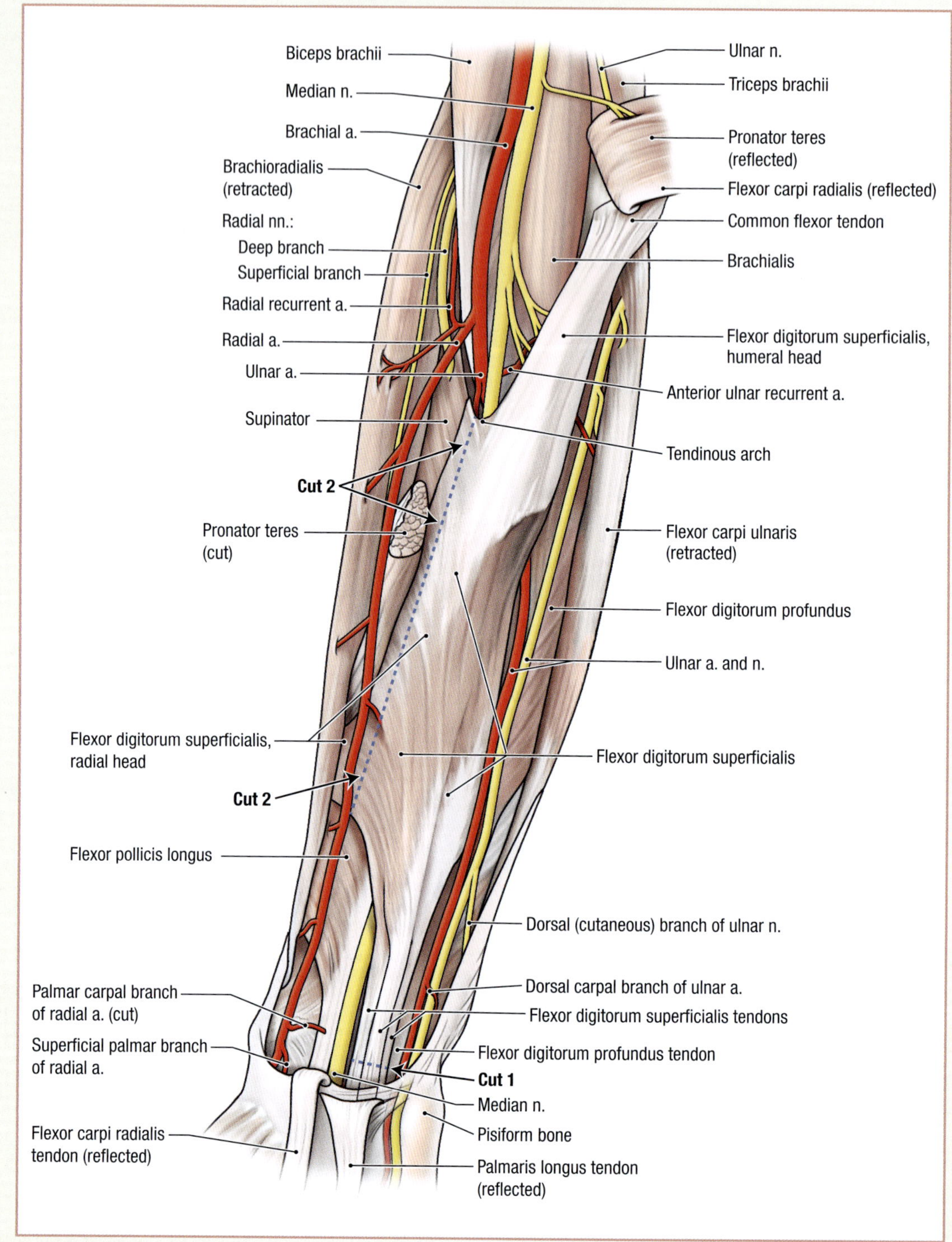

FIGURE 2.27 ● Intermediate layer of anterior compartment of right forearm. Anterior view.

attach to the middle phalanges of digits 2 to 5, resulting in flexion at the proximal interphalangeal (PIP) joints.

10. Proximal to the wrist, observe that the four tendons of the flexor digitorum superficialis lie between the median nerve and the ulnar artery and nerve.
11. Review the attachments and actions of the flexor digitorum superficialis (see **TABLE 2.5**).

Neurovasculature of Anterior Forearm

ATLAS 2.68, 2.69; VIDEO 2.7.3

1. Refer to FIGURE 2.27.
2. On the lateral side of the proximal forearm, clean the brachioradialis muscle and tendon.
3. At the point where the pronator teres passes deep to the brachioradialis, use blunt dissection to open the

connective tissue plane and identify the **superficial branch of the radial nerve**.

4. Follow the superficial branch of the radial nerve to the distal one-third of the forearm and confirm that it emerges on the posterior side of the brachioradialis tendon and distributes to the dorsum of the hand.
5. In the cubital fossa, use blunt dissection to follow the **brachial artery** distally until it bifurcates into the **radial** and **ulnar arteries**.
6. Clean the radial artery and follow it distally as far as the level of the wrist. The radial veins and their tributaries may be removed to clear the dissection field. *Note that the radial artery gives rise to several unnamed muscular branches in the forearm.*
7. Find the **radial recurrent artery** arising from the radial artery near its origin from the brachial artery.
8. Observe that the radial recurrent artery courses superiorly in the connective tissue plane between the brachioradialis and brachialis to meet the radial collateral branch of the profunda brachii artery forming part of the anastomotic network around the elbow.
9. Identify the **median nerve** in the cubital fossa and observe that it is positioned medial to the brachial artery and passes deep to the flexor digitorum superficialis. *Note that the median nerve innervates all but one and a half muscles of the anterior compartment of the forearm.*
10. To expose the distal part of the median nerve, the flexor digitorum superficialis must be cut and retracted. On one upper limb only, use sharp dissection to cut the four tendons of the flexor digitorum superficialis proximal to the wrist (**Cut 1**). On the contralateral limb, use blunt dissection to separate the layers and tendons of the muscles but do not cut them.
11. Detach the flexor digitorum superficialis from its attachment on the anterior oblique line of the radius (**Cut 2**), paying attention to not cut the radial artery.
12. Retract the flexor digitorum superficialis medially, leaving it attached to the ulna and medial epicondyle of the humerus.
13. Refer to FIGURE 2.28.
14. Use blunt dissection to free the median nerve from the loose connective tissue that lies between the intermediate and deep layers of anterior forearm muscles.
15. Observe that the median nerve gives small muscular branches to the palmaris longus, flexor carpi radialis, flexor digitorum superficialis, and pronator teres.
16. Identify the **anterior interosseous nerve**, which arises from the median nerve to innervate the deep layer of anterior forearm muscles.
17. Identify the **ulnar artery** in the cubital fossa and insert a probe along its anterior surface to observe that it passes posterior to the deep head of the pronator teres.
18. Using the inserted probe as a guide, use a scalpel to cut the deep head of the pronator teres and reflect the now fully transected muscle to broaden the dissection field.
19. Clean the ulnar artery from the cubital fossa to the wrist by removing the ulnar veins. *Note that several muscular branches arise from the ulnar artery in the forearm.*
20. Observe that the ulnar artery passes posterior to the median nerve in the cubital fossa between the flexor digitorum superficialis and flexor digitorum profundus and that it is joined by the **ulnar nerve** about one-third of the way down the forearm.
21. Observe that the ulnar artery and nerve lie deep to the flexor carpi ulnaris in the distal forearm and pass into the hand on the lateral side of the pisiform bone at the wrist (see **Clinical Correlation 2.5**).

CLINICAL CORRELATION 2.5

Median and Ulnar Nerve Injuries

ATLAS 2.5, 2.6, 2.53

The median nerve is vulnerable to trauma in the cubital fossa, where it passes between the two heads of the pronator teres, in the carpal tunnel, or within the lateral palm. Depending on the location of the injury, the patient may present with weakness or loss of wrist flexion, impaired flexion of digits 1 and 2 (hand of benediction), lack of opposition of the thenar muscles (thenar wasting), or sensory deficits in the palm and first 3½ digits.

The ulnar nerve is vulnerable to trauma where it courses posterior to the medial epicondyle, at the wrist within Guyon's canal, or in the hand. Depending on the site of trauma, the patient may present with loss or weakness of wrist adduction, impaired adduction and abduction of the digits (claw hand), weakness of flexion of digits 4 and 5, or sensory deficits in the medial palm and last 1½ digits.

22. Identify and clean the **common interosseous artery**, a branch of the ulnar artery arising about 3 cm distal to the elbow.
23. Observe that the common interosseous artery courses posterolaterally toward the interosseous membrane before dividing into the anterior posterior interosseous arteries. *Note that the common interosseous artery is usually quite short and may be absent, in which case the anterior and posterior interosseous arteries arise directly from the ulnar artery.*
24. Identify the **anterior interosseous artery** and follow it distally on the anterior surface of the interosseous membrane between the muscles of the deep layer of anterior forearm muscles.

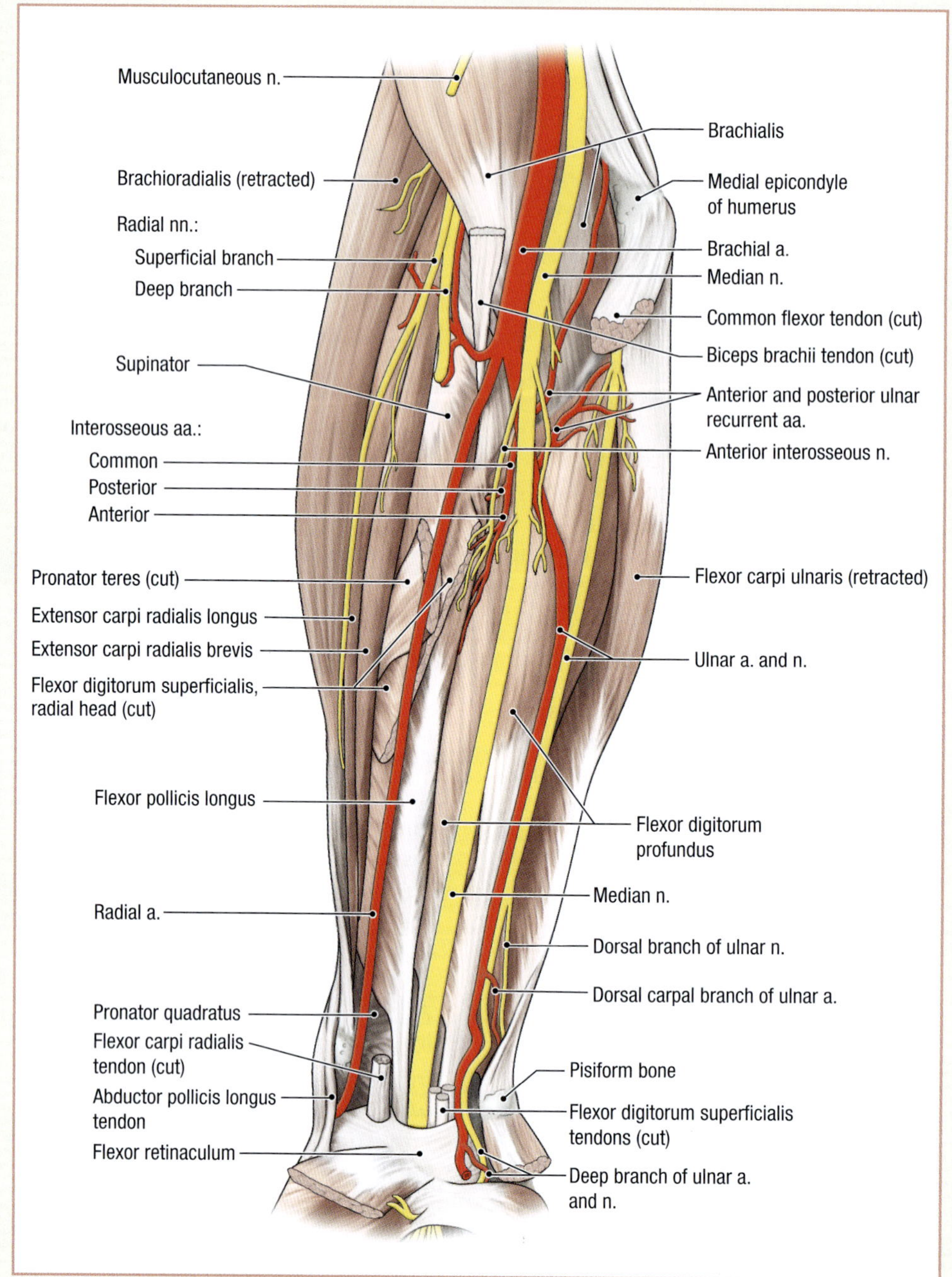

FIGURE 2.28 ● Deep layer of anterior compartment of right forearm. Anterior view.

25. At the proximal end of the interosseous membrane, identify the **posterior interosseous artery** and observe that it passes posteriorly to enter the posterior compartment of the forearm. Do not attempt to follow it into the posterior compartment at this time.
26. Identify the **anterior ulnar recurrent artery** coursing anterior to the medial epicondyle to anastomose with the inferior ulnar collateral artery.
27. Identify the **posterior ulnar recurrent artery** coursing posterior to the medial epicondyle to anastomose with the superior ulnar collateral artery.
28. Identify the ulnar nerve in the distal forearm and follow it proximally.
29. Near the elbow, observe that the ulnar nerve courses posterior to the medial epicondyle of the humerus to penetrate the proximal attachment of the flexor carpi ulnaris. *Note that the ulnar nerve innervates the flexor carpi ulnaris and medial half of the flexor digitorum profundus.*

Deep Layer of Anterior Forearm

ATLAS 2.69, 2.70; VIDEO 2.7.4

1. Refer to FIGURE 2.28.
2. Three muscles comprise the deep layer of the anterior forearm: flexor digitorum profundus, flexor pollicis longus, and pronator quadratus.
3. Deep to the reflected flexor digitorum superficialis, identify and clean the surface of the **flexor digitorum profundus**. *Note that the flexor digitorum profundus has two sources of motor innervation: the anterior interosseous branch of the median nerve to the lateral half of the muscle, and the ulnar nerve to its medial half.*
4. Observe that distally, the flexor digitorum profundus gives rise to four individual tendons which attach to the distal phalanges of digits 2 to 5, resulting in flexion at the distal interphalangeal (DIP) joints.
5. Review the attachments and actions of the flexor digitorum profundus (see **TABLE 2.5**).
6. On the radial side of the forearm, identify and clean the **flexor pollicis longus**, readily identifiable due to its "feather-like" appearance as all the muscle fibers attach to one side of the tendon.
7. Review the attachments and actions of the flexor pollicis longus (see **TABLE 2.5**).
8. Refer to FIGURE 2.29.
9. Retract the tendons of the flexor digitorum profundus and flexor pollicis longus medially and laterally, respectively, and identify the **pronator quadratus**.
10. Observe that the fibers of the pronator quadratus run transversely from the ulna to the radius.
11. In the distal forearm, observe that the anterior interosseous artery and nerve pass between the pronator quadratus and interosseous membrane.

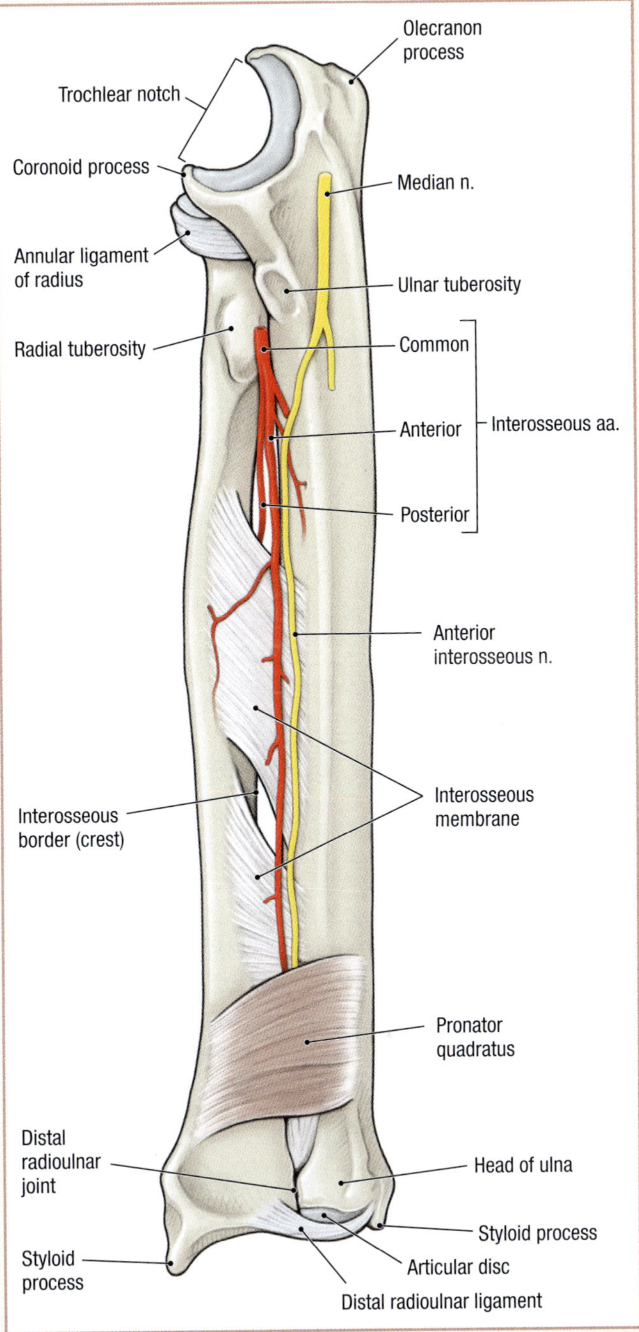

FIGURE 2.29 Interosseous neurovasculature of right forearm. Anterior view.

Dissection Follow-up

1. Review the attachments and actions of the superficial, intermediate, and deep muscles in the anterior compartment of the forearm in **TABLE 2.5**.
2. Follow the brachial artery from its origin in the arm to its bifurcation in the cubital fossa.
3. Review the branches and paths of the radial and ulnar arteries from the elbow to the wrist.
4. Review the course, branches, and pattern of motor innervation of the median nerve.
5. Review the course, branches, and pattern of motor innervation of the ulnar nerve.
6. Replace the anterior forearm muscles in their correct anatomical positions, taking care to align the cut tendons correctly on the limb where they were cut.

TABLE 2.5 Muscles of Anterior Compartment of Forearm

Muscle	*Proximal Attachments*	*Distal Attachments*	*Actions*	*Innervation*
SUPERFICIAL (FIRST) LAYER				
Pronator teres	Medial epicondyle of humerus and coronoid process of ulna	Lateral midshaft of radius	Pronates and flexes the forearm	Median n.
Flexor carpi radialis	Medial epicondyle of humerus	Base of metacarpals 2–3	Flexes and abducts the wrist	
Palmaris longus		Palmar aponeurosis	Flexes the wrist	
Flexor carpi ulnaris		Pisiform bone and base of metacarpal 5	Flexes and adducts the wrist	Ulnar n.
INTERMEDIATE (SECOND) LAYER				
Flexor digitorum superficialis	Medial epicondyle of humerus and oblique line of radius	Middle phalanges of digits 2–5	Flexes the PIP of digits 2–5	Median n.
DEEP (THIRD) LAYER				
Flexor digitorum profundus	Anterior and medial surface of ulna and interosseous membrane	Distal phalanges of digits 2–5	Flexes the DIP of digits 2–5	Lateral half—anterior interosseous n.; medial half—ulnar n.
Flexor pollicis longus	Anterior surface of radius and interosseous membrane	Base of distal phalanx of thumb	Flexes the IP of thumb	Anterior interosseous branch of median n.
Pronator quadratus	Distal radius	Distal ulna	Pronates the forearm	

Abbreviations: DIP, distal interphalangeal; IP, interphalangeal; n., nerve; PIP, proximal interphalangeal.

PALM OF HAND

Dissection Overview

The hand may be divided into five fascial compartments (hypothenar, thenar, central, adductor, and interosseous) separated by two potential spaces (thenar and midpalmar). The more superficially located thenar and hypothenar compartments contain intrinsic muscles of the hand to the thumb and little digit, respectively. The central compartment contains the extrinsic tendons arising from the forearm which reach the hand after passing through the carpal tunnel. The deeply located adductor and interosseous compartments contain intrinsic muscles of the hand and are located deep to the potential spaces.

In the palm, two arterial arches course between the muscle layers. The superficial palmar arch is mainly derived from the ulnar artery, whereas the deep palmar arch arises from the radial artery. The nerve supply of the palmar aspect of the hand is from the median and ulnar nerves.

The order of dissection will be as follows: The skeletal anatomy of the hand will be reviewed. The palmar aponeurosis will be studied and removed. The superficial palmar arch will be dissected, followed by the tendons of the muscles of the anterior compartment of the forearm. The transverse carpal ligament will be cut, and the flexor tendons will be released from the palm. The flexor tendons will be followed into the palm, and the lumbricals studied. The muscles of the thenar and hypothenar groups will be dissected. The deep palmar arch will be dissected along with the deep branch of the ulnar nerve. The adductor pollicis and interossei will be studied.

Skeletal Anatomy

Refer to a skeleton or an articulated hand and identify the following skeletal features.

Skeleton of Hand

ATLAS 2.72, 2.76D, 2.94A

1. Refer to FIGURE 2.30.
2. Identify the **eight carpal bones** in the proximal hand and observe that they are positioned in essentially two rows of four.
3. In the proximal row of carpal bones from lateral to medial, identify the **scaphoid, lunate, triquetrum,** and **pisiform**.
4. In the distal row of carpal bones from lateral to medial, identify the **trapezium, trapezoid, capitate,** and **hamate**.
5. Identify the 5 **metacarpals**, numbered from 1 to 5 from lateral to medial with the thumb counting as the 1st digit and the "pinky" or little finger counting as the 5th.
6. Observe that digit 1 (the thumb) has two phalanges: **proximal** and **distal**.
7. Observe that digits 2 to 5 (the fingers) have three phalanges: **proximal, middle,** and **distal**.
8. Medially, identify the pisiform and **hook of the hamate** forming the medial wall of the **carpal tunnel**.
9. Laterally, identify the **tubercle of the scaphoid** and **tubercle of the trapezium** forming the lateral wall of the carpal tunnel. *Note that a portion of the flexor retinaculum, the transverse carpal ligament, bridges the carpal bones forming the roof of the carpal tunnel which allows passage of nine flexor tendons and the median nerve from the forearm into the hand.*

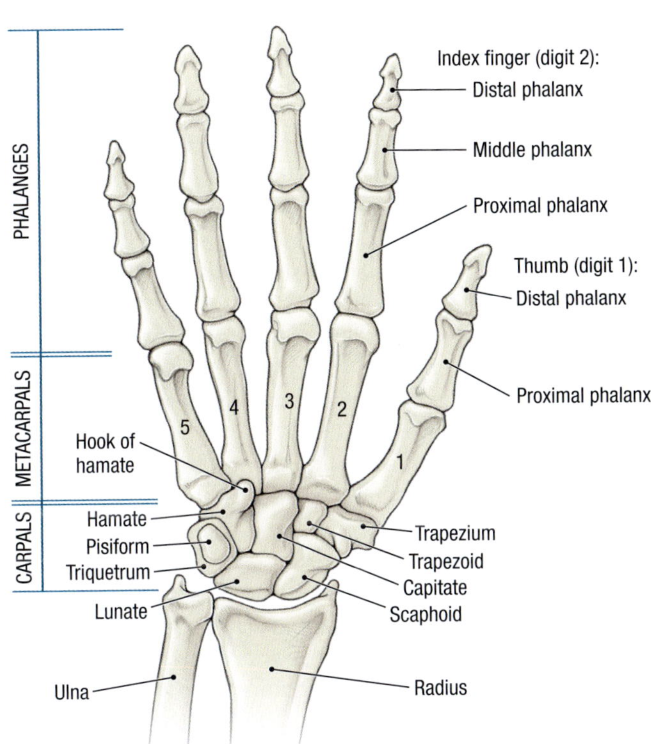

FIGURE 2.30 ● Skeleton of right wrist and hand. Anterior (palmar) view.

Dissection Instructions

Skin Incisions of Palm

VIDEO 2.8.1

Dissection Note: In some cadavers, the hands may be stuck in a clenched position after the embalming process making it difficult to dissect the palm. If the hand is clenched, flex the wrist and gently force open the digits, and have a dissection partner hold it open or use string to maintain the position.

1. Refer to FIGURE 2.31.
2. With the cadaver in the supine position, make a longitudinal incision from the midline of the wrist (E) along the palm to a point near the base of the 3rd digit (M), the midline of the hand.

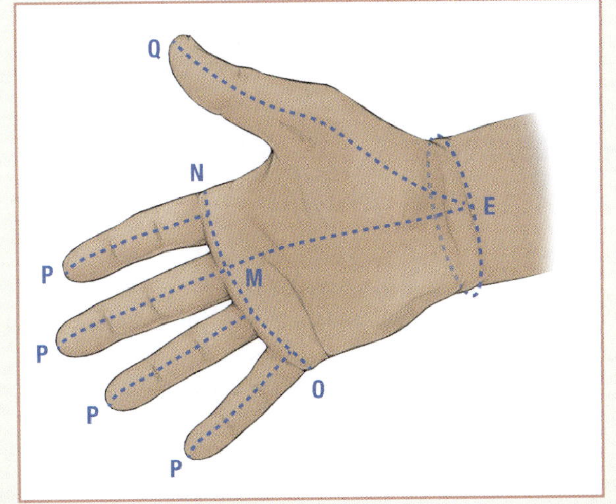

FIGURE 2.31 ● Skin incisions of hand. Anterior (palmar) view.

3. Make a transverse incision proximal to the level of the webs of the fingers beginning laterally at the base of the 2nd digit (N) to the base of the 5th digit (O).
4. Make a longitudinal incision on the anterior surface of digits 2 to 5 from the transverse palm incision (N to O) to the tip of each digit (P). *Note that the subcutaneous tissue on the palmar surface of the digits is very thin, especially at the skin creases; thus, it is recommended to proceed with caution while making incisions in this region.*
5. Make a longitudinal incision from the midline of the wrist (E) along the palmar surface of the thumb to the tip of the 1st digit (Q).
6. Beginning in the midline of the palm and working toward the periphery, remove the thick skin from the palmar surface of the hand staying superficial to the palmar aponeurosis.
7. Remove the skin by cutting along the medial and lateral aspects of the hand and carefully freeing it from the underlying aponeurosis and place it in the tissue container.
8. Reflect the skin of the digits away from the midlines, paying attention to not damage the underlying fibrous digital sheaths, and work peripherally, taking care to avoid damaging the digital nerves and vessels coursing along the length of each digit.
9. Remove the palmar skin of the digits by cutting along the periphery of each digit.
10. Turn the hand over and remove the skin on the dorsum of the hand. *Note that the skin on the dorsum of the hand is much thinner and more loosely attached than the skin on the palm. Exercise caution while removing the thin skin to not damage the underlying superficial veins on the dorsum of the hand.*
11. Remove the skin on the dorsum of the hand distal to the carpometacarpal joints, leaving the skin on the posterior surface of the digits intact at this point in the dissection.

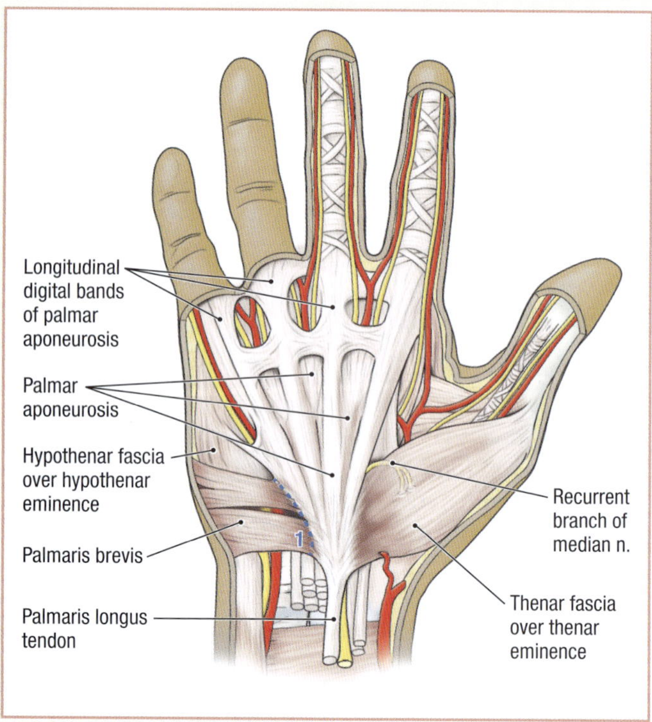

FIGURE 2.32 ■ Superficial palm of right hand. Anterior (palmar) view.

Superficial Palm

ATLAS 2.73, 2.75, 2.78; VIDEO 2.8.2

1. Refer to FIGURE 2.32.
2. On the palmar surface of the hand, identify the **palmar fascia**, a continuation of the antebrachial fascia in the forearm.
3. Observe that the palmar fascia thickens centrally as the **palmar aponeurosis** and serves as the distal attachment of the palmaris longus if present. *Note that although the palmaris longus may be absent, the palmar aponeurosis is always present.*
4. Carefully use scraping motions with a scalpel blade to clean the fat from the palmar aponeurosis. Observe that the palmar aponeurosis has four bands of **longitudinal fibers**, one band to each of the digits 2 to 5, which end by attaching to the fibrous digital sheath near the base of the proximal phalanx of each digit.
5. Identify the thin palmar fascia covering the **thenar eminence** lateral to the palmar aponeurosis and **hypothenar eminence** medial to the palmar aponeurosis.
6. Identify the **palmaris brevis**, a thin, fragile muscle responsible for contracting the skin at the base of the medial palm. *Note that the palmaris brevis may not be readily visible in some cadavers.*
7. Detach the palmaris brevis from the palmar aponeurosis (**Cut 1**) and reflect it medially.
8. Use a probe to elevate the palmar aponeurosis near its distal attachments away from the underlying structures in the palm.
9. In the forearm where the palmaris longus tendon was cut, use sharp dissection to carefully detach the palmar aponeurosis from the underlying structures. Grasp the distal palmaris longus tendon with hemostats to apply traction to the palmar aponeurosis during its removal.

10. While reflecting the palmar aponeurosis, do not cut too deeply as the **superficial palmar arch** is in contact with its deep surface. Similarly, be careful to preserve the **recurrent branch of the median nerve** entering the thenar eminence along its distal margin.
11. Near the proximal end of digits 2 and 3, remove the band of longitudinal fibers of the palmar aponeurosis.
12. On the upper limb with the superficial dissection, detach the palmar aponeurosis beginning distally. Using the same techniques with the scalpel, carefully detach the palmar aponeurosis from the underlying structures and reflect it toward the forearm, leaving it attached to the tendon of the palmaris longus.
13. Refer to FIGURE 2.33.
14. Identify the **ulnar artery** in the forearm and use blunt dissection to follow it into the palm lateral to the pisiform bone with the ulnar nerve to where it divides into superficial and deep branches.
15. Observe that the **superficial branch of the ulnar artery** crosses the palm to form the **superficial palmar arterial arch.** The superficial palmar arterial arch is completed by a smaller contribution from the **superficial palmar branch of the radial artery**.

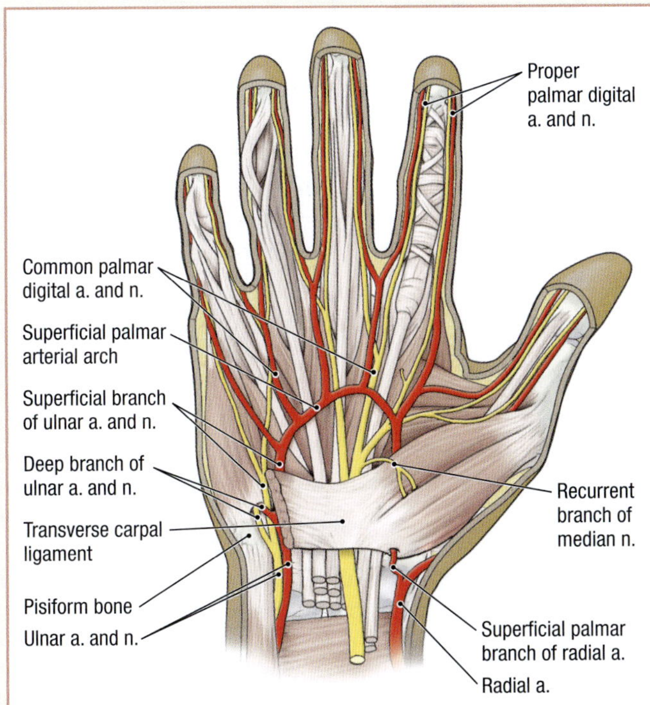

FIGURE 2.33 ● Superficial palm of right hand with removed palmar aponeurosis. Anterior (palmar) view.

16. Use blunt dissection to clean the superficial palmar arterial arch as well as the vessels arising from it, the **common palmar digital arteries**.
17. Trace one or two common palmar digital arteries distally and observe that they divide into two **proper palmar digital arteries** supplying the adjacent sides of two digits.
18. Find the ulnar nerve lateral to the pisiform bone and use a probe to dissect the **superficial branch of the ulnar nerve**, which supplies cutaneous innervation to digit 5 and the medial side of digit 4.
19. Identify the **deep branch of the ulnar nerve** and follow it a short distance until it disappears between the muscles of the hypothenar eminence.

Carpal Tunnel

ATLAS 2.69, 2.78, 2.80, 2.82; VIDEO 2.8.3

1. Refer to FIGURE 2.34.
2. Identify the **transverse carpal ligament**, the roof of the carpal tunnel, between the thenar and hypothenar eminences.
3. Insert a probe deep to the transverse carpal ligament from proximal to distal.
4. Use a scalpel to cut through the transverse carpal ligament superficial to the probe and open the carpal tunnel (**Cut 1**).
5. Refer to FIGURE 2.35.
6. Examine the contents of the carpal tunnel: median nerve, four tendons of the flexor digitorum superficialis, four tendons of the flexor digitorum profundus, and the tendon of the flexor pollicis longus.

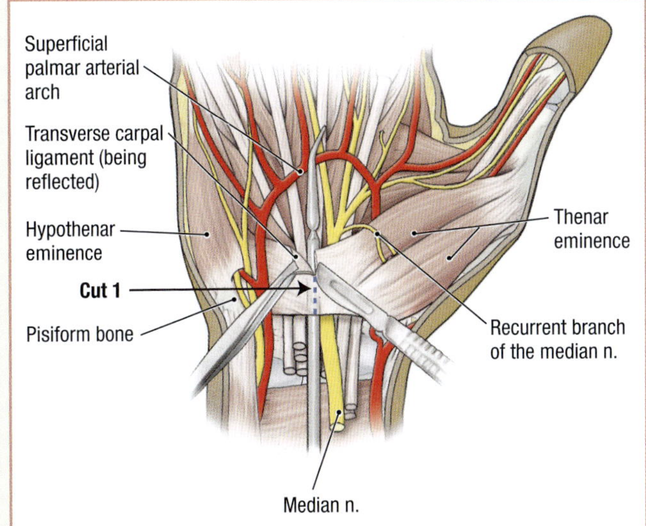

FIGURE 2.34 ● Opening right carpal tunnel. Anterior (palmar) view.

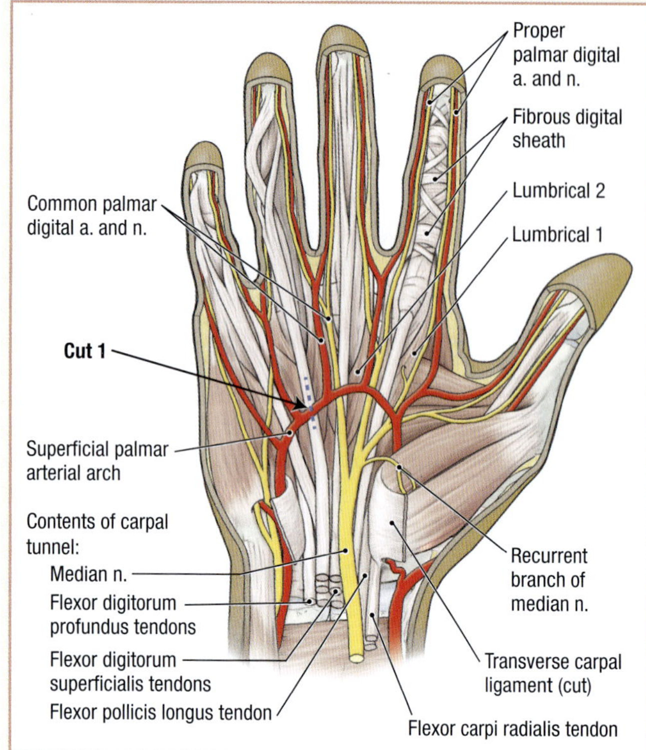

FIGURE 2.35 ● Contents of right carpal tunnel in intermediate palm. Anterior (palmar) view.

CLINICAL CORRELATION 2.6

Carpal Tunnel Syndrome

ATLAS 2.69, 2.71

A common flexor sheath surrounds the tendons of the flexor digitorum profundus and superficialis, but not the tendon of the flexor pollicis longus as they pass through the carpal tunnel as shown in FIGURE B2.1. A swelling of the common flexor synovial sheath, commonly caused by repetitive movement, may encroach on the available space in the carpal tunnel resulting in compression of the contents. As a result of the swelling, the median nerve may be compressed resulting in pain and paresthesia of the thumb, index, and middle fingers and weakness of the thenar muscles.

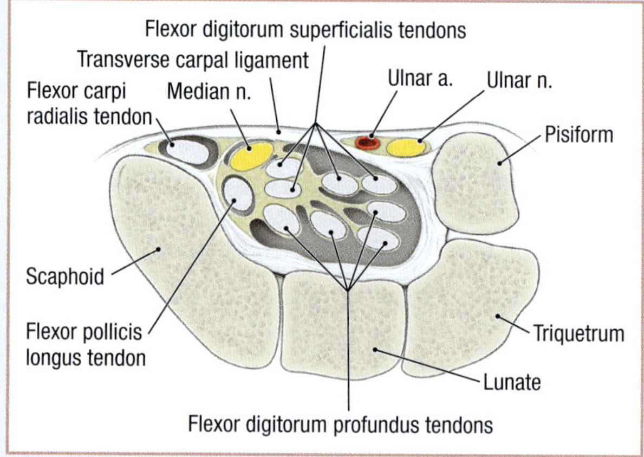

FIGURE B2.1 ● Axial section of right carpal tunnel. Inferior view.

7. Find the median nerve at the level of the wrist and follow it through the carpal tunnel. Gently slide a probe along the lateral aspect of the median nerve to identify the **recurrent branch of the median nerve** supplying the thenar muscles.
8. Identify and clean the median nerve in the hand as well as its various branches. *Note that the median nerve innervates five muscles in the hand: lumbricals 1 and 2 via common palmar digital nerves, and the thenar muscles via the recurrent branch of the median nerve.*
9. Follow the **common palmar digital branches** of the median nerve toward the lateral 3½ digits. Observe that the common palmar digital nerves typically divide to give rise to two **proper palmar digital nerves**, which accompany the proper palmar digital arteries. *Use an illustration to study the cutaneous distribution of the median nerve in the hand.*
10. Identify and clean the flexor tendons that pass through the carpal tunnel (see **Clinical Correlation 2.6**). Observe that the flexor tendons pass through the palm of the hand deep to the superficial palmar arch and digital nerves and then enter the fibrous digital sheaths on the anterior surfaces of the digits.

Dissection Note: Perform the following dissection steps only on the upper limb with the deep dissection already performed in the forearm.

11. Refer to FIGURE 2.36.
12. In the distal forearm, use blunt dissection to separate the tendons of the flexor digitorum superficialis from the tendons of the flexor digitorum profundus.
13. Use scissors to cut the superficial palmar arch in the midline of the palm (**Cut 1**) and retract the common digital branches of the median and ulnar nerves laterally and medially, respectively.
14. Pull the tendons of the flexor digitorum superficialis anteriorly to free them from the carpal tunnel. *Note that during this procedure, the common flexor synovial sheath will be destroyed.*

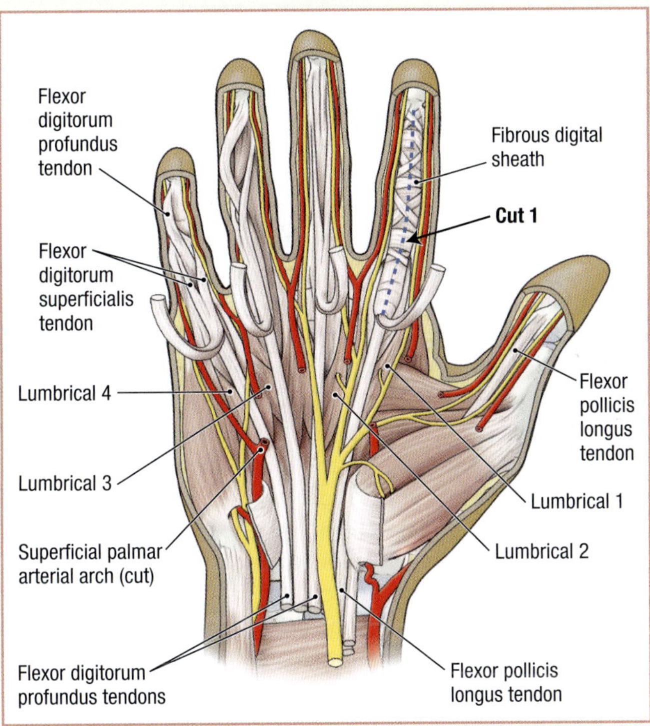

FIGURE 2.36 ■ Intermediate palm of right hand. Anterior (palmar) view.

15. Clean the surface of the tendons of the flexor digitorum superficialis near the base of each digit.
16. In the palm, identify and clean the tendons of the flexor digitorum profundus and observe the relationship of the four attached **lumbricals** on the lateral aspect of each tendon.
17. Clean the surface of the lumbricals but do not disrupt their points of attachment to the flexor digitorum profundus.
18. Review the attachments and actions of the flexor digitorum profundus and lumbricals (see **TABLE 2.5** and **TABLE 2.6**).
19. Use a scalpel to carefully make a midline incision through the **fibrous digital sheath** on the flexor surface of at least one digit (**Cut 1**) and remove it from the digit.
20. Study the relationship of the tendons of the flexor digitorum superficialis and flexor digitorum profundus. Verify that the flexor digitorum superficialis tendon splits to attach to the middle phalanx on each side and that the flexor digitorum profundus tendon passes through the split to attach to the distal phalanx for digits 2 to 5.
21. Identify the flexor pollicis longus in the forearm and follow its tendon distally through the carpal tunnel into the palm. Gently pull on the tendon to confirm that the flexor pollicis longus flexes the distal phalanx of the thumb.

Thenar Eminence

ATLAS 2.71C, 2.75, 2.78; VIDEO 2.8.4

1. Refer to FIGURE 2.37.
2. Remove the thin layer of palmar fascia off the thenar eminence, making an effort to preserve the recurrent branch of the median nerve.
3. Identify and clean the two superficially located muscles of the thenar group: **abductor pollicis brevis** and **flexor pollicis brevis**.
4. Use a probe to follow the recurrent branch of the median nerve and separate the abductor pollicis brevis from the flexor pollicis brevis (see **Clinical Correlation 2.7**).

CLINICAL CORRELATION 2.7

Recurrent Branch of Median Nerve Injury

ATLAS 2.73, 2.78

The recurrent branch of the median nerve is superficial and can easily be severed by "minor" cuts over the thenar eminence. If the recurrent branch of the median nerve is injured, the thenar muscles are paralyzed and the thumb cannot be opposed. Commonly, the recurrent branch of the median nerve is referred to as the thenar branch, or "the million-dollar nerve," due to its importance and potential value if severed.

5. Elevate the abductor pollicis brevis and transect it and the flexor pollicis brevis with sharp dissection near their distal attachments.
6. Identify the **opponens pollicis** deep to the abductor and flexor pollicis brevis. *Note that the opponens pollicis attaches to the lateral side of the entire length of the shaft of the 1st metacarpal bone.*
7. Review the attachments and actions of the **thenar group of muscles** (see **TABLE 2.6**).

Hypothenar Eminence

ATLAS 2.78, 2.81; VIDEO 2.8.5

1. Refer to FIGURE 2.37.
2. Clean the thin layer of palmar fascia off the hypothenar eminence.
3. Identify the three muscles of the hypothenar group: abductor digiti minimi, flexor digiti minimi brevis, and opponens digiti minimi.

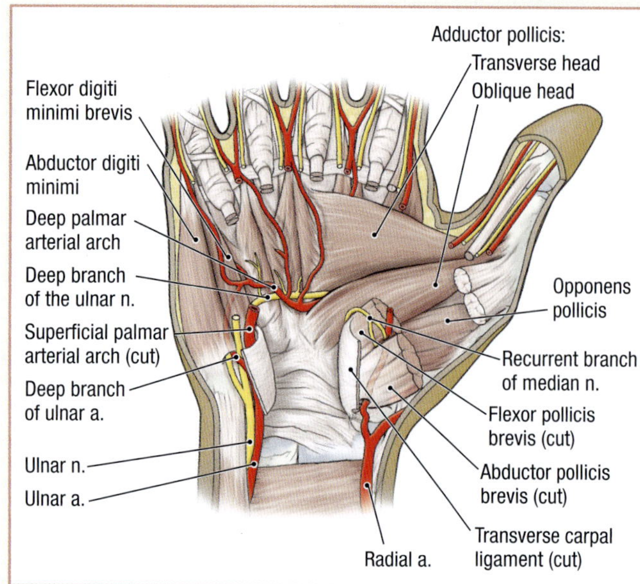

FIGURE 2.37 ● Deep palm of right hand. Anterior (palmar) view.

4. Find the tendons of the abductor digiti minimi and flexor digiti minimi brevis near their distal attachments on the base of the proximal phalanx of digit 5. Use blunt dissection to separate and define the borders of the muscles along their tendons.
5. Use a probe to elevate the abductor digiti minimi and identify the underlying **opponens digiti minimi**.
6. If the opponens digiti minimi is not visible, detach the abductor digiti minimi from its distal attachment and reflect the muscle toward its attachment on the flexor retinaculum while preserving the deep branches of the ulnar artery and ulnar nerve.
7. Review the attachments and actions of the hypothenar group of muscles (see **TABLE 2.6**).

Deep Palm

ATLAS 2.77, 2.81, 2.82, 2.84; VIDEO 2.8.6

Dissection Note: Perform the following dissection sequence only on one upper limb.

1. Refer to FIGURE 2.37.
2. Transect the flexor digitorum profundus in the distal forearm proximal to the carpal tunnel.
3. Reflect the tendons of the flexor digitorum profundus and associated lumbricals distally as far as possible to expose the deep palm.
4. Find the ulnar nerve and the ulnar artery on the lateral side of the pisiform and identify the **deep branch of the ulnar nerve** and the **deep palmar branch of the ulnar artery**.
5. Follow the deep branches of the ulnar artery and nerve to the proximal attachments of the flexor digiti minimi brevis and abductor digiti minimi.
6. Push a probe parallel to the deep branch of the ulnar nerve where it pierces the opponens digiti minimi to course within the **ulnar (Guyon's) canal**.
7. Use a scalpel to cut down to the inserted probe and release the branches of the ulnar nerve.
8. Use blunt dissection to follow the deep branch of the ulnar nerve laterally across the palm and observe that it lies on the anterior surface of the interossei to reach the adductor pollicis.
9. Identify the **deep palmar arterial arch** and observe that it arises from the radial artery laterally and the deep branch of the ulnar artery medially.
10. Identify the **palmar metacarpal arteries** and use an illustration to study the branches of the deep palmar arch.
11. Identify the **adductor pollicis** in the deep palm and use blunt dissection to define its borders.
12. Identify the two heads of the adductor pollicis muscle: **oblique** and **transverse**.
13. Review the attachments and actions of the **adductor pollicis** (see **TABLE 2.6**).
14. Refer to FIGURE 2.38.
15. Identify the three **palmar interossei** and observe their unipennate appearance. Observe that the three **P**almar interossei are **Ad**ductors (**PAD**), which adduct digits 2, 4, and 5 toward the midline of the hand, an imaginary axial line drawn through the long axis of digit 3.
16. The **dorsal interossei** are bipennate muscles and will be seen on the dorsal surface of the hand occupying the intervals between the metacarpal bones. *Note that dorsal interossei are considered intrinsic muscles of the palm of the hand despite their visibility on the dorsal surface.*
17. The four **D**orsal interossei are **Ab**ductors (**DAB**), which move digits 2, 3, and 4 away from the midline of the hand. The two dorsal interossei attaching to digit 3 move it to either side of midline back and forth. *Note that all of the interossei are innervated by the deep branch of the ulnar nerve.*

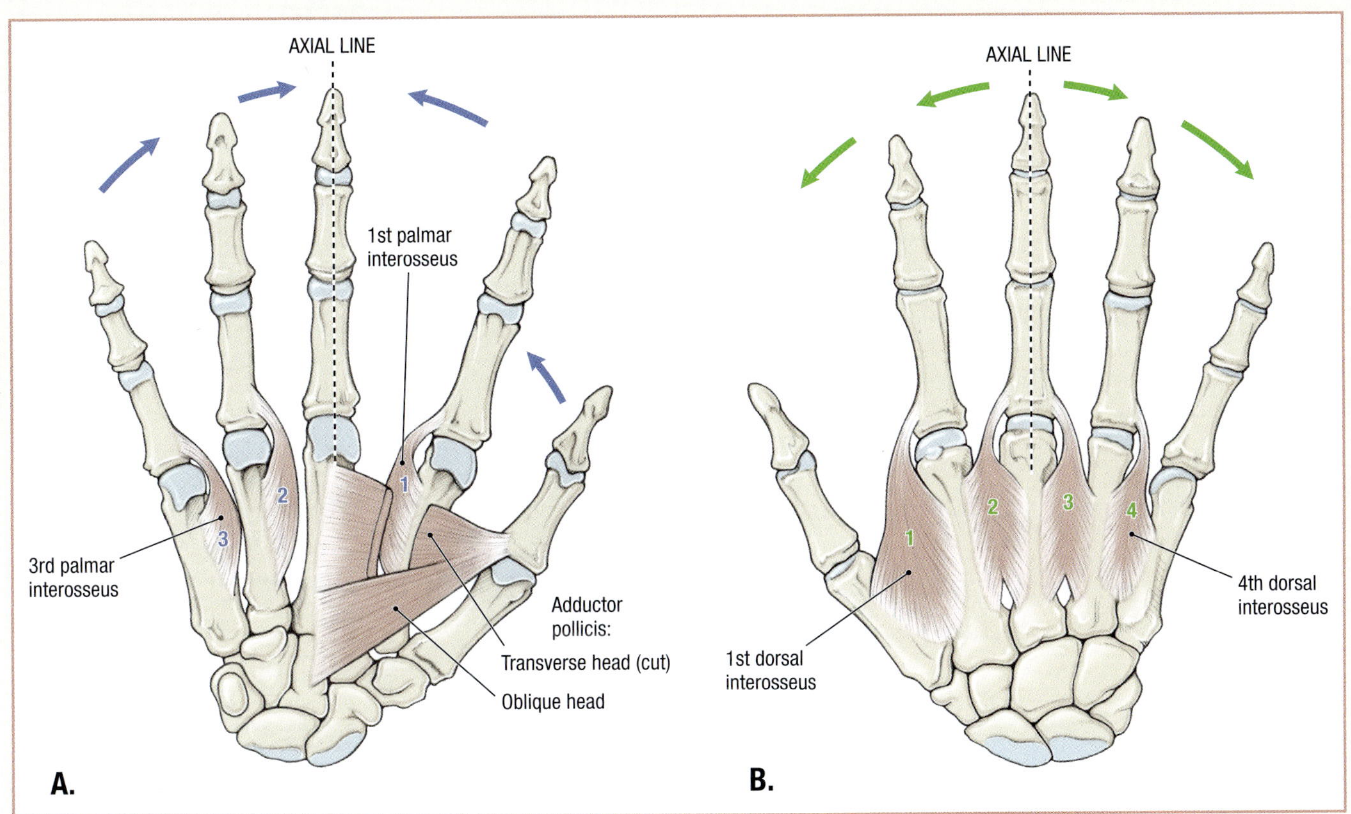

FIGURE 2.38 ● **A.** Palmar interossei of right hand. Anterior (palmar) view. **B.** Dorsal interossei of right hand. Posterior (dorsal) view.

Dissection Follow-up

1. Review the movements of the fingers and thumb defining flexion, extension, abduction, and adduction and the muscles responsible for each using **TABLE 2.6**.
2. Review the path of the median nerve from the forearm into the hand and review its pattern of motor and cutaneous innervation.
3. Review the path of the ulnar artery from the elbow to the hand and review the formation of the palmar arterial arches.
4. Review the path of the ulnar nerve from posterior to the medial epicondyle of the humerus to the hand and review its pattern of motor and cutaneous distribution.
5. Place the dissected muscles, tendons, and nerves back into their correct anatomical positions.
6. Familiarize yourself with the cutaneous distribution of the ulnar and median nerves in the hand.

TABLE 2.6 Muscles of Hand

<table>
<tr><th>Muscle</th><th>Proximal Attachments</th><th>Distal Attachments</th><th>Actions</th><th>Innervation</th></tr>
<tr><td colspan="5">SUPERFICIAL PALM</td></tr>
<tr><td>Palmaris brevis</td><td>Medial aspect of the palmar aponeurosis</td><td>Skin over the hypothenar eminence</td><td>Wrinkle skin of the medial palm</td><td>Ulnar n.</td></tr>
<tr><td colspan="5">THENAR GROUP OF MUSCLES</td></tr>
<tr><td>Abductor pollicis brevis</td><td rowspan="3">Transverse carpal ligament and tubercle of the scaphoid and trapezium</td><td>Lateral side, base of proximal phalanx of the thumb</td><td>Abducts the thumb</td><td rowspan="3">Recurrent branch of the median n.</td></tr>
<tr><td>Flexor pollicis brevis</td><td>Volar side, base of proximal phalanx of the thumb</td><td>Flexes the thumb</td></tr>
<tr><td>Opponens pollicis</td><td>Lateral side of the shaft of the 1st metacarpal bone</td><td>Rotates the 1st metacarpal toward the palm</td></tr>
<tr><td colspan="5">HYPOTHENAR GROUP OF MUSCLES</td></tr>
<tr><td>Abductor digiti minimi</td><td rowspan="3">Pisiform, hamate, and transverse carpal ligament</td><td>Medial side, base of the proximal phalanx of digit 5</td><td>Abducts digit 5</td><td rowspan="3">Deep branch of the ulnar n.</td></tr>
<tr><td>Flexor digiti minimi brevis</td><td>Volar side, base of the proximal phalanx of digit 5</td><td>Flexes digit 5</td></tr>
<tr><td>Opponens digiti minimi</td><td>Medial border of the 5th metacarpal bone</td><td>Rotates 5th metacarpal toward the palm</td></tr>
<tr><td colspan="5">DEEP PALM</td></tr>
<tr><td>Lumbricals</td><td>Flexor digitorum profundus tendons</td><td>Radial side of the extensor expansions of digits 2–5</td><td>Flexes MCP and extends PIP and DIP of digits 2–5</td><td>1 and 2—median n.; 3 and 4—deep branch of ulnar n.</td></tr>
<tr><td>Adductor pollicis</td><td>Transverse head—anterior surface of the shaft of 3rd metacarpal
Oblique head—2nd and 3rd metacarpals and adjacent carpal bones</td><td>Medial side of base of the proximal phalanx of the thumb</td><td>Draws the thumb toward the plane of the palm (adduction)</td><td rowspan="3">Deep branch of the ulnar n.</td></tr>
<tr><td>Palmar interossei</td><td>Palmar surface of metacarpals of digits 2, 4, and 5</td><td>Base of the proximal phalanges and the extensor expansion of digits 2, 4, and 5</td><td>Adducts digits 2, 4, and 5 and assists lumbricals in MCP flexion and extension of PIP and DIP of digits 2–5</td></tr>
<tr><td>Dorsal interossei</td><td>Metacarpal bones 1–5</td><td>Base of the proximal phalanges and the extensor expansion of digits 2–4</td><td>Abducts digits 2–4 and assists lumbricals in MCP flexion and extension of PIP and DIP of digits 2–5</td></tr>
</table>

Abbreviations: DIP, distal interphalangeal; MCP, metacarpophalangeal; n., nerve; PIP, proximal interphalangeal.

POSTERIOR FOREARM AND DORSUM OF HAND

Dissection Overview

The posterior compartment of the forearm contains the extensor and supinator muscles of the hand and digits and can be divided into superficial and deep layers. The muscles of the superficial layer extend the wrist and the digits. The muscles of the deep layer cause supination of the forearm, extension of the index finger, and abduction and extension of the thumb with a group of "outcropping" muscles. Innervation to the muscles of the posterior forearm is by branches of the radial nerve. The nerves and vessels of the posterior compartment run in the connective tissue plane dividing the superficial and deep layers.

In the dorsum of the hand, the skin is thinner and looser than the palm, intrinsic muscles are absent, and the bones are relatively superficial making them easily palpable. As there are no intrinsic muscles in the dorsum of the hand, no motor innervation is required, and the radial, ulnar, and median nerves share the cutaneous innervation.

The order of dissection will be as follows: The subcutaneous tissue will be removed from the elbow to the wrist. The muscles of the superficial layer will be identified and followed to their distal attachments in the hand. On the side where the deep dissection of the flexor muscles was performed, the tendons of the superficial muscles of the posterior forearm will be released from the extensor retinaculum and retracted to expose the muscles of the deep layer. The contents and boundaries of the anatomical snuffbox will be studied.

Dissection Instructions

Dorsum of Hand

ATLAS 2.89, 2.90; VIDEO 2.9.1

1. Refer to FIGURE 2.39.
2. With the cadaver in the supine position, flex the elbow and rotate the upper limb to achieve increased visibility of the posterior compartment of the forearm and dorsum of the hand, and use string to hold it in this position or have a dissection partner assist in orienting the upper limb throughout the dissection.
3. Remove any remaining skin from the posterior aspect of the forearm and hand as well as the posterior surface of at least one digit.
4. Use blunt dissection to remove the remnants of the subcutaneous tissue from the posterior forearm and dorsum of the hand, taking care to preserve the **dorsal venous arch** and its contributions to the **basilic** and **cephalic veins**.
5. Identify and clean the **superficial branch of the radial nerve** on the dorsum of the hand.
6. Identify and clean the **dorsal cutaneous branch of the ulnar nerve** on the dorsum of the hand.
7. Follow the dorsal venous network toward the digits and verify that the **dorsal digital veins** drain into this network on the dorsum of the hand.
8. Identify the **extensor retinaculum**, a transversely oriented specialization of the antebrachial fascia, on the posterior surface of the distal forearm.
9. Use scissors to incise the posterior surface of the **antebrachial fascia** from the olecranon to the wrist while preserving the extensor retinaculum (**Cut 1**).
10. Use blunt dissection to separate the antebrachial fascia from the underlying muscles, detach it from its attachments to the radius and ulna, and place it in the tissue container. *Note that in the proximal posterior forearm, the fascia may be difficult to separate from the muscles and it may be necessary to use sharp dissection.*

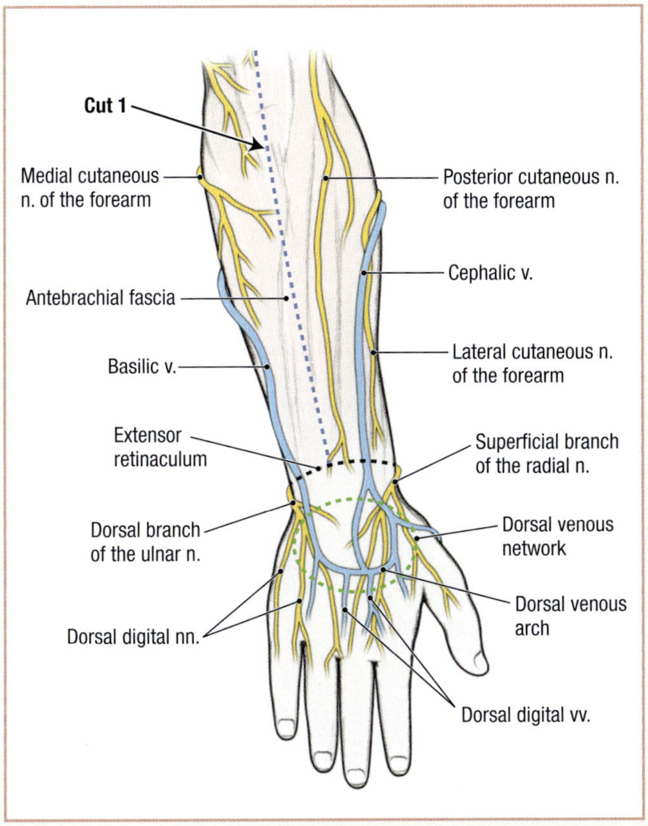

FIGURE 2.39 ● Superficial veins and cutaneous nerves of posterior forearm and dorsum of right hand. Posterior view.

Superficial Layer of Posterior Forearm

ATLAS 2.87A, 2.88A, 2.91; VIDEO 2.9.2

1. Refer to FIGURE 2.40.
2. Identify and clean the **anconeus** near the olecranon process of the ulna. Recall that the anconeus is a muscle of the posterior compartment of the arm and innervated by the radial nerve along with the triceps brachii (see **Clinical Correlation 2.8**).

CLINICAL CORRELATION 2.8

Radial Nerve Injury

ATLAS 2.7, 2.88

The radial nerve is vulnerable to injury within the radial groove at the lateral aspect of the elbow where it crosses anterior to the lateral epicondyle or as it pierces the supinator. Distal trauma or compression of the radial nerve affects the extensor compartment of forearm, resulting in a weakened ability to extend the wrist or digits (wrist drop), whereas proximal injury may also affect the triceps brachii resulting in weakness of elbow extension and sensory loss to the region superficial to the snuffbox.

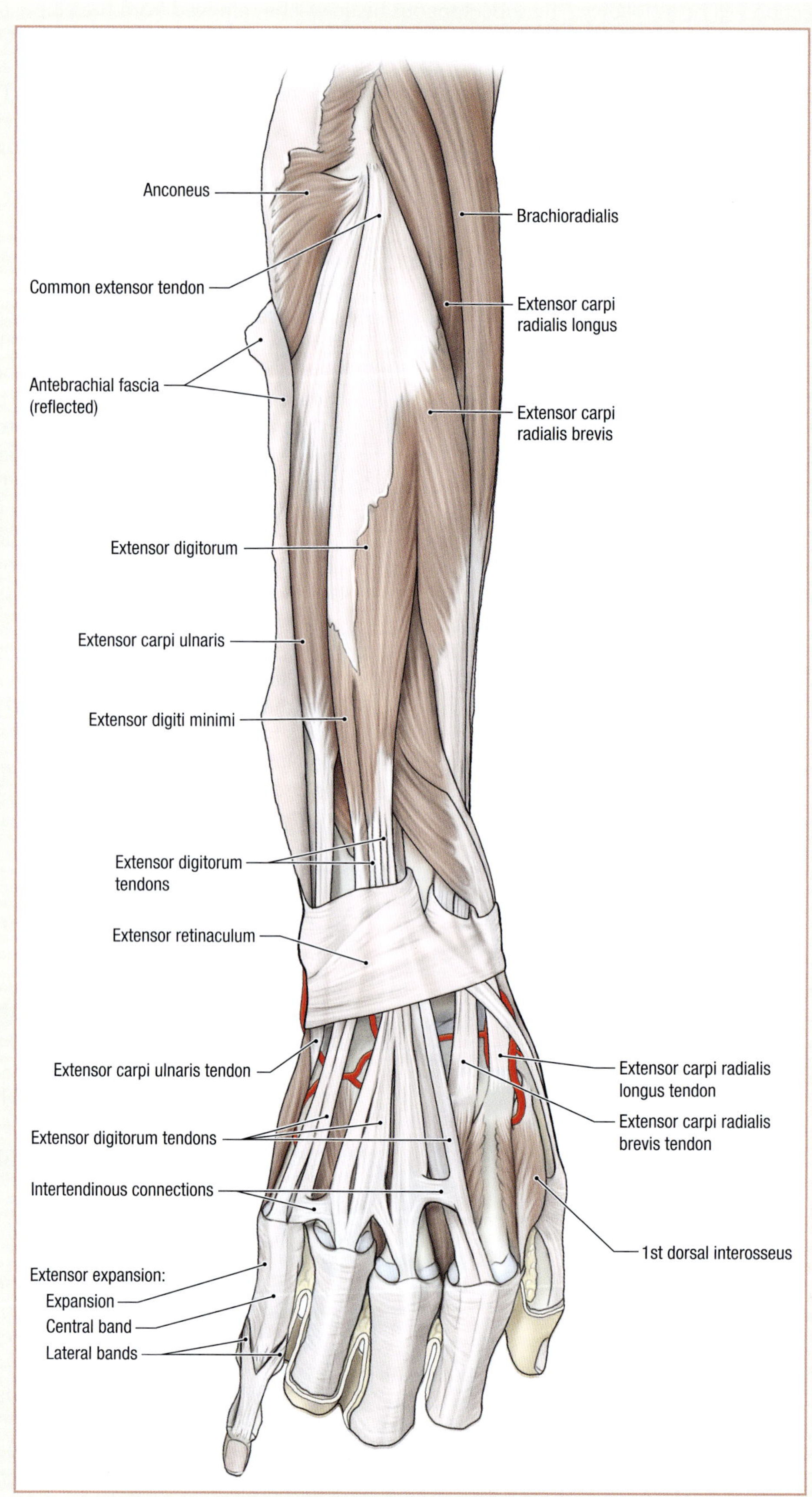

FIGURE 2.40 ■ Superficial layer of posterior compartment of right forearm. Posterior (dorsal) view.

3. Review the attachments and actions of the **anconeus** (see **TABLE 2.7**).
4. Identify and clean the **brachioradialis** on the lateral aspect of the forearm. Recall that the brachioradialis originates in the posterior compartment of the arm and forms the lateral border of the cubital fossa.
5. Adjacent to the brachioradialis, identify and clean the **extensor carpi radialis longus** and the **extensor carpi radialis brevis**.
6. In the middle of the posterior forearm, identify and clean the **extensor digitorum**.
7. Observe that the extensor digitorum splits distally into four tendons that pass deep to the **extensor retinaculum** to reach digits 2 to 5. *Note that all of the extensor tendons travel across the dorsal wrist deep to the extensor retinaculum within synovial tendon sheaths.*
8. Observe that the tendons of the extensor digitorum are connected to each other by **intertendinous connections** on the posterior surface of the hand near the metacarpophalangeal (MCP) joints.
9. Identify and clean the **extensor digiti minimi** on the ulnar side of the extensor digitorum muscle belly. *Note that the extensor digiti minimi often sends two tendons distally to digit 5.*
10. On the ulnar side of the forearm, identify and clean the **extensor carpi ulnaris**.
11. Observe that four of the muscles in the superficial layer of the posterior forearm (extensor carpi radialis brevis, extensor digitorum, extensor digiti minimi, and extensor carpi ulnaris) originate on the lateral epicondyle of the humerus by way of a **common extensor tendon**.
12. Review the attachments, actions, and innervations of the muscles in the superficial layer of the posterior forearm (see **TABLE 2.7**).
13. Refer to FIGURE 2.41.
14. Identify the **extensor expansion** on the dorsum of the digits on which the skin was removed. Observe that the "hoodlike" expansion retains the extensor tendon in the midline of the digit.
15. On the peripheral sides of a skinned digit, observe that the extensor expansion wraps around the dorsum and sides of the proximal phalanx and distal end of the metacarpal bone.
16. Turn the palm and follow the tendon of a lumbrical to the extensor expansion and verify that it attaches from the flexor digitorum profundus tendon to the extensor expansion proximally.
17. Follow the tendon of an interosseus muscle distally and verify that it attaches to the extensor expansion.
18. Observe that the extensor expansion continues across both the PIP and DIP joints to insert on the base of the distal phalanx.
19. Gently pull on the extensor digitorum tendon and verify that pulling on the extensor expansion results in extension of both the PIP and DIP joints; thus, contraction of the extensor digitorum, the lumbricals, or the interossei will all result in extension of the digit at the PIP and DIP joints.
20. On the palmar surface of the digit, retract the tendons of the flexor digitorum superficialis and profundus from the phalanges and observe that the tendons are anchored to the bone by short and long extensions from the synovial sheaths of the digit, the **vincula brevia** and **vincula longa**, respectively. *Note that the vincula longa and brevia are the primary route of blood vessels to supply the distal portion of the flexor tendons.*

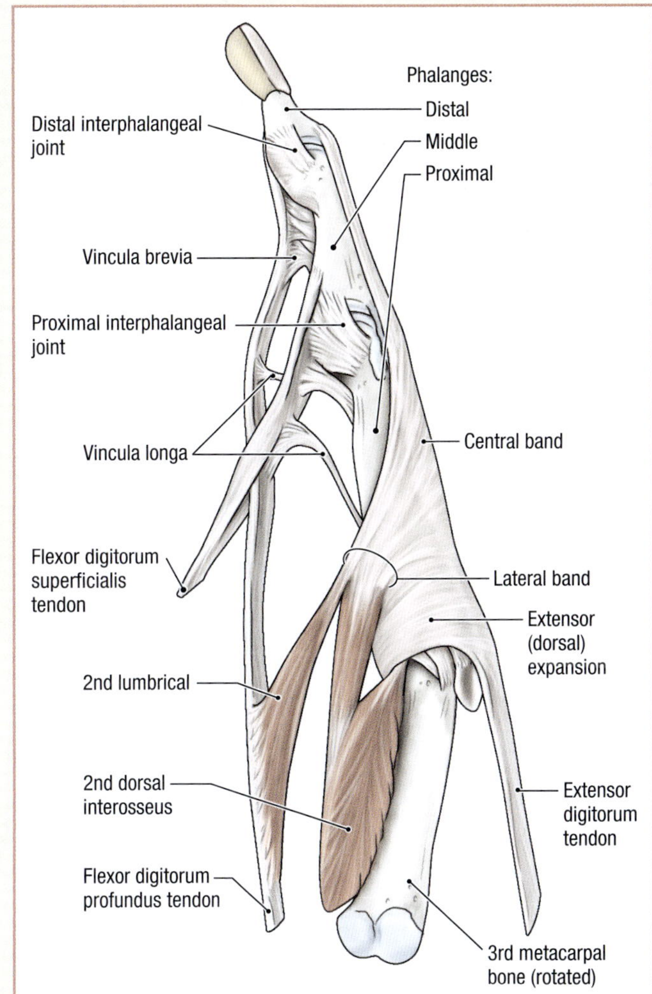

FIGURE 2.41 ● Extensor expansion of right third digit. Lateral view.

Deep Layer of Posterior Forearm

ATLAS 2.87B, 2.88B, 2.92; VIDEO 2.9.3

Dissection Note: Perform the following dissection sequence only on one upper limb.

1. Refer to FIGURE 2.42.
2. On the upper limb with the deep anterior forearm dissection, use sharp dissection to cut through the

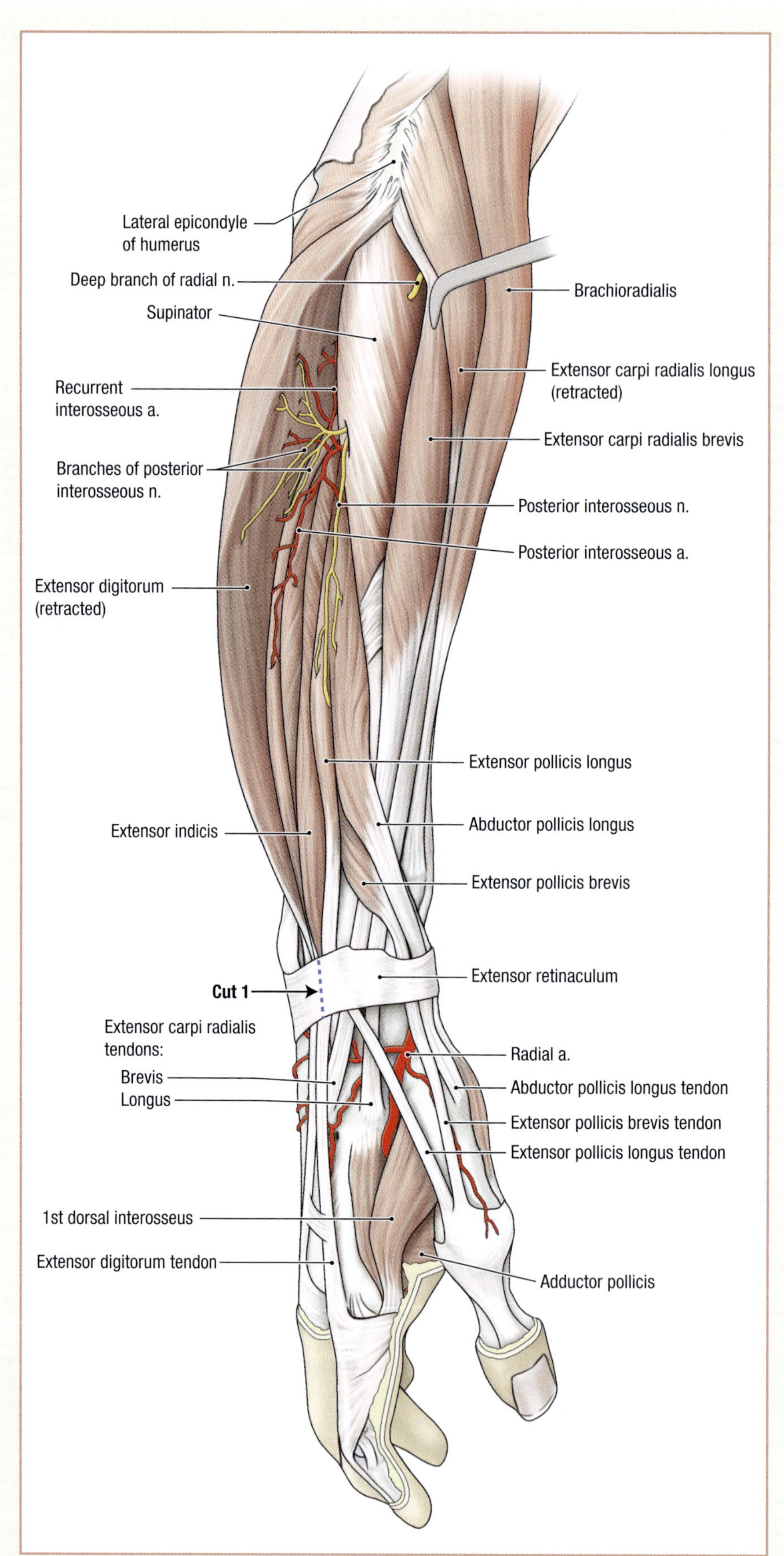

FIGURE 2.42 ● Deep layer of posterior compartment of right forearm. Lateral view.

extensor retinaculum to release the tendons of the extensor digitorum (**Cut 1**).

3. Use blunt dissection to separate the muscles of the superficial layer of the posterior forearm from the muscles comprising the **deep layer of the posterior forearm**.
4. Near the elbow, retract the brachioradialis and identify the **supinator** wrapped around the proximal end of the radius.
5. On the lateral aspect of the elbow, find the radial nerve in the connective tissue plane between the brachioradialis and brachialis deep to the brachioradialis.
6. Observe that the radial nerve divides into a **superficial branch** coursing deep to the brachioradialis, and a **deep branch** which enters the supinator.
7. Look for the deep branch of the radial nerve where it emerges from the distal border of the supinator as the **posterior interosseous nerve**.
8. Observe that the posterior interosseous nerve is accompanied by the **posterior interosseous artery**, a branch of the common interosseous artery.
9. Identify and clean the "outcropping" muscles of the of the thumb: **abductor pollicis longus**, **extensor pollicis brevis**, and **extensor pollicis longus**. Observe that the tendons of these three muscles emerge from the interval between the extensor digitorum and the extensor carpi radialis brevis.
10. Use blunt dissection to identify and clean the **extensor indicis** deep to the extensor digitorum. *Note that its tendon travels with the tendon of the extensor digitorum to reach the 2nd digit, or "index" finger, for which it is named.*
11. Review the attachments, actions, and innervations of the muscles in the deep layer of the posterior forearm (see **TABLE 2.7**).
12. Refer to FIGURE 2.43.
13. Identify the **anatomical snuffbox**, a depression on the posterolateral surface of the wrist bound laterally by the abductor pollicis longus and the extensor pollicis brevis tendons and posteriorly by the extensor pollicis longus tendon.
14. Within the anatomical snuffbox, identify the **radial artery**.
15. Use blunt dissection to clean the radial artery and follow it distally until it disappears between the two heads of the **first dorsal interosseus**. *Note that the radial artery supplies arterial blood to the dorsum of the hand via a branch to the dorsal carpal arch arising in the anatomical snuffbox.*
16. Deep to the radial artery, clean the distal attachments of the extensor carpi radialis longus and brevis onto the bases of the 2nd and 3rd metacarpals, respectively.

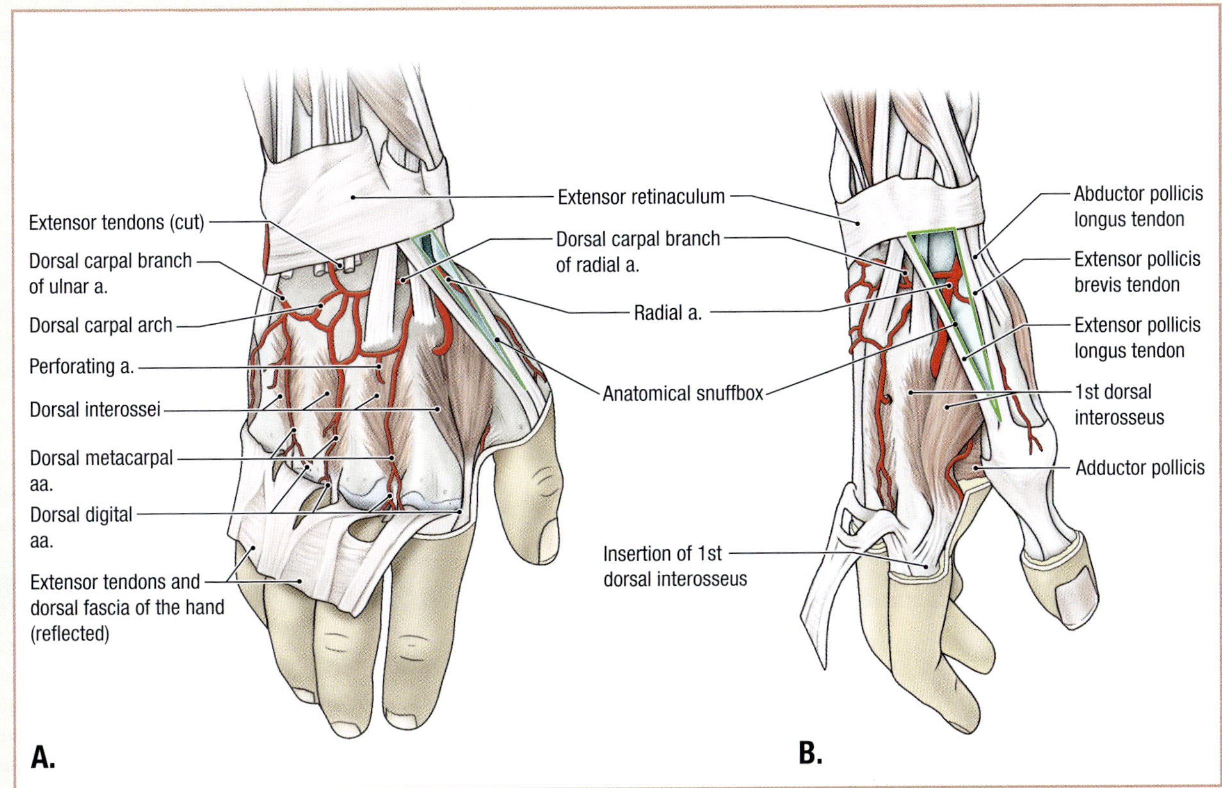

FIGURE 2.43 A. Dorsum of right hand. Posterior (dorsal) view. B. Anatomical snuffbox. Lateral view.

Dissection Follow-up

1. Review the actions and attachments of each muscle in the posterior compartment of the forearm in **TABLE 2.7**.
2. Review the muscles that insert into the extensor expansion and the actions of each.
3. Review the course of the common interosseous branch of the ulnar artery and its branches.
4. Review the boundaries and contents of the anatomical snuffbox, noting the path of the radial artery from the cubital fossa to the deep palmar arterial arch via this space.
5. Review the path and pattern of motor and cutaneous innervation of the radial nerve.
6. Replace the muscles of the posterior compartment of the forearm into their correct anatomical positions.

TABLE 2.7 Muscles of Posterior Compartment of Forearm

<table>
<tr><th>Muscle</th><th>Proximal Attachments</th><th>Distal Attachments</th><th>Actions</th><th>Innervation</th></tr>
<tr><td colspan="5">SUPERFICIAL LAYER</td></tr>
<tr><td>Anconeus (posterior arm)</td><td>Lateral epicondyle of humerus</td><td>Lateral surface of olecranon and posterior surface of proximal ulna</td><td>Assists triceps in extension of the elbow</td><td rowspan="3">Radial n.</td></tr>
<tr><td>Brachioradialis</td><td>Proximal two-thirds of lateral supracondylar ridge</td><td>Lateral surface of distal radius (radial styloid process)</td><td>Flexes the forearm in neutral (midpronated) position</td></tr>
<tr><td>Extensor carpi radialis longus</td><td>Distal lateral supracondylar ridge</td><td>Base of 2nd metacarpal</td><td rowspan="2">Extends and abducts the hand</td></tr>
<tr><td>Extensor carpi radialis brevis</td><td rowspan="4">Lateral epicondyle of humerus via common extensor tendon</td><td>Base of 3rd metacarpal</td><td>Deep branch of radial n.</td></tr>
<tr><td>Extensor digitorum</td><td>Extensor expansions of digits 2–5</td><td>Extends digits 2–5</td><td rowspan="3">Posterior interosseous n.</td></tr>
<tr><td>Extensor digiti minimi</td><td>Extensor expansion of digit 5</td><td>Extends fifth digit</td></tr>
<tr><td>Extensor carpi ulnaris</td><td>Base of 5th metacarpal</td><td>Extends and adducts the hand</td></tr>
<tr><td colspan="5">DEEP LAYER</td></tr>
<tr><td>Supinator</td><td>Lateral epicondyle of humerus, radial collateral and annular ligaments, crest of ulna</td><td>Lateral, posterior, and anterior surfaces of proximal ulna</td><td>Supinates forearm</td><td>Deep branch of the radial n.</td></tr>
<tr><td colspan="5">"OUTCROPPING" MUSCLES OF DEEP LAYER</td></tr>
<tr><td>Abductor pollicis longus</td><td rowspan="4">Posterior surfaces of the radius, ulna, and interosseous membrane</td><td>Base of 1st metacarpal</td><td>Abducts and extends CMC of the thumb</td><td rowspan="4">Posterior interosseous n.</td></tr>
<tr><td>Extensor pollicis brevis</td><td>Base of the proximal phalanx of digit 1</td><td>Extends MCP of the thumb</td></tr>
<tr><td>Extensor pollicis longus</td><td>Base of the distal phalanx of digit 1</td><td>Extends MCP and IP of the thumb</td></tr>
<tr><td>Extensor indicis</td><td>Extensor expansion of digit 2</td><td>Extends digit 2</td></tr>
</table>

Abbreviations: CMC, carpometacarpal; IP, interphalangeal; MCP, metacarpophalangeal; n., nerve.

JOINTS OF UPPER LIMB

Dissection Overview

In order to dissect the joints in the upper limb, it will be necessary to reflect or remove the majority of the surrounding muscles. Because the joint dissections will make it difficult to review key muscular relationships later, it is recommended to limit the joint dissections to one upper limb and to keep the soft tissue structures of the other limb intact for review purposes. While removing the muscles of the selected upper limb, take advantage of this opportunity to review the attachments, actions, and innervation of each muscle as it is removed.

The order of dissection will be as follows: The SC and AC joints will be dissected. The glenohumeral joint will be dissected. The elbow joint and radioulnar joints will be studied. The wrist joint will be dissected. Finally, the joints of the digits will be studied.

Dissection Instructions

Dissection Note: Perform the following joint dissections only on one upper limb, preferably the side where the deeper dissections of the forearm occurred previously.

Sternoclavicular Joint

ATLAS 2.48; VIDEO 2.10.1

1. Refer to FIGURE 2.44.
2. On an articulated skeleton, identify the **jugular notch of the manubrium** between the **medial (sternal) ends of the clavicles.**
3. With the cadaver in the supine position, identify the **SC joint**. Observe that the clavicles articulate with the manubrium at each **clavicular notch** and the adjacent part of the **1st costal cartilage**.
4. Observe that the tendon of the **sternocleidomastoid** attaches to the anterior surface of the SC joint.
5. Identify and clean the **anterior sternoclavicular ligament**, which spans from the sternum to the clavicle.
6. Identify and clean the **costoclavicular ligament**, which runs obliquely from the 1st costal cartilage to the inferior surface of the clavicle near its medial end.
7. Use a scalpel to remove the anterior sternoclavicular ligament to expose the joint cavity.
8. Identify the **articular disc** within the SC joint cavity. Observe that inferomedially, the articular disc is attached to the 1st costal cartilage, whereas superolaterally, it is attached to the clavicle to resist medial displacement of the clavicle.
9. Palpate the movements of the SC joint either on yourself or on the cadaver. Circumduct the upper limb and observe that the SC joint allows a limited amount of movement in every direction.

Acromioclavicular Joint

ATLAS 2.48, 2.49; VIDEO 2.10.2

1. Refer to FIGURE 2.45.
2. On an articulated skeleton, identify the **AC joint** and observe that the AC joint is located where the **lateral (acromial) end of the clavicle** articulates with the **acromion of the scapula.**
3. Inferomedial to the acromion, identify the **coracoid process of the scapula** and observe its proximity to the **suprascapular notch.**
4. Use sharp dissection to cut the anterior attachment of the deltoid to the clavicle and acromion and reflect the muscle laterally.
5. Detach the trapezius from the lateral end of the clavicle and supraclavicular fascia superiorly if it was previously not done.
6. Detach the pectoralis minor from its attachment to the coracoid process and reflect it inferiorly. If the pectoralis minor was previously detached from its inferior attachment to the ribs, remove the muscle and place it in the tissue container.

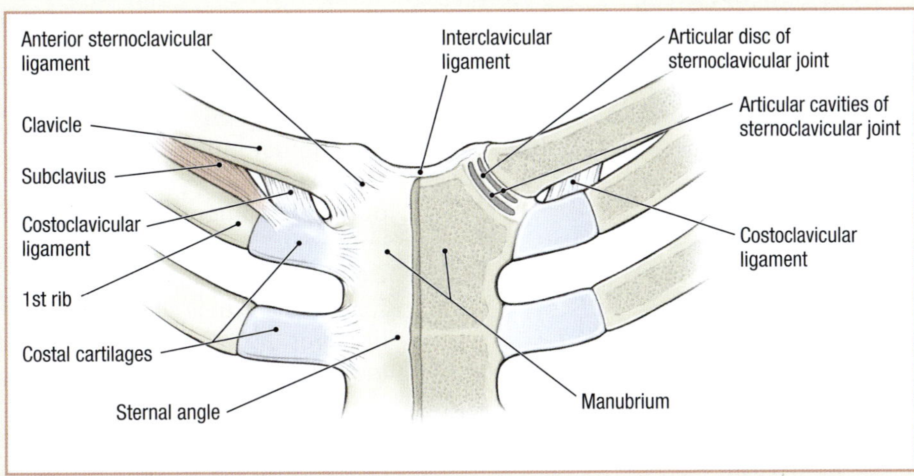

FIGURE 2.44 ■ Surface (*right*) and sectional (*left*) views of sternoclavicular joints. Anterior view.

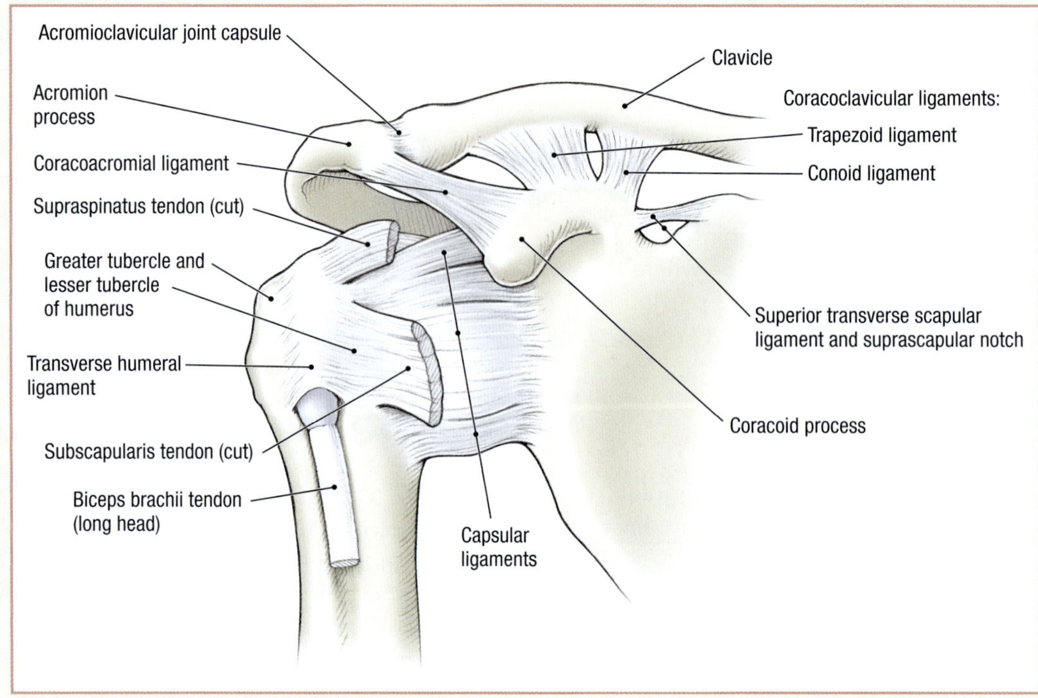

FIGURE 2.45 ● Right acromioclavicular and glenohumeral joints. Anterior view.

7. Identify the AC joint, a plane synovial joint between the acromion and the lateral end of the clavicle.
8. Identify and clean the **coracoclavicular ligament** located between the clavicle and coracoid process. Observe that the coracoclavicular ligament has two parts: the **trapezoid ligament** more anterolaterally and the **conoid ligament** more posteromedially.
9. Open the AC joint by completely removing the joint capsule.
10. Separate the acromion from the lateral end of the clavicle and observe the shape of the articulating surfaces, which causes the acromion to slide inferior to the distal end of the clavicle when the acromion is forced medially. *Note that the conoid and trapezoid ligaments prevent the acromion from moving inferiorly relative to the clavicle.*

Glenohumeral Joint

ATLAS 2.50, 2.51, 2.52; VIDEO 2.10.3

1. Refer to FIGURE 2.45.
2. On an articulated skeleton, identify the **glenohumeral (shoulder) joint** and observe that it is the articulation between the **glenoid fossa of the scapula** and the **head of the humerus**.
3. Identify the **anatomical neck of the humerus** and note its oblique orientation distal to the smooth articulating surface of the head of the humerus.
4. On the cadaver, reflect the pectoralis major laterally and make an incision through its tendon near the attachment to the intertubercular sulcus. Cut any adhering neurovascular structures and place the muscle and associated tissue in the tissue container.
5. Cut through the proximal attachment of the coracobrachialis to the coracoid process, detach any adhering neurovascular structures, and reflect the muscle inferiorly.
6. Detach the short head of the biceps brachii from the coracoid process.
7. Cut the tendon of the long head of the biceps approximately 3 cm inferior to the transverse humeral ligament and reflect the biceps brachii inferiorly.
8. Elevate and cut the tendons of the supraspinatus and subscapularis near their lateral attachments to the humerus.
9. Identify the **capsule of the glenohumeral joint** and remove the muscles and tendons overlying the capsule on its superior and anterior surfaces (see **Clinical Correlation 2.9**).

CLINICAL CORRELATION 2.9

Shoulder Injuries

ATLAS 2.50, 2.51

The glenohumeral (shoulder) joint has a greater degree of movement than any other joint in the body and is thus prone to injury because the mobility comes at the cost of stability. Shoulder dislocations, a complete separation of the head of the humerus from the glenoid fossa, commonly occur inferiorly between the gap in rotator cuff muscles to lie either anterior or posterior to the infraglenoid tubercle and long head of the triceps. Subluxations, temporary displacements of the humeral head, are also common at the shoulder. A blow to the superior aspect of the shoulder may lead to a separated shoulder, displacement of the acromial end of the clavicle with the acromion process at the AC joint.

10. Verify that the joint capsule is attached to the anatomical neck of the humerus. Recall that posteriorly, the tendons of the infraspinatus and teres minor blend with and reinforce the joint capsule.
11. Observe that the **glenohumeral ligament** strengthens the anterior wall of the fibrous capsule. The glenohumeral ligament can be divided into three portions: superior, middle, and inferior. *Note that the three portions of the glenohumeral ligament may not be easily identifiable.*
12. Refer to FIGURE 2.46.
13. Use a scalpel to carefully open the anterior surface of the joint capsule by making an oblique cut medial to the anatomical neck of the humerus.
14. Within the capsule, identify the **tendon of the long head of the biceps brachii** and observe that the tendon passes through the glenoid cavity to attach to the supraglenoid tubercle.
15. Palpate the relative thickness of the capsule and make horizontal incisions or remove portions of the capsule to increase visibility within the space while sparing the biceps tendon.
16. Abduct and rotate the upper limb to increase visibility of the humeral head and use a saw or a chisel to remove the head of the humerus at the anatomical neck. Make an effort to preserve the attachment of the capsule while removing the humeral head.
17. Use a probe to explore the **glenoid cavity** and identify the **glenoid labrum**.

Elbow and Proximal Radioulnar Joints

ATLAS 2.59, 2.60, 2.61, 2.62; VIDEO 2.10.4

1. Refer to FIGURE 2.47.
2. On an articulated skeleton, verify that the elbow joint consists of three bones and three distinct joints that allow flexion and extension as well as pronation and supination.
3. Identify the **hinge joint** between the trochlea of the humerus and the trochlear notch of the ulna.

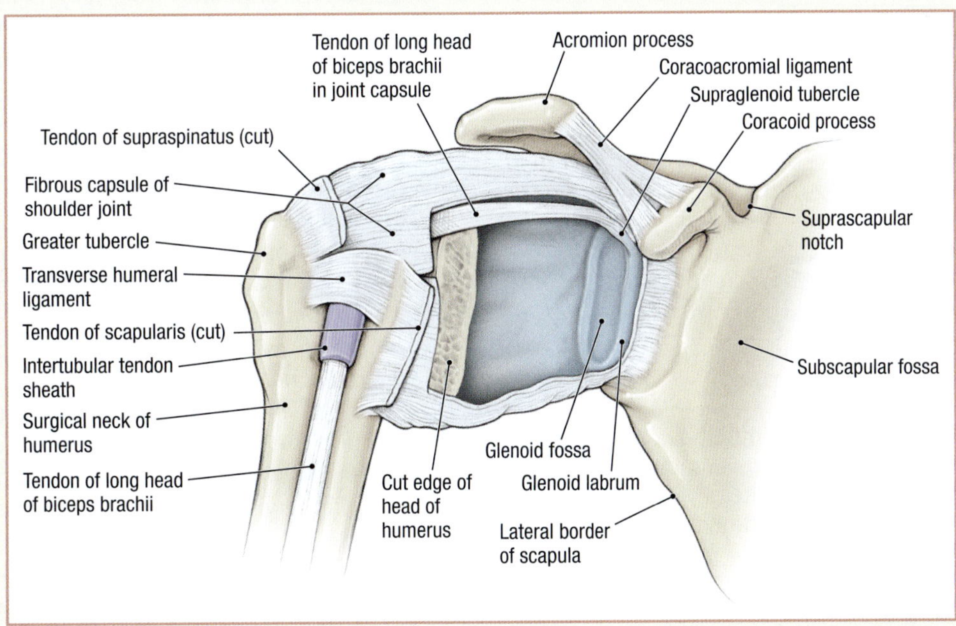

FIGURE 2.46 ● Opened glenohumeral joint with head of humerus removed. Anterior view.

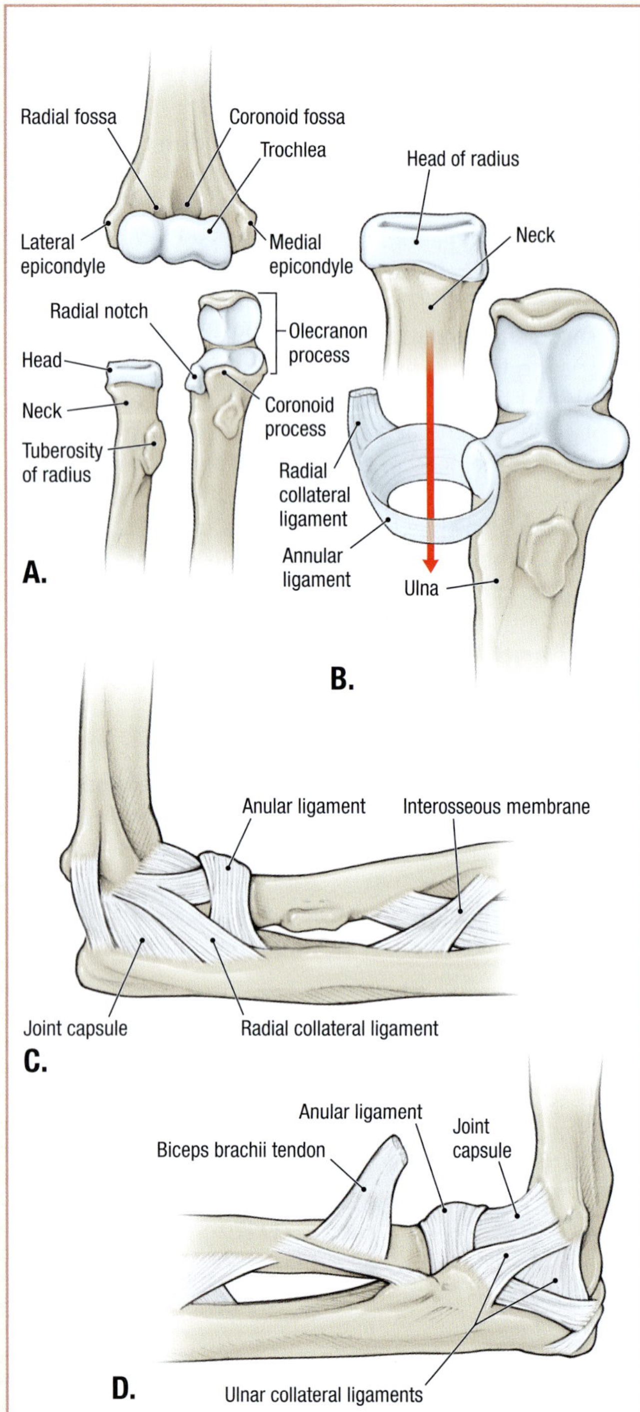

FIGURE 2.47 ■ **A.** Disarticulated right elbow. Anterior view. **B.** Disarticulated proximal radioulnar joint. Anterior view. **C.** Ligaments of right elbow. Lateral view. **D.** Ligaments of right elbow and biceps tendon. Medial view.

4. Identify the **gliding joint** between the capitulum of the humerus and the head of the radius.
5. Identify the **pivot joint** between the head of the radius and the radial notch of the ulna.
6. With the cadaver in the supine position, cut the biceps brachii tendon where it crosses the cubital fossa and remove the muscle from the dissection field.
7. Remove the brachialis from the anterior surface of the joint capsule.
8. Rotate the upper limb either laterally or medially and detach the triceps brachii tendon from the olecranon and the posterior surface of the joint capsule and reflect the muscle superiorly.
9. If all the joint dissections are being performed on one upper limb, increase the mobility and decrease the weight of the upper limb by removing the bulk of the triceps brachii.
10. Cut and detach the muscles of the anterior forearm by cutting through the common flexor tendon at the medial epicondyle and reflect the muscles inferiorly.
11. Identify the **ulnar collateral ligament** on the medial side of the elbow joint and observe that it consists of a strong anterior cord and a fanlike posterior portion.
12. Cut the brachioradialis proximally near its attachment to the lateral supracondylar ridge and reflect the muscle inferiorly.
13. Cut and reflect the superficial muscles of the posterior forearm by cutting through their attachment to the lateral epicondyle of the humerus.
14. Take a moment to observe the attachments of the supinator. Observe its role in supination while actively pronating and supinating the forearm. Recall that the biceps brachii also supinates the forearm by pulling on the radial tuberosity while the forearm is pronated.
15. Detach the supinator from its proximal and distal attachments and place it in the tissue container.
16. Identify and clean the **radial collateral ligament** and observe that it fans out from the lateral epicondyle of the humerus to the **annular ligament**.
17. On an articulated skeleton, verify that the **proximal radioulnar joint** is a pivot joint between the head of the radius and the radial notch of the ulna.
18. Actively pronate and supinate the forearm and observe that the head of the radius can freely rotate in the annular ligament. *Note that the annular ligament completely encircles the head of the radius along with the radial notch of the ulna.*
19. Open the elbow joint by making a transverse cut through the anterior surface of the joint capsule between the ulnar and the radial collateral ligaments. To increase visibility, remove a portion of the joint capsule anteriorly.
20. Use a probe to explore the extent of the **synovial cavity** and observe the smooth articular surfaces of the humerus, ulna, and radius.
21. Use the dissected specimen to perform the movements of the elbow joint: flexion, extension, pronation, and supination. Observe the joint surfaces and the collateral ligaments during these movements.

Intermediate and Distal Radioulnar Joints

ATLAS 2.63, 2.64, 2.95, 2.96; VIDEO 2.10.5

1. Refer to FIGURE 2.48.
2. In the forearm, identify the **interosseous membrane** between the radius and ulna creating a strong fibrous (syndesmosis) joint and observe its attachments along the interosseous margins of the radius and ulna.
3. To better visualize the interosseous membrane, carefully use sharp dissection to remove any remaining portions of muscular tissue adhered on its anterior surface.
4. Observe that the interosseous membrane does not connect to the elbow and has a gap proximally allowing for passage of the nerves and vessels from the anterior compartment of the forearm to the posterior compartment.
5. Confirm the path of the anterior interosseous artery along the anterior aspect of the interosseous membrane until it passes deep to the pronator quadratus.
6. On an articulated skeleton, observe that the distal radioulnar joint is a pivot joint between the head of the ulna and the ulnar notch of the radius.
7. Verify that the **wrist (radiocarpal) joint** is the articulation between the distal end of the **radius** and the proximal row of **carpal bones**. The wrist is a condyloid joint and allows for movement in two planes: flexion/extension in the sagittal plane and abduction/adduction in the coronal plane.

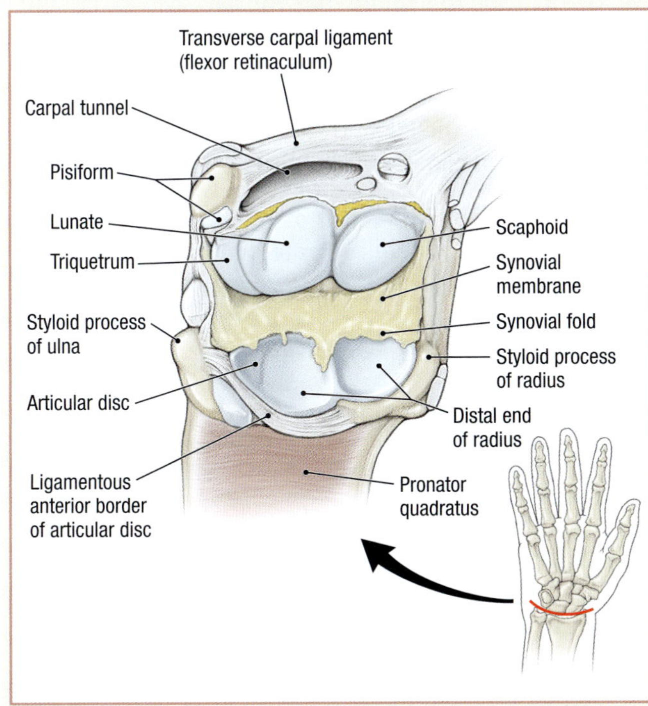

FIGURE 2.48 ● Disarticulated right radiocarpal joint. Anterior view.

8. Identify the **midcarpal joint**, the articulation between the two rows of carpal bones. Observe that the proximal row of carpal bones articulates with the radius proximally at the wrist and that the distal row of carpal bones articulates distally at the carpometacarpal joint.
9. In the anterior compartment of the forearm, remove all the tendons and soft tissue structures crossing the wrist. Review the distal attachments, actions, and innervations of each muscle during removal.
10. Observe that the anterior and posterior surfaces of the wrist joint are reinforced by the **radiocarpal ligaments**. *Note that each ligament is named according to its specific sites of attachment.*
11. Extend the wrist and cut transversely through the radiocarpal ligaments on the anterior surface of the joint capsule proximal to the transverse carpal ligament and carpal tunnel. Do not cut completely through the joint capsule; rather, leave the hand attached to the forearm posteriorly.
12. Use a probe to explore the distal radioulnar joint and identify the joint space between the radius and ulna.
13. Identify the **articular surface of the radius** on its distal end and verify that it articulates with the **scaphoid** and **lunate** carpal bones.
14. Identify the smooth proximal surfaces of the **scaphoid, lunate,** and **triquetrum**. *Note that the scaphoid and lunate bones are positioned to transmit forces from the hand to the forearm and therefore are the ones most frequently fractured in a fall on the outstretched hand.*
15. Identify the **articular disc of the wrist**. Verify that the articular disc holds the distal ends of the radius and the ulna together and articulates with the triquetrum when the hand is adducted.
16. Use the dissected specimen to perform the movements of the wrist joint: flexion, extension, adduction, abduction, and circumduction. Observe the articular surfaces during these movements.

Metacarpophalangeal and Interphalangeal Joints

ATLAS 2.91, 2.98; VIDEO 2.10.6

1. Refer to FIGURE 2.49.
2. On an articulated skeleton, identify the **MCP joints**. Confirm that the MCP joints are condyloid joints like the wrist and support flexion/extension and abduction/adduction.
3. Identify the **PIP** and **DIP joints** of digits 2 to 5, and the **interphalangeal (IP) joint** of the thumb. Confirm that the IP joints are hinge joints and allow only flexion and extension.
4. Select a digit to use as a representative example for the other digits.

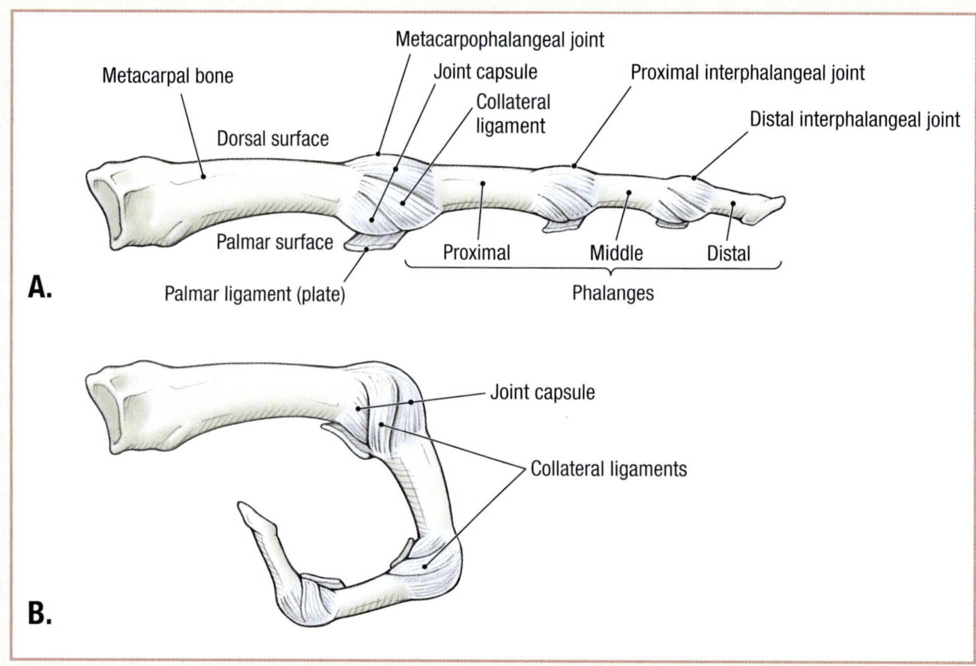

FIGURE 2.49 ● Metacarpophalangeal and interphalangeal joints of right 3rd digit in extension (**A**) and flexion (**B**). Medial view.

5. Cut the attachments of the flexor digitorum superficialis from the middle phalanx and the flexor digitorum profundus from the distal phalanx.
6. Remove the associated lumbrical, palmar and dorsal interossei, and the extensor expansion to expose the MCP joint capsule of the selected digit.
7. Identify and clean the **collateral ligaments of the MCP joint.**
8. Move the digit to confirm that the collateral ligaments are slack in extension and taut in flexion. Therefore, the digits cannot be spread (abducted) unless they are extended.
9. Use the dissected specimen to perform the movements of the digit at the MCP joint: flexion, extension, abduction, and adduction.
10. Identify and clean the **collateral ligaments of the PIP and DIP joints** of the selected digit.
11. Use a scalpel to make an incision along the anterior surface of one PIP joint.
12. Use a probe to explore the synovial cavity of the **PIP** joint and inspect the articular surfaces covered with smooth cartilage.
13. Use the dissected specimen to perform flexion and extension of the PIP and DIP joints and confirm that the collateral ligaments limit the range of motion.

Dissection Follow-up

1. Review the names of the bones articulating at each joint of the upper limb.
2. Review the movements permitted at each joint of the upper limb.
3. Identify the key ligaments associated with each joint and review their respective points of attachment.
4. Return any reflected muscles of the upper limb back to their anatomical positions.

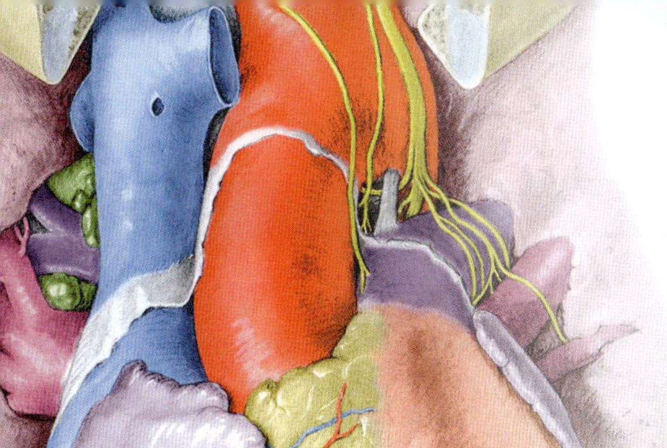

CHAPTER 3
Thorax

REFERENCES

ATLAS = *Grant's Atlas of Anatomy*, 16th ed., figure number

VIDEO = *Grant's Dissection Videos*, video sequence number

The thorax is the superior part of the trunk of the body, and as it is located between the neck, abdomen, upper limb, and back, it shares structures with each of these regions. The thoracic wall functions to house and protect the heart, lungs, and upper abdominal organs; support the weight of the upper limb; and serve as site of muscle attachment from the surrounding regions. The protective function of the thoracic wall is combined with mobility to accommodate volume changes during respiration. These two dissimilar functions, protection and mobility, are accomplished by the alternating arrangement of the ribs and intercostal muscles.

To allow communication with the vital organs to other regions, the thorax has two apertures that allow the passage of structures either superiorly or inferiorly. Structures pass between the thorax, neck and head, and upper limb through the superior thoracic aperture (e.g., trachea, esophagus, vagus nerves, thoracic duct, and major blood vessels). The diaphragm attaches to the structures forming the boundaries of the inferior thoracic aperture and separates the thoracic and abdominal cavities. Several large structures (e.g., aorta, thoracic duct, inferior vena cava, esophagus, and vagus nerves) pass between the thorax and abdomen through openings in the diaphragm.

CLINICAL CORRELATIONS

During your dissection protocol, you may encounter anatomical variations, clinical conditions, disease processes, or medical devices in your cadaveric donor. The following select clinical correlations are described in more detail throughout this chapter.

Thorax

3.1. Pneumothorax and Hemothorax, see the **Pleural Cavities** sequence. ATLAS 3.27
3.2. Pulmonary Embolism, see the **Right Lung** sequence. ATLAS 3.36, 3.37
3.3. Cardiac Tamponade and Pericardiocentesis, see the **Heart in Mediastinum** sequence. ATLAS 3.28
3.4. Myocardial Infarction, see the **Surface Features and Valves of Heart** sequence. ATLAS 3.48
3.5. Heart Dominance, see the **Coronary Arteries** sequence. ATLAS 3.50, 3.51
3.6. Septal Defects, see the **Right Atrium** sequence. ATLAS 3.54
3.7. Recurrent Laryngeal Nerve Injury, see the **Superior Mediastinum** sequence. ATLAS 3.60, 3.63
3.8. Bronchoscopy, see the **Superior Mediastinum** sequence. ATLAS 3.36

PECTORAL REGION

The subcutaneous tissue of the pectoral region contains the usual elements common to all body regions: blood vessels, lymph vessels, cutaneous nerves, superficial fat, fascia, and sweat glands. In addition, the subcutaneous tissue of the anterior thoracic wall contains mammary glands in all individuals, although the modified sweat glands responsible for milk production are typically more developed in lactating females.

If the thorax is your first dissection, or if you have not yet completed dissection of the upper limb, place the cadaver in a supine position and follow the dissection protocols outlined in the **Pectoral Region and Subcutaneous Tissue of Upper Limb** section of **Chapter 2**. Following completion of dissection of the pectoral region, return to this page.

INTERCOSTAL SPACE

Dissection Overview

An intercostal space is the interval between adjacent ribs and is truly a space only in a skeleton as three layers of muscle and neurovascular structures fill these spaces in the body. From superficial to deep, the three layers of muscle are external intercostal, internal intercostal, and innermost intercostal. The 11 intercostal spaces on each side of the thorax are numbered according to the rib that forms its superior boundary.

The order of dissection will be as follows: The skeletal anatomy of the ribs and thoracic cage will be studied. The surface anatomy of the pectoral region will be reviewed. The external and internal intercostals will be studied and reflected in the 5th intercostal space. Branches of intercostal nerves and vessels will be identified. The innermost intercostal will be identified.

Skeletal Anatomy

Refer to a skeleton or isolated ribs and sternum and identify the following skeletal features.

Rib

ATLAS 3.12, 3.14

1. Refer to FIGURE 3.1.
2. On an isolated **6th** or **7th rib**, identify the **head** and **neck of the rib** and observe that the head of the rib has **articular facets (surfaces)**.
3. Lateral to the neck of the rib, identify the **tubercle**, a bony prominence on its inferior surface, and the associated **articular facet (surface)**.
4. Lateral to the tubercle, identify the **costal angle** where the rib changes direction along the **shaft (body)**, as well as the **costal groove** along its inferior surface.
5. Identify the **sternal end** of the rib, the distal extremity of the bone.
6. Refer to FIGURE 3.2.
7. On an articulated skeleton, observe that the **head** of a rib usually articulates with two vertebral bodies and their intervertebral (IV) disc. For example, the head of rib 5 articulates with vertebral bodies T4 and T5. *Note that the 1st, 10th, 11th, and 12th ribs are exceptions to this rule because their heads articulate with only one vertebral body.*
8. Identify the **tubercle** of a rib and observe that it articulates with the **transverse costal facet** on the transverse process of the thoracic vertebra of the same number.
9. Inferior to the articulation of the rib and transverse process, identify an **IV foramen** and observe that the corresponding spinal nerve would exit through this space inferior to the corresponding rib in the thoracic region.
10. Recall that the IV foramen is formed by aspects from two adjacent vertebrae: the **inferior vertebral notch** from the more superiorly located vertebra and the **superior vertebral notch** from the more inferiorly located vertebra.

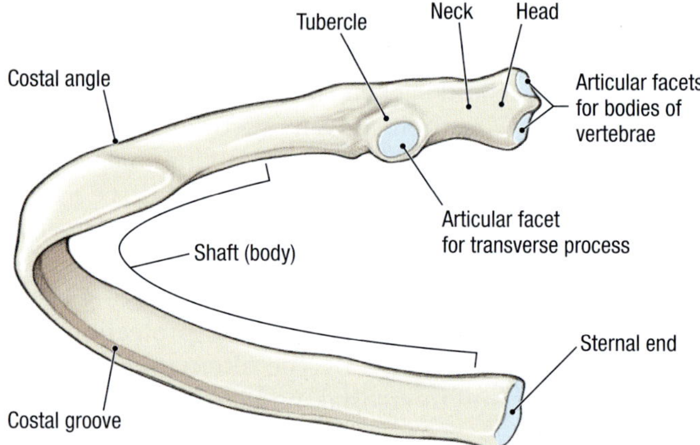

FIGURE 3.1 ■ Typical left rib. Posterior view.

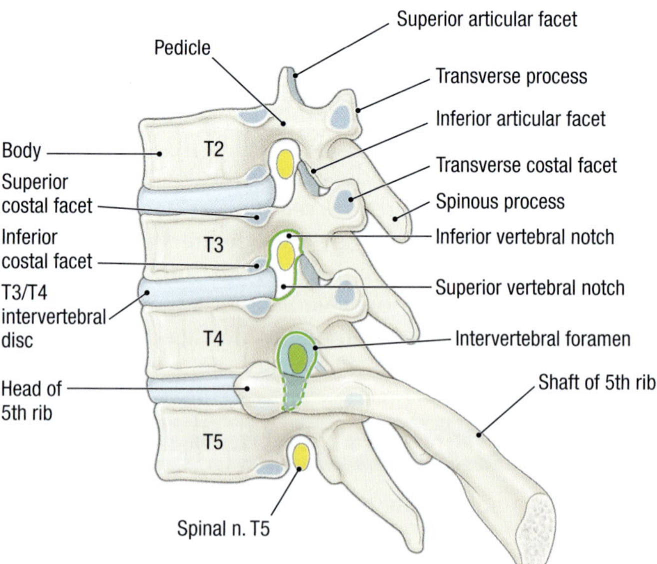

FIGURE 3.2 ■ Portion of thoracic vertebral column (T2–T5). Lateral view.

Sternum and Clavicle

ATLAS 3.10A, 3.11

1. Refer to FIGURE 3.3.
2. On the **sternum** from superior to inferior, identify the **manubrium, body of the sternum**, and **xiphoid process.**
3. Examine the sternum and observe that the **sternal angle** is at the level of the **2nd costal cartilage** anteriorly and the level of the **T4/T5 IV disc** posteriorly.
4. On a clavicle, identify the **medial (sternal) end** and the **lateral (acromial) end.**
5. On an articulated skeleton, identify the **jugular (suprasternal) notch**, the space between the two sternal ends of the clavicles where they articulate with the manubrium of the sternum forming the bilateral **sternoclavicular (SC) joints.**
6. Observe that the lateral end of the clavicle articulates with the **acromion process** of the scapula to create the **acromioclavicular (AC) joint** laterally.

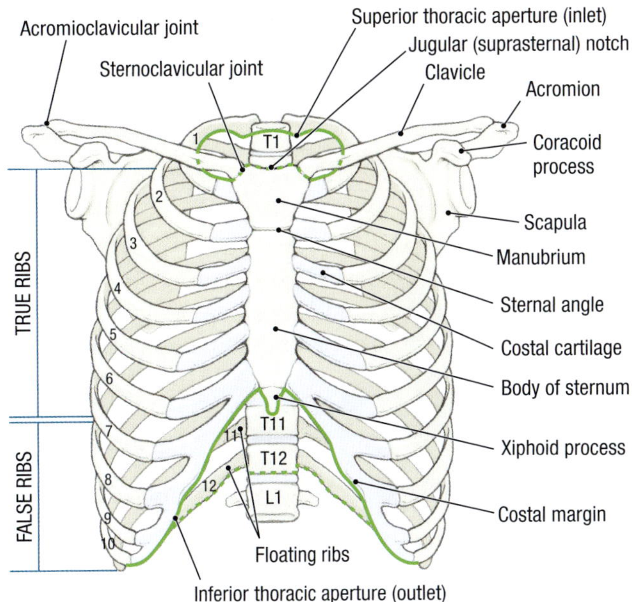

FIGURE 3.3 ● Thoracic cage. Anterior view.

Thoracic Cage

ATLAS 3.10

1. Refer to FIGURE 3.3.
2. Identify the **superior thoracic aperture (thoracic inlet)**, the opening at the superior extent of the thoracic cage.
3. Identify the boundaries of the superior thoracic aperture: anteriorly by the superior portion of the manubrium of the sternum, laterally by the right and left 1st ribs, and posteriorly by the body of vertebra T1.
4. Identify the **inferior thoracic aperture (thoracic outlet)**, the opening at the inferior extent of the thoracic cage, and observe that it is larger than the superior thoracic aperture.
5. Identify the boundaries of the inferior thoracic aperture: anteriorly by the xiphisternal joint and the costal margin, laterally by ribs 11 and 12, and posteriorly by the body of vertebra T12.
6. Anteriorly along the lateral aspect of the sternum, observe that **costal cartilage** is attached to the anterior end of some ribs. *Note that ribs are classified by the way their costal cartilages articulate medially.*
7. Identify the **true ribs (ribs 1 to 7)**, in which the costal cartilages articulate directly to the sternum.
8. Observe that the **1st rib** is the highest, shortest, broadest, and most sharply curved rib.
9. Identify the **false ribs (ribs 8 to 10)**, in which the costal cartilages articulate with the costal cartilage of the superiorly located rib, as seen along the **costal margin.**
10. Identify the two **false or floating ribs (ribs 11 and 12)**, which do not articulate anteriorly with a skeletal element but end in the abdominal musculature.
11. Observe that the ribs angle inferiorly approximately two vertebral levels as they wrap laterally and anteriorly around the thorax.

Surface Anatomy

Review the surface anatomy features outlined in the **Pectoral Region** of **Chapter 2** (see FIGURE 2.6). Following completion of your review of the pectoral region, return to this page.

Dissection Instructions

Intercostal Space

ATLAS 3.16, 3.17, 3.18; VIDEO 3.1.1

1. Refer to FIGURE 3.4.
2. Turn the cadaver to the supine position and palpate the jugular notch (suprasternal notch) on the superior aspect of the manubrium between the sternal ends of the clavicles.
3. Palpate the inferior extent of the **sternocleidomastoid (SCM)**, a large diagonally oriented muscle of the neck attaching to either side of the jugular notch. Observe that the SCM has two heads inferiorly: a **clavicular head** attaching to the clavicle and a **sternal head** attaching to the manubrium of the sternum.
4. Deep and medial to the SCM, identify the inferior extent of the infrahyoids (strap muscles), attaching to the superior extent of the **manubrium** along its deep surface.

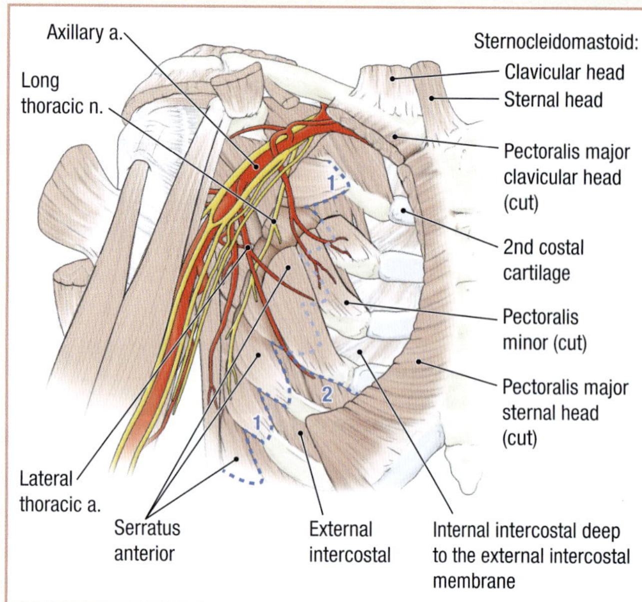

FIGURE 3.4 External aspect of right anterior thoracic wall. Anterior view.

5. Palpate the **sternal angle (manubriosternal junction)** between the manubrium and **body of the sternum** and confirm that it is at the height of the **2nd costal cartilage**.
6. Inferior to the body of the sternum, palpate the **xiphoid process** just below the **xiphisternal junction** and progress bilaterally along the **costal margins**.
7. Palpate the ribs and intercostal spaces beginning at the level of the sternal angle and identify each intercostal space by number.
8. Use a scalpel to remove any remaining muscular tissue of the clavicular and sternal heads of the pectoralis major along the inferior aspect of the clavicle and lateral aspects of the sternum bilaterally.
9. Remove any remaining muscular tissue of the **pectoralis minor** attaching to the ribs.
10. Review the locations of the serratus anterior, lateral thoracic artery arising from the axillary artery, and long thoracic nerve.
11. Detach the serratus anterior one attachment at a time from its proximal attachments on the upper eight or nine ribs (**Cut 1**).
12. Reflect the serratus anterior, along with the long thoracic nerve and lateral thoracic artery laterally.
13. Identify the **external intercostal** in the 5th intercostal space. Observe that the fibers of the external intercostal course from superolateral to inferomedial.
14. Identify the **external intercostal membrane** located at the anterior end of the intercostal space, between the **costal cartilages** where the fibers of the external intercostal end.
15. Insert a probe deep to the external intercostal membrane lateral to the border of the sternum in the 5th intercostal space and push the probe laterally deep to the external intercostal membrane and muscle.
16. With the probe as a guide, cut the external intercostal membrane and muscle from the inferior surface of the 5th rib (**Cut 2**). Continue the cut laterally toward the midaxillary line and reflect the external intercostal membrane and muscle inferiorly.
17. Identify the **internal intercostal** and observe that the fibers course superomedial to inferolateral, perpendicular to the fiber direction of the external intercostal.
18. Observe that the internal intercostal fibers occupy the intercostal space all the way to the sternum and are visible deep to the external intercostal membrane.
19. Refer to FIGURE 3.5.
20. Begin at the lateral border of the sternum and detach the internal intercostal from the superior surface of the 6th rib. Continue to detach the internal intercostal as far laterally as the midaxillary line and reflect the muscle superiorly.
21. Look for the 5th **intercostal nerve, artery,** and **vein** inferior to the 5th rib, observing that small **collateral vessels** may occupy the inferior aspect of an intercostal space. *Note that often the neurovascular structures course within the intercostal space with the pattern of VAN from superior to inferior (vein, **a**rtery, and **n**erve).*
22. Deep to the intercostal neurovascular structures, identify the **innermost intercostal** and observe that it has the same fiber direction as the internal intercostal but does not extend as far anteriorly in the intercostal space.
23. Observe that the intercostal neurovasculature runs in the plane between the internal intercostal and innermost intercostals.

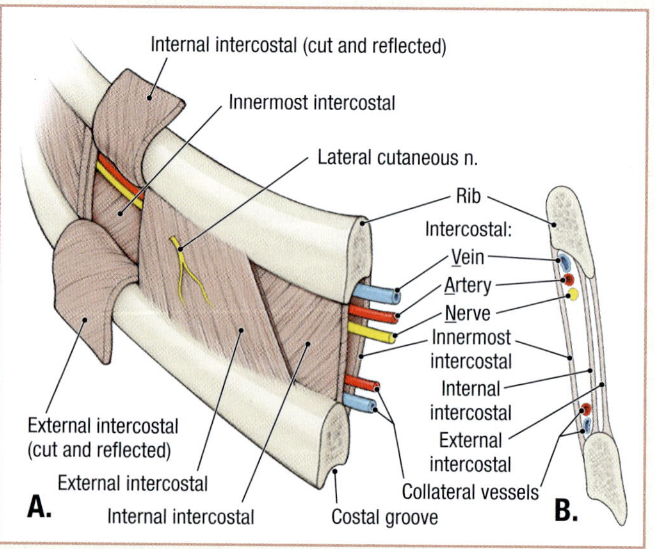

FIGURE 3.5 **A.** Intercostal muscles and contents of intercostal space. **B.** Coronal section of adjacent ribs and intercostal space at midaxillary line. Anterior views.

Dissection Follow-up

1. Review the muscles of the intercostal space with their respective actions in **TABLE 3.1**.
2. Review the origin, course, and branches of the intercostal neurovasculature with their respective relationships in the intercostal space.
3. Replace the internal and external intercostals in their correct anatomical positions.
4. Consult a dermatome chart and compare the dermatome pattern to the distribution of the intercostal nerves.

TABLE 3.1 Intercostal Muscles

Muscle	*Superior Attachment*	*Inferior Attachment*	*Actions*	*Innervation*
External intercostal	Inferior border of the rib above	Superior border of the rib below	Elevates the rib below	Intercostal nn.
Internal intercostal			Depresses the rib above	
Innermost intercostal				

Abbreviation: nn., nerves.

ANTERIOR THORACIC WALL AND PLEURAL CAVITIES

Dissection Overview

The body cavities (thoracic, pericardial, abdominal, and pelvic) are lined by regionally named serous membranes, which secrete a small amount of fluid to lubricate the movements of organs. In the thoracic cavity, there is a bilayer serous membrane around the lungs (pleura) and another around the heart (pericardial). The parietal pleura lines the inner surfaces of the thoracic wall, the superior aspect of the diaphragm, and the centrally located mediastinum, while the visceral pleura covers the surfaces of the lungs. Between the two layers of pleura is a potential space called the pleural cavity.

The thorax contains two pleural cavities (right and left) and the mediastinum. The pleural cavities occupy the lateral aspect of the thoracic cavity and contain one lung each. The mediastinum, the region between the two pleural cavities, contains the heart and other contents of the thorax.

Two methods of thoracic wall dissection will be described, and either method may be followed depending on the needs of the course. The first dissection sequence creates a window through the thoracic wall to preserve the relationships at the root of the neck. The second dissection sequence involves complete removal of the thoracic wall to increase visibility of the thoracic structures and facilitate lung removal. Depending on the approach, the SCM and infrahyoid muscles may be detached from the sternum and clavicle, and the clavicles cut at their midpoint. The costal cartilages and sternum may be cut at the level of the xiphisternal joint, or the costal margin may be elevated and the underlying diaphragm detached. In either approach, the ribs and intercostal structures will be cut at the midaxillary line.

The order of dissection will be as follows: The thoracic wall will be cut and opened in either window or removal approach along with the associated costal parietal pleura. The inner surface of the thoracic wall and the contents of the pleural cavities will be studied.

Dissection Instructions

Dissection Note: Various techniques may be implemented to expose the thoracic contents, two of which are described in the following dissection sequences. It is recommended to familiarize yourself with the instructions for each approach and then to follow the instructions of only one approach throughout the dissection that correlates best to your course objectives.

Window through Thoracic Wall

ATLAS 3.21, 3.23; VIDEO 3.2.1

Dissection Note: The window technique preserves the relationships of the root of the neck superiorly and the thoracic outlet inferiorly. Removal of the lungs and dissection of the mediastinum, however, are more difficult due to the smaller region of access, and the bones may need to be cut further to increase visibility.

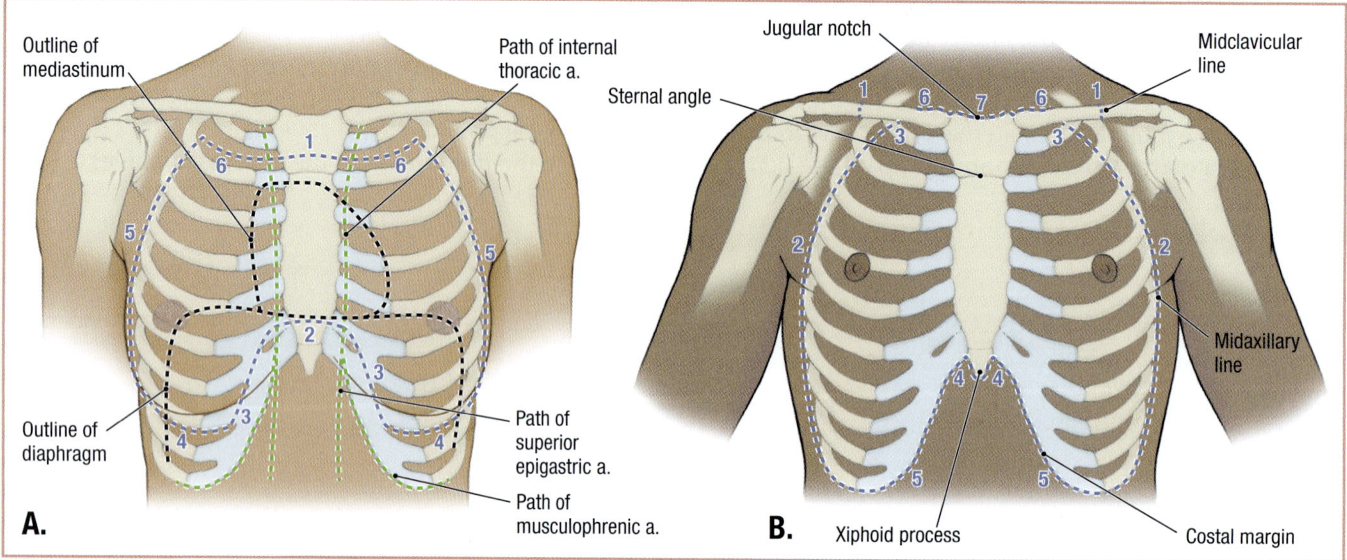

FIGURE 3.6 ● **A.** Removal of anterior thoracic wall in window approach. **B.** Removal of full anterior thoracic wall approach. Anterior views.

1. Refer to FIGURE 3.6A.
2. Reflect the pectoralis major laterally, the pectoralis minor superiorly, and the serratus anterior laterally.
3. Use the bone saw to make a horizontal incision midway between the jugular notch and the sternal angle through the manubrium (**Cut 1**). *Note that for all cuts using the bone saw, eye protection should be worn, and you must only allow the saw to pass through the bone and cartilage but not into the deeper tissues within the thorax.*
4. At the level of the xiphisternal joint, approximately at the level of the 6th costal cartilage, use the bone saw to make a transverse cut across the sternum and costal cartilages (**Cut 2**).
5. Continue the saw cut bilaterally, approximately 4 cm superior to the inferior border of the **costal margin** following its curve inferolaterally (**Cut 3**).
6. Use scissors to cut through the intercostal muscles to the midaxillary line at approximately the 8th intercostal space (**Cut 4**).
7. Use a saw or bone cutters to make vertical cuts through ribs 2 to 8 in the midaxillary line on both sides of the thorax, beginning inferiorly and progressing superiorly (**Cut 5**). Elevate the cut portion of ribs or push against the cut rib one at a time to verify you have cut completely through each rib.
8. Use sharp dissection to make a series of vertical cuts through the muscles in intercostal spaces 1 to 8 in the midaxillary line. The cuts should be aligned with the cut ribs and deep enough to cut the parietal pleura but not the surface of the lungs.
9. Use scissors to cut through the muscles within the 1st intercostal space from the vertical cut along the midaxillary line to the horizontal cut through the manubrium (**Cut 6**).
10. Gently elevate the inferior end of the cut sternum along with the attached portions of the costal cartilages and ribs.
11. Near the inferior end of the cut sternum, identify the **right and left internal thoracic (mammary) vessels,** and if they have not already been severed, use scissors to cut them inferiorly.
12. Continue to elevate the inferior end of the window of the anterior thoracic wall and use scissors to cut any adhesions of parietal pleura from the inner surface of the thoracic wall onto the mediastinum.
13. Cut the internal thoracic vessels superiorly at the level of the 1st rib.
14. Remove the window of the anterior thoracic wall along with the attached portions of the internal thoracic vessels.

Removal of Anterior Thoracic Wall

ATLAS 3.21, 3.22, 3.23

Dissection Note: Removing the entire anterior thoracic wall makes lung removal and mediastinal dissection easier and begins the transition into both the neck and abdomen. A full removal of the anterior thoracic wall disrupts some relationships of the root of the neck as well as the anterior border of the diaphragm and anterior abdominal wall.

1. Refer to FIGURE 3.6B.
2. Reflect the pectoralis major laterally, the pectoralis minor superiorly, and the serratus anterior laterally.
3. Use a probe to gently push the contents of the axilla away from the inferior aspect of the clavicle.
4. Use a saw to cut both clavicles at their midpoint (**Cut 1**). *Note that for all cuts using the bone*

saw, eye protection should be worn, and you must only allow the saw to pass through the bone and cartilage but not into the deeper tissues within the thorax.

5. Use a saw or bone cutters to cut ribs 2 to 8 in the midaxillary line on both sides of the thorax (**Cut 2**), beginning inferiorly and progressing superiorly. Elevate the cut portion of ribs or push against the cut rib one at a time to verify you have cut completely through each rib.
6. Palpate the 1st rib and use blunt dissection to push the contents of the axilla away from the rib.
7. Use the saw or bone cutters to cut through the 1st rib near the costal cartilage (**Cut 3**). While making the cut, pay attention to not damage any of the neurovascular structures passing into the axilla, in particular the subclavian vein.
8. Use sharp dissection to make a series of vertical cuts through the muscles in intercostal spaces 1 to 8 in the midaxillary line. The cuts should be aligned with the cut ribs and deep enough to cut the parietal pleura but not the surface of the lungs.

Dissection Note: The inferior cuts in this approach may either replicate steps 4 through 6 as described in the **Window through Thoracic Wall** approach or steps 9 through 13 below.

9. Elevate the superior attachment of the **rectus abdominis** with a probe.
10. Using the probe as a guide, transect the rectus abdominis horizontally superior to the curve of the costal margin (**Cut 4**).
11. Continue the cut following the costal margin through the anterolateral abdominal wall muscles until you reach the midaxillary line (**Cut 5**). *Note that care must be taken to not cut too deeply and thus enter the abdominal cavity.*
12. Gently elevate the inferior end of the sternum along with the attached portions of the costal margin and ribs superiorly and identify the muscular fibers of the diaphragm attaching along its deep surface.
13. Use a scalpel to trace along the curve of the costal margin to detach the diaphragm from its deep surface.
14. Near the inferior end of the sternum, identify the **right and left internal thoracic vessels**. If they have not already been severed, use scissors to cut the internal thoracic vessels inferiorly.
15. Continue to elevate the inferior end of the anterior thoracic wall using scissors to cut any adhesions of parietal pleura from the inner surface of the thoracic wall reflecting posteriorly onto the mediastinum.
16. Cut the internal thoracic vessels superiorly at the level of the 1st rib.
17. Detach the two heads of the SCM from the superior margin of the sternum and the superior surface of the clavicle, respectively (**Cut 6**).
18. Use blunt dissection to loosen the distal portion of the SCM and reflect it superiorly.
19. Use your fingers or a probe to push the **infrahyoid muscles** posteriorly. Follow the infrahyoid muscles inferiorly and detach them from the deep surface of the sternum (**Cut 7**).
20. Remove the anterior thoracic wall along with the attached portions of the internal thoracic vessels.

Anterior Thoracic Wall

ATLAS 3.22; VIDEO 3.2.2

1. Refer to FIGURE 3.7.
2. Identify the **costal parietal pleura** on the internal surface of the anterior thoracic wall.
3. Peel off a portion of the costal parietal pleura from the inner surface of the anterior thoracic wall and pay attention to the distinct tearing sound as you separate the pleura from the thoracic wall. The sound is the tearing of the fibers of the **endothoracic fascia**, the loose connective tissue attaching the costal parietal pleura to the thoracic wall.
4. Identify the **transversus thoracis** on the deep surface of the sternum and costal cartilages. Observe that the inferior attachment of the transversus thoracis is on the sternum, and its superior attachments are on costal cartilages 2 to 6.
5. Identify the **manubrium**, **body**, and **xiphoid process** of the sternum from the posterior view.
6. Identify and clean the **internal thoracic artery** and **veins** between the transversus thoracis and costal cartilages.
7. Follow the internal thoracic artery inferiorly and identify at least one of its **anterior intercostal branches**.
8. Observe that **anterior intercostal arteries** arise from the internal thoracic artery to supply the anterior aspect of the intercostal space. *Note that the posterior aspect of the intercostal space is supplied by posterior intercostal arteries arising directly from the thoracic aorta to create an anastomosis with the anterior intercostal branches.*
9. Observe that posterior to the 6th or 7th costal cartilage, the internal thoracic artery terminates by dividing into the **superior epigastric artery** and the **musculophrenic artery**.
10. Study the course and distribution of a typical intercostal nerve and note that it supplies the intercostal muscles, the skin of the thoracic wall, and the parietal pleura.
11. If a full anterior thoracic wall approach was implemented, identify the cut edge of the **diaphragm** inferiorly and the cut edges of the two visible infrahyoid muscles, the **sternothyroid** and **sternohyoid**.

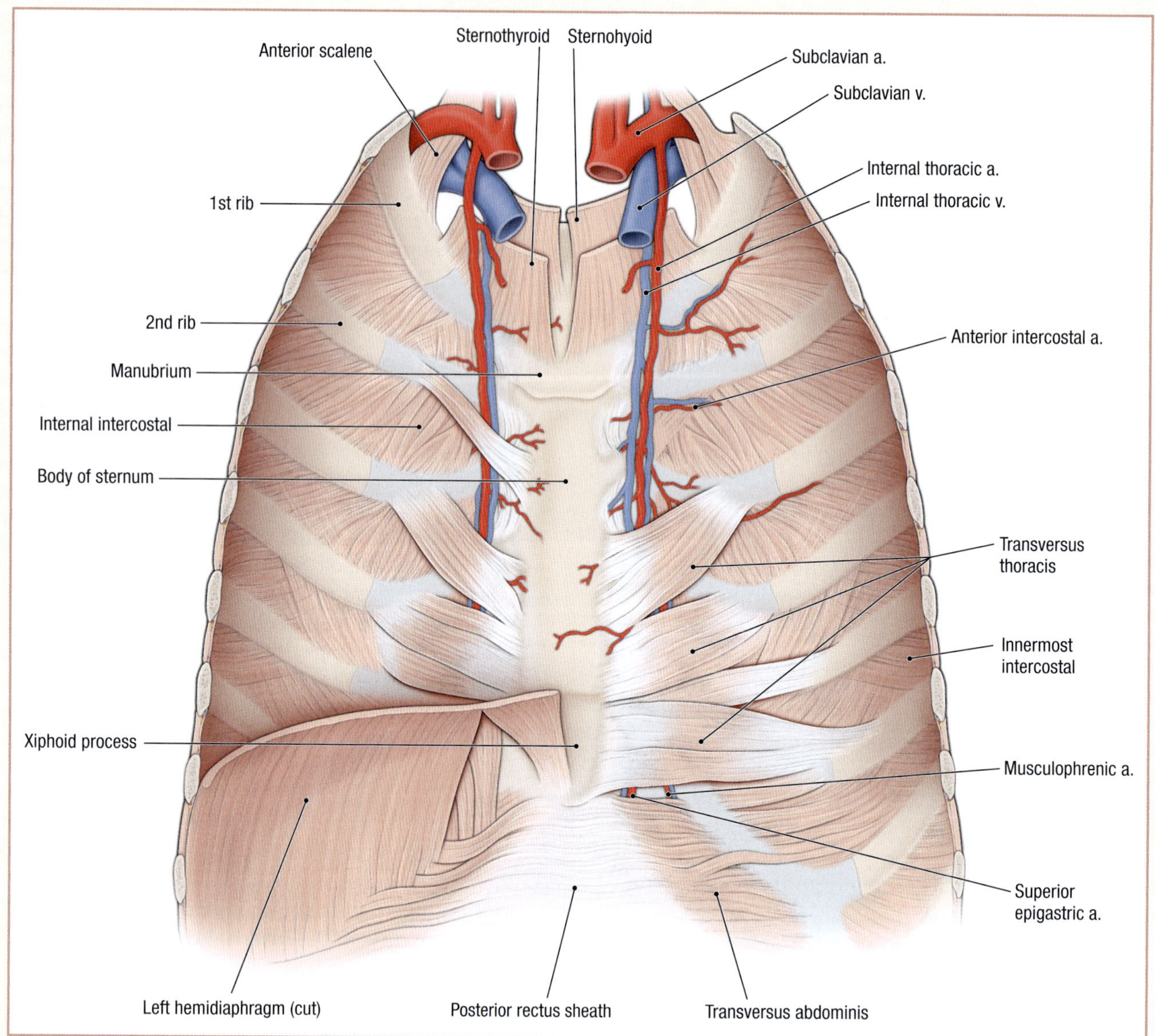

FIGURE 3.7 ● Anterior thoracic wall. Posterior view.

Pleural Cavities

ATLAS 3.24, 3.27; VIDEO 3.2.3

1. Refer to FIGURE 3.8.
2. Use your hands to carefully explore the right and left pleural cavities, paying attention as the cut ends of the ribs are sharp and can easily cut you or your gloves. To reduce the risk of injury, fold the serratus anterior into the thoracic cavity over the cut ends of the ribs before you begin palpating the pleural cavities.
3. Use paper towels or suction to remove fluid that may have collected during the embalming process in the **pleural cavity** (see **Clinical Correlation 3.1**). *Note that in the living body, the pleural cavity is a potential space as only a thin layer of serous fluid separates the visceral and parietal layers.*

CLINICAL CORRELATION 3.1

Pneumothorax and Hemothorax

ATLAS 3.27

Under pathologic conditions, the potential space of the pleural cavity may become a real space. With trauma, air may enter the pleural cavity causing the lung to collapse due to changes in intrathoracic pressure and the elasticity of the lung tissue as seen in pneumothorax. Excess fluid may also accumulate in the pleural cavity and compress the lung, producing breathing difficulties. The fluid could be excess serous fluid from pleural effusion or blood accumulation resulting in hemothorax. Chest tubes may be inserted through the thoracic wall to drain air or fluid from the pleural cavity, typically through the 5th or 6th intercostal spaces in the midaxillary line.

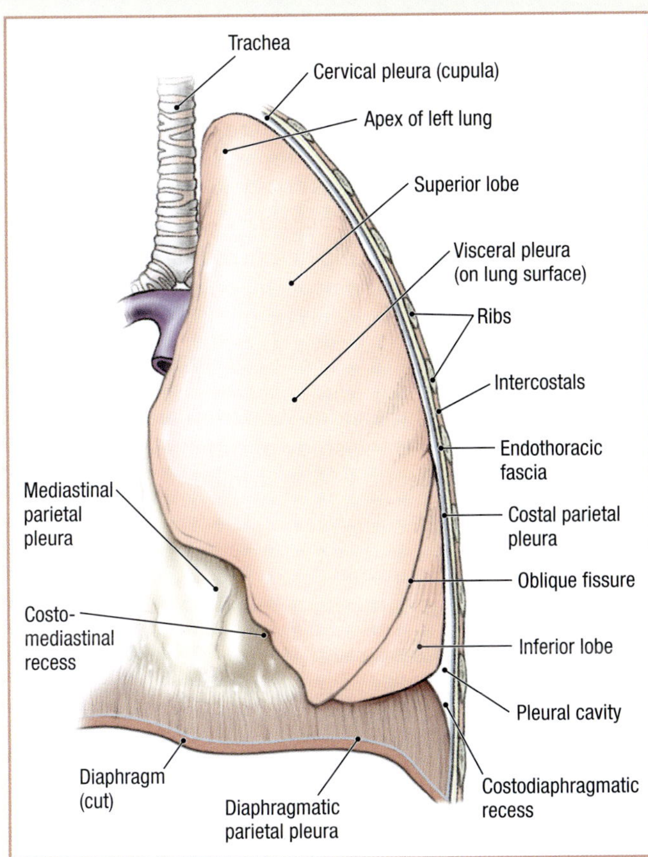

FIGURE 3.8 ● Pleural cavity and pleurae of left lung. Anterior view.

4. Identify the subdivisions of the **parietal pleura**, the outer lining of the serous membrane enclosing the pleural cavities, beginning with the **costal parietal pleura** on the inner surface of the thoracic wall. Observe that some of the costal parietal pleura was cut and removed with the anterior thoracic wall.
5. Identify the **mediastinal parietal pleura** lining the mediastinum medially, and the **diaphragmatic parietal pleura** covering the superior surface of the diaphragm inferiorly.
6. Identify the **cervical parietal pleura (pleural cupula)** extending superior to the 1st rib. *Note that endothoracic fascia underlies all the subdivisions of parietal pleura.*
7. Observe that the parietal pleura is folded sharply at the **lines of pleural reflection** where the costal parietal pleura meets the diaphragmatic parietal pleura and where the costal parietal pleura meets the mediastinal parietal pleura.
8. The areas where one parietal pleura contacts another parietal pleura are called **pleural recesses.** Identify the two **costodiaphragmatic recesses** (left and right) located at the most inferior limits of the parietal pleura between the ribs and diaphragm.
9. Inferiorly along the lateral border of the diaphragm, place your fingers in the **costodiaphragmatic (costophrenic) recess** and follow it posteriorly, observing the acute angle that the diaphragm makes with the inner surface of the thoracic wall. *Note that during quiet inspiration, the inferior border of the lung does not extend into the costodiaphragmatic recess.*
10. Using the removed portion of the anterior thoracic wall, appreciate the relative location of the two **costomediastinal recesses** (larger on the left than the right), which occur posterior to the sternum where costal parietal pleura meets mediastinal parietal pleura.
11. Place your hand between the lung and the mediastinum and palpate the **root of the lung**, composed of the physical structures passing from the mediastinum in and out of the lung.
12. Observe that at the root of the lung, the mediastinal parietal pleura is continuous with the visceral pleura and demarcates the boundary of the **hilum** of the lung. *Note that the root of the lung is attached to the mediastinum, but all other parts of the lung should slide freely against the parietal pleura as the lung moves within the pleural cavity.*
13. Identify the **pulmonary ligament**, the inferior extension of the pleural reflection around the root of the lung anchoring the inferior lobe of each lung to the mediastinum.
14. Observe that each lung is completely covered with **visceral (pulmonary) pleura**. Make no attempt to remove the visceral pleura as this will destroy the lung tissue.
15. Use your fingers to trace the periphery of the lung within the pleural cavity and break any pleural adhesions between visceral and parietal pleurae that may be present because of embalming or disease processes.

Dissection Follow-up

1. Review the attachments and the actions of the pectoralis major and minor, serratus anterior, and transversus thoracis.
2. Use the dissected specimen to project the lines of pleural reflection to the anterior thoracic wall.
3. Review the course and branches of the internal thoracic artery from its origin on the subclavian artery to its terminal bifurcation.
4. Review the course of the intercostal nerves and the pattern of somatic innervation (including pain fibers) to the costal pleura.
5. Replace the anterior thoracic wall, serratus anterior, and pectoralis major and minor and in their correct anatomical positions.

LUNGS

Dissection Overview

The respiratory system can be subdivided into conducting and respiratory portions. The lungs are the primary respiratory organs in humans and form part of the lower aspect of the conducting portion. The alveoli are the gas exchange portion of the lungs within the respiratory portion and are not visible without the aid of a microscope. The lungs and other structures of the conducting system are readily visible for study.

Although the lungs are bilateral organs, the right and left lungs have distinct anatomical differences that will be studied. Structures entering and exiting the medial surface of the lung at the hilum include the bronchi, pulmonary artery, pulmonary veins, bronchiole arteries, nerves, and lymphatics. The hilum is a space demarcated by the reflection of the parietal and visceral serous membranes of the lung, while the root consists of the physical tubes entering and leaving the lung as shown in FIGURE 3.9.

The order of dissection will be as follows: The surface features and relationships of the lungs seen from an anterior view will be studied with the lungs in the thorax. The lungs will then be removed, and the study of surface features and relationships of the lungs will be completed. The mediastinal surface and root of the lung will be studied.

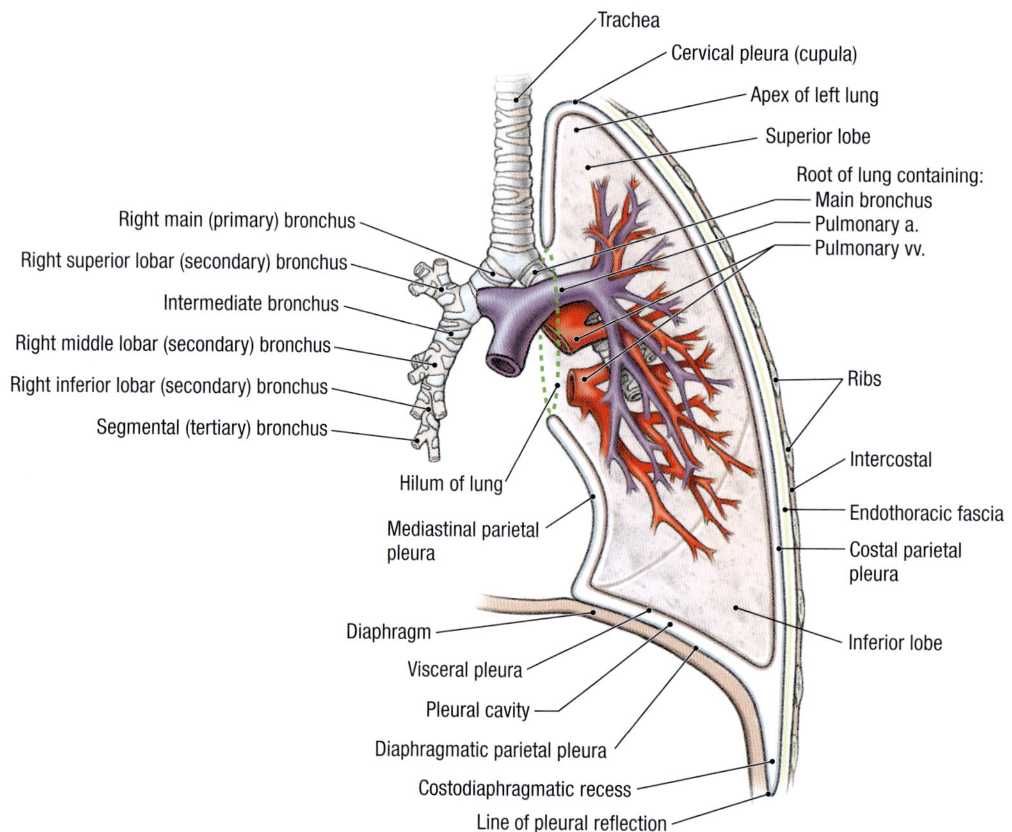

FIGURE 3.9 Coronal (frontal) section through left thoracic cavity near midaxillary line. Anterior view.

Dissection Instructions

Lungs in Thorax

ATLAS 3.24, 3.25, 3.29; VIDEO 3.3.1

1. Refer to FIGURE 3.10.
2. Observe the lungs in situ and identify their three surfaces beginning with the **costal surface**, which, as its name infers, is the surface of the lung adjacent to the ribs.
3. Gently pull a lung laterally and identify the **mediastinal surface**, which rests in contact with the centrally located mediastinum.
4. Elevate the inferior aspect of the lung and identify the **diaphragmatic surface** lying directly over the diaphragm. *Note that contraction of diaphragmatic muscle fibers pulls the diaphragm inferiorly, which increases the volume of the thoracic cavity consequently lowering the pressure in the lungs to draw in air.*

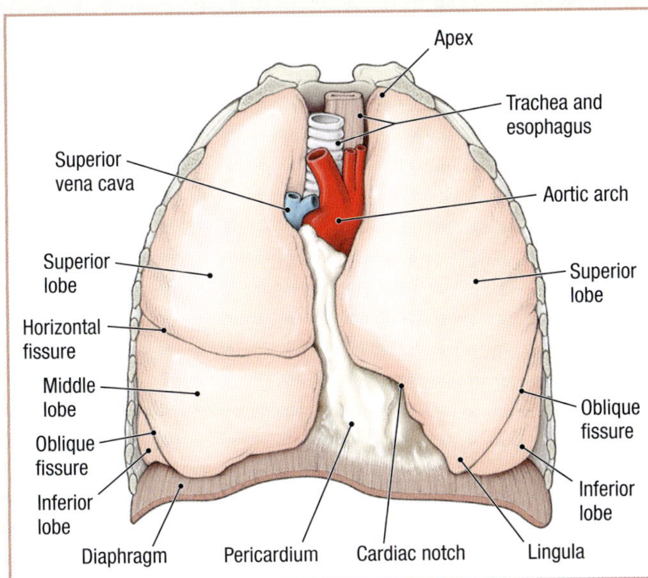

FIGURE 3.10 ● Thoracic cavity with lungs in situ. Anterior view.

5. Identify the three lobes of the right lung: **superior**, **middle**, and **inferior**.
6. Identify the two lobes of the left lung: **superior** and **inferior**. *Note that variations in the number of lobes may occur.*
7. Observe the **oblique fissure (major fissure)** on both lungs just superior to the inferior lobe. Using the anterior thoracic wall as a guide, observe that the oblique fissure lies deep to the 5th rib laterally and deep to the 6th costal cartilage anteriorly.
8. Identify the **horizontal fissure (minor** or **transverse fissure)** on the right lung between the superior and middle lobes.
9. Using the anterior thoracic wall as a guide, observe that the horizontal fissure lies deep to the 4th rib and 4th costal cartilage.
10. Observe that the **apex** of the lung lies superior to the body of the 1st rib along with the associated cervical pleura and therefore lies superior to the plane of the superior thoracic aperture in the neck.
11. Between the right and left pleural cavities, identify the **pericardium (pericardial sac)**. The pericardium occupies the midline between the lungs, lies posterior to the sternum and costal cartilages, and contains the heart.
12. Insert your hand into the pleural cavity between the pericardium and the lung and palpate the structures within the **root of the lung**. Each root of the lung consists of the pulmonary vessels and the main or primary bronchus.
13. On the lateral surface of the pericardium, identify the **phrenic nerve** and the **pericardiacophrenic vessels** travelling together deep to the mediastinal pleura.
14. Observe that the phrenic nerve and pericardiacophrenic vessels pass anterior to the root of the lung. Do not dissect the phrenic nerve or pericardiacophrenic vessels at this time because they will be dissected with the mediastinum.

Right Lung

ATLAS 3.30, 3.32; VIDEO 3.3.2

1. Refer to FIGURE 3.10.
2. Retract the right lung laterally to stretch the root of the lung while preserving the phrenic nerve and pericardiacophrenic vessels medially.
3. While retracting the lung, use sharp dissection to carefully transect the root of the lung halfway between the lung and the mediastinum. Take care not to cut into the mediastinal structures or the lung.
4. Gently pull the lung laterally and use a probe or your fingers to determine that the root of the lung is completely transected, ensuring the pulmonary ligament has been cut.
5. Slide your hands completely under the right lung, ensuring you are not within the oblique fissure and lift it from the pleural cavity. Pay particular attention not to cut yourself on the sharp edges of the ribs while doing so. *Note that the lung tissue is quite delicate and the lungs must be removed gently to avoid damaging the tissue or separating the lobes.*
6. Refer to FIGURE 3.11.
7. On the removed right lung, identify the superior, middle, and inferior lobes as well as the horizontal and oblique fissures.
8. Identify the costal, mediastinal, and diaphragmatic surfaces of the right lung.
9. Identify the anterior, posterior, and inferior borders of the right lung.
10. On the mediastinal surface of the right lung, identify the shallow **cardiac impression** anterior to the **esophageal impression**.
11. Identify the **impression of the azygos arch** arching superior to the root of the lung anteriorly to the **superior vena cava impression**.
12. Identify the cut edge of parietal pleura forming the hilum of the lung surrounding the root of the lung, and the thin inferior extension of the cut **pulmonary ligament**.
13. Examine the cut edges of the root of the right lung and identify the **right main (primary) bronchus**, **right pulmonary artery**, and **right pulmonary veins** (see **Clinical Correlation 3.2**).

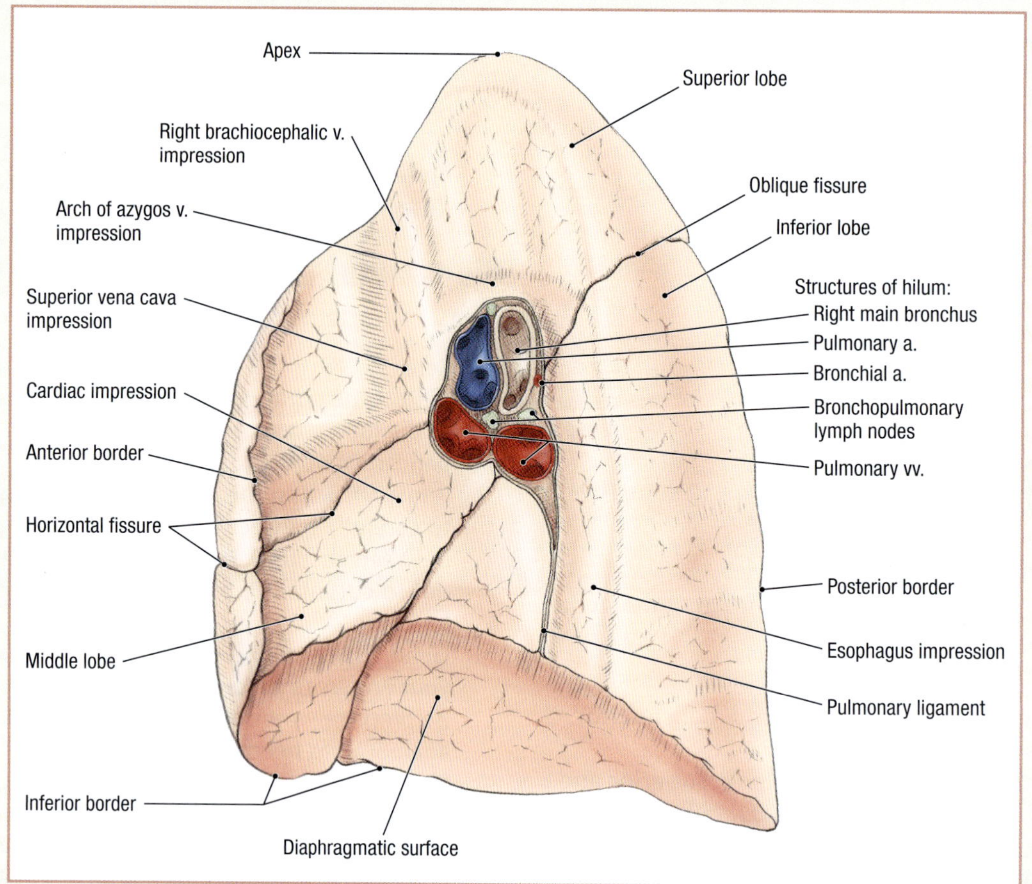

FIGURE 3.11 ■ Mediastinal surface of right lung. Medial view.

CLINICAL CORRELATION 3.2

Pulmonary Embolism

ATLAS 3.36, 3.37

A pulmonary embolism is a blockage of a pulmonary artery or its branches by a blood clot (embolus), fat, or air. Blockage of a pulmonary artery results in decrease or loss of blood to a portion of the lung tissue rendering it incapable of gas exchange despite air flowing into the region. If the clot is large enough, it may lead to pulmonary infarct or tissue death known as necrosis, resulting in decreased blood oxygen levels and respiratory distress. Often, the blood clots originate in the veins of the lower limb as a deep vein thrombosis (DVT) which pass to the right side of the heart via venous return through the caval system and then pass into the lungs via a pulmonary artery, resulting in a blockage as the diameter of the vessels narrow.

14. Observe that the right pulmonary artery is usually superior to the pulmonary veins. *Note that the pulmonary artery contains oxygen-poor blood, and the pulmonary veins contain oxygen-rich blood.*
15. Observe that the right main bronchus lies posterior to the right pulmonary artery.
16. Insert a probe into the lumen of the right main bronchus and verify its pattern of branching into each lobe. *Note that the right main bronchus may have already divided within the mediastinum.*
17. In the right lung, identify the **superior, middle,** and **inferior lobar (secondary) bronchi.** *Note that the right superior lobar bronchus passes superior to the right pulmonary artery and therefore is also called the "eparterial bronchus."*

Left Lung

ATLAS 3.31, 3.33; VIDEO 3.3.3

1. Observe that the heart is positioned more to the left-hand side of the thoracic cavity and the thoracic aorta descends on the left, which combine to often make the left lung more difficult to remove despite its smaller size.
2. Repeat steps 1 to 4 from the **Right Lung** instructions, ensuring that you are not grasping only the superior lobe of the left lung and are posterior to the entire lung. Pay particular attention not to cut yourself on the sharp edges of the ribs while doing so.
3. Refer to FIGURE 3.12.
4. On the removed left lung, identify the costal, mediastinal, and diaphragmatic surfaces.

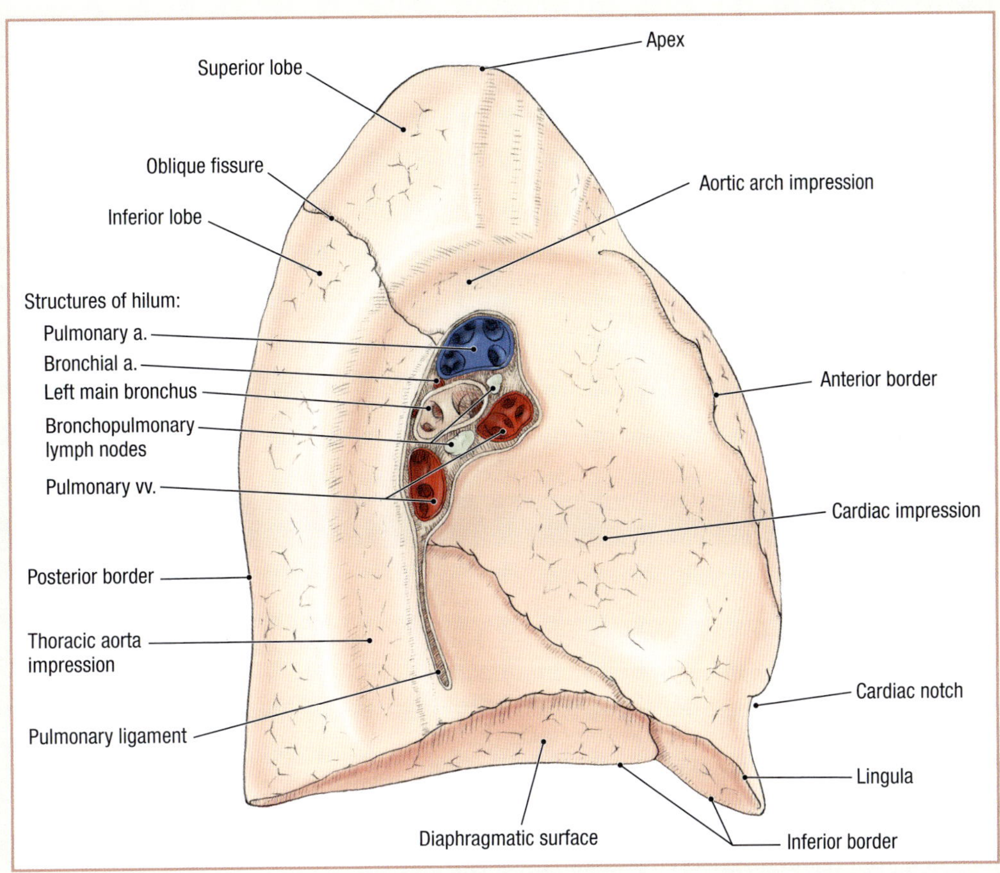

FIGURE 3.12 ● Mediastinal surface of left lung. Medial view.

5. Identify the anterior, posterior, and inferior borders of the left lung.
6. On the mediastinal surface of the left lung, identify the more prominent **cardiac impression** inferior to the **aortic arch impression** and anterior to the **thoracic aorta impression.**
7. Identify the **cardiac notch** along the anterior border of the superior lobe and verify that in anatomical position it is positioned anterior to the heart.
8. Identify the **lingula**, the inferior, medial portion of the superior lobe, and verify that it is the homolog of the middle lobe of the right lung.
9. Identify the cut edge of parietal pleura forming the hilum of the lung surrounding the root of the lung, and the thin inferior extension of the cut **pulmonary ligament.**
10. Examine the cut edges of the **root of the left lung** and identify the **left main (primary) bronchus, left pulmonary artery**, and **left pulmonary veins.**
11. Observe that the left pulmonary artery is usually superior to the left pulmonary veins.
12. Observe on the left lung that the left main bronchus contains cartilage and commonly lies inferior to the left pulmonary artery.
13. Insert a probe into the lumen of the left main bronchus and verify its pattern of branching into each lobe. *Note that the left main bronchus may have already divided within the mediastinum.*
14. Identify the **superior** and **inferior lobar (secondary) bronchi.**
15. Compare the two lungs and observe that the right lung is typically shorter but has greater volume than the left lung.
16. Verify that each lung has a **superior** and **inferior lobe** separated by the **oblique fissure** and observe that most of the inferior lobe lies posteriorly and that most of the superior lobe lies anteriorly in the thorax.
17. Use blunt dissection to follow one lobar bronchus approximately 3 to 4 cm deeper into the lung tissue until it branches into several **segmental (tertiary) bronchi.** *Note that the right lung contains 10 segmental bronchi, and the left lung contains either 9 or 10, each of which supply one bronchopulmonary segment of the lung.*
18. Identify a **bronchial artery** coursing along the surface of the main or lobar bronchi.
19. In addition to the already identified structures, at the hilum of the lung, briefly look for bronchial veins, lymph nodes, lymph vessels, and autonomic nerves. *Note that the lungs have a rich nerve supply via the anterior and posterior pulmonary plexuses with sympathetic contributions from the right and left sympathetic trunks and parasympathetic contributions from the right and left vagus nerves.*

Dissection Follow-up

1. Review the surfaces, borders, and component parts of each lung.
2. Review the structures of the root of the lung and the respective location of the bronchus and pulmonary artery for the right and left lungs.
3. Review the regional naming pattern of the parietal pleura and review the relationship of the pleural reflections to the thoracic wall, diaphragm, and mediastinum to create the costomediastinal and costodiaphragmatic recesses.
4. Review the regional parts of the parietal pleura and the locations of reflection to create spaces within the pleural cavities.
5. Review the relationship of the phrenic nerves to the root of the lung.
6. Replace the lungs in their correct anatomical positions within the pleural cavities or place them in a container following your labs protocol for removed organs.
7. Replace the anterior thoracic wall and project the borders, surfaces, and fissures of the lungs to the surface of the thoracic wall.

MEDIASTINUM

Dissection Overview

The mediastinum is the region between the two pleural cavities. For descriptive purposes, the mediastinum can be divided into four parts based on their relative locations as shown in FIGURE 3.13. An imaginary transverse plane at the level of the sternal angle intersects the T4/T5 IV disc and separates the superior mediastinum from the inferior mediastinum. The inferior mediastinum is further subdivided by the pericardium into three parts. The anterior mediastinum lies between the sternum and the pericardium and, in children and adolescents, contains part of the thymus. The middle mediastinum is centrally located and contains the pericardium, the heart, and the roots of the great vessels. The posterior mediastinum lies posterior to the pericardium and anterior to the bodies of vertebrae T5–T12 and contains structures that pass between the neck, thorax, and abdomen (esophagus, vagus nerves, azygos system of veins, thoracic duct, and thoracic aorta). It is worth noting that some structures that course through the mediastinum (esophagus, vagus nerve, phrenic nerve, and thoracic duct) pass through more than one mediastinal subdivision.

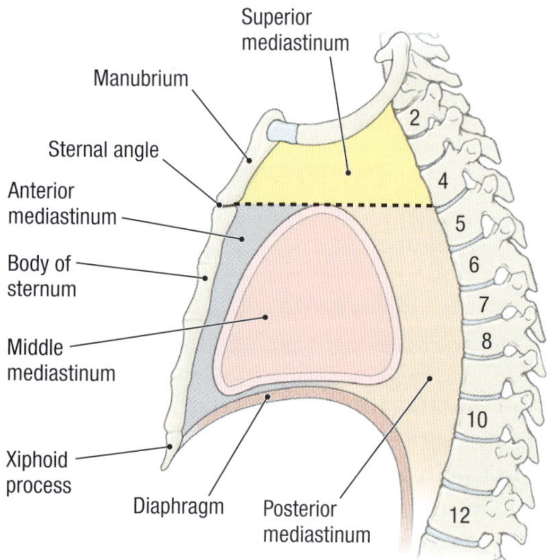

FIGURE 3.13 ● Boundaries and subdivisions of mediastinum. Lateral view.

The order of dissection will be as follows: The mediastinal pleura will be examined, and the mediastinal structures will be palpated. The costal and mediastinal pleurae will then be removed. The pericardium will be opened, and its relationship to the heart and great vessels will be explored. The characteristics of the parietal serous pericardium will then be studied. The heart will be removed by cutting the great vessels.

Dissection Instructions

Inferior Mediastinum

ATLAS 3.28, 3.73, 3.74; VIDEO 3.4.1

1. Refer to FIGURE 3.13.
2. Observe that the **mediastinum** has a **superior boundary** of the superior thoracic aperture, an **inferior boundary** of the diaphragm, an **anterior boundary** of the sternum, a **posterior boundary** of vertebral bodies T1–T12, and **lateral boundaries** of mediastinal pleurae (left and right).
3. Use the anterior thoracic wall to identify the location of the sternal angle relative to the mediastinum. Verify that the sternal angle is at the same height as the T4/T5 IV disc and that a plane intersecting these points would subdivide the mediastinum into superior and inferior portions.
4. Palpate the **mediastinal parietal pleura** and observe that the plane of the sternal angle is at the level of the superior border of the pericardium, the bifurcation of the trachea, the end of the ascending aorta, the beginning *and* end of the arch of the aorta, and the beginning of the thoracic aorta.

5. Observe that as you move from anterior to posterior, the mediastinal parietal pleura is in contact with the **pericardium**, **root of the lung**, and either the **esophagus** on the right side or the **thoracic aorta** on the left side.
6. Identify the left and right **phrenic nerves** and the left and right **pericardiacophrenic vessels** coursing deep to the mediastinal pleura. Observe that the phrenic nerve and pericardiacophrenic vessels are located between the mediastinal pleura and pericardium about 1.5 cm anterior to the root of the lung.
7. Clean and follow the phrenic nerve and pericardiacophrenic vessels inferiorly toward the diaphragm. Recall that the phrenic nerves arise from vertebral levels C3–C5 and that each phrenic nerve is the only motor innervation to the ipsilateral half of the diaphragm as well as sensory innervation to the mediastinal and diaphragmatic parietal pleurae.

Heart in Mediastinum

ATLAS 3.24, 3.45; VIDEO 3.4.2

1. Refer to FIGURE 3.14.
2. Identify the **pericardial sac (pericardium)** enclosing the heart and observe that it is pierced by the **aorta**, **pulmonary trunk**, and **superior vena cava** superiorly; the **four pulmonary veins** posterolaterally; and the **inferior vena cava** inferiorly.
3. Observe that the pericardial sac lies deep to the **mediastinal parietal pleura** and consists of two layers: the **fibrous pericardium** externally and the **parietal pericardium** internally.

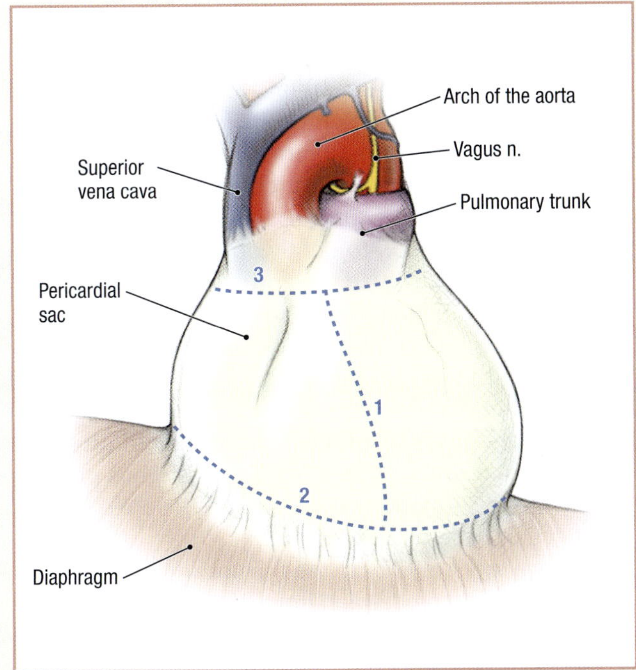

FIGURE 3.14 ● Incisions to open pericardial sac. Anterior view.

4. Remove the mediastinal parietal pleura and associated fat covering the anterior surface of the pericardial sac between the right and left phrenic nerves and pericardiacophrenic vessels.
5. Observe that the pericardial sac is attached to the **central tendon of the diaphragm** inferiorly and thus can move up and down during inspiration and expiration carrying the heart with it.
6. Use forceps to elevate the anterior surface of the pericardium and use scissors to make a vertical incision through the pericardium, starting 2 cm superior to the diaphragm inferiorly and extending to 2 cm inferior to the great vessels superiorly (**Cut 1**).
7. Make a transverse cut around the periphery of the pericardium inferiorly 2 cm superior to the point of reflection of the pericardium with the diaphragm (**Cut 2**).
8. Make a transverse cut around the periphery of the pericardium superiorly 2 cm inferior to the point of reflection of the pericardium with the great vessels (**Cut 3**). Take care to not cut the phrenic nerves and accompanying vessels.
9. Open the flaps of pericardium widely.
10. Refer to FIGURE 3.15.
11. On the inner surface of the pericardial sac, identify the smooth surface of the **parietal layer of serous pericardium**.
12. Observe that the parietal layer of serous pericardium reflects onto the heart as the **visceral layer of serous pericardium (epicardium)** at the roots of the great vessels.
13. Use your fingers to palpate and explore the now-visible **pericardial cavity**, the potential space between the parietal and visceral layers of serous pericardium (see **Clinical Correlation 3.3**). *Note that normally, the pericardial cavity contains only a thin film of serous fluid that lubricates the serous surfaces and allows free movement of the heart within the pericardium.*

CLINICAL CORRELATION 3.3

Cardiac Tamponade and Pericardiocentesis

ATLAS 3.28

Inflammatory diseases can cause fluid to accumulate in the pericardial cavity (pericardial effusion). Bleeding into the pericardial cavity (hemopericardium) may result from penetrating heart wounds or from perforation of weakened heart muscle following myocardial infarction. As the pericardium is composed of fibrous connective tissue, it cannot stretch; thus, fluid collected in the pericardial cavity will compress the heart resulting in cardiac tamponade. To relieve cardiac tamponade, fluid from the pericardial cavity can be drained by inserting a needle into the pericardial cavity (pericardiocentesis) either in the left subcostal angle or at the left 5th or 6th intercostal spaces near the sternum.

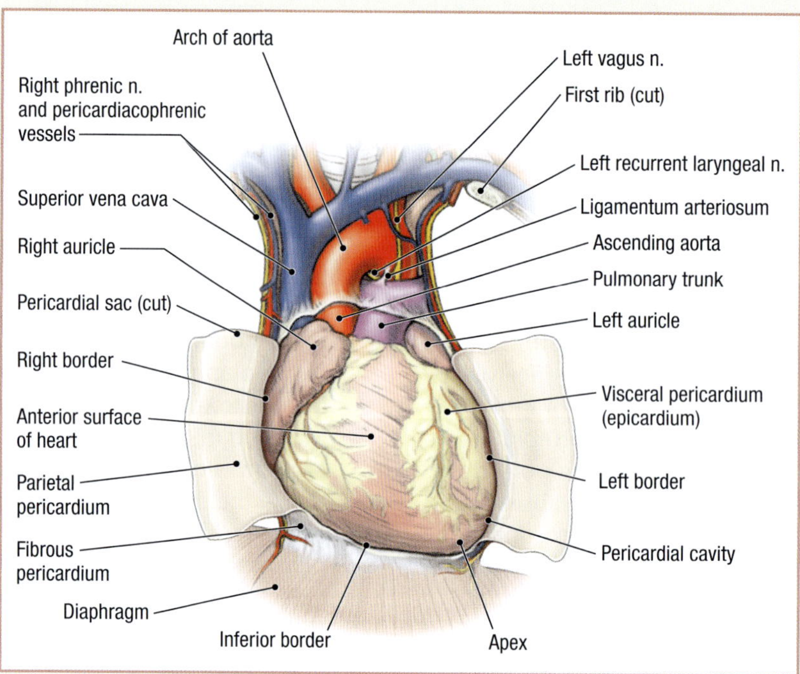

FIGURE 3.15 ● Heart in situ with reflected pericardial sac. Anterior view.

14. Within the pericardial cavity, identify the **superior vena cava, ascending aorta, pulmonary trunk, pulmonary veins**, and the **inferior vena cava.**
15. Examine the surface of the heart and observe that the **right border of the heart** is formed by the **right atrium.**
16. Observe that the majority of the anterior surface of the heart and the **inferior border** are formed by the **right ventricle** and a small part of the **left ventricle** and that the **left border** is formed by the left ventricle.
17. The **superior border of the heart** is formed by the **right** and **left atria** and **auricles.** *Note that the right, inferior, and left borders of the heart are typically readily identifiable on a chest radiograph, while the superior border of the heart is often difficult to identify.*
18. Identify the **apex of the heart** on the inferior left side of the heart and observe that it is part of the left ventricle. *Note that the apex of the heart is normally located deep to the left 5th intercostal space, approximately 9 cm lateral to the midline.*
19. Identify the **base of the heart** formed by the left atrium and part of the right atrium. *Note that clinicians often refer to the emergence of the great vessels from the heart as its base.*
20. Place the anterior thoracic wall into its correct anatomical position and use the cadaver to project the outline of the heart to the surface of the thoracic wall.

Removal of Heart

ATLAS 3.45, 3.46; VIDEO 3.4.3

1. Refer to FIGURE 3.16.
2. External and superior to the pericardium, identify the **arch of the aorta.**
3. Use blunt dissection to identify and clean the **left vagus nerve** where it crosses the left side of the aortic arch.
4. Observe that the **vagus nerve** descends within the thorax posterior to the root of the lung, whereas the phrenic nerve passes anterior to the root of the lung.
5. Identify the initial portion of the **left recurrent laryngeal nerve** where it branches from the left vagus nerve inferior to the aortic arch and posterior to the **ligamentum arteriosum.**
6. Use blunt dissection to gently open the interval between the concavity of the aortic arch and pulmonary trunk and identify the **ligamentum arteriosum,** connecting the left pulmonary artery to the inferior aspect of the arch of the aorta.
7. Place a hand in the pericardial cavity so that your fingers are posterior to the heart in the **oblique pericardial sinus.** Lift the heart gently while pushing your fingers superiorly until they are stopped by the reflection of serous pericardium.
8. Push a finger posterior to the pulmonary trunk and ascending aorta, proceeding from left to right, until your fingertip emerges between the superior vena cava and the ascending aorta in the **transverse pericardial sinus.**
9. Use your fingers to explore the lines of reflection of the serous pericardium where the great vessels (aorta,

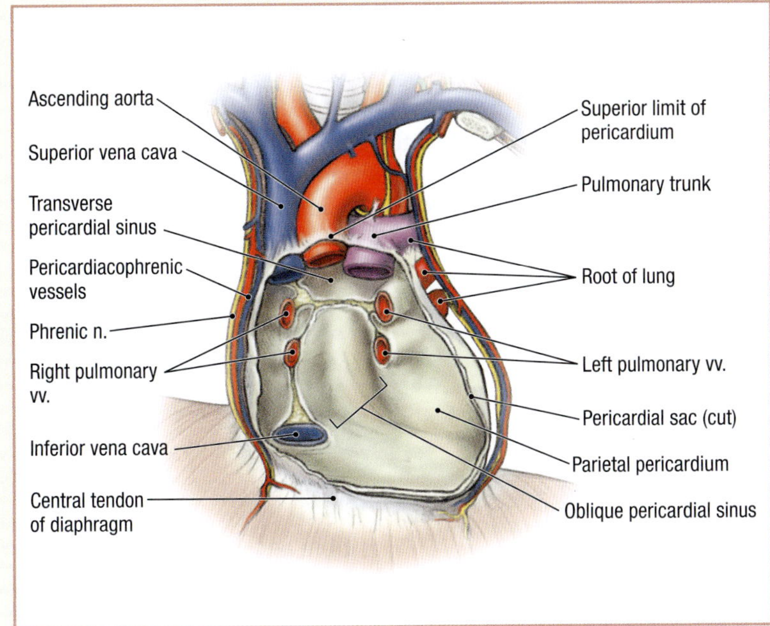

FIGURE 3.16 ● Pericardial cavity and sinuses with heart removed. Anterior view.

pulmonary trunk, superior vena cava, inferior vena cava, and four pulmonary veins) enter and exit the heart.

10. Place a probe through the transverse pericardial sinus.
11. Cut the **ascending aorta** and **pulmonary trunk** anterior to the probe about 1.5 cm superior to the point where the aorta and pulmonary trunk emerge from the heart.
12. Cut the **superior vena cava** about 1 cm superior to its junction with the right atrium.
13. Lift the apex and inferior surface of the heart superiorly and cut the **inferior vena cava** close to the surface of the diaphragm.
14. Continue lifting the heart and cut the **four pulmonary veins** close to the inner surface of the pericardial sac where they form the lateral boundaries of the oblique pericardial sinus.
15. Cut any remaining reflections of the serous pericardium from the posterior surface of the heart to the inner surface of the pericardial sac and remove the heart from the pericardial sac.
16. With the heart removed, examine the posterior aspect of the pericardium and identify the openings of eight vessels and the lines of pericardial reflection.

Dissection Follow-up

1. Review the parts of the mediastinum and state their boundaries.
2. Review the attachments of the pericardium to the diaphragm and roots of the great vessels.
3. Compare the appearance and functional properties of the parietal and visceral layers of serous pericardium to those of the parietal and visceral pleurae.
4. Return the reflected tissue back to anatomical position.
5. Review the embryonic origin of the transverse and oblique pericardial sinuses.

EXTERNAL FEATURES OF HEART

Dissection Overview

The heart is a vital organ responsible for circulating blood throughout the human body by contraction of its muscular wall. The heart wall consists of three layers, which from superficial to deep are the epicardium (visceral pericardium), the myocardium, and the endocardium. During systole, the heart contracts and functions as a two-pump system with one side devoted to circulating oxygen-poor blood, and the other circulating oxygen-rich blood. As the blood circulates, it collects within four different chambers separated from one another by septa and valves.

Blood supply to the heart itself occurs during diastole, or the resting phase, as the blood pressure in the ventricles drops, causing a slight reversal of blood in the aorta to close the aortic valve, fill the aortic sinuses, and allow blood to passively flow into the coronary arteries. The right and left coronary arteries form a circle or "crown" around the circumference of the heart to supply the heart tissue. Venous drainage of the heart approximately parallels the main arterial branches and returns blood directly to the right atrium.

The order of dissection will be as follows: The surface features of the heart will be examined from both anterior and superior perspective. The valves and cusps of the aortic and pulmonary semilunar valves will be studied. The coronary veins will be cleaned and isolated. The coronary arteries will be cleaned and isolated.

Dissection Instructions

Surface Features and Valves of Heart

ATLAS 3.43, 3.46A, 3.58; VIDEO 3.5.1

1. Refer to FIGURE 3.17.
2. Examine the external surface of the heart and identify the **coronary (atrioventricular) sulcus** coursing around the circumference of the heart, separating the atria from the ventricles.
3. Identify the **anterior interventricular sulcus** separating the right and left ventricles on the **sternocostal (anterior) surface** of the heart and observe that the right ventricle predominantly forms the anterior surface of the heart. *Note that the interventricular sulci indicate the location of the interventricular septum internally, which lies at a right angle to the coronary sulcus.*
4. On the anterior surface of the heart, identify the **right auricle** extending from the right atrium and the **left auricle** extending from the left atrium.
5. Observe that left ventricle predominantly forms the **diaphragmatic (inferior) surface** of the heart.
6. On the inferior surface of the heart, identify the **opening of the inferior vena cava** and the **posterior interventricular sulcus** running from the apex of the heart to the coronary sulcus. *Note that the coronary arteries and cardiac veins are in the coronary and interventricular sulci.*
7. Observe that the **left pulmonary surface** of the heart is formed mainly by the left ventricle and aligned with the cardiac impression of the left lung.
8. Observe that the **right pulmonary surface** of the heart is formed mainly by the right atrium.
9. Insert a probe into the lumen of the ascending aorta and gently open the **aortic valve** to view the connection of the aorta to the left ventricle through the aortic valve.
10. Identify the **right cusp of the aortic valve** and **opening of the right coronary artery (RCA)** and observe that they are positioned somewhat anteriorly due to the rotation of the vessels during embryonic development.
11. Identify the **left cusp of the aortic valve** and **opening of the left coronary artery (LCA)** and observe that they are positioned somewhat posteriorly (see **Clinical Correlation 3.4**).
12. Identify the **posterior cusp of the aortic valve,** often called the noncoronary cusp as no coronary artery arises in this location, and observe that it lies toward the right border of the heart.
13. Observe that behind each valve cusp is a small pocket called an **aortic sinus** (**right**, **left**, and **posterior,** respectively).
14. Place a probe within the lumen of the pulmonary trunk and gently open the pulmonary valve to view the connection of the pulmonary trunk to the right ventricle.
15. Identify the **right cusp of the pulmonary valve** and observe that it lies somewhat anteriorly in line with the right cusp of the aortic valve.
16. Identify the **left cusp of the pulmonary valve** and observe that it lies somewhat posteriorly in line with the left cusp of the aortic valve.
17. Identify the **anterior cusp of the pulmonary valve** and observe that it lies toward the left border of the heart.
18. Identify the **superior vena cava** on the right side of the heart and observe that it is vertically aligned with the inferior vena cava on the inferior aspect of the right atrium.
19. Identify the openings of the **four pulmonary veins,** two on the right and two on the left, on the posterior surface of the heart draining into the **left atrium**.

CLINICAL CORRELATION 3.4

Myocardial Infarction

ATLAS 3.48

Restricted blood flow to the heart tissue leading to necrosis may occur rapidly, as seen in occlusion of a vessel by an embolus (blood clot), or gradually over time as seen in atherosclerosis, resulting in ischemia. Once the tissue has become necrotic and nonfunctioning, it is classified as having undergone a myocardial infarction (MI), often simply referred to as a "heart attack." The most common procedures to restore blood flow to the affected area are the insertions of stents (tubes placed within the occluded coronary vessel) or coronary bypass grafts (the attachment of a "new vessel," often a vein or the left internal thoracic artery, to both a point before and after the blockage to literally "bypass" the point of blockage). A bypass may be done on a single vessel or on multiple vessels as needed to return blood flow to the heart.

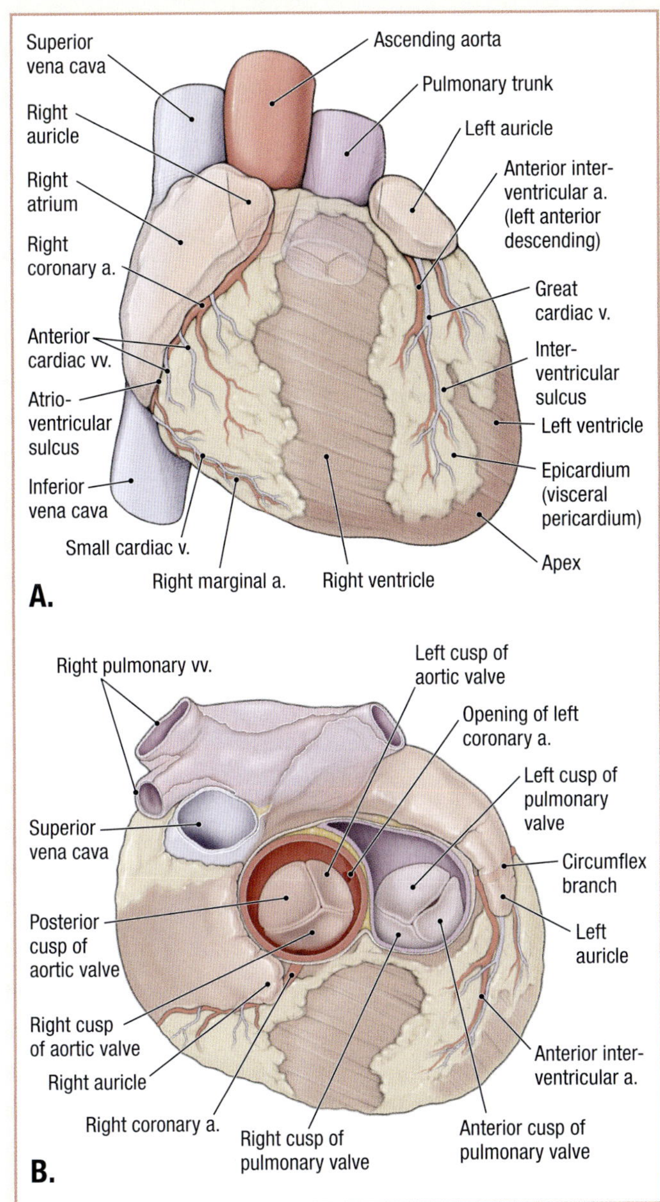

FIGURE 3.17 ● Surface anatomy of heart. **A.** Anterior view. **B.** Superior view.

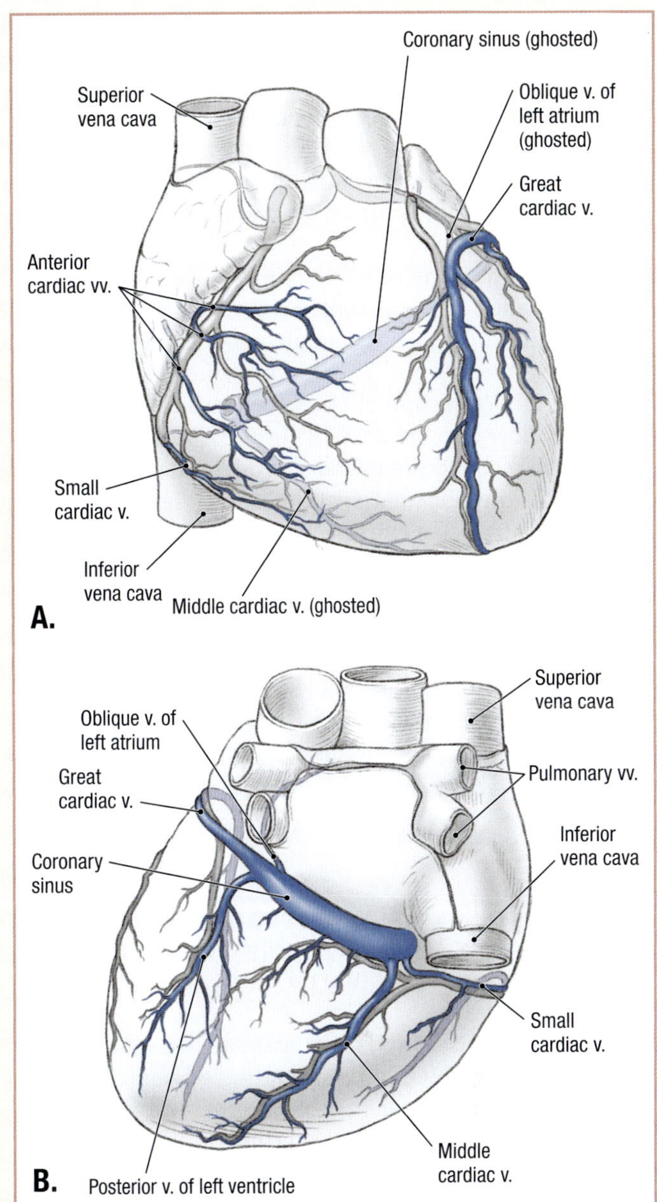

FIGURE 3.18 ● Cardiac veins and coronary sinus. **A.** Anterior view. **B.** Posterior view.

Cardiac Veins

ATLAS 3.49; VIDEO 3.5.2

Dissection Note: As you study the vessels of the heart, realize that they (and the fat that surrounds them) are located between the visceral pericardium (epicardium) and the muscular wall of the heart. Because the cardiac veins course superficial to the coronary arteries, they will be dissected first.

1. Refer to FIGURE 3.18.
2. Identify the **coronary sinus** on the diaphragmatic surface of the heart. Observe that the coronary sinus is a dilated portion of the venous system of the heart located in the coronary sulcus.
3. Use blunt dissection to clean the fat and portions of the epicardium overlying the coronary sinus. Observe that the coronary sinus is about 2 to 2.5 cm in length and opens into the right atrium. *Note that the opening of the coronary sinus will be seen when the internal features of the right atrium are dissected.*
4. Define the borders and surface of the coronary sinus and follow its path around the heart in the coronary sulcus to the point where it receives the **great cardiac vein**.
5. Follow and clean the great cardiac vein onto the sternocostal surface of the heart. Observe that the great cardiac vein often passes deep to the arteries on the anterior aspect of the heart.

6. Clean the great cardiac vein sufficiently to verify its course from the apex of the heart toward the coronary sinus in the anterior interventricular sulcus. *Note that additional veins assist in draining the left ventricle back to the great cardiac vein or coronary sinus.*
7. In the posterior interventricular sulcus, identify and clean the **middle cardiac vein** and trace it to the coronary sinus.
8. Near the location of inferior vena cava, toward the termination of the coronary sinus, identify the **small cardiac vein** coursing laterally around the heart from the right.
9. Use blunt dissection to clean the small cardiac vein and follow it to the anterior surface of the heart where it courses along the inferior border of the heart.
10. On the anterior surface of the heart, identify the **anterior cardiac veins**, which bridge the atrioventricular (AV) sulcus between the right atrium and the right ventricle, and pass superficial to the RCA.
11. Observe that most veins of the heart are tributaries to the coronary sinus with the exception of the anterior cardiac veins, which drain the anterior wall of the right ventricle directly into the right atrium.

Coronary Arteries

ATLAS 3.48, 3.50; VIDEO 3.5.3

1. Refer to FIGURE 3.19.
2. Place a probe within the lumen of the aorta into the left aortic sinus and identify the **opening of the LCA** by inserting the tip of the probe into the opening.
3. On the surface of the heart, palpate the tip of the probe inside the LCA between the left auricle and the pulmonary trunk.
4. Use blunt dissection to clean the LCA, beginning at the ascending aorta for a short distance inferior to the left auricle. Observe that the LCA is quite short and divides into the **anterior interventricular branch** and **circumflex branch** within the coronary sulcus.
5. Use blunt dissection to clean and follow the path of the **anterior interventricular branch** in the anterior interventricular sulcus toward the apex of the heart. Do not disrupt the great cardiac vein. *Note that clinicians call the anterior interventricular branch of the LCA the left anterior descending (LAD) artery.*
6. Use blunt dissection to clean and follow the **circumflex branch of the left coronary artery** in the coronary sulcus around the left side of the heart.
7. Observe that the circumflex branch of the LCA accompanies the coronary sinus in the coronary sulcus and has several branches that supply the wall of the left ventricle.

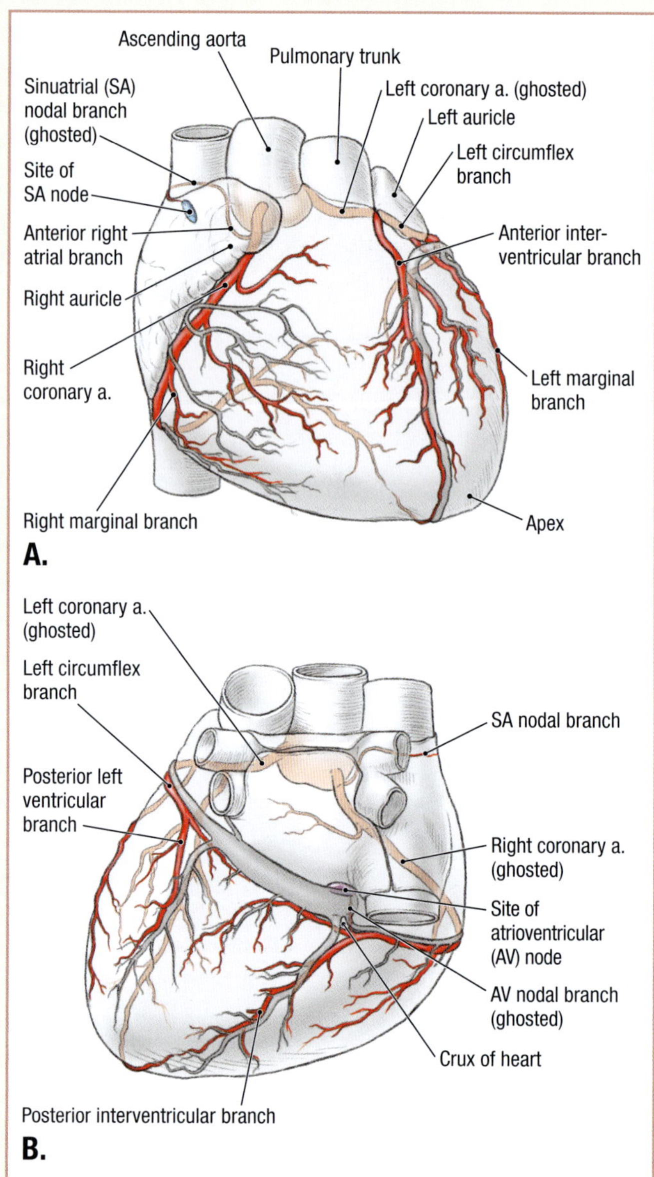

FIGURE 3.19 ● Right and left coronary arteries and branches. **A.** Anterior view. **B.** Posterior view.

8. Place a probe within the lumen of the aorta into the right aortic sinus and identify the **opening of the RCA** by inserting the tip of the probe into the opening.
9. On the surface of the heart, palpate the tip of the probe inside the RCA in the coronary sulcus between the right auricle and ascending aorta.
10. Elevate the right auricle and use blunt dissection to clean the RCA for a short distance.
11. Identify the **sinuatrial (SA) nodal branch**, which arises close to the origin of the RCA and ascends along the anterior wall of the right atrium toward

the superior vena cava to supply the SA node. *Note that the SA nodal branch may be quite small and difficult to find.*

12. Follow the RCA in the coronary sulcus while making efforts to preserve the anterior cardiac veins arching over the artery toward the right atrium.
13. Identify and clean the **right marginal branch** of the RCA, which usually arises near the inferior border of the heart where it accompanies the small cardiac vein.
14. Continue to follow and clean the RCA in the coronary sulcus onto the diaphragmatic (inferior) surface of the heart until it reaches the posterior interventricular sulcus to give rise to the **posterior interventricular branch**, which accompanies the middle cardiac vein.
15. Follow and clean the posterior interventricular branch toward the apex of the heart.
16. Identify the **crux of the heart**, the point where the posterior interventricular sulcus meets the coronary sulcus and observe that the **artery to the AV node** arises from the RCA near this location (see **Clinical Correlation 3.5**).

CLINICAL CORRELATION 3.5

Heart Dominance

ATLAS 3.50, 3.51

Heart dominance refers to the pattern of arterial supply to the heart tissue, predominantly in the left ventricle. Consideration of the branching pattern of a patient's coronary arteries is of clinical importance as these vessels are true end arteries, meaning the region lacks collateral supply from other large branches and thus is at risk if the vessel is occluded or compromised. Compromise of coronary arteries may occur suddenly with an embolus or gradually due to atherosclerosis. Occlusion of the vessels causes chest pain (angina) and may require a bypass or angioplasty to correct arterial flow.

Right dominance (67%) is the most common with the RCA and LCA sharing distribution to the cardiac tissue (FIGURE B3.1). In right dominance, the RCA gives rise to the posterior interventricular branch to supply the left ventricular wall and posterior portion of the interventricular septum. In left dominance (15%), the circumflex branch of the LCA gives rise to the posterior interventricular branch. Other variations in the branching pattern of the coronary vessels may also occur including co-dominance where both the RCA and LCA give rise to branches reaching the crux of the heart, or when the circumflex branch arises from the RCA and not LCA.

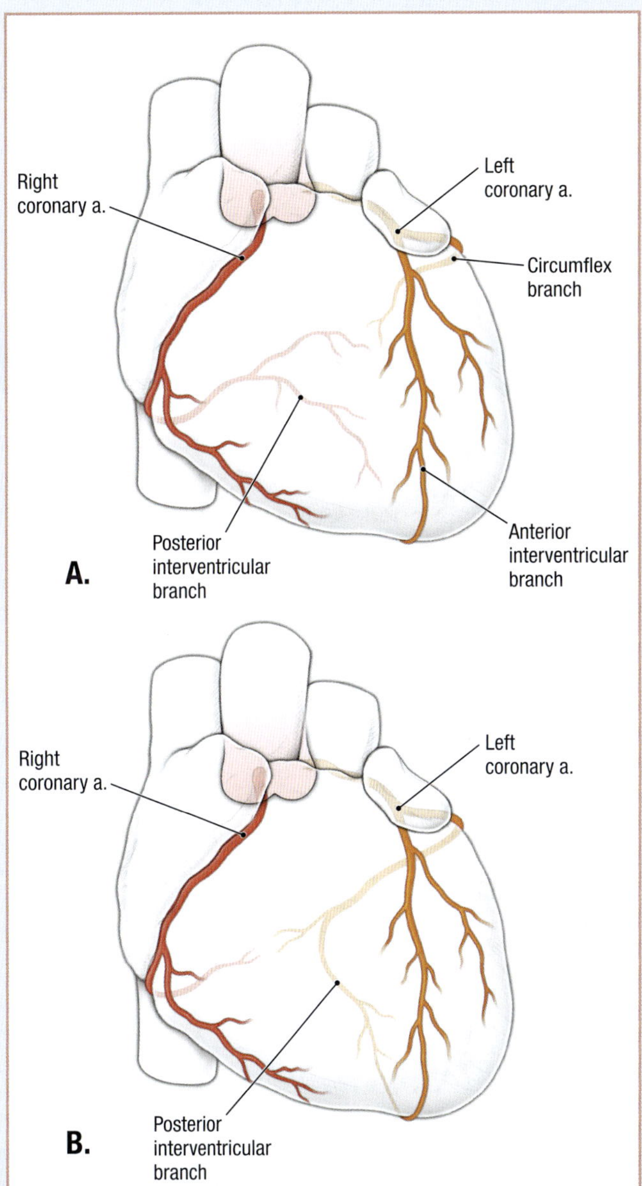

FIGURE B3.1 ● **A.** Right coronary artery dominance. **B.** Left coronary artery dominance. Anterior views.

17. Remove the remaining fat and visceral pericardium from the surface of the heart to better visualize the heart vasculature.

Dissection Follow-up

1. Review the borders and surfaces of the heart.
2. On the surface of the heart, review the boundaries and locations of the four chambers.
3. Review the location of the coronary sulcus and interventricular sulci of the heart and name the vessels that course within them.
4. Trace the path of blood from the right aortic sinus to the coronary sinus, naming all vessels that are involved.
5. Trace the path of blood from the left aortic sinus to the apex of the heart and follow the venous return to the coronary sinus, naming all vessels that are involved.
6. Return the heart to the pericardial cavity and position all reflected tissue back to anatomical position.

INTERNAL FEATURES OF HEART

Dissection Overview

Cardiac muscle tissue within the walls of the heart is regulated by the conducting system of the heart. The "pacemaker" of the heart is the SA node located within the wall of the right atrium near the superior vena cava at the superior end of the crista terminalis. Impulses from the SA node pass through the wall of the right atrium to the AV node, which then pass in the AV bundle through the membranous part of the interventricular septum. Subsequently, the AV bundle divides into right and left bundles, which lie within the muscular part of the interventricular septum and stimulate the ventricles to contract via Purkinje fibers.

Corresponding to the relaxation and contraction of the chambers of the heart, blood passes through the heart from the right atrium to the right ventricle to reach the lungs. After receiving oxygen from the lungs, the blood returns to the heart via the left atrium to then pass to the left ventricle to pump to the heart itself and remainder of the body. The cuts that will be performed to investigate the chambers of the heart are designed to preserve most of the vessels that have previously been dissected on the surface of the heart.

The order of dissection will be as follows: The right atrium will be opened, and the internal features examined. The right ventricle will be opened, and the internal features examined. The left atrium will be opened, and the internal features examined. The left ventricle will be opened, and the internal features examined.

Dissection Instructions

Dissection Note: Remove the heart from the dissection field to perform the following dissection sequence leaving the remainder of the thorax covered to prevent desiccation of the tissue. The chambers of the heart will contain clotted blood that must be removed to study their internal features more clearly. The clots will be hard and may need to be broken before they can be extracted. Observe the lab rules and regulations for discarding the clotted blood in the proper tissue containers.

Right Atrium

ATLAS 3.43A, 3.54; VIDEO 3.6.1

1. Refer to FIGURE 3.20.
2. Gently elevate the right auricle with a pair of forceps and use scissors to make a cut through its free edge along the superior border. Insert one blade of the scissors through the opening and make a short horizontal cut toward the right, below the junction of the superior vena cava and the right atrium (**Cut 1**).

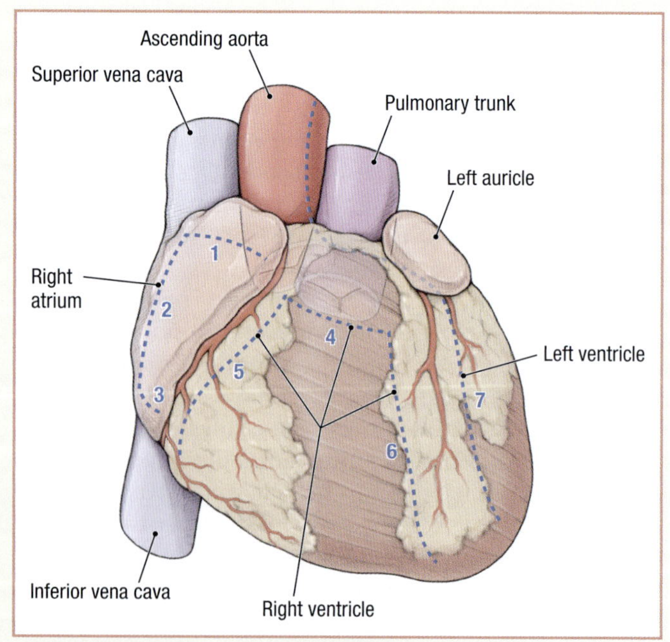

FIGURE 3.20 ● Incisions to open heart chambers. Anterior view.

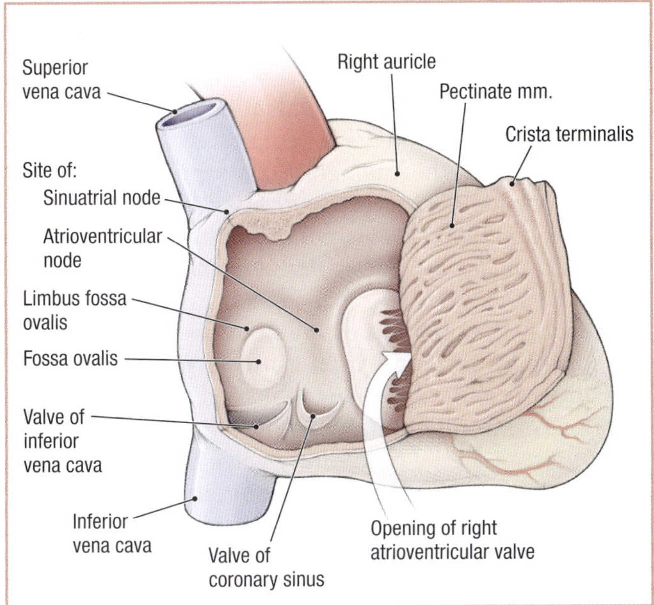

FIGURE 3.21 ● Internal features of right atrium. Anterior view.

3. At the right extent of the horizontal incision through the right atrium (**Cut 1**), make a vertical incision through the lateral edge of the right atrium, stopping superior to the junction with the inferior vena cava (**Cut 2**).
4. At the inferior extent of the vertical incision through the right atrium (**Cut 2**), make a short horizontal cut toward the left, stopping just short of the coronary sulcus (**Cut 3**).
5. Refer to FIGURE 3.21.
6. Use a pair of forceps to grasp the free edge of the flap of atrial wall and gently pull it to the left to open the right atrium widely.
7. Remove the blood clots from the right atrium using forceps and, if permitted, take the heart to the sink to rinse the right atrium with water.
8. On the inner surface of the **anterior wall of the right atrium**, identify the **pectinate muscles** forming horizontal ridges directed at the **crista terminalis**, a vertical ridge of muscle connecting the pectinate muscle fibers.
9. On the superior aspect of the right atrium, identify the **opening of the superior vena cava**.
10. Identify the **opening** and **valve of the inferior vena cava** on the inferior aspect of the right atrium.
11. On the posterior wall of the right atrium, identify the **opening** and **valve of the coronary sinus**. Insert a probe into the opening of the coronary sinus and verify its location within the coronary sulcus.
12. On the medial aspect of the right atrium, identify the **fossa ovalis**, a small depression on the **interatrial septum**, and observe its relative location inferior to the thickened ridge of the **limbus fossa ovalis** (see **Clinical Correlation 3.6**).

CLINICAL CORRELATION 3.6

Septal Defects

ATLAS 3.54

Developmental defects may occur in the interatrial or interventricular septa. Atrial septal defects (ASDs) usually relate to incomplete closure of the foramen ovale, a shunt in fetal circulation allowing the oxygen- and nutrient-rich blood from the placenta to pass from the right atrium to the left atrium without passing through the developing lungs. Small ASDs are quite common and often clinically insignificant. Large ASDs allow oxygen-rich blood from the lungs to pass from the left atrium to the right atrium leading to increased pressure and enlargement of the right atrium, right ventricle, and pulmonary trunk.

Ventricular septal defects (VSDs) typically occur in the membranous portion of the septum and often relate to other anomalies near the base of the pulmonary trunk or aorta due to common embryological origin of these tissues. VSDs are one of the most common congenital anomalies and of significant concern as they allow for a left-to-right shunting of blood between the ventricles resulting in pulmonary hypertension or heart failure.

13. Parts of the conducting system of the heart are in the walls of the right atrium but cannot be seen in dissection. *Note that the SA node lies at the superior end of the crista terminalis at the junction between the right atrium and the superior vena cava, whereas the AV node is in the interatrial septum superior to the opening of the coronary sinus.*
14. Identify the opening of the **right AV valve** leading to the right ventricle and use a probe to observe the path of blood from the right atrium to the right ventricle.

Right Ventricle

ATLAS 3.43, 3.55; VIDEO 3.6.2

1. Refer back to FIGURE 3.20.
2. Use a probe or finger to determine the level of the **pulmonary valve** in the pulmonary trunk.
3. Use sharp dissection to make a short horizontal cut through the **anterior wall of the right ventricle** immediately inferior to the level of the pulmonary valve (**Cut 4**).
4. Make an incision about 1 cm away from the coronary sulcus beginning at the right end of horizontal incision (**Cut 4**) superiorly and ending at the margin of the right ventricle inferiorly (**Cut 5**). While making the cut, verify the thickness of the ventricular wall to

ensure the cusps of the AV valve are not cut on the deep surface.

5. Insert your finger through the opening in the ventricular wall and palpate the **interventricular septum** using the LAD as a guide.
6. From the left end of the horizontal incision (**Cut 4**), make a cut toward the apex of the heart about 2 cm to the right of the anterior interventricular sulcus parallel to the right side of the interventricular septum, to a level just above the right margin of the heart (**Cut 6**).
7. Refer to FIGURE 3.22.
8. Reflect the cut portion of the right ventricular wall inferiorly.
9. Within the right ventricle, use forceps to carefully remove blood clots. Once the clots have been removed, gently rinse the right ventricle with water to remove any remaining loose material.
10. Identify the **opening of the right AV (tricuspid) valve** and observe that it has **three cusps: anterior**, **septal**, and **posterior**, which are named for their respective locations.
11. Identify the **chordae tendineae** and observe that these delicate tendons pass from the valve cusps to the apices of **papillary muscles** arising from the walls of the right ventricle.
12. Identify the **three papillary muscles** beginning with the **anterior papillary muscle**, which is the largest and easiest to identify. The **septal papillary muscle** is very small and may actually be multiple smaller muscles arising from the interventricular septum, whereas the **posterior papillary muscle** lies deep within the chamber. *Note that the chordae tendineae of each papillary muscle attach to the adjacent sides of two valve cusps.*
13. Identify the **trabeculae carneae**, the roughened muscular ridges on the inner surface of the wall of the right ventricle.
14. Identify the **septomarginal trabecula (moderator band)** near the inferior extent of the right ventricle arching from the interventricular septum to the base of the anterior papillary muscle. *Note that the septomarginal trabecula contains the part of the right bundle of the conducting system that stimulates the anterior papillary muscle.*
15. Identify the **opening of the pulmonary trunk** superiorly within the right ventricle and observe the smooth cone-shaped region named the **conus arteriosus (infundibulum)** inferior to the opening.
16. Observe that the **pulmonary valve** consists of **three semilunar cusps: anterior**, **right**, and **left**.
17. Look into the pulmonary trunk from a superior view and examine the superior surface of the pulmonary valve. Observe that each semilunar valve cusp has one fibrous **nodule** and two **lunules**, which help to seal the valve cusps and prevent backflow of blood during diastole.

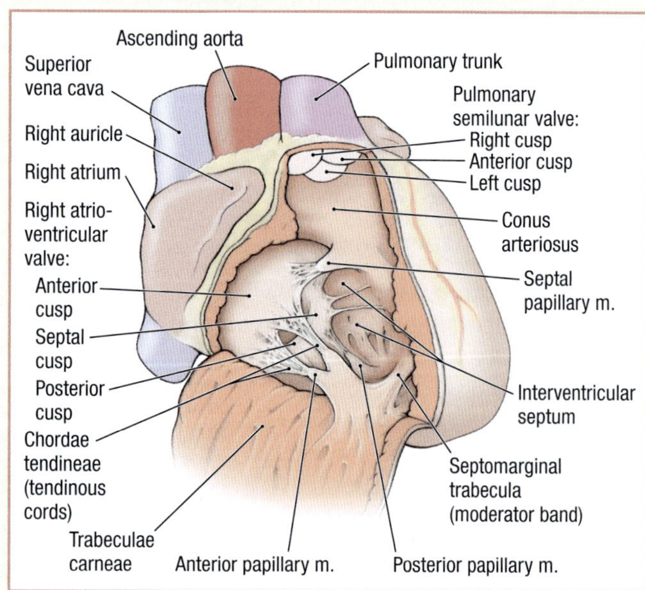

FIGURE 3.22 ● Internal features of right ventricle. Anterolateral view.

Left Atrium

ATLAS 3.46A, 3.56; VIDEO 3.6.3

1. Refer to FIGURE 3.23.
2. Examine the posterior surface of the heart and identify the openings of the **four pulmonary veins** into the left atrium. The pulmonary veins are usually

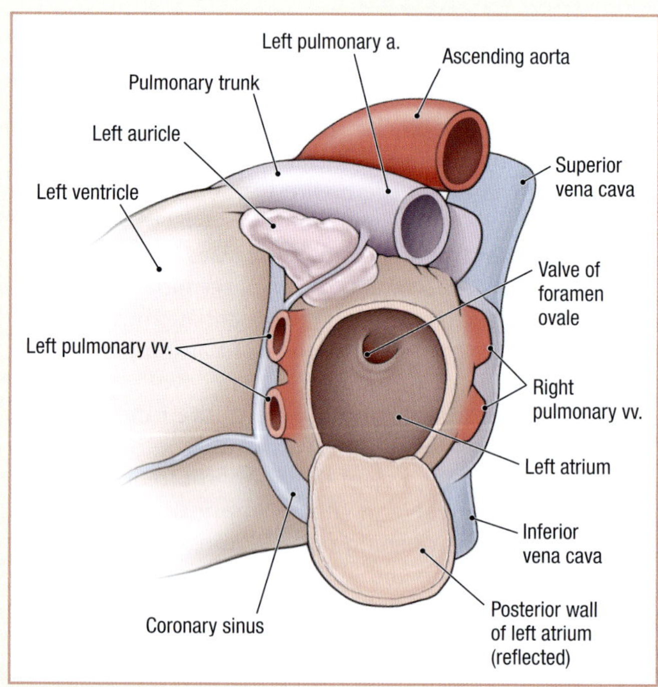

FIGURE 3.23 ● Internal features of left atrium. Posterolateral view.

arranged in pairs: two from the right lung and two from the left lung.
3. Use scissors to make an inverted U-shaped cut through the posterior wall of the left atrium using the openings of the pulmonary veins as reference points laterally.
4. Use a pair of forceps to grasp the free edge of the flap and gently pull it inferiorly.
5. Remove the large blood clots within the left atrium and then gently rinse out any remaining clots with water.
6. Identify the **opening into the left auricle**, observing that its inner surface is covered with pectinate muscle, while the rest of the inner surface of the left atrium is smooth.
7. Identify the **valve of the foramen ovale** on the **interatrial septum** in the left atrium.
8. Place your finger on the surface of the interatrial septum within the left atrium and your thumb on the surface of the interatrial septum within the right atrium and verify the relative thinness of the fossa ovalis compared to the rest of the interatrial septum.
9. Identify the **opening of the left AV valve** and use a probe to observe the path of blood from the left atrium to the left ventricle.

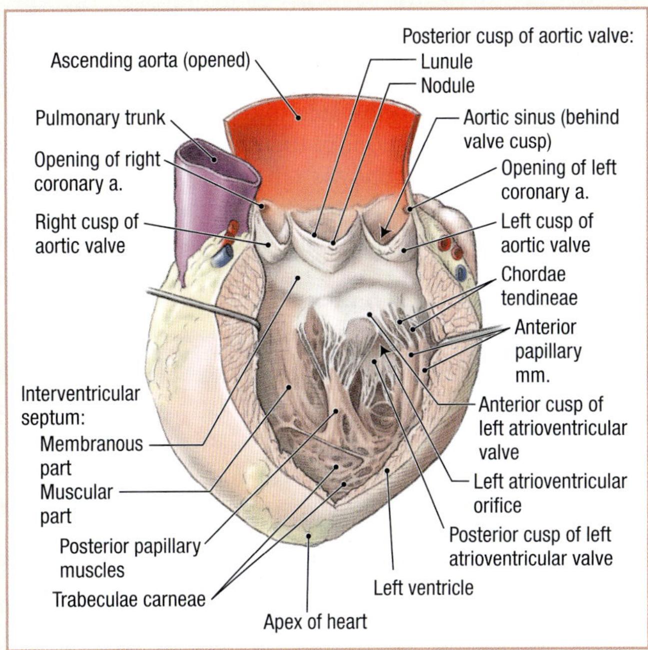

FIGURE 3.24 ■ Internal features of left ventricle. Oblique anterior view.

Left Ventricle

ATLAS 3.56, 3.57; VIDEO 3.6.4

Dissection Note: The following procedure will cut the anterior interventricular branch of the LCA and the great cardiac vein. Alternate approaches may be taken to spare these vessels.

1. Refer back to FIGURE 3.20.
2. Look into the aorta from a superior view and identify the **aortic valve** and its **three semilunar valve cusps: right**, **left**, and **posterior**.
3. Insert one blade of the scissors between the left and right semilunar cusps and make a cut inferiorly through the anterior wall of the ascending aorta anterior and parallel to the LCA (**Cut 7**).
4. Cut through the junction of the ascending aorta and left ventricle and bisect the anterior interventricular branch of the LCA and the great cardiac vein.
5. Continue the cut to the apex of the heart about 2 cm to the left of the anterior interventricular sulcus, making it parallel to the left side of the interventricular septum.
6. Refer to FIGURE 3.24.
7. Open the left ventricle and the ascending aorta widely.
8. Use forceps to carefully remove blood clots in the left ventricle. Once the majority of clots have been removed, gently rinse the left ventricle with water to remove the remaining clots.
9. In the left ventricle, identify the **left AV valve (bicuspid valve, mitral valve)**. Distinguish the **anterior cusp** from the **posterior cusp**.
10. Identify the **anterior papillary muscle** and the **posterior papillary muscle** and observe that the **chordae tendineae** of each papillary muscle attach to both valve cusps.
11. Observe that the inner surface of the wall of the left ventricle is roughened by **trabeculae carneae**.
12. Examine the split **aortic valve** and identify its **right**, **left**, and **posterior semilunar cusps**, observing that each has one nodule and two lunules.
13. Superior to the aortic valve, identify the openings of the **coronary arteries** and study their relationship to the semilunar valve cusps and the **aortic sinuses**. *Note that the posterior cusp is also called the noncoronary cusp because there is no coronary artery arising from its sinus.*
14. Palpate the **muscular part of the interventricular septum** and observe its thickness by placing the thumb of your right hand in the right ventricle and your index finger in the left ventricle.
15. Move your thumb and index finger superiorly along the interventricular septum and palpate the thin **membranous part of the interventricular septum** inferior to the attachment of the right cusp of the aortic valve.

Dissection Follow-up

1. Review the internal features of each of the chambers of the heart.
2. Review the course of blood as it passes through the chambers and valves of the heart beginning in the superior vena cava and ending in the ascending aorta.
3. Review the connections of the great vessels to the various chambers of the heart.
4. Review the conducting system of the heart.
5. Return the heart to the thorax and place the anterior thoracic wall in anatomical position.
6. Locate the auscultation point for each heart valve on the anterior thoracic wall.

SUPERIOR MEDIASTINUM

Dissection Overview

The superior mediastinum is located superior to the plane connecting the sternal angle anteriorly and T4/T5 IV disc posteriorly. The superior mediastinum contains structures passing between the thorax and neck, the thorax and upper limb, or the thorax and abdomen. The superior mediastinum contains portions of the great vessels with their branches, the thymus, trachea, esophagus, thoracic duct, vagus nerve, phrenic nerves, and cardiac plexus.

The order of dissection will be as follows: The brachiocephalic veins will be cleaned and studied to expose the aortic arch. The aortic arch and the proximal ends of its branches will be identified and cleaned. The trachea and its bifurcation will be studied. The portion of the esophagus in the superior mediastinum will be identified along with the vagus nerves.

Dissection Instructions

Superior Mediastinum

ATLAS 3.60, 3.61, 3.63; VIDEO 3.7.1

1. Refer back to FIGURE 3.13.
2. Review the **boundaries of the superior mediastinum** beginning superiorly with the **superior boundary** of the superior thoracic aperture and the **inferior boundary** of the plane intersecting the sternal angle and T4/T5 IV disc. The **anterior boundary** is the manubrium of the sternum, and **posterior boundary** is the bodies of vertebrae T1–T4. The **lateral boundaries** of the superior mediastinum are the right and left mediastinal pleurae.
3. Remove the anterior thoracic wall.
4. Identify the **thymus**, an organized fatty mass that lies immediately posterior to the manubrium of the sternum. The thymus can be recognized in the cadaver by the thymic veins on its posterior surface which drain to the brachiocephalic veins. *Note that the thymus may be absent or difficult to identify in the adult; however, in the newborn, it is an active lymphatic organ that can be easily visualized on a chest radiograph.*
5. Reflect the infrahyoid muscles superiorly, the thin layer of muscles extending from the neck into the superior aspect of the superior mediastinum.
6. If present, remove the thymus from the superior mediastinum.
7. Refer to FIGURE 3.25.
8. Identify and clean the **superior vena cava** and follow it superiorly until its two tributaries, the **left and right brachiocephalic veins**, are visible. *Note that the two brachiocephalic veins meet to form the superior vena cava posterior to the inferior border of the right 1st costal cartilage.*
9. Use blunt dissection to clean the left and right brachiocephalic veins and free them from the structures that lie posteriorly.
10. Follow the superior vena cava inferiorly and observe that it passes anterior to the superior aspect of the root of the right lung.
11. Identify and clean the superior aspect of **azygos vein** on the right side of the mediastinum.
12. Identify the **arch of the azygos vein** and observe that it passes superior to the root of the right lung to drain into the posterior aspect of the superior vena cava.
13. Cut the left brachiocephalic vein just lateral to where it drains into the superior vena cava and reflect it superiorly and to the left. Reflect the superior vena cava and attached right brachiocephalic and azygos veins to the right.
14. Identify the **right** and **left phrenic nerves** where they were previously dissected in the middle mediastinum. Recall that the phrenic nerves pass anterior to the roots of the right and left lungs.
15. Follow the phrenic nerves superiorly and observe that they pass posterior to the brachiocephalic veins.
16. Clean the phrenic nerves from the level of the thoracic inlet to where they enter the superior surface of the diaphragm along with accompanying pericardiacophrenic vessels.
17. Identify and clean the **arch of the aorta** and observe that it begins and ends at the level of the sternal angle.

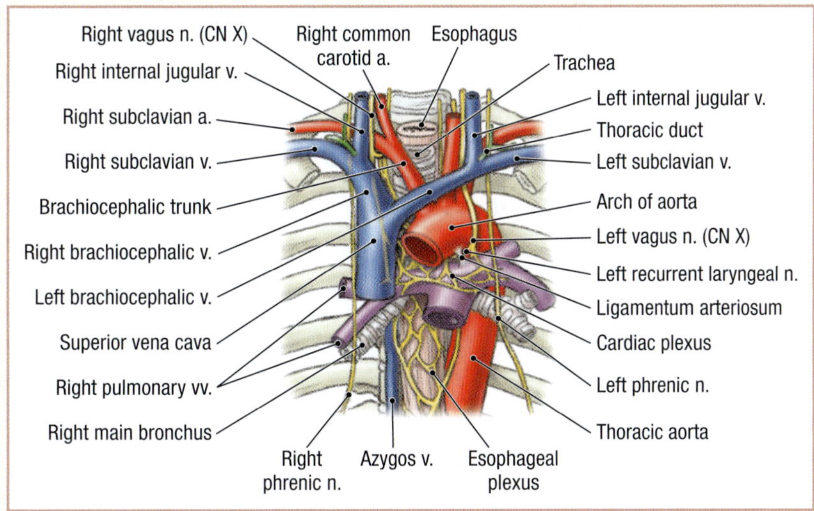

FIGURE 3.25 ■ Contents of superior mediastinum. Anterior view.

18. On the superior aspect of the arch of the aorta, identify and clean its branches from anterior to posterior, the **brachiocephalic trunk**, **left common carotid artery**, and **left subclavian artery**.
19. Identify the ligamentum arteriosum, the fibrous cord connecting the concavity of the arch of the aorta to the left pulmonary artery. *Note that the ligamentum arteriosum is the remnant of the ductus arteriosus, a fetal shunt diverting blood to the aorta from the outflow to the lungs.*

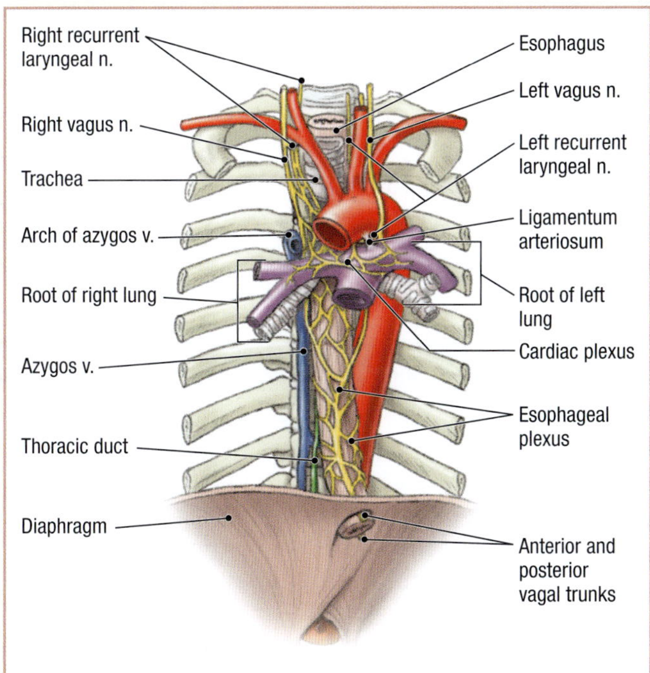

FIGURE 3.26 ■ Branches of arch of aorta with brachiocephalic veins removed. Anterior view.

20. Identify the **left vagus nerve** and **left recurrent laryngeal nerve** on the left side of the arch of the aorta. Observe that the left recurrent laryngeal nerve passes posterior to the ligamentum arteriosum as it loops around the arch of the aorta.
21. Follow and clean the left vagus nerve inferiorly as it passes posterior to the root of the left lung toward the **esophagus**.
22. Refer to FIGURE 3.26.
23. On the right side of the superior mediastinum, observe that the **right vagus nerve** passes posterior to the root of the right lung toward the esophagus.
24. Identify and clean the inferior aspect of the **right recurrent laryngeal nerve**, a branch of the right vagus nerve, where it loops around the right subclavian artery (see **Clinical Correlation 3.7**). *Note that if the right upper limb has not been dissected, the right subclavian artery will not be readily visible.*

CLINICAL CORRELATION 3.7

Recurrent Laryngeal Nerve Injury

ATLAS 3.60, 3.63

The recurrent laryngeal nerves innervate the intrinsic muscles of the larynx except for the cricothyroid and are thus responsible for proper vocal function. Compression of the recurrent laryngeal nerves may result in paralysis of the vocal folds and hoarseness, a possible clinical symptom for disease processes at the root of the neck or superior mediastinum. The left recurrent laryngeal nerve has a close relationship to the aortic arch as it passes through the superior mediastinum and may be compressed or stretched due to mediastinal tumors from bronchial or esophageal carcinoma, enlarged lymph nodes, or an aortic arch aneurysm.

25. Identify the **trachea** near the midline in the superior mediastinum.
26. At the plane of the sternal angle, identify the **bifurcation of the trachea** into the **right main bronchus** and **left main bronchus**. Use blunt dissection to clean the bifurcation of the trachea and main bronchi and identify any **tracheobronchial lymph nodes** if present.
27. Observe that the arch of the azygos vein passes superior to the right main bronchus and the arch of the aorta passes superior to the left main bronchus.
28. Palpate the trachea near its bifurcation and identify the C-shaped **tracheal cartilaginous rings**. *Note that the open part of the "C" is directed posteriorly, with the posterior aspects connected by the trachealis.*
29. Observe that the esophagus is located posterior to the trachea in close relationship to the open part of the tracheal cartilages.
30. Observe that the right main bronchus is typically larger in diameter, shorter, and oriented more vertically than the left main bronchus.
31. Carefully make an inverted "Y"-shaped cut following the branching pattern of the main bronchi. Observe that inside the trachea, at the inferior border of the tracheal bifurcation, is a ridge of cartilage called the **carina** (see **Clinical Correlation 3.8**).

CLINICAL CORRELATION 3.8

Bronchoscopy

ATLAS 3.36

A bronchoscopy is an endoscopic technique to visualize the internal features of the trachea and bronchi for diagnosis and treatment. The carina serves as an important landmark to locate the termination of the trachea and superior ends of the right and left main bronchi. The carina is usually positioned slightly to the left of the median plane of the trachea. The carina may shift due to enlarged tracheobronchial lymph nodes and appear wider, pushed posteriorly, or be immobile on examination. When food or foreign bodies are aspirated, they usually enter the right main bronchus because it is wider and more vertically oriented than the left main bronchus.

32. Identify and clean the pulmonary trunk to its bifurcation point into the **right and left pulmonary arteries**.
33. Observe that the right pulmonary artery passes posterior to the superior vena cava and that the left pulmonary artery passes anterior to the **descending (thoracic) aorta**.

Dissection Follow-up

1. Review the tributaries of the superior vena cava and position of the arch of the azygos vein.
2. Review the position of the ascending aorta, the arch of the aorta, and its branches.
3. Compare the positions of the phrenic and vagus nerves relative to the root of the lung.
4. Compare the course of the right and left recurrent laryngeal nerves and relate these differences to the embryonic origin of the associated arteries.
5. Replace the contents of the superior mediastinum into their correct anatomical positions.
6. Return the anterior thoracic wall to its correct anatomical position and project the structures of the superior mediastinum to the surface of the thoracic wall.

POSTERIOR MEDIASTINUM

Dissection Overview

The posterior mediastinum lies posterior to the pericardium and contains structures that course between the neck and thorax and between the thorax and abdomen. To emphasize their close relationship to the heart, the structures in the posterior mediastinum will be approached through the posterior wall of the pericardium. The posterior mediastinum contains the thoracic aorta, thoracic duct, azygos and hemiazygos veins, lymph nodes, and autonomic branches.

The order of dissection will be as follows: The pericardium will be reviewed, and its posterior wall removed. The esophagus will be studied. The azygos vein and its tributaries will be studied. The thoracic duct will be identified. The descending aorta and its branches will be dissected. The thoracic portion of the sympathetic trunk and its branches will be dissected.

Dissection Instructions

Posterior Mediastinum

ATLAS 3.46B, 3.46C, 3.69, 3.70; VIDEO 3.8.1

1. Refer back to FIGURE 3.13.
2. Review the **boundaries of the posterior mediastinum** beginning superiorly with its **superior boundary** at the plane of the sternal angle and its **inferior boundary** at the diaphragm. The **anterior boundary** is the pericardium, and its posterior boundary is the bodies of vertebrae T5–T12. The **lateral boundaries** of the posterior mediastinum are the right and left mediastinal pleurae.
3. Place the heart in the pericardial cavity and observe that the esophagus lies immediately posterior to the left atrium and part of the left ventricle.
4. Remove the heart from the pericardial cavity.
5. Identify the cut edge of the mediastinal parietal pleura and follow it further posteriorly until it contacts the sides of the vertebral bodies where it transitions to **costal parietal pleura**.
6. Detach the costal parietal pleura in the midaxillary line near the cut ends of ribs 1 to 5 and peel the pleura off the inner surface of the posterior thoracic wall, moving from lateral to medial. Observe that the **endothoracic fascia** provides a natural cleavage plane for separation of costal parietal pleura from the thoracic wall.
7. Remove the costal parietal pleura up to the point where it covers the vertebral column.
8. From the right side of the thorax, use blunt dissection from a lateral approach to gently separate the esophagus from the posterior aspect of the pericardium.
9. Refer to FIGURE 3.27.
10. Use scissors to carefully make a vertical cut through the posterior wall of the pericardium in the oblique pericardial sinus.
11. Spread the cut edges of the posterior wall of the pericardium and identify the **esophagus**, the muscular tube to the right of the midline.
12. Identify the **thoracic (descending) aorta** on the left side of the thorax slightly posterior to the esophagus coursing inferiorly through the posterior mediastinum.
13. Use blunt dissection to elevate and reflect the remainder of the posterior wall of the pericardium, leaving the portion adhering to the diaphragm undisturbed.
14. Use scissors to cut the pericardium near its attachments to the great vessels and diaphragm and place the pericardium in the tissue container.
15. Use blunt dissection to clean the **esophagus** and observe that its surface is covered by the **esophageal plexus of nerves** innervating the inferior portion of the esophagus.

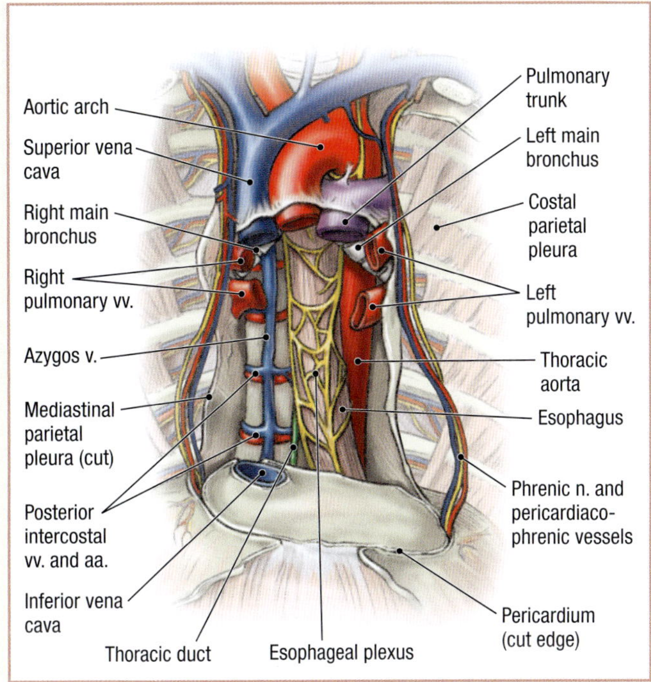

FIGURE 3.27 ● Contents of posterior mediastinum. Anterior view.

16. Locate the **left vagus nerve** on the left side of the arch of the aorta and use blunt dissection to demonstrate that the fibers of the left vagus nerve spread out on the anterior surface of the esophagus to contribute to the esophageal plexus.
17. Locate the **right vagus nerve** where it courses through the superior mediastinum and use blunt dissection to demonstrate that it spreads out on the posterior surface of the esophagus to contribute to the esophageal plexus.
18. Observe that the esophageal plexus condenses to form the **anterior vagal trunk** on the anterior surface of the esophagus and the **posterior vagal trunk** on the posterior surface of the esophagus, just superior to the esophageal hiatus in the diaphragm. *Note that due to the curvature of the diaphragm, the vagal trunks may not be visible at this stage of the dissection.*
19. Identify the **azygos vein** where it arches superior to the root of the right lung and follow it inferiorly to the level of the diaphragm.
20. Refer to FIGURE 3.28.
21. Clean the azygos vein on the right side of the thorax as well as the **posterior intercostal veins** which drain into it.
22. Retract the esophagus to the left and explore the area between the **azygos vein** and the **thoracic aorta** to identify the **thoracic duct**, which has the appearance of a small vein without blood in it.

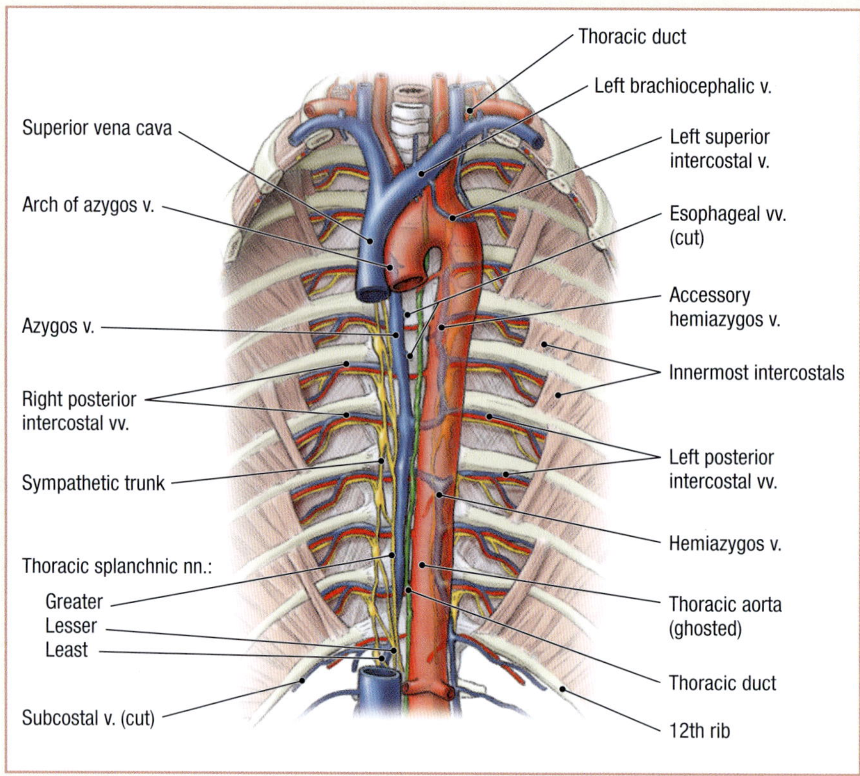

FIGURE 3.28 ■ Azygos system and sympathetic trunk. Anterior view.

23. Use blunt dissection to clean the thoracic duct, paying attention as it is thin walled and easily torn. *Note that the thoracic duct may be a network of several smaller ducts instead of a single duct posterior to the esophagus.*
24. Follow the thoracic duct inferiorly to where it passes through the diaphragm with the thoracic aorta.
25. Observe that the thoracic duct crosses the anterior surface of the right posterior intercostal arteries, the hemiazygos vein, and the accessory hemiazygos vein. *Note that superiorly, the thoracic duct terminates by draining into the left venous angle, the junction of the left internal jugular vein and left subclavian vein. Do not attempt to demonstrate its superior termination at this time.*
26. On the left side of the posterior thorax, clean the **hemiazygos vein** inferiorly and the **accessory hemiazygos vein** superiorly. Identify and clean a few posterior intercostal veins that drain into the azygos system.
27. Follow the accessory hemiazygos and hemiazygos veins across the T8 and T9 vertebral bodies, respectively, and observe that they terminate by draining into the azygos vein. *Note that variations of the azygos system are common.*
28. Examine the branches of the **thoracic aorta.** Identify and clean the **esophageal arteries** on the deep surface of the esophagus and the **left bronchial arteries** coursing along the main bronchi (if visible). *Note that the left bronchial arteries arise from the anterior surface of the aorta, whereas the right bronchial arteries may arise from intercostal arteries, the thoracic aorta, or the left bronchial arteries and are distinguished by their area of distribution.*
29. Dissect one pair of **posterior intercostal arteries** (right and left) and follow them to their intercostal space. Observe that the right posterior intercostal arteries cross the midline on the anterior surface of the vertebral bodies and pass posterior to all other contents of the posterior mediastinum.
30. On both sides of the thorax, identify and clean an **intercostal nerve** and follow it laterally until it disappears posterior to the **innermost intercostal muscle.**
31. On both sides of the thorax, identify the **sympathetic trunk (chain).**
32. Starting superiorly in the thorax, clean and follow the sympathetic trunk inferiorly and observe that it crosses the heads of ribs 2 to 9.
33. Inferior to rib 9, observe that the sympathetic trunk courses anteriorly to lie on the sides of the thoracic vertebral bodies.
34. Observe that the sympathetic trunk has one **sympathetic ganglion** for each thoracic vertebral level.
35. Demonstrate that two **rami communicantes (white ramus communicans** and **gray ramus communicans)** connect each intercostal nerve with its

corresponding thoracic sympathetic ganglion. *Note that white rami are myelinated and contain presynaptic sympathetic axons. During dissection, it is not possible to distinguish white and gray rami from each other based on appearance; however, the more lateral of the two rami is the white ramus communicans.*

36. Use blunt dissection to clean the contributions to the **greater splanchnic nerves** arising from the sympathetic trunk at vertebral levels T5–T9 bilaterally and observe that the greater splanchnic nerves are not completely formed until lower thoracic levels.
37. The **lesser splanchnic nerves** arise from the sympathetic trunk at vertebral levels T10–T11 and the **least splanchnic nerves** from T12 bilaterally. Due to the curvature of the diaphragm, these two pairs of nerves cannot be easily seen at this time.

Dissection Follow-up

1. Review the boundaries of the anterior, middle, and posterior mediastina.
2. Study a transverse section through the midlevel of the thorax and identify the contents of the posterior mediastinum and observe the relationship of the contents of the posterior mediastinum to the heart and vertebral bodies.
3. Review the course and distribution of an intercostal nerve.
4. Review the parts of the aorta (ascending, arch, and thoracic), naming all branches derived from each region and their areas of distribution.
5. Review the origin and course of the right and left posterior intercostal arteries.
6. Name the structures in the posterior mediastinum that cross anterior to the right posterior intercostal arteries.
7. Replace the contents of the posterior mediastinum, the heart, the lungs, and the anterior thoracic wall to anatomical position.

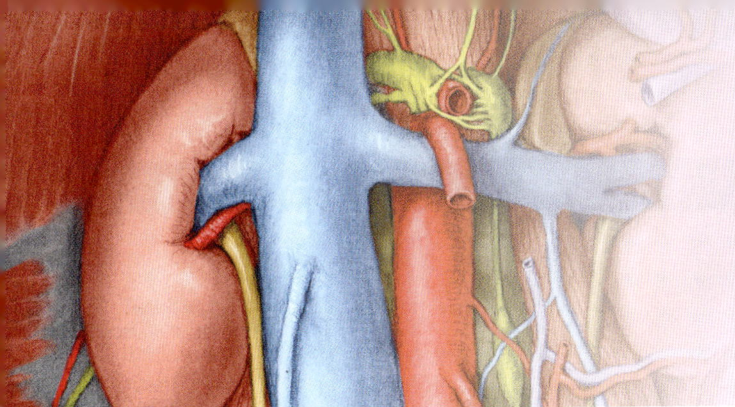

CHAPTER 4
Abdomen

REFERENCES	
ATLAS = *Grant's Atlas of Anatomy*, 16th ed., figure number	VIDEO = *Grant's Dissection Videos*, video sequence number

The abdomen is the central portion of the trunk between the thorax and pelvis. Superiorly, the abdominal cavity is physically divided from the thoracic cavity by the diaphragm. Inferiorly, the abdominal cavity is continuous with the pelvic cavity, and thus, the two regions are commonly referred to as the abdominopelvic cavity. As the abdominal organs (viscera) are not bilaterally symmetrical, it is worth noting that use of the words "right" and "left" in names and instructions refers to the right and left sides of the cadaver in anatomical position.

The contents of the abdominal cavity are partially protected by the thoracic cage, a muscular abdominal wall, anterolaterally, and by the vertebral column, lower ribs, and pelvic bones posteriorly. Although the muscular anterolateral abdominal wall offers less protection than the thoracic cage, it adds the benefit of increased range of motion along with the ability to increase intraabdominal pressure to assist in voiding of the bowels, vomiting, childbirth, and respiration.

CLINICAL CORRELATIONS

During your dissection protocol, you may encounter anatomical variations, clinical conditions, disease processes, or medical devices in your cadaveric donor. The following select clinical correlations will be described in more detail throughout this chapter.

Abdomen

4.1. Caput Medusae, see the **Subcutaneous Tissue of Abdomen** sequence. ATLAS 4.7
4.2. Epigastric Artery Anastomoses, see the **Epigastric Vessels and Deep Inguinal Ring** sequence. ATLAS 4.5
4.3. Inguinal Hernias, see the **Anterior Abdominal Wall** sequence. ATLAS 4.18
4.4. Lacerated Spleen and Splenomegaly, see the **Spleen** sequence. ATLAS 4.35
4.5. Liver Enlargement, see the **Liver** sequence. ATLAS 4.50, 4.54
4.6. Cystic Artery Variants, see the **Gallbladder** sequence. ATLAS 4.57A, 4.62
4.7. Appendicitis, see the **Midgut Derivatives** sequence. ATLAS 4.43
4.8. Superior Mesenteric Artery Syndrome, see the **Superior Mesenteric Artery and Vein** sequence. ATLAS 4.68
4.9. Portal Hypertension, see the **Hepatic Portal Vein** sequence. ATLAS 4.66
4.10. Testicular Varicocele, see the **Retroperitoneal Vasculature** sequence. ATLAS 4.19, 4.68
4.11. Kidney Stones, see the **Kidneys** sequence. ATLAS 4.72
4.12. Suprarenal Gland Development, see the **Suprarenal Glands** sequence. ATLAS 4.70
4.13. Diaphragmatic Hernias and Paralysis, see the **Diaphragm** sequence. ATLAS 4.79

SUBCUTANEOUS TISSUE OF ABDOMEN

Dissection Overview

The subcutaneous tissue in the abdominal region is continuous with the thoracic region superiorly and the back posteriorly. Anteriorly in the inguinal region inferior to the umbilicus, it forms two distinct layers: a superficial fatty layer (Camper's fascia) and a deep membranous layer (Scarpa's fascia). The membranous layer is continuous with the fascia lata of the thigh and the fasciae in the perineum.

The anterolateral abdominal wall lies deep to the subcutaneous tissue and is formed laterally by three broad flat muscles which attach to the midline via thin aponeurotic extensions surrounding the vertically oriented fibers of the anterior muscles. On the deep surface of the muscular wall, the transversalis fascia surrounds the abdominal cavity with a layer of fatty tissue and the parietal peritoneum as illustrated in FIGURE 4.1.

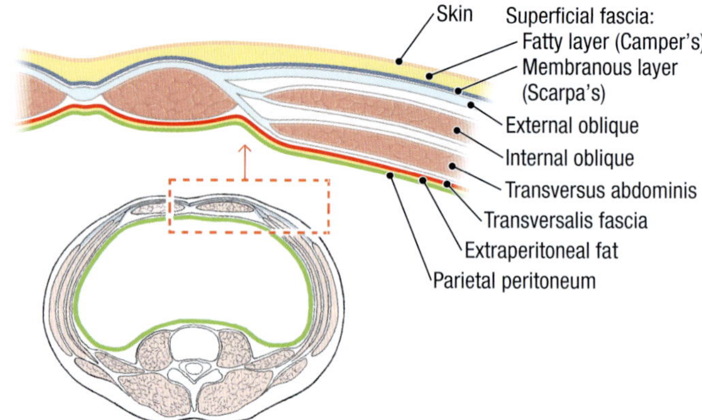

FIGURE 4.1 ■ Axial section of lower abdomen demonstrating layers of anterior abdominal wall. Inferior view.

The order of dissection will be as follows: The skeletal anatomy of the abdomen will be studied. The surface anatomy of the abdomen and the abdominal subdivisions into either quadrants or regions will be studied. The skin will be either reflected or removed from the abdomen. The subcutaneous tissue will either be removed or reflected in a full- or partial-thickness approach. Neurovascular structures in the abdomen will be studied.

Skeletal Anatomy

Use an articulated skeleton to identify the following structures.

Sternum and Costal Margin

ATLAS 3.10

1. Refer to FIGURE 4.2.
2. In the midline, identify the **xiphoid process**, the extension of bone inferior to the **body of the sternum.** *Note that although the xiphoid is often triangular, it may appear bifid or split in some individuals.*
3. Identify the location of the **xiphisternal junction (joint)** at the intersection of the body of the sternum and the xiphoid process near the level of the 6th costal cartilage.
4. On the lateral aspects of the xiphisternal junction, identify the **costal cartilages** of the false ribs merging to form the **costal margin.**

Bony Pelvis

ATLAS 5.3, 5.4

1. Refer to FIGURE 4.2.
2. In the midline of the bony pelvis, identify the **pubic symphysis** at the junction of the **right** and **left pubic bones** anteriorly.
3. Identify the **pubic crest** coursing laterally from the pubic symphysis on the superior aspect of the pubic bones.
4. On the lateral aspect of the pubic crest, identify the **pubic tubercle**, the medial attachment of the **inguinal ligament.**
5. Identify the **anterior superior iliac spine (ASIS)** along the anterior aspect of the **ilium.**

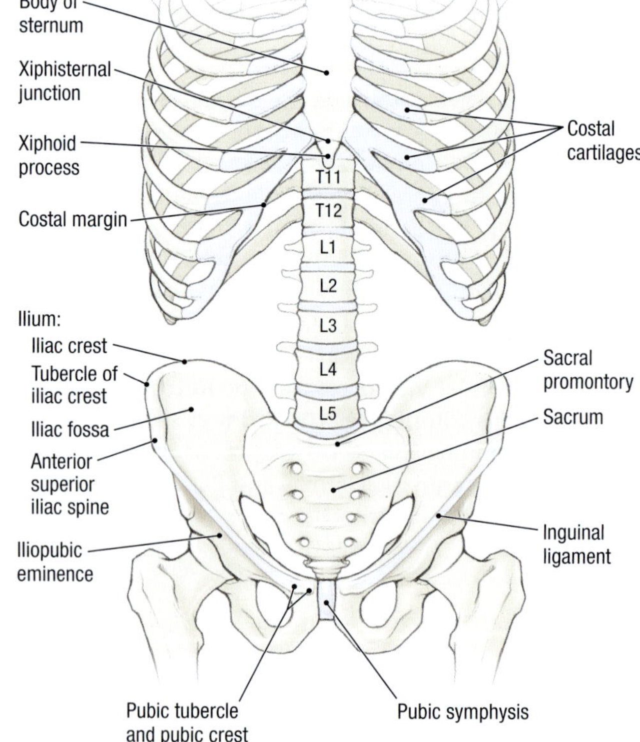

FIGURE 4.2 ■ Abdominal skeleton. Anterior view.

6. Beginning at the ASIS, follow the bony ridge of the **iliac crest** posteriorly toward the midaxillary line.
7. Identify the **iliac tubercle** approximately midway along the length of the iliac crest near the midaxillary line.

Surface Anatomy

The surface anatomy of the abdomen may be studied on a living subject or on a cadaver. On the cadaver, note that fixation of tissue during embalming may make it difficult to distinguish bone from well-preserved soft tissues in some specimens.

Abdomen

ATLAS 4.2

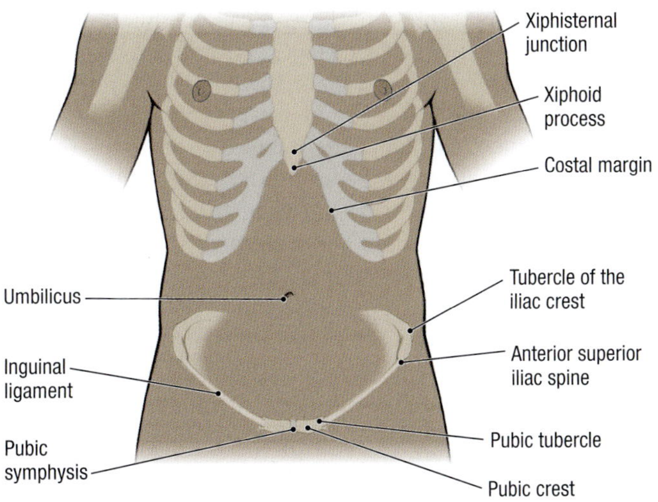

FIGURE 4.3 ● Surface anatomy of abdomen. Anterior view.

1. Refer to FIGURE 4.3.
2. With the cadaver in the supine position, palpate the **xiphoid process** in the midline, just inferior to the **xiphisternal junction**.
3. At the midpoint of the abdomen, identify the **umbilicus**.
4. Trace your finger inferiorly along the midline from the umbilicus to the **pubic symphysis**.
5. Palpate laterally from the pubic symphysis along the **pubic crest** to the **pubic tubercle**.
6. Trace the path of the **inguinal ligament** from the pubic tubercle medially to the ASIS on the anterior aspect of the hip laterally.

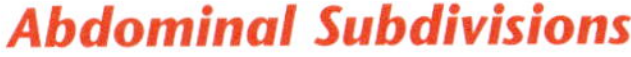

Abdominal Subdivisions

ATLAS 4.3

The quadrant and regional systems are both commonly used and rely on surface anatomy for proper orientation. The quadrant system is suitable for general descriptions and will be used to describe the position of organs in this dissection guide.

1. Refer to FIGURE 4.4.
2. Use your fingers to trace the planes used in the **quadrant system** to subdivide the abdomen.
3. Identify the location of the **median plane** beginning superiorly at the body of the sternum and xiphoid process.
4. Progress inferiorly along the **linea alba** past the umbilicus until you reach the pubic symphysis. *Note that depending on the amount of abdominal subcutaneous tissue, the linea alba and pubic symphysis may not be easily palpable.*
5. Return to the umbilicus and identify the location of the horizontally oriented **transumbilical plane**.
6. Identify the **right** and **left upper quadrants** superior to the transumbilical plane to the right and left sides of the median plane, respectively.
7. Identify the **right** and **left lower quadrants** inferior to the transumbilical plane to the right and left sides of the median plane, respectively.
8. Refer to FIGURE 4.5.
9. Use your fingers to trace the planes used in the **regional system** to subdivide the abdomen.

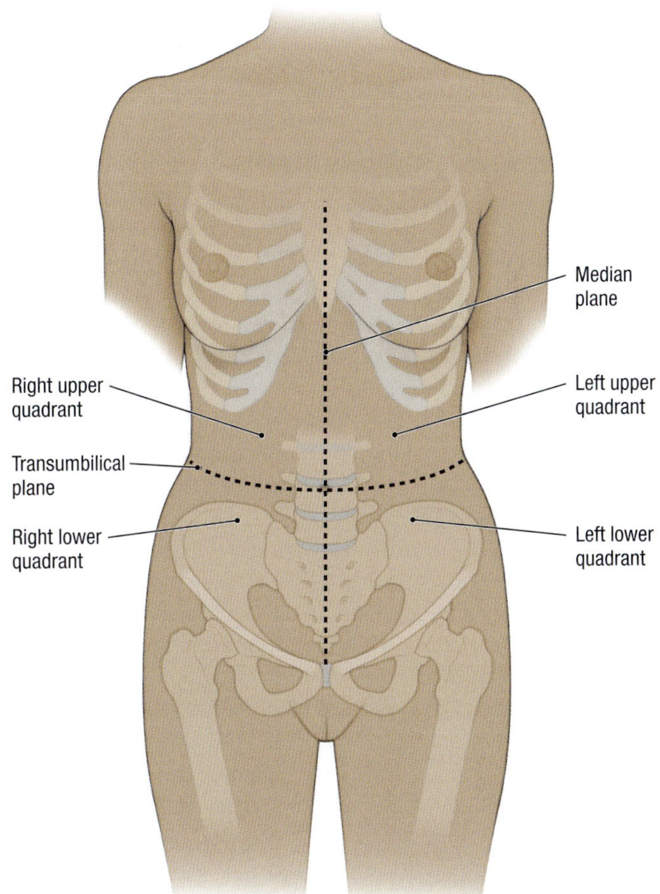

FIGURE 4.4 ● Four abdominal quadrants. Anterior view.

10. Identify the location of the vertically oriented **midclavicular lines**, which intersect the midpoint of each clavicle superiorly and the midpoint between the ASIS and the pubic tubercle inferiorly, effectively the midpoint of each inguinal ligament.
11. Palpate the **iliac crest** and **iliac tubercle** on the superolateral aspect of the ilium about 5 cm posterior to the ASIS to identify the location of the horizontally oriented **transtubercular plane**, passing through the right and left iliac tubercles.
12. Return to the xiphoid process and palpate bilaterally along the **costal margin** to the lowest palpable level to identify the location of the horizontally oriented **subcostal plane**.
13. Identify the nine abdominal regions beginning superiorly with the **right** and **left hypochondriac regions** deep to the thoracic cage to either side of the **epigastric region**.
14. Progress inferiorly to the **right** and **left lumbar regions** to either side of the centrally located **umbilical region**.
15. Continue inferiorly to the **right** and **left inguinal regions** to either side of the **hypogastric (pubic) region**. *Note that clinical complaints may be more specifically described using the regional system than the quadrant system, and thus, you should be familiar with both descriptive methods.*

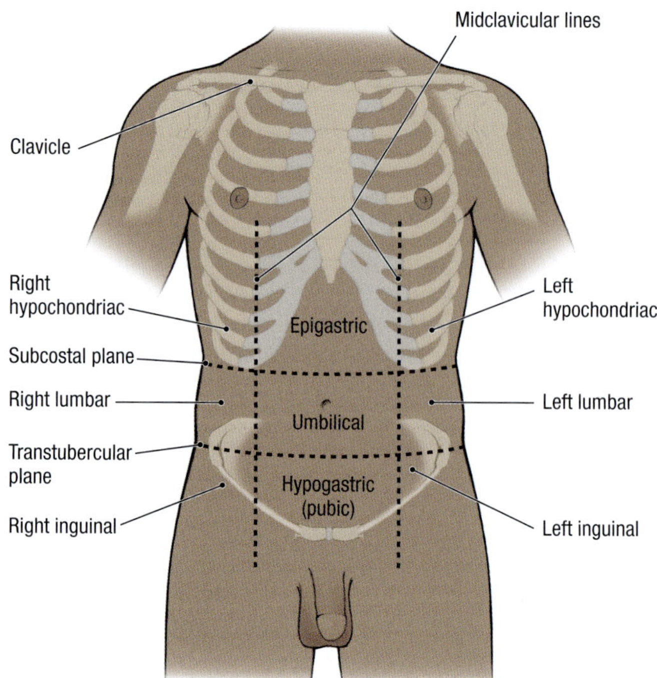

FIGURE 4.5 Nine abdominal regions. Anterior view.

Dissection Instructions

Skin Incisions of Abdomen

VIDEO 4.1.1

Dissection Note: Prior to commencing with skin incisions, decide to either perform a full- or partial-thickness approach and to either reflect or remove the skin from the dissection field. See **Removing Skin** in the **Introduction Chapter** for descriptions.

1. Refer to FIGURE 4.6.
2. Make a midline skin incision from the xiphisternal junction (C) to the pubic symphysis (E), encircling the umbilicus (U).
3. Make an incision from the xiphisternal junction (C) along the costal margin laterally to a point on the midaxillary line (V). *Note that if the thorax has been dissected previously, this incision has already been made.*
4. Make a skin incision beginning 3 cm inferior to the pubic crest (E) running parallel to the line of the inguinal ligament to a point 3 cm inferior to the ASIS. *Note that care must be made along this incision line as superficial structures in the thigh may easily be damaged, particularly in cadavers with little adipose tissue.*
5. Continue the incision posteriorly, 3 cm below the iliac crest to a point on the midaxillary line (F).
6. Make a transverse skin incision from the encircling cut around the umbilicus to each midaxillary line.

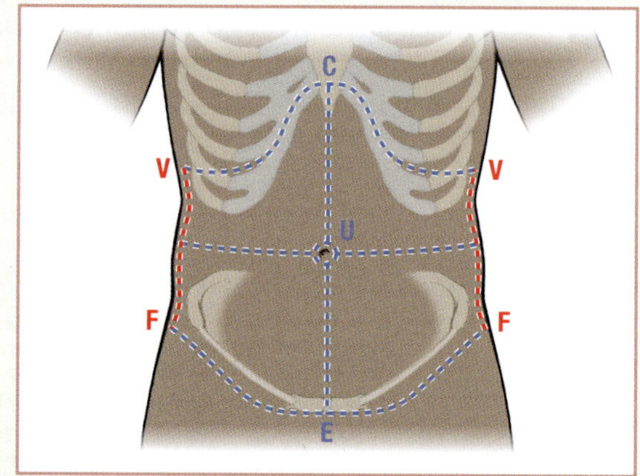

FIGURE 4.6 Abdominal skin incisions. Anterior view.

7. If reflecting the skin, use the uncut sections of skin laterally as hinge points to leave the skin attached along the peripheral aspect of the abdomen and reflect the skin only as far laterally as the midaxillary line.
8. If removing the skin, make a vertical skin incision along the midaxillary line in the thorax (V) to the tubercle of the iliac crest (F). *Note that if the back has been dissected previously, this incision has already been made.*
9. If using a partial-thickness removal method, remove the skin, but not the subcutaneous tissue, from medial to lateral using either a pair of locking forceps or the

buttonhole technique. At any point, the portions of skin may be cut into smaller segments to facilitate removal.

10. If using a full-thickness skin removal method, skip the following dissection instructions on the subcutaneous tissue of the abdomen.
11. If the skin is to be removed, detach the skin along the periphery and place it in the tissue container.

Subcutaneous Tissue of Abdomen

ATLAS 4.6, 4.7, 4.11; VIDEO 4.1.2

1. Refer to FIGURE 4.7.
2. Just lateral to the midclavicular line in the abdominal region, create a vertical cut through the subcutaneous tissue, about 7.5 cm lateral to the midline. *Note that the superficial epigastric artery and vein course in the superficial fascia in this area but do not make a special effort to find them.*
3. Dissect through the subcutaneous tissue down to the **aponeurosis of the external oblique**.
4. On the medial side of the vertical cut, use blunt dissection to separate the subcutaneous tissue from the aponeurosis of the external oblique (**Arrow 1**).
5. As you remove the subcutaneous tissue inferior to the umbilicus, observe that superficially, the **fatty layer (Camper's fascia)** is intimately connected on its deep surface to the **membranous layer (Scarpa's fascia)**.

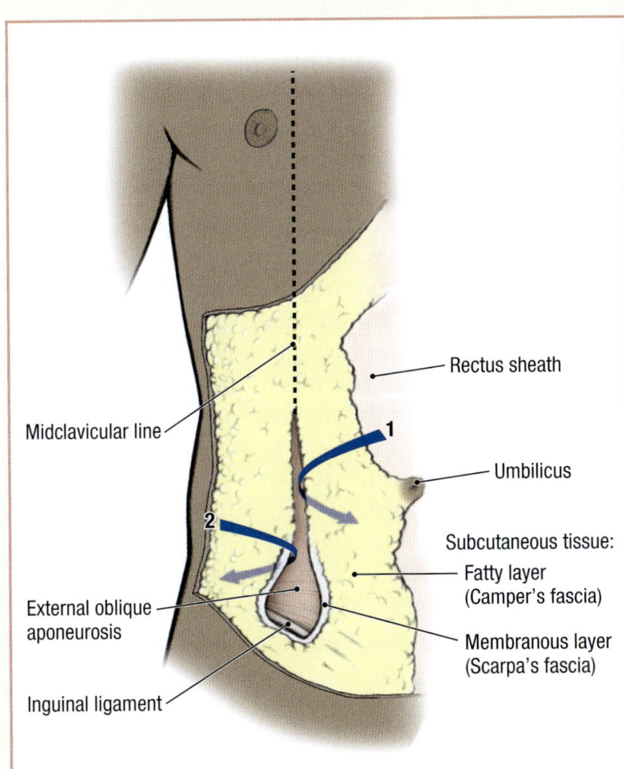

FIGURE 4.7 ● Subcutaneous tissue of abdomen. Anterior view.

6. Observe that the membranous layer may be separated from the underlying deep or investing fascia surrounding the muscles of the region with minimal effort.
7. Near the umbilicus, make a brief effort to identify branches of the **superficial epigastric vein** coursing within the subcutaneous tissue of the region (see **Clinical Correlation 4.1**).

CLINICAL CORRELATION 4.1

Caput Medusae

ATLAS 4.7

In patients who have obstruction of the inferior vena cava or the hepatic portal vein, the superficial veins of the abdominal wall may become engorged as they accommodate increased venous return. The dilated superficial veins may be visible around the umbilicus in a condition commonly referred to as caput medusae due to the "snake-like" appearance of the vessels resembling the hair of Medusa. The dilated vessels are branches of the superficial epigastric vein, which anastomose with the lateral thoracic vein in the subcutaneous tissue of the abdomen creating an important collateral venous channel from the femoral vein to the axillary vein.

8. As you approach the midline, identify one or two **anterior cutaneous nerves** that enter the subcutaneous tissue 2 to 3 cm lateral to the midline. *Note that the abdominal cutaneous nerves are branches of the intercostal nerves (T7–T11), subcostal nerve (T12), and iliohypogastric nerve (L1).*
9. While removing the subcutaneous tissue, consult a dermatome chart and note that T6 innervates the skin overlying the xiphoid process, T10 innervates the skin of the umbilicus, T12 innervates the skin superior to the pubic symphysis, and L1 innervates the skin overlying the pubic symphysis.
10. Lateral to the vertical cut made paralleling the midclavicular line in step 2, use blunt dissection to separate the subcutaneous tissue from the external oblique (**Arrow 2**).
11. As you near the midaxillary line, identify the **lateral cutaneous nerves** entering the subcutaneous tissue and clean the branches of at least one lateral cutaneous nerve.
12. Remove the subcutaneous tissue from superior to inferior and clearly demonstrate the inferior border of the external oblique where it terminates as the **inguinal ligament**.
13. Detach the subcutaneous tissue from the midline, midaxillary line, and proximal thigh and place it in the tissue container.

Dissection Follow-up

1. Familiarize yourself with the distribution of the superficial epigastric vessels.
2. Review the abdominal distribution of the anterior rami of spinal nerves T6–L1.
3. If a full- or partial-thickness skin reflection was performed, replace the reflected portions of skin back to anatomical position.

ANTEROLATERAL ABDOMINAL WALL

Dissection Overview

Three flat muscles (external oblique, internal oblique, and transversus abdominis) form most of the lateral abdominal wall. The three flat muscles have broad, fleshy proximal attachments (to the ribs, vertebrae, and pelvis) and broad, aponeurotic distal attachments (to the ribs, linea alba, and pubis). The rectus abdominis forms the bulk of the anterior abdominal wall from the fifth rib superiorly to the pubic crest inferiorly. Between the right and left rectus abdominis lies the midline tendinous structure of the linea alba. The lateral muscle aponeuroses wrap around the rectus abdominis to reach the linea alba forming the rectus sheath.

The inguinal canal is located at the inferior extent of the abdominal wall superior to the medial half of the inguinal ligament and extends from the deep (internal) inguinal ring to the superficial (external) inguinal ring. In the female, the round ligament of the uterus passes through the deep inguinal ring. During development of the male, the testis and all its related vessels, nerves, and ducts passed through the deep inguinal ring on the way to the scrotum, essentially an outpouching of the anterolateral abdominal wall.

The order of dissection will be as follows: The three flat muscles of the anterolateral abdominal wall will be studied and reflected bilaterally. The superficial inguinal ring and inguinal canal will be studied. The composition and contents of the rectus sheath will be explored. The anterior abdominal wall will be reflected.

Dissection Instructions

External Oblique

ATLAS 4.8A, 4.9A, 4.11A, 4.15A; VIDEO 4.2.1

1. Refer to FIGURE 4.8A.
2. Clean any remnants of the superficial fat and fascia from the surface of the anterior abdominal wall and place it in the tissue container.
3. Identify the **external oblique** and observe that its fibers course from superolateral to inferomedial.
4. Remove a portion of the investing fascia from the surface of the external oblique to better visualize the fiber direction and extent of the muscle. *Note that in thinner cadavers, removal of the overlying investing fascia may compromise the stability of the muscle.*
5. Use blunt dissection to clean the aponeurosis of the external oblique and clearly delineate the **semilunar line (linea semilunaris)** coursing vertically near the midclavicular line.
6. Observe that the inferior border of the aponeurosis of the external oblique curves posteriorly and thickens to form the **inguinal ligament** attaching from the ASIS to the pubic tubercle. *Note that large vessels and nerves coursing between the abdominal cavity and lower limb pass deep to the inguinal ligament but will not be dissected at this time.*
7. Review the attachments and actions of the external oblique (see **TABLE 4.1**).
8. Refer to FIGURE 4.8B and C.
9. Clean the inferomedial portion of the external oblique aponeurosis and identify the opening of the **superficial (external) inguinal ring** formed in the external oblique aponeurosis.
10. Observe that the superficial inguinal ring permits the **round ligament of the uterus** in the female, and **spermatic cord** in the male, to pass from the inguinal canal to the suprapubic region.
11. Identify the **ilioinguinal nerve** emerging through the superficial inguinal ring. *Note that the ilioinguinal nerve supplies sensory innervation to the skin on the anterior surface of the external genitalia and medial surface of the thigh after providing motor innervation to the anterolateral abdominal wall.*
12. Observe that in the female, the ilioinguinal nerve lies anterior to the round ligament of the uterus, which may be quite small and difficult to identify.
13. Observe that in the male, the ilioinguinal nerve lies anterior to the spermatic cord.

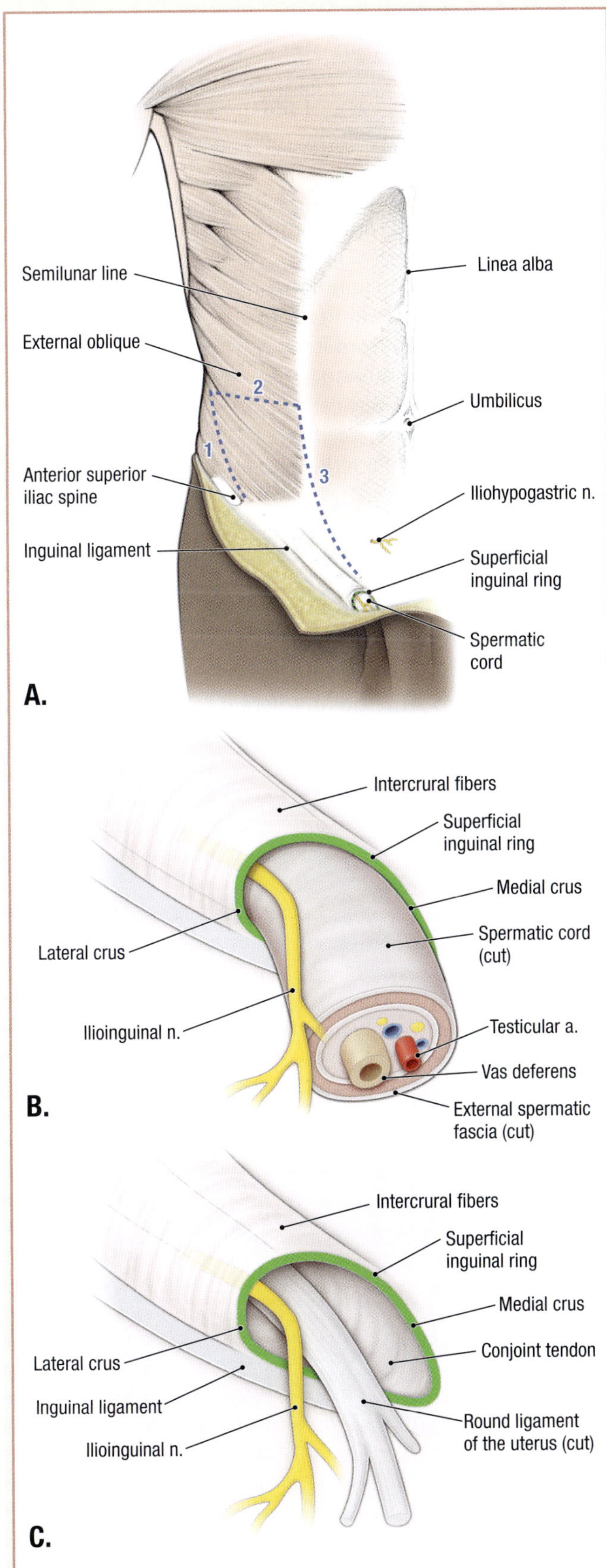

FIGURE 4.8 ● **A.** Opening abdominal wall. **B.** Right superficial inguinal ring in male. **C.** Right superficial inguinal ring in female. Anterior views.

14. At the margins of the superficial inguinal ring, identify the **external spermatic fascia**, the thin layer of fascia extending from the external oblique aponeurosis to the spermatic cord.
15. Use a probe to identify the **lateral (inferior) crus** attaching to the pubic tubercle and defining the lateral margin of the superficial inguinal ring.
16. Identify the **medial (superior) crus** attaching to the pubic crest and defining the medial margin of the superficial inguinal ring.
17. Identify the **intercrural fibers**, the delicate fibers spanning the crura superolateral to the superficial inguinal ring. *Note that intercrural fibers prevent the crura from spreading apart.*
18. Insert a probe through the superficial inguinal ring into the **inguinal canal** and observe that the external oblique aponeurosis forms the anterior wall of the inguinal canal, and that the inguinal ligament forms its floor.
19. Identify the **lacunar ligament** inferior to the contents of the inguinal canal and observe that it is formed at the medial end of the inguinal ligament by fibers that turn posteriorly and attach to the pecten pubis. *Note that the lacunar ligament is oriented medial to the femoral vein, artery, and nerve and will be more visible after opening the inguinal canal.*

Internal Oblique

ATLAS 4.8B, 4.9B, 4.12, 4.15B; VIDEO 4.2.2

Dissection Note: To expose the internal oblique, the external oblique will be partially transected and reflected inferiorly.

1. Refer to FIGURE 4.8A.
2. Make a vertical incision through the external oblique beginning at the ASIS and ending at the level of the umbilicus (**Cut 1**). Cut only the external oblique layer and none of the underlying layers by proceeding slowly and cautiously.
3. Use blunt dissection to carefully elevate the external oblique and identify the underlying **internal oblique** laterally.
4. Make a horizontal incision across the external oblique stopping at the **semilunar line** (**Cut 2**). *Note that your fingers or a probe cannot pass medial to the semilunar line because the external oblique aponeurosis fuses to the underlying internal oblique aponeurosis at this location.*
5. Use blunt dissection to carefully separate the external oblique from the underlying internal oblique layer superiorly.
6. Make a vertical cut through the external oblique aponeurosis just lateral to the semilunar line. Continue the cut inferiorly toward the superficial inguinal ring but do not connect the cut through the superficial ring perimeter (**Cut 3**).

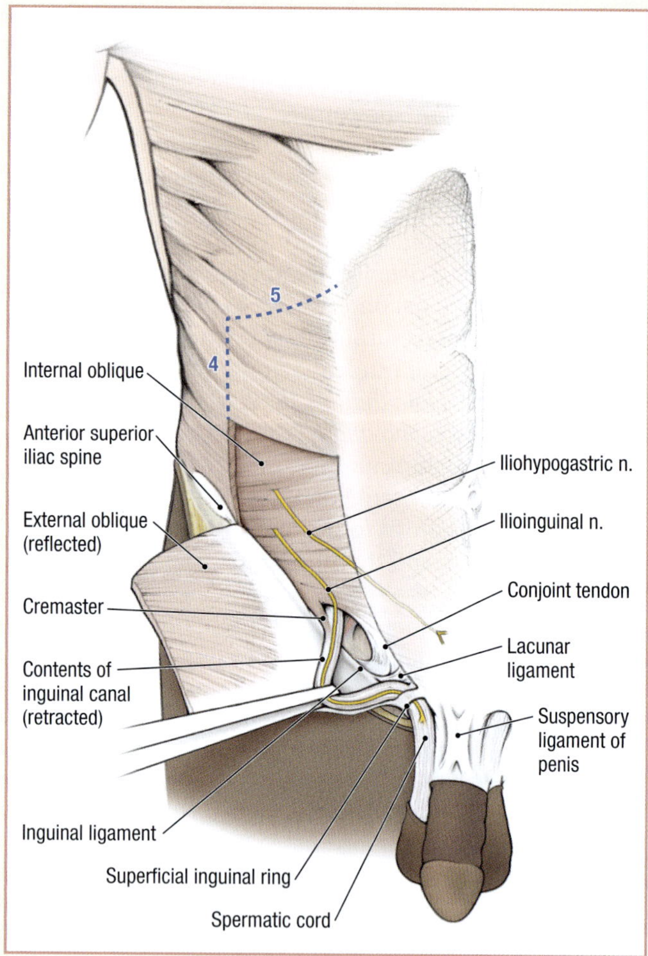

FIGURE 4.9 ● Exposed inguinal canal and internal oblique. Anterior view.

7. Refer to FIGURE 4.9.
8. Reflect the flap of external oblique inferiorly using the inguinal ligament as a hinge to reveal the inguinal portion of the internal oblique.
9. Examine the exposed upper portion of the internal oblique fibers and observe that they are arranged perpendicularly to the external oblique fibers and course from superomedial to inferolateral.
10. Examine the exposed lower portion of the internal oblique and observe that from the lateral half of the inguinal ligament, the fibers arch over the contents of the canal (round ligament or spermatic cord) to join with the aponeurosis of the **transversus abdominis** forming the **conjoint tendon**. *Note that the arching fibers of the internal oblique form parts of the anterior wall of the inguinal canal laterally, roof centrally, and posterior wall medially.*
11. Review the attachments and actions of the internal oblique (see **TABLE 4.1**).
12. Within the inguinal canal, make an effort to identify the fibers of the **cremaster** and its associated **cremasteric fascia** connecting from the internal oblique to the round ligament of the uterus in the female or the spermatic cord in the male.
13. Identify the ilioinguinal nerve coursing in the intermuscular plane between the external oblique and internal oblique within the inguinal canal.
14. Observe that the ilioinguinal nerve runs parallel and inferior to the **iliohypogastric nerve** and can be differentiated from it, as it emerges through the superficial inguinal ring.
15. Using the lateral vertical cut through the external oblique as a guide, continue to cut through the external oblique superiorly to a point just above the costal margin (**Cut 4**). *Note that the easiest point of separation of the anterolateral abdominal wall muscle layers is laterally near the midaxillary line where the muscles are thickest.*
16. Make an incision through the external oblique about 2 cm superior to the inferior edge of the costal margin and cut medially, keeping the cut parallel to its curvature until the point where it becomes aponeurotic (**Cut 5**).
17. Refer to FIGURE 4.10.
18. Grasp the free edge of the external oblique and use blunt dissection to separate it from the underlying

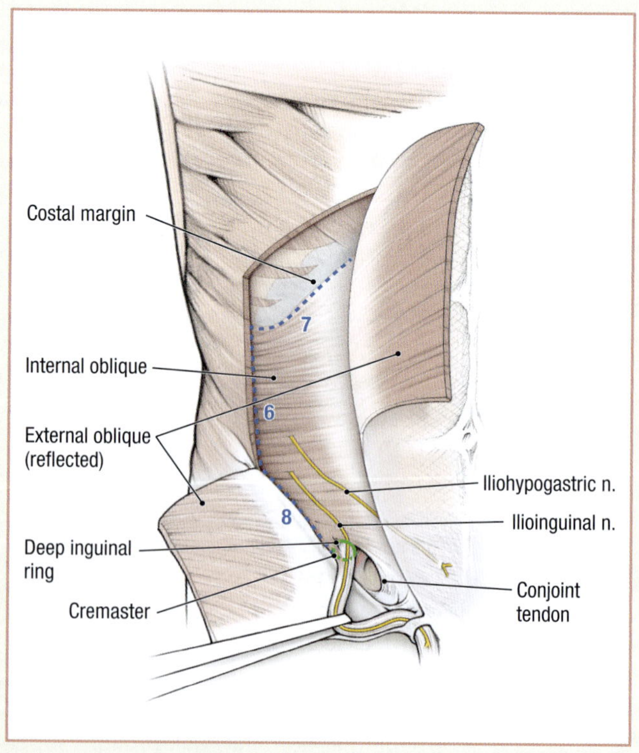

FIGURE 4.10 ● Reflection of internal oblique. Anterior view.

internal oblique and reflect the superior portion of the muscle medially.

19. Follow the ilioinguinal nerve proximally to find where it pierces the internal oblique and follow it into the plane of separation between the internal oblique and transversus abdominis.
20. Gently push a probe through the opening where the ilioinguinal nerve pierces the internal oblique to increase the separation of the muscular layers at this location.
21. Make a vertical incision through the internal oblique following the path of the lateral cut through the external oblique (**Cut 6**), sparing the ilioinguinal and iliohypogastric nerves.
22. Near the ASIS, use blunt dissection to separate the internal oblique from the underlying transversus abdominis. *Note that the transversus abdominis is difficult to separate from the internal oblique medially where their tendons fuse to form the conjoint tendon.*
23. Cut the internal oblique along the costal margin continuing its separation from the underlying transversus abdominis (**Cut 7**).
24. Cut the internal oblique about 2 cm superior to the inguinal ligament and reflect the muscle medially (**Cut 8**).

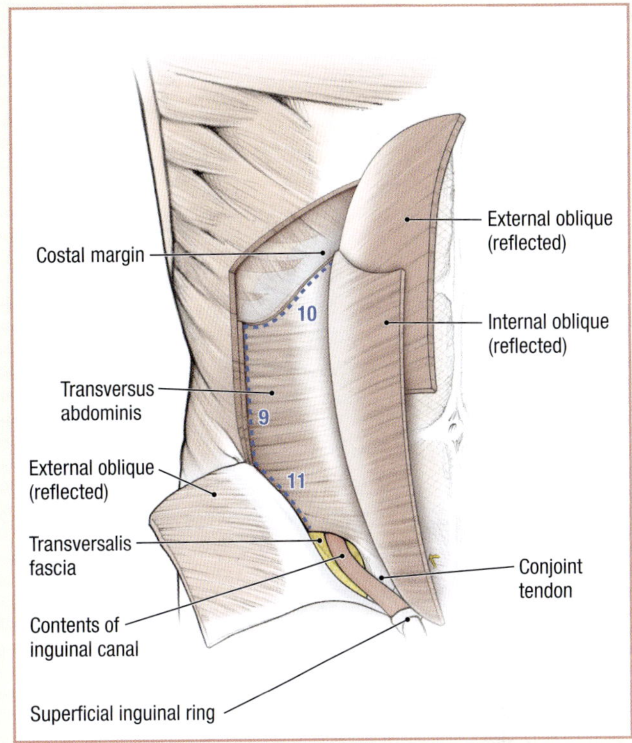

FIGURE 4.11 ● Reflection of transversus abdominis. Anterior view.

Transversus Abdominis

ATLAS 4.8B, 4.9C, 4.13, 4.15D; VIDEO 4.2.3

1. Refer to FIGURE 4.11.
2. Deep to the reflected internal oblique, identify the **transversus abdominis**.
3. Examine the exposed upper portion of the transversus abdominis and observe that it has predominantly horizontally oriented fibers.
4. Observe that the arching fibers of the inferior part of the transversus abdominis form part of the roof of the inguinal canal, and its aponeurotic insertion forms part of the posterior wall.
5. Identify the **transversalis fascia** inferior and deep to the arching fibers of the internal oblique and transversus abdominis.
6. Review the attachments and actions of the transversus abdominis (see **TABLE 4.1**).
7. Carefully incise the transversus abdominis along the same vertical line as used to cut the external and internal obliques (**Cut 9**) and use blunt dissection to separate the underlying transversalis fascia and parietal peritoneum from its deep surface. Take care to not pierce the peritoneum and enter the abdominal cavity or cut the thoracoabdominal nerves in the region.
8. Cut the transversus abdominis along the costal margin continuing its separation from the underlying transversalis fascia (**Cut 10**).
9. Cut through the transversus abdominis about 2 cm superior to the inguinal ligament and reflect the muscle medially (**Cut 11**).

Rectus Abdominis

ATLAS 4.8A, 4.9D; VIDEO 4.2.4

Dissection Note: Perform the following dissection sequence on only one side.

1. Refer to FIGURE 4.12.
2. On the anterior abdominal wall, identify the **rectus sheath** formed by the aponeuroses of the three pairs of anterolateral abdominal wall muscles (external oblique, internal oblique, and transversus abdominis) as they fuse toward their medial attachment at the **linea alba** around the **rectus abdominis**.
3. Observe that in the upper three-fourths of the abdomen, the aponeuroses from the external oblique and the anterior lamina of the internal oblique form the **anterior rectus sheath**, while the posterior lamina of the internal oblique and the transversus abdominis form the **posterior rectus sheath**.
4. Observe that approximately halfway between the umbilicus and the pubic symphysis, all layers of the lateral muscle aponeuroses course anterior to the rectus abdominis as the anterior rectus sheath, and there is no longer a posterior rectus sheath below this level.

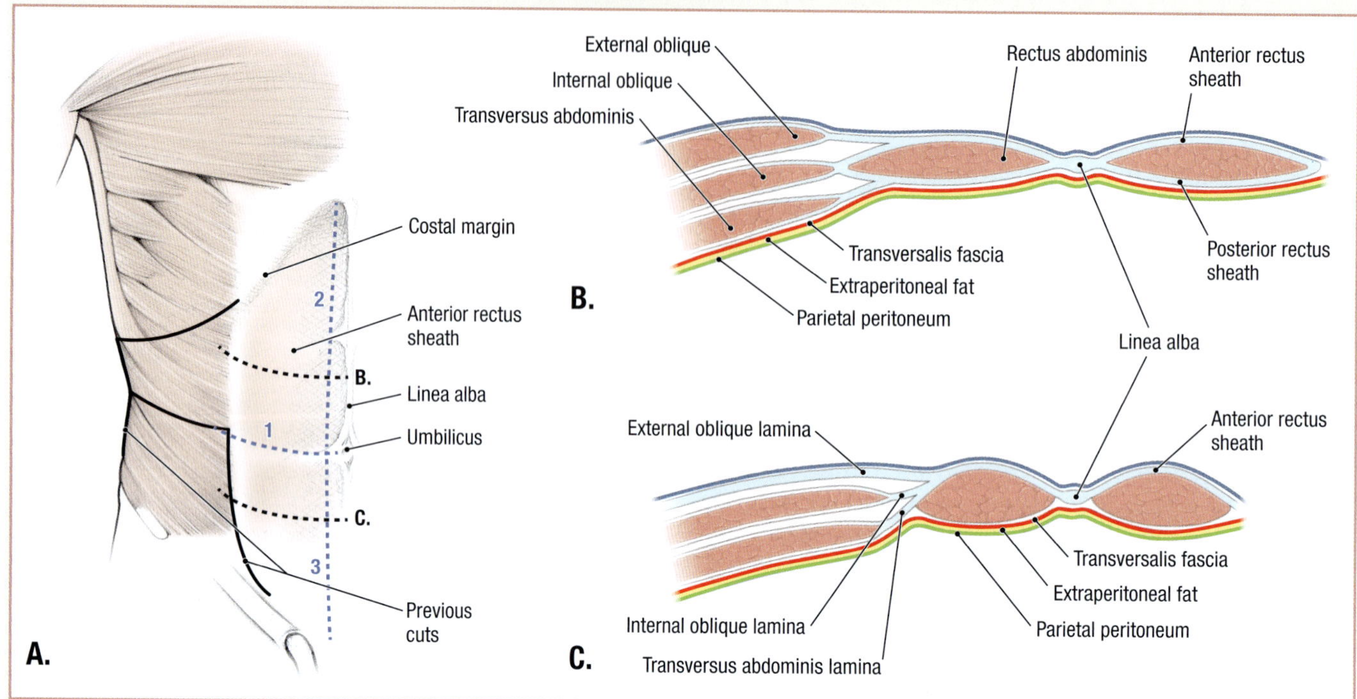

FIGURE 4.12 ● **A.** Opening of anterior rectus sheath. Anterior view. **B.** Axial section through anterior abdominal wall superior to arcuate line. Inferior view. **C.** Axial section through anterior abdominal wall inferior to arcuate line. Inferior view.

5. Make a transverse cut through the anterior rectus sheath on the right side beginning at the semilunar line laterally and ending approximately 2.5 cm lateral to the umbilicus. Use a probe to lift the free edge of the rectus sheath as you cut, ensuring you do not cut through the underlying rectus abdominis (**Cut 1**).
6. Make a vertical incision through the rectus sheath extending in a superior direction along the medial border of the rectus abdominis to the costal margin lateral to the **linea alba** (**Cut 2**).
7. Extend the vertical cut inferiorly along the medial border of the rectus abdominis to the level of the pubic crest (**Cut 3**).
8. Refer to FIGURE 4.13.
9. Observe that the anterior rectus sheath is firmly attached to the anterior surface of the rectus abdominis by several **tendinous intersections**.
10. Separate the anterior rectus sheath from the anterior surface of the rectus abdominis between the tendinous intersections.
11. Carefully detach the tendinous intersections from the anterior rectus sheath, by keeping your cutting instrument along the anterior surface of the rectus abdominis, and reflect the rectus sheath laterally.
12. To increase visibility of the rectus abdominis, additional cuts may be made through the anterior rectus sheath both superiorly and inferiorly to allow for further reflection of the sheath.

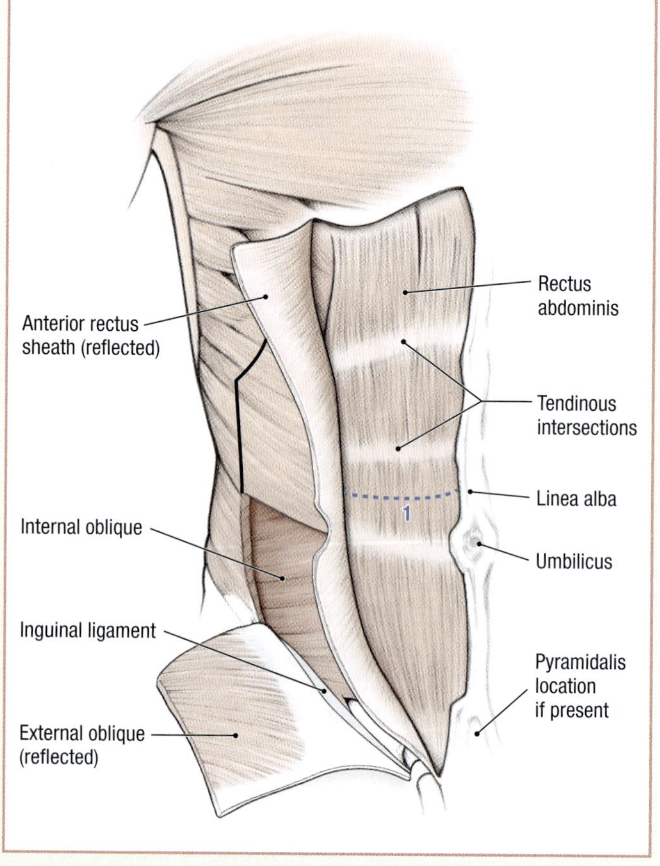

FIGURE 4.13 ● Rectus abdominis. Anterior view.

13. Observe that the subdivisions of the **rectus abdominis** by the tendinous intersections are responsible for the appearance of the "six pack."
14. Review the attachments and actions of the rectus abdominis (see **TABLE 4.1**).
15. Anterior to the inferior aspect of the rectus abdominis, look for the **pyramidalis** attaching from to the anterior surface of the pubis to the linea alba. *Note that the pyramidalis is frequently absent.*

Epigastric Vessels and Deep Inguinal Ring

ATLAS 4.8B, 4.14, 4.15D, 4.16A; VIDEO 4.2.5

1. Refer to FIGURE 4.13.
2. Use blunt dissection to mobilize the medial border of the rectus abdominis.
3. Near the level of the umbilicus, transect the rectus abdominis on one side (**Cut 1**).
4. Refer to FIGURE 4.14.
5. Along the lateral side of the rectus abdominis, observe that branches of six nerves (T7–T12) enter the rectus sheath to penetrate the deep surface of the muscle to then emerge from the sheath as **anterior cutaneous branches**.
6. Reflect the two halves of the cut rectus abdominis superiorly and inferiorly. If the cutaneous nerves prevent full reflection of the rectus abdominis, cut them where they enter the deep surface of the muscle.
7. Identify the **superior epigastric artery** and accompanying veins on the posterior surface of the rectus abdominis superiorly.
8. Identify the much larger **inferior epigastric artery** and accompanying veins on the posterior surface of the rectus abdominis inferiorly.
9. Deep to the reflected rectus abdominis, examine the posterior rectus sheath and identify the **arcuate line** at its inferior limit midway between the pubic symphysis and the umbilicus.
10. Identify the thin, fibrous **transversalis fascia** inferior to the arcuate line. *Note that the transversalis fascia is reinforced on its deep surface by the parietal peritoneum lining the abdominal cavity.*
11. Identify the **inferior epigastric vessels** where they enter the rectus sheath at the level of the arcuate line within the layer of extraperitoneal fat (see **Clinical Correlation 4.2**).

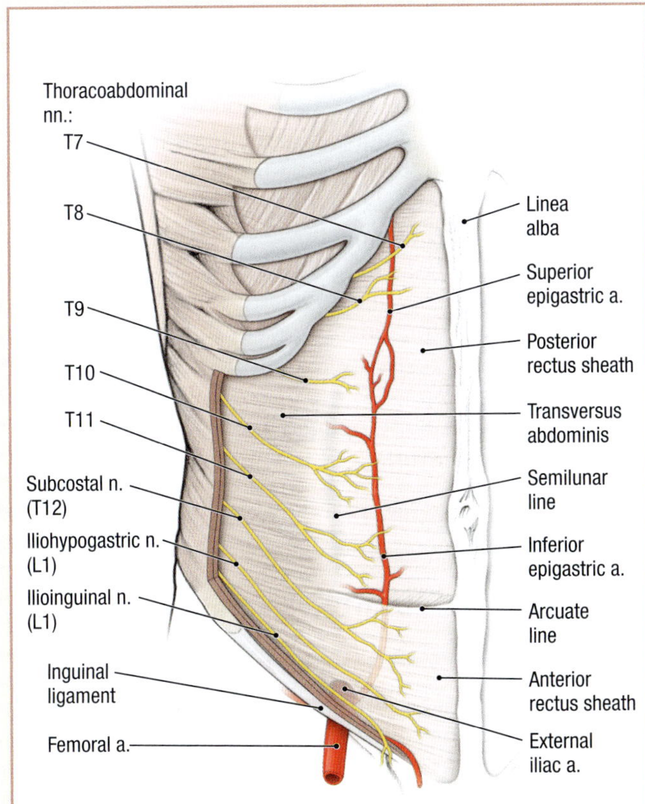

FIGURE 4.14 ● Posterior rectus sheath. Anterior view.

CLINICAL CORRELATION 4.2

Epigastric Artery Anastomoses

ATLAS 4.5

The superior epigastric vessels anastomose with the inferior epigastric vessels within the rectus sheath. If the inferior vena cava becomes obstructed, the anastomosis between the inferior epigastric and superior epigastric veins provides a collateral venous channel that drains into the superior vena cava. If the aorta is occluded, collateral arterial circulation to the lower part of the body occurs through the superior and inferior epigastric arteries.

12. Observe that the deep inguinal ring is lateral to the inferior epigastric vessels and identified by the presence of the **round ligament of the uterus** in the female, or **ductus (vas) deferens** in the male, coursing through it.
13. Use a probe to verify that the anterior wall of the inguinal canal is formed by the external oblique (whole length) and the internal oblique (lateral half).
14. Observe that the posterior wall of the inguinal canal is formed by the transversalis fascia (whole length) and conjoint tendon (medial half).
15. Observe that the inferior wall (floor) of the inguinal canal is the inguinal ligament and that the superior wall (roof) is the transversalis fascia laterally, arching fibers of the internal oblique centrally, and the transversus abdominis medially.

Dissection Follow-up

1. Review the attachments and action of each muscle in **TABLE 4.1**.
2. Review the structures that form the layers of the abdominal wall.
3. Use the dissected specimen to review, compare, and contrast the rectus sheath just superior to the level of the umbilicus and just superior to the pubic symphysis.
4. Review the blood and nerve supply to the anterior abdominal wall.
5. Replace the muscles of the anterior abdominal wall in their correct anatomical positions.
6. Familiarize yourself with the orientation and location of the inguinal canal.

TABLE 4.1 Muscles of Anterolateral Abdominal Wall

Muscle	*Proximal Attachments*	*Distal Attachments*	*Actions*	*Innervation*
External oblique	External surfaces of ribs 5–12	Linea alba, pubic crest and tubercle, and anterior half of the iliac crest	Compresses and supports abdominal viscera; flexes and rotates the trunk	Thoracoabdominal nn. T7–T11 and subcostal n.
Internal oblique	Thoracolumbar fascia, iliac crest, and lateral half of inguinal ligament	Inferior borders of ribs 10–12, linea alba, pubic crest, and pecten pubis via conjoint tendon		Thoracoabdominal nn. T7–T11, subcostal n., and L1
Transversus abdominis	Internal surfaces of costal cartilages 7–12, thoracolumbar fascia, and iliac crest	Linea alba with internal oblique, pubic crest, and pecten pubis via conjoint tendon		
Rectus abdominis	Xiphoid process, costal cartilages 5–7	Pubic symphysis and pubic crest	Flexes trunk, assists in pelvic tilt, and compresses abdominal viscera	Thoracoabdominal nn. T7–T11 and subcostal n.

Abbreviations: n., nerve; nn., nerves.

REFLECTION OF ABDOMINAL WALL

Dissection Overview

As the abdominal cavity is commonly described in both quadrant and regional subdivisions, two methods of abdominal wall dissection will be described and either method may be followed depending on the needs of the course. The first dissection sequence subdivides the anterior abdominal wall into quadrants. Direct reference to the position of the abdominal organs within the abdominal quadrants will thus be given with the quadrant technique; however, the portions of reflected abdominal wall may become a hindrance later in the dissection protocol.

The second dissection sequence involves reflecting the entire anterior abdominal wall in one large piece. Reflecting the entire wall maintains the anatomical relations of the structures coursing along the inner aspect of the anterior abdominal wall inferiorly. The entire anterior abdominal wall can be repositioned for reviewing either the quadrant or the regional approach to subdividing the abdominal cavity and contents.

The order of dissection will be as follows: The anterior abdominal wall will be cut and opened in either the abdominal quadrant reflection approach or the abdominal wall reflection approach. The inner surface of the anterior abdominal wall will be studied.

Dissection Instructions

Dissection Note: Select either the **Abdominal Quadrant Reflections** or **Abdominal Wall Reflection** approach for your study of the anterior abdominal wall and disregard the dissection sequence for the other approach. When you have finished with the selected approach, continue to the **Peritoneum and Peritoneal Cavity** section.

Abdominal Quadrant Reflections

ATLAS 4.8, 4.10; VIDEO 4.3.1

Dissection Note: If performing the **Abdominal Wall Reflection**, skip the following instructional sequence.

1. Refer to FIGURE 4.15A.
2. Reflect the cut halves of the rectus abdominis superiorly and inferiorly.

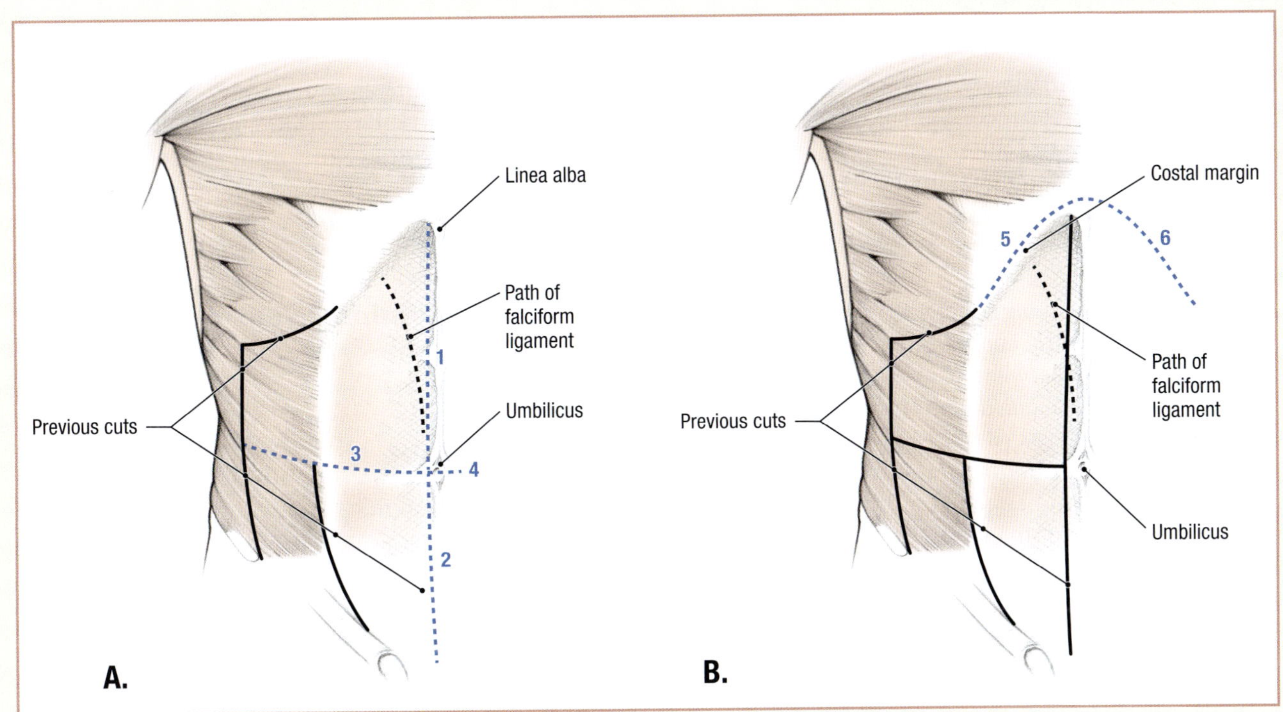

FIGURE 4.15 ■ Opening anterior abdominal wall using quadrant approach (**A**) or reflection approach (**B**). Anterior views.

3. On the right side of the umbilicus, use scissors to create a small hole (2.5 cm) through the abdominal wall to the abdominal cavity.
4. Insert your finger or a blunt probe through the hole into the abdominal cavity and pull the posterior wall of the rectus sheath, associated extraperitoneal fascia, and peritoneum anteriorly to create a space between the anterior abdominal wall and the abdominal viscera.
5. Make a vertical cut from the umbilicus to the xiphoid process 1 cm to the right of the midline to preserve the falciform ligament (**Cut 1**).
6. Extend the midline cut inferiorly as far as the pubic symphysis, staying 1 cm to the right of the midline to preserve the median umbilical fold (**Cut 2**).
7. Return the rectus abdominis halves to their correct anatomical positions.
8. At the level of the umbilicus, raise the abdominal wall creating a space between it and the abdominal contents.
9. Make a horizontal incision through the entire abdominal wall in the transumbilical plane on the right side (**Cut 3**). The scissors should pass through the previous transverse cut made in the rectus abdominis and external oblique.
10. Extend the transverse incision through the abdominal wall muscles and tissue laterally to the midaxillary line.
11. Repeat the transverse cut on the left side of the abdomen to the midaxillary line (**Cut 4**).
12. Open the flaps of the abdominal wall and identify the **falciform ligament** on the inner surface of the right upper quadrant flap. Observe that the falciform ligament connects the parietal peritoneum on the posterior aspect of the anterior abdominal wall to the visceral peritoneum on the anterior surface of the liver.

Abdominal Wall Reflection

ATLAS 4.8, 4.10; VIDEO 4.3.2

Dissection Note: If the abdominal quadrant reflection dissection approach was performed, skip ahead to the instructional sequence entitled **Anterior Abdominal Wall.**

1. Refer to FIGURE 4.15B.
2. Reflect the transected portion of the rectus abdominis superiorly on the right side.
3. Make a horizontal cut through the posterior rectus sheath superiorly to free the anterior abdominal wall from the costal margin and xiphoid process (**Cut 5**).
4. Make an incision through the transversalis fascia and parietal peritoneum beginning at the midline around the circumference of the entire cut edge of anterolateral abdominal wall musculature to the right until you reach the iliac crest.

5. On the left, make an incision through anterior rectus sheath following the curve of the costal margin and reflect the sheath to expose the underlying rectus abdominis fibers.
6. Use a probe to elevate the superior portion of the left rectus abdominis along its superior attachment and transect the muscle fibers superior to the curve of the costal margin.
7. Continue the transverse cut laterally through the attached portions of anterolateral abdominal wall muscles following the curve of the costal margin toward the midaxillary line (**Cut 6**). *Note that a portion of this cut was made during the reflection of the abdominal oblique.*
8. Make an incision through the transversalis fascia and parietal peritoneum beginning at the midline around the circumference of the entire cut edge of anterolateral abdominal wall musculature to the left until you reach the iliac crest.
9. Begin reflection of the entire anterolateral abdominal wall in the upper right-hand quadrant of the abdomen.
10. Cut through the falciform ligament attaching the anterior surface of the liver to the deep surface of the anterior abdominal wall.
11. Reflect the entire anterior abdominal wall inferiorly using the inferior attachments of the muscles to the suprapubic region as a hinge.
12. To increase mobility of the flap of abdominal wall, it may be helpful to make short lateral incisions just above the inguinal ligament to the lateral umbilical folds to free the musculature and reflected wall.

Anterior Abdominal Wall

ATLAS 4.21; VIDEO 4.3.3

1. Refer to FIGURE 4.16.
2. On the inner surface of the lower abdominal wall, identify the **median umbilical fold**, which lies in the midline inferior to the umbilicus. *Note that the median umbilical fold contains the urachus, the remnant of the allantois from embryological development.*
3. Identify the **medial umbilical fold** located lateral to the median umbilical fold, angling inferolaterally away from the midline. *Note that the medial umbilical fold contains the remnant of the obliterated umbilical artery from embryological development.*

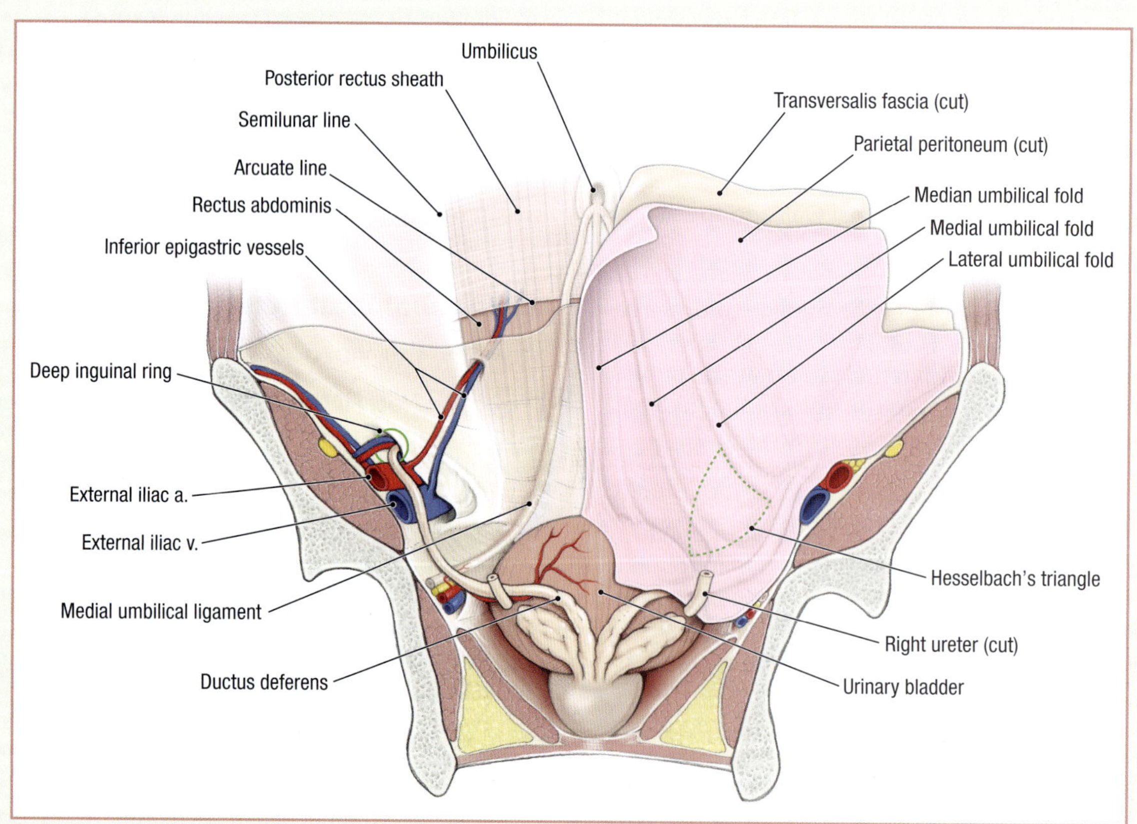

FIGURE 4.16 Anterior abdominal wall. Posterior view.

4. Identify the **lateral umbilical fold** located lateral to the medial umbilical fold, overlying the inferior epigastric artery and vein. *Note that the lateral fold contains the only functional contents of the umbilical folds.*
5. Lateral to the lateral umbilical fold, observe a small depression in the peritoneum marking the location of the **deep inguinal ring** in the transversalis fascia. *Note that in the male, this depression is more readily visible due to the presence of the testicular vessels and vas deferens passing through the deep inguinal ring to the inguinal canal.*
6. Observe that the inferior abdominal wall medial to the inferior epigastric vessels is less supported internally by the aponeuroses, thus creating a natural weak point in the posterior wall of the inguinal canal known as **Hesselbach's (inguinal) triangle**.
7. Hesselbach's triangle is bound laterally by the inferior epigastric vessels, medially by the lateral edge of the rectus abdominis, and inferiorly by the inguinal ligament (see **Clinical Correlation 4.3**).

CLINICAL CORRELATION 4.3

Inguinal Hernias

ATLAS 4.18

The inguinal canal is a weak area of the anterior abdominal wall through which abdominal viscera may protrude as an inguinal hernia. An inguinal hernia is classified according to its position relative to the inferior epigastric vessels as shown in FIGURE B4.1. An indirect inguinal hernia exits the abdominal cavity through the deep inguinal ring lateral to the inferior epigastric vessels and follows the inguinal canal (an indirect course through the abdominal wall). In contrast, a direct inguinal hernia exits the abdominal cavity medial to the inferior epigastric vessels through Hesselbach's (inguinal) triangle and follows a relatively direct course through the abdominal wall.

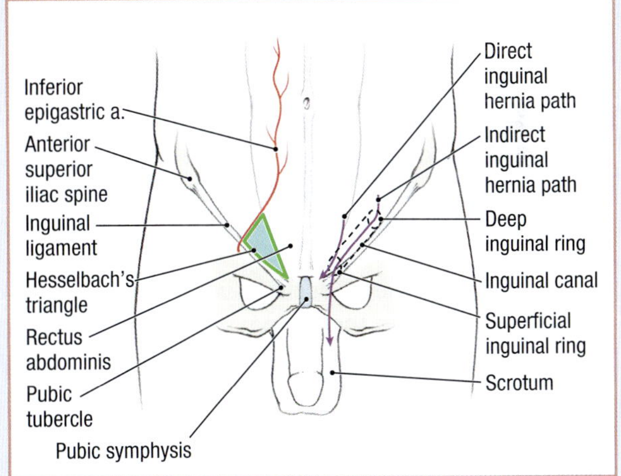

FIGURE B4.1 ■ Anatomical pathways and relationships of inguinal hernias. Anterior view.

Dissection Follow-up

1. Review the location of the falciform ligament.
2. Review the location and contents forming each umbilical fold.
3. Compare the contents entering the deep inguinal ring in female and male cadaveric specimens.
4. Replace the muscles of the anterior abdominal wall in their correct anatomical positions.

PERITONEUM AND PERITONEAL CAVITY

Dissection Overview

The thoracic, pericardial, abdominal, and pelvic cavities are lined by regionally named serous membranes which secrete a small amount of fluid to lubricate the movements of organs. In the abdominal and pelvic cavities, this bilayer membrane is called peritoneum. The parietal peritoneum lines the inner surfaces of the abdominal and pelvic walls, while the visceral peritoneum covers the surfaces of the abdominal and pelvic organs. Between the two layers of peritoneum is a potential space called the peritoneal cavity.

During embryological development, intraperitoneal (peritoneal) organs grow away from the posterior abdominal wall and end up suspended by peritoneum within the peritoneal cavity carrying their neurovascular supply with them. Intraperitoneal organs include the stomach, first part of the duodenum, jejunum, ileum, cecum, appendix, transverse colon, sigmoid colon, upper one-third of the rectum, liver, tail of the pancreas, and spleen.

Retroperitoneal (extraperitoneal) organs develop posterior to the peritoneum and are not suspended in the peritoneal cavity. Retroperitoneal organs include the kidneys, ureters, suprarenal glands, and inferior two-thirds of the rectum. Secondarily retroperitoneal organs begin as intraperitoneal organs during development but end in a location behind the peritoneum. Secondarily retroperitoneal organs include the duodenum (second through fourth parts), pancreas (head, neck, and uncinate process), and colon (ascending and descending). Infraperitoneal refers to organs located inferior to the parietal peritoneum within the pelvic region.

The order of dissection will be as follows: The abdominal viscera will be identified in situ and localized by abdominal quadrant. The named specializations of the peritoneum will be studied. For a more complete understanding, review the development of the gastrointestinal tract before examining the peritoneal specializations.

Dissection Instructions

Abdominal Viscera

ATLAS 4.22, 4.31A; VIDEO 4.4.1

1. Refer to FIGURE 4.17.
2. Reflect the anterior abdominal wall to expose the **peritoneal cavity**.
3. Inspect the abdominal cavity observing how some organs are suspended within the cavity (intraperitoneal), whereas others lie posterior to the peritoneum (retroperitoneal).
4. As you perform the inspection, you may encounter adhesions between the abdominal wall and organs or between parts of organs. If adhesions are present, separate them gently with your fingers or carefully cut them with scissors to mobilize the organs. Take care while detaching adhesions to not puncture the intestinal organs.

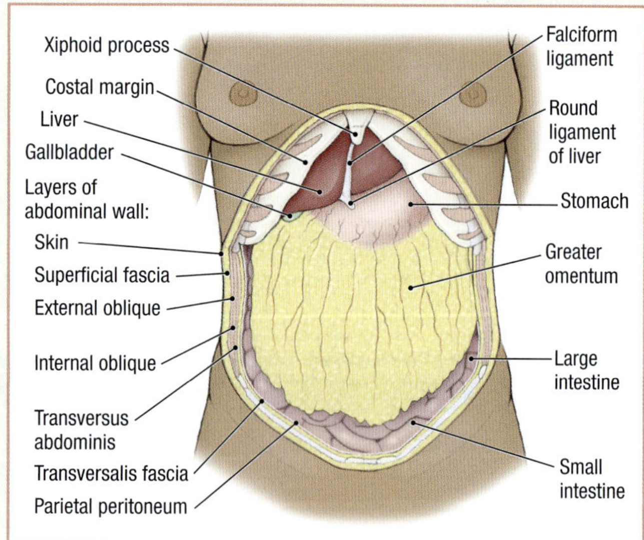

FIGURE 4.17 ● Abdominal cavity contents in situ. Anterior view.

5. As you examine the organs in the abdominal cavity, particularly those related to the **gastrointestinal tract**, relate the organs to the four abdominal quadrants.
6. Identify the **liver** in the right upper quadrant extending across the midline into the left upper quadrant.
7. Identify the **gallbladder** in the right upper quadrant where it extends below the inferior border of the liver. *Note that commonly the gallbladder is found at the tip of the right 9th costal cartilage in the midclavicular line.*
8. Identify the **stomach** in the left upper quadrant. Observe that the stomach lies deep to the liver, which partially covers its anterior surface. Verify that the stomach is continuous with the esophagus proximally and the duodenum distally.
9. Find the **spleen** in the left upper quadrant posterior to the stomach.
10. Identify the **greater omentum** attached to the greater curvature of the stomach.
11. Refer to FIGURE 4.18.
12. Reflect the greater omentum superiorly over the costal margin and identify the **small intestine**.
13. The small intestine has three parts and begins at the pyloric end of the stomach with the **duodenum**, followed by the **jejunum**, and ending as the **ileum**. *Note that the duodenum lies posterior to the other parts of the gastrointestinal tract and will be dissected and studied with the pancreas.*
14. The jejunum and ileum extend from the left upper quadrant to the right lower quadrant but due to their length and mobility occupy all four abdominal quadrants. Beginning in the left upper quadrant, pass the jejunum and ileum between your hands and appreciate their length, position, comparative thickness, and termination.
15. Identify the **large intestine** beginning in the right lower quadrant where the terminal end of the ileum drains into it at the **ileocecal junction**. Use your hands to trace the large intestine from the right lower quadrant around the peritoneal cavity to the

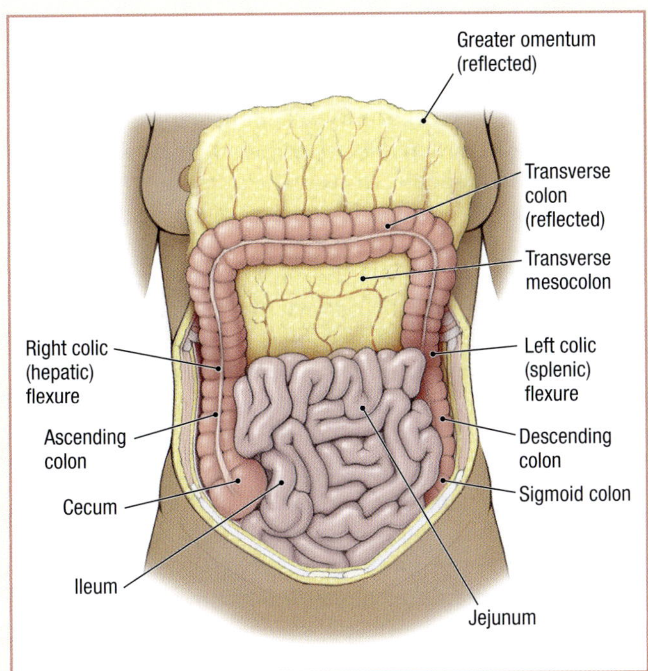

FIGURE 4.18 ■ Abdominal cavity contents with reflected transverse colon and greater omentum. Anterior view.

left lower quadrant, noting the position (quadrant) and mobility of each of its six parts.

16. Identify the **cecum**, the first of six portions of the large intestine, in the right lower quadrant.
17. Identify the **appendix**, the "worm-like" outgrowth on the inferior end of the cecum. *Note that the appendix has a variety of orientations and may or may not be present because it commonly becomes inflamed and is removed surgically.*
18. Follow the cecum superiorly and identify the **ascending colon**, which extends from the right lower quadrant to the right upper quadrant, where it ends at the **right colic (hepatic) flexure**.
19. At the right colic flexure, the large intestine changes direction and courses horizontally as the **transverse colon**, which extends from the right upper quadrant to the left upper quadrant ending at the **left colic (splenic) flexure**.
20. At the left colic flexure, the large intestine curves inferiorly as the **descending colon**, which extends from the left upper quadrant to the left lower quadrant.
21. Identify the **sigmoid colon** in the left lower quadrant, the portion of the large intestine coursing from the abdominal cavity into the pelvic cavity and ending at the level of the third sacral vertebra.
22. Identify the last portion of the large intestine, the **rectum**, inferior to the level of the third sacral vertebra. *Note that the superior one-third of the rectum will be dissected with the abdominal viscera, while the inferior two-thirds will be dissected with the pelvic viscera.*

Reflection of Diaphragm

ATLAS 4.22A; VIDEO 4.4.2

Dissection Note: Depending on the cadaver, some of the structures within the abdominal cavity may or may not be readily visible. If the thorax has previously been dissected but visibility of the upper abdominal cavity remains limited and mobility of the contents is difficult, use the following dissection steps to increase visibility of the abdominal contents. If organ visibility is clear, proceed to the **Peritoneum** sequence.

1. On the left side of the torso, use bone cutters to detach the costal cartilages of ribs 6 and 7 from the xiphisternal junction and lateral border of the sternum.
2. Working through the opening just created, use your hands to elevate the left side of the costal cartilage and use scissors to detach the diaphragm from its anterior attachment on the posterior surface of the costal cartilages.
3. Continue to reflect the left portion of the costal cartilage laterally toward the midaxillary line leaving the lateral aspect connected to act as a hinge.
4. Repeat steps 2 and 3 on the right side and reflect the right costal cartilage laterally.
5. Beginning near the midaxillary line, use scissors to make an incision through the muscular portions of the left and right hemidiaphragms arching medially toward the central tendon of the diaphragm while sparing the central tendon and phrenic nerves.
6. Reflect the anterior aspect of the diaphragm superiorly into the thoracic cavity using the ligamentous attachments to the liver as a hinge.

Peritoneum

ATLAS 4.22B, 4.23, 4.24, 4.27; VIDEO 4.4.3

1. Refer to FIGURE 4.19.
2. Identify the **visceral peritoneum** on the surface of the stomach, small intestine, large intestine, and liver and observe that it is smooth and slippery.
3. Identify the **parietal peritoneum** on the inner surface of the abdominal wall. Observe that the parietal peritoneum is continuous with the visceral peritoneum but changes names due to location.
4. Identify the **greater omentum** and observe that it attaches to the greater curvature of the stomach, extends out into the abdominal cavity, and then doubles back on itself deeply to attach to the transverse colon. *Note that the greater omentum typically lies between the intestines and the anterior abdominal wall but may shift in location or become partially fused to surrounding structures.*
5. Spread out the "apron-like" greater omentum and identify the dominant portion, the **gastrocolic ligament**, as well as the **gastrosplenic** and

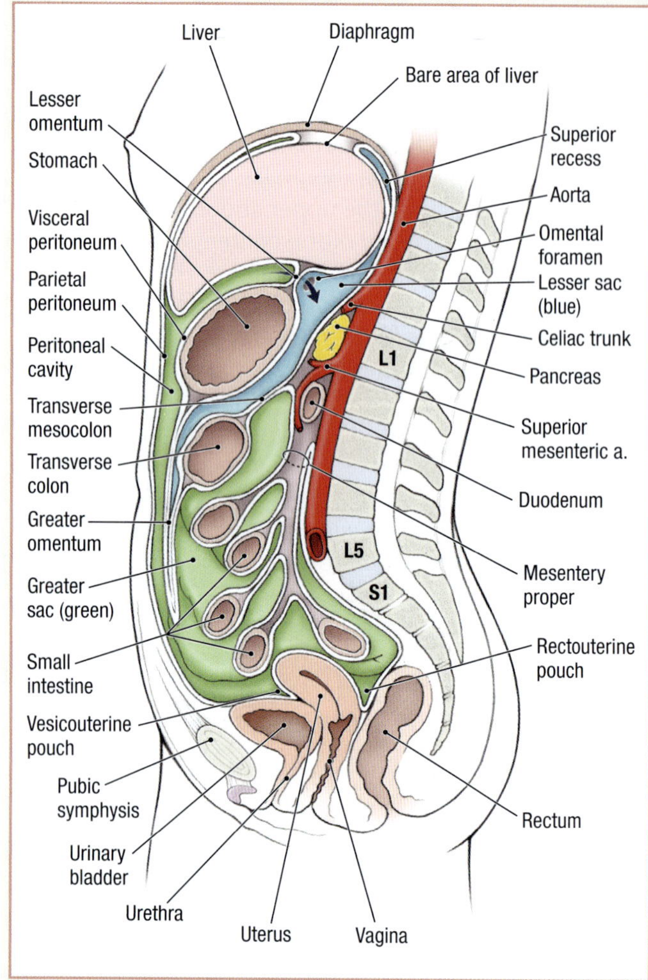

FIGURE 4.19 ● Midsagittal section of female peritoneal cavity. Lateral view.

gastrophrenic ligaments. *Note that the gastrosplenic and gastrophrenic ligaments will be more visible later.*

6. Elevate the inferior border of the liver and identify the **lesser omentum** attaching from the inferior surface of the liver to the lesser curvature of the stomach and first part of the duodenum. *Note that the subdivisions of the lesser omentum will be studied with the visceral surface of the liver.*
7. Reflect the greater omentum superiorly over the costal margin and identify the **transverse mesocolon** attaching from the transverse colon to the anterior surface of the duodenum and pancreas along the posterior abdominal wall.
8. Follow the transverse mesocolon to the left and identify the **phrenicocolic ligament** attaching between the left colic flexure and diaphragm.
9. Identify the **mesentery proper** suspending the jejunum and ileum from the posterior abdominal wall at the **root of the mesentery**, an oblique line from the left upper quadrant to the right lower quadrant.
10. Observe that the parietal peritoneum lines the posterior abdominal wall superior to the root of the mesentery to fill the **right inframesocolic compartment** in the region medial to the ascending colon.
11. On the lateral side of the ascending colon, identify the **right paracolic gutter**, the point of reflection of peritoneum from the lateral wall of the abdominal cavity to the organ.
12. Elevate the small intestine with the mesentery proper and observe that the parietal peritoneum lines the posterior abdominal wall inferior to root of the mesentery to fill the **left inframesocolic compartment** in the region medial to the descending colon.
13. On the lateral side of the descending colon, identify the **left paracolic gutter**, the point of reflection of peritoneum from the lateral wall of the abdominal cavity to the organ.
14. Identify the **mesoappendix**, which attaches the appendix to the distal ileum and cecum and contains the appendicular artery.
15. Identify the **sigmoid mesocolon** in the lower left quadrant, which suspends the sigmoid colon from the posterior abdominal wall.
16. Refer to FIGURE 4.20.
17. Observe that the liver lies against the inferior surface of the diaphragm to which it is attached by ligaments made of peritoneum.
18. On the anterior surface of the liver, identify the **falciform ligament**, connecting from the parietal peritoneum on the anterior abdominal wall to the visceral peritoneum on the surface of the liver.

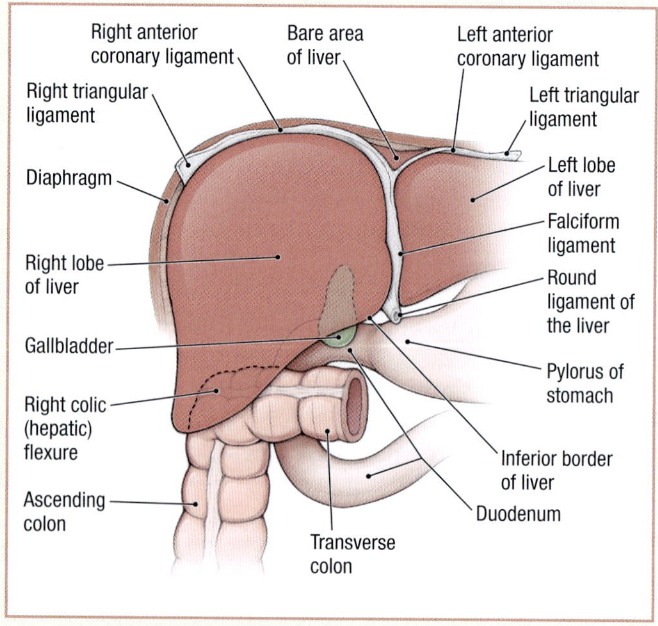

FIGURE 4.20 ● Ligaments of liver. Anterior view.

19. Identify the **round ligament of the liver (ligamentum teres hepatis)** in the inferior edge of the falciform ligament. *Note that the round ligament of the liver is the remnant of the left umbilical vein from fetal development.*
20. Follow the falciform ligament superiorly and observe that it is continuous with the **coronary ligament** attaching the liver to the inferior aspect of the diaphragm. The coronary ligament bounds the region of the liver known as the **bare area** and can be subdivided into **right** and **left anterior** and **right** and **left posterior** portions.
21. The lateral aspects of the coronary ligaments fuse as the **left triangular ligament**, between the left lobe of the liver and the diaphragm, and the **right triangular ligament**, between the right lobe of the liver and the diaphragm.
22. Refer to FIGURE 4.21.
23. The previously identified peritoneal structures are found in a part of the peritoneal cavity called the **greater sac**. Posterior to the stomach and lesser omentum is a smaller part of the peritoneal cavity called the **lesser sac (omental bursa)**.
24. The **omental (epiploic) foramen** connects the greater and lesser peritoneal sacs posterior to the hepatoduodenal ligament.
25. Study a diagram of the lesser sac to appreciate that its lowest part, the inferior recess, extends inferiorly as far as the greater omentum. *Note that during development, the inferior recess extended between the layers of the greater omentum.*
26. The highest part of the lesser peritoneal sac, the **superior recess**, extends superiorly between the diaphragm and the caudate lobe of the liver. *Note that the posterior wall of the lesser peritoneal sac is the peritoneum overlying the pancreas.*

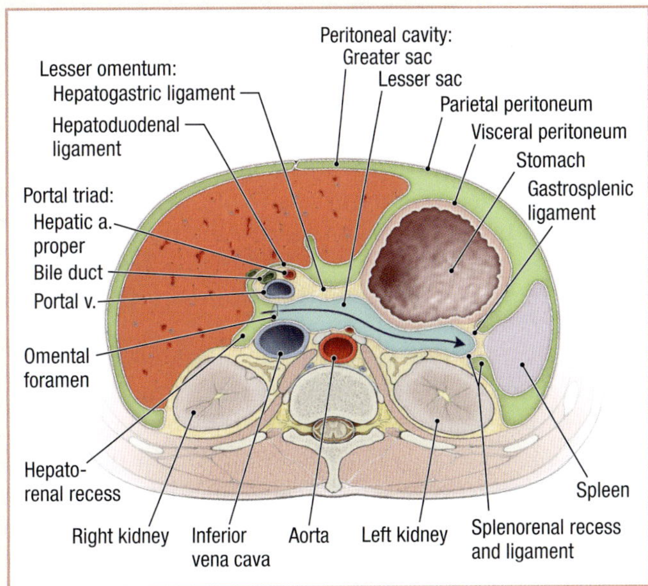

FIGURE 4.21 Axial section through abdominal cavity. Inferior view.

Dissection Follow-up

1. Review all parts of the gastrointestinal tract proximal to distal in order.
2. State the quadrant(s) in which each abdominal organ is typically found.
3. List the intraperitoneal organs and name the specialized peritoneal structures suspending each.
4. Review the locations of the paracolic and mesenteric gutters and discuss how these channels can assist in the spread of infection or disease.
5. Review the list of retroperitoneal and secondarily retroperitoneal organs.
6. Replace the abdominal organs and muscles of the anterior abdominal wall in their correct anatomical positions.

FOREGUT DERIVATIVES

Dissection Overview

During embryonic development, the primitive gut tube subdivides into three distinct components based on location and vascular supply. Foregut derivatives will receive vascular supply from branches of the celiac trunk, midgut derivatives from branches of the superior mesenteric artery, and hindgut derivatives from branches the inferior mesenteric artery.

The celiac trunk arises from the anterior surface of the abdominal aorta near its entrance into the abdominal cavity via the aortic hiatus at vertebral level T12 and is approximately encircled by the lesser curvature of the stomach. The celiac trunk supplies intraperitoneal organs (stomach, spleen, liver, and gallbladder) and retroperitoneal organs (aspects of the duodenum and pancreas).

The order of dissection will be as follows: The surface features of the stomach will be studied. The portal triad in the hepatoduodenal ligament will be dissected. Branches of the celiac trunk supplying the stomach, spleen, liver, and gallbladder will be dissected. The hepatic portal vein will be studied. The surface features of the spleen, liver, and gallbladder will be studied.

Dissection Instructions

Stomach and Visceral Surface of Liver

ATLAS 4.28, 4.29, 4.32, 4.51; VIDEO 4.5.1

1. Refer to FIGURE 4.22.
2. Identify the **greater curvature** of the stomach on the left lateral margin of the **body of the stomach** and observe that the **gastrocolic ligament** of the **greater omentum** attaches along this curve.
3. Observe that the body of the stomach is inferior to the rounded superior protrusion of the **fundus**.
4. Observe that the fundus of the stomach connects to the inferior aspect of the diaphragm by the **gastrophrenic ligament** of the greater omentum, and that the body of the stomach along the greater curvature also connects to the spleen by the **gastrosplenic (gastrolienal) ligament** of the greater omentum.
5. Identify the **cardial (cardiac) notch**, which delineates the fundus from the **cardia** of the stomach. Observe that the cardia contains the inlet of the stomach connecting to the esophagus.
6. Identify the **lesser curvature** of the stomach on the right margin and observe the change of direction of the curvature at the **angular incisure (notch)**, where the body of the stomach transitions to the **pyloric part**.
7. Within the pyloric region of the stomach, palpate the **pyloric sphincter**, the circular muscle responsible for controlling the passage of food from the stomach to the duodenum.
8. Refer back to FIGURE 4.20 and refer to FIGURE 4.23.
9. On the anterior surface of the liver, identify the **right lobe** and **left lobe** on either side of the **falciform ligament**.

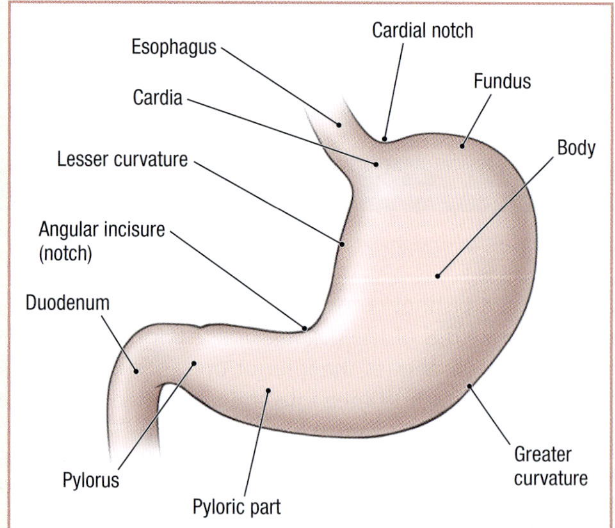

FIGURE 4.22 ● Parts of stomach. Anterior view.

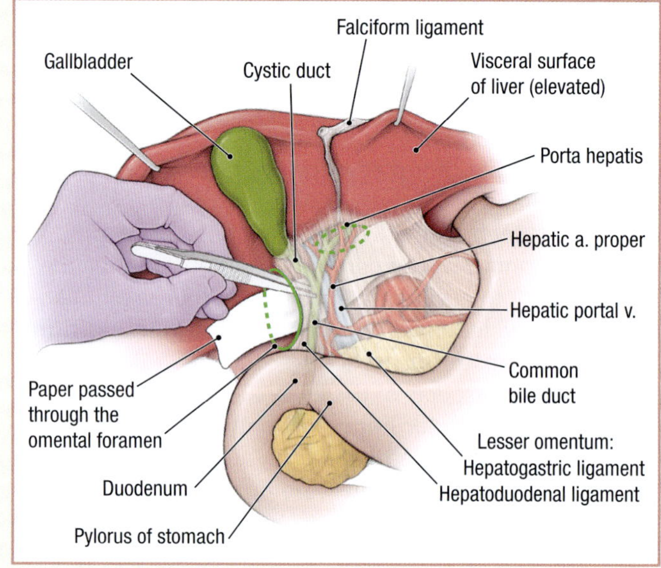

FIGURE 4.23 ● Lesser omentum and omental foramen. Anterior view.

10. Follow the right or left lobe superiorly to identify the **diaphragmatic surface of the liver**, the portion in contact with the diaphragm, and inferiorly to identify the **inferior border of the liver** on the free edge of the anterior surface.
11. Raise the inferior border of the liver and identify the **visceral surface of the liver**. Observe that the visceral surface of the liver is in contact with the gallbladder and the peritoneum covering the stomach, duodenum, colon, right kidney, and right suprarenal gland.
12. On the visceral surface of the liver, identify the **porta hepatis**, the fissure through which vessels, ducts, lymphatics, and nerves enter and leave the liver.
13. Identify the **gallbladder** along the inferior border of the liver and observe that it is directed posteriorly toward the porta hepatis. *Note that the gallbladder may have been surgically removed; however, the depression marking its location should still be visible on the visceral surface of the liver.*
14. Identify the subdivisions of the **lesser omentum**: the **hepatogastric ligament**, from the liver to the lesser curvature of the stomach, and the **hepatoduodenal ligament**, from the liver to the first part of the duodenum.
15. Insert your finger into the **omental foramen** and review its boundaries beginning with the **anterior boundary** formed by the hepatoduodenal ligament containing the **portal triad**, autonomic nerves, and lymphatic vessels.
16. Identify the **posterior boundary** of the omental foramen, the parietal peritoneum overlying the **inferior vena cava** and right crus of the diaphragm.

17. Identify the superior boundary of the omental foramen, the caudate lobe of the liver, and the inferior boundary, the **first part of the duodenum**, and observe that both are covered with visceral peritoneum.

Portal Triad

ATLAS 4.29, 4.30, 4.56; VIDEO 4.5.2

Dissection Note: As you dissect the branches of the celiac trunk, realize that the arteries are named by their region of distribution and not by their point of origin or branching pattern.

1. Refer to FIGURE 4.23.
2. Gently elevate the liver and diaphragm superiorly to expose the lesser omentum.
3. To aid dissection, a strip of white paper may be placed into the omental foramen to increase visibility of the surrounding structures.
4. Use blunt dissection to separate the peritoneum of the hepatoduodenal ligament anterior to the vessels and ducts.
5. Within the hepatoduodenal ligament, identify the **portal triad**: the **bile (common bile) duct** laterally, **hepatic artery proper** medially, and **hepatic portal vein** posteriorly.
6. Use blunt dissection to trace the bile duct superiorly and identify the **cystic duct** and **common hepatic duct**.
7. Follow the common hepatic duct superiorly until it receives its tributaries, the **right** and **left hepatic ducts**, which exit the **porta hepatis** on the visceral surface of the liver.
8. Return to the hepatoduodenal ligament and use blunt dissection to clean the **hepatic artery proper**, removing the tough "connective tissue" around this vessel containing the autonomic nerve plexus.
9. Refer to FIGURE 4.24.
10. Follow the hepatic artery proper toward the liver until it branches into the **left hepatic artery** and the **right hepatic artery** near the porta hepatis.
11. Identify the **cystic artery**, commonly arising from the right hepatic artery in the hepatoduodenal ligament, and follow it toward the gallbladder for a short distance.
12. Identify the **right gastric artery**, commonly arising from the hepatic artery proper, and follow it to the lesser curvature of the stomach.
13. Identify the large **hepatic portal vein** lying posterior to the hepatic artery proper and bile duct.
14. Follow the hepatic portal vein superiorly toward the porta hepatis where it divides into **right and left portal veins**. *Note that the hepatic portal vein usually receives the left and right gastric veins as tributaries.*
15. Follow the hepatic portal vein inferiorly and observe that it passes posterior to the first part of the duodenum.

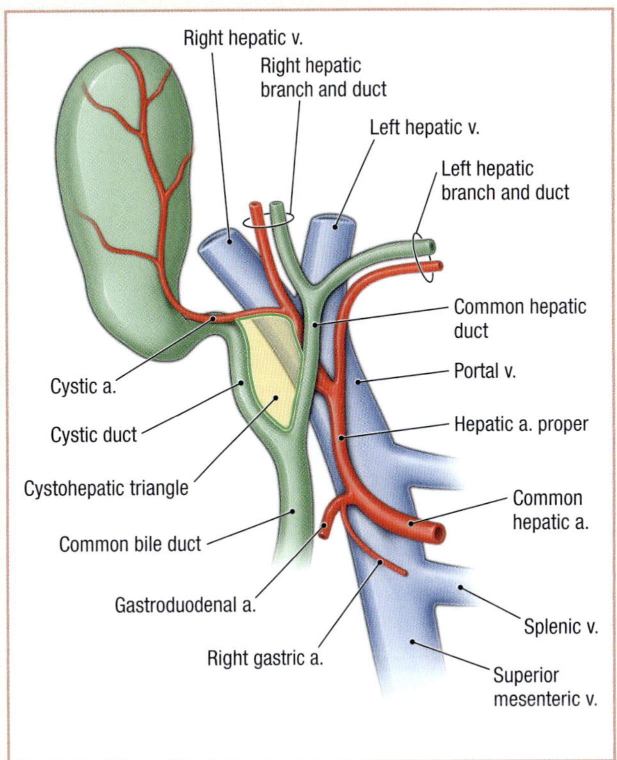

FIGURE 4.24 ● Portal triad in isolation. Anterior view.

16. Identify and remove any visible lymph nodes within the hepatoduodenal ligament. *Note that the lymphatic vessels accompanying the lymph nodes are typically too small to see in embalmed specimens and no effort should be made to identify them.*

Celiac Trunk

ATLAS 4.33, 4.58; VIDEO 4.5.3

Dissection Note: The following dissection descriptions reference a common pattern of branching of the celiac trunk and associated vessels, although variations in the arteries of this region are common.

1. Refer to FIGURE 4.25.
2. Use blunt dissection to gently split the hepatogastric ligament near its attachment to the liver.
3. Follow the hepatic artery proper inferiorly and confirm that it is the continuation of the **common hepatic artery**.
4. Observe that the common hepatic artery gives rise to the **gastroduodenal artery**, which passes posterior to the first part of the duodenum.
5. Follow the gastroduodenal artery inferiorly and identify the **supraduodenal artery** supplying the first part of the duodenum, the **right gastroomental (gastroepiploic) artery** supplying the greater curvature of the stomach, and the proximal aspect of the

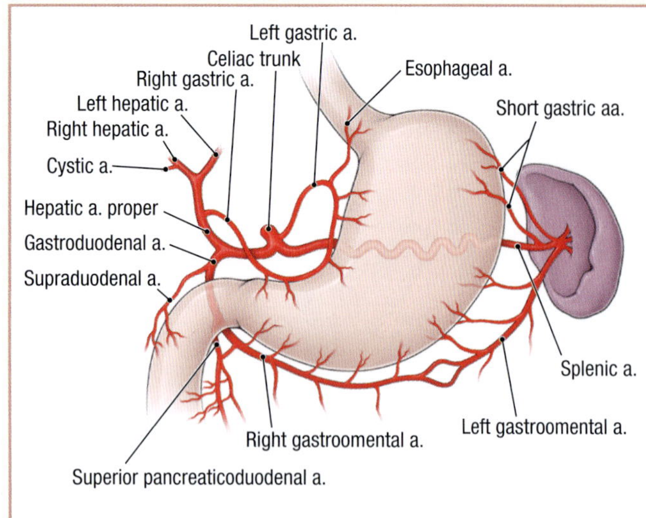

FIGURE 4.25 ■ Branches of celiac trunk (artery) isolated. Anterior view.

superior pancreaticoduodenal artery supplying the head of the pancreas.

6. Follow the common hepatic artery to the left side of the body toward its origin from the **celiac trunk.** *Note that the celiac trunk arises from the anterior surface of the abdominal aorta at the level of the 12th thoracic vertebra.*
7. Observe that the celiac trunk also gives rise to the **left gastric artery** and the **splenic artery** in addition to the common hepatic artery.
8. Use blunt dissection to follow the **left gastric artery** superiorly toward the esophagus and stomach and then to the lesser curvature of the stomach.
9. Observe that the left gastric artery forms an anastomosis with the right gastric artery along the lesser curvature of the stomach within the lesser omentum. *Note that branches of the gastric arteries distribute to both the anterior and posterior surfaces of the stomach.*
10. Reflect the gastrocolic portion of the greater omentum superiorly and use blunt dissection to separate it from its attachment to the transverse colon while sparing its attachment to the greater curvature of the stomach.
11. Reflect the stomach superiorly with the greater omentum and follow the **splenic artery** to the left for about 5 cm, verifying that it lies against the posterior abdominal wall, is tortuous, and courses along the superior border of the pancreas where it may be partially imbedded. *Do not dissect the branches arising from the middle portion of the splenic artery at this time.*
12. Locate the portion of the splenic artery posterior to the stomach and identify the **short gastric arteries** supplying the fundus of the stomach within the gastrosplenic ligament.
13. Observe that near its distal end, the splenic artery gives rise to the **left gastroomental (gastroepiploic) artery,** which courses in the greater omentum about 2 cm away from the greater curvature of the stomach.
14. Find the **right gastroomental artery** from its origin off the gastroduodenal artery and follow it along its path within the greater omentum near the right end of the greater curvature of the stomach to the point where it anastomoses with the left gastroomental artery.

Spleen

ATLAS 4.30, 4.33, 4.35; VIDEO 4.5.4

Dissection Note: The spleen is the largest hematopoietic organ in the body and its size and weight may vary considerably depending on the volume of blood it contained and the health of the individual during life.

1. Refer to FIGURE 4.26.
2. Retract the fundus of the stomach to the right and gently pull the spleen anteriorly.
3. Observe that the spleen has a smooth **diaphragmatic surface** and sharp anterior, inferior, and superior borders. *Note that the superior border of the spleen is often notched due to its pattern of embryological development.*
4. Observe that the **visceral surface of the spleen** is related to four organs: **stomach, left kidney, colon** (at the left colic flexure), and **pancreas.**
5. Observe that the diaphragmatic surface of the spleen is related to the diaphragm and **ribs 9, 10,** and **11** (see **Clinical Correlation 4.4**).

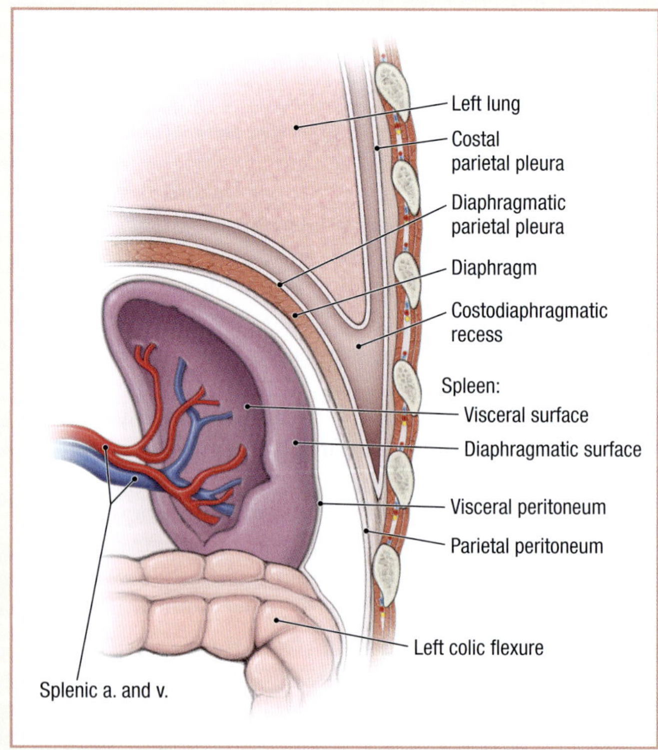

FIGURE 4.26 ■ Relationships of spleen to thoracic wall. Anterior view.

CLINICAL CORRELATION 4.4

Lacerated Spleen and Splenomegaly

ATLAS 4.35

The relationship of the spleen to left ribs 9, 10, and 11 is of clinical importance in evaluating rib fractures due to blunt trauma or penetrating wounds as shown in FIGURE B4.2. A lacerated spleen bleeds profusely into the abdominal cavity and may have to be removed surgically (splenectomy). During thoracentesis (pleural tap), the invasive removal of air or fluid from the pleural cavity, there is a risk of puncturing the spleen on the left side of the torso.

Splenomegaly is enlargement of the spleen due to infection, liver disease, or some cancers. The spleen is considered enlarged when it can be palpated inferior to the costal margin during physical examination.

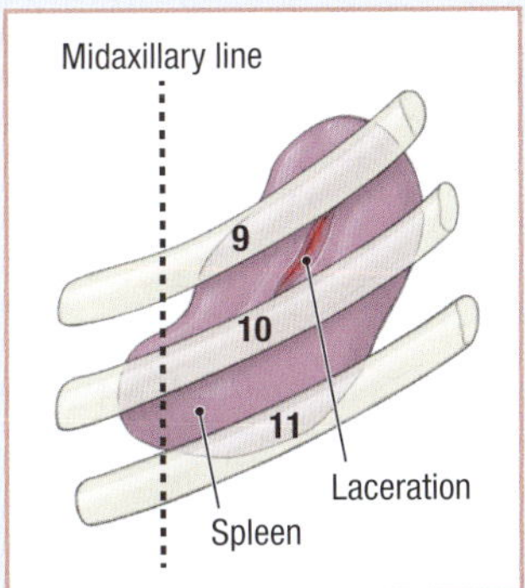

FIGURE B4.2 ● Lacerated spleen. Lateral view.

6. Observe that the spleen is an intraperitoneal organ suspended within the abdominal cavity by the gastrosplenic ligament from the greater curvature of the stomach and splenorenal (lienorenal) ligament to the body wall anterior to the left kidney.
7. Identify the visceral peritoneum along the diaphragmatic surface of the spleen and observe its proximity to the parietal peritoneum along the inferior aspect of the left hemidiaphragm.
8. Observe the proximity of the spleen to the **inferior lobe of the left lung**, **costodiaphragmatic recess**, and left lower **ribs** through the respiratory diaphragm.

Liver

ATLAS 4.50, 4.51; VIDEO 4.5.5

Dissection Note: To study the surface features of the liver, it will first be detached from the diaphragm.

1. Refer to FIGURE 4.27.
2. Use scissors to cut the **falciform ligament** between the liver and diaphragm, extending the incision superiorly to the level of the **anterior coronary ligament**.
3. Gently pull the liver inferiorly and extend the cut bilaterally through the coronary ligaments along the inferior surface of the diaphragm toward the **right** and **left triangular ligaments**.
4. Roll the liver anteriorly and use scissors to cut the **inferior vena cava** between the superior aspect of the liver and the inferior aspect of the diaphragm.
5. Insert your fingers between the liver and diaphragm and gently tear the connective tissue attaching the liver to the diaphragm at the **bare area** of the liver.
6. Continue to roll the superior aspect of the liver anteroinferiorly and cut the **posterior coronary ligament** on the posterior aspect of the liver, freeing it from the diaphragm.
7. Elevate the inferior border of the liver and cut the inferior vena cava close to the inferior surface of the liver. *Note that the two cuts through the inferior vena cava will leave a short segment of vena cava within the liver.*
8. The liver should now be freely mobile but attached to the other abdominal viscera by the **portal triad**: bile duct, hepatic artery proper, and hepatic portal vein. Move the liver carefully to avoid tearing the vessels of the portal triad.
9. Examine the **liver** and observe that the **right lobe** is approximately six times larger than the **left lobe** and that the sharp **inferior border** of the liver separates its **visceral surface** from its **diaphragmatic surface** (see **Clinical Correlation 4.5**).

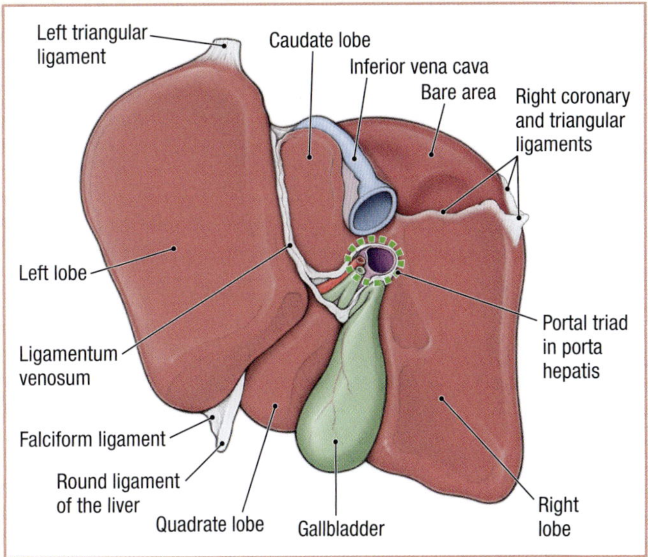

FIGURE 4.27 ● Visceral surface of liver. Inferior view.

CLINICAL CORRELATION 4.5

Liver Enlargement

ATLAS 4.50, 4.54

The liver may undergo pathologic changes that could be encountered during dissection. The liver may be enlarged, which happens in liver congestion due to cardiac insufficiency (cardiac cirrhosis), or it may be small and have fibrous nodules indicating cirrhosis of the liver. Because the liver is essentially a capillary bed downstream from the gastrointestinal tract, metastatic tumor cells are often trapped within it, resulting in secondary tumors.

10. Identify the **bare area** on the posterior aspect of the diaphragmatic surface of the liver and observe that it is bound by the cut edges of the coronary ligaments. *Note that in this location, the liver was immediately adjacent to the diaphragm and not covered by peritoneum.*
11. Examine the **visceral surface** of the liver and identify the approximately H-shaped set of fissures and fossae defining its four lobes. Observe that the **ligamentum venosum** and **falciform ligament** occupy the left fissure of the "H" and that the **gallbladder** and **inferior vena cava** occupy the fossae that form the right side of the "H."
12. Identify the **porta hepatis** forming the horizontal bar of the "H," the location where structures passing through the hepatoduodenal ligament (bile ducts, hepatic arteries, hepatic portal vein, lymphatics, and autonomic nerves) enter or leave the liver.
13. Identify the **caudate lobe** between the inferior vena cava and ligamentum venosum and the **quadrate lobe** between the round ligament of the liver and gallbladder.
14. Examine the small segment of the **inferior vena cava** attached to the liver and remove any coagulated blood from within its lumen. Observe that several **hepatic veins** drain directly from the liver into the inferior vena cava.
15. Two common conventions are used to divide the liver. The first divides the liver into **right** and **left anatomical lobes** using the falciform ligament as a guide. The second divides the liver by the pattern of bile drainage and vascular supply into **functional lobes**. In this convention, the right and left sides are separated by the inferior vena cava and ultimately divided into eight hepatic segments.
16. The liver has a substantial lymphatic drainage system. At the porta hepatis, small lymph vessels drain into **hepatic lymph nodes** which connect to lymphatic vessels accompanying the hepatic arteries toward **celiac lymph nodes** located around the celiac trunk. Lymph from the liver also drains posteriorly into **phrenic nodes**.

Gallbladder

ATLAS 4.56, 4.57, 4.59A; VIDEO 4.5.6

Dissection Note: The gallbladder and surrounding tissue is commonly stained dark green by bile leakage through its wall postmortem.

1. Refer to FIGURE 4.28.
2. With the liver into its correct anatomical position, confirm that the gallbladder is located near the tip of the 9th costal cartilage in the midclavicular line.

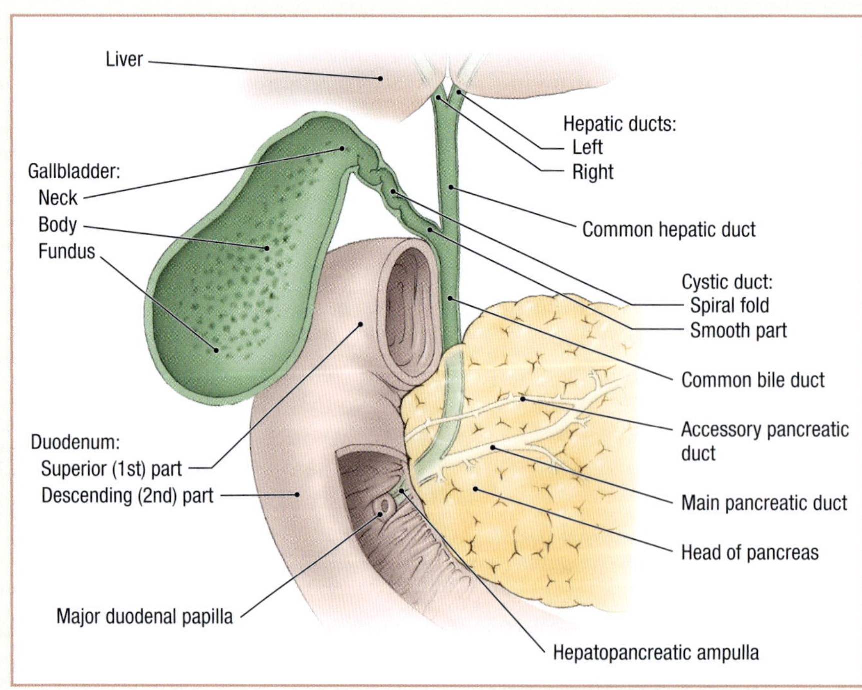

FIGURE 4.28 ● Gallbladder and biliary tree. Anterior view.

3. Identify the **fundus** of the gallbladder, the anteriorly directed distal end of the organ extending past the free edge of the liver. The attached portion of the gallbladder is the **body**, whereas the **neck** is the narrow portion leading toward the biliary tree.
4. Lift the inferior border of the liver to expose its visceral surface and use blunt dissection to carefully detach the gallbladder from its fossa.
5. Review the course of the **cystic artery** from the hepatic vessels (see **Clinical Correlation 4.6**). *Note that the cystic artery is often stained green by bile rendering it fragile and difficult to dissect.*

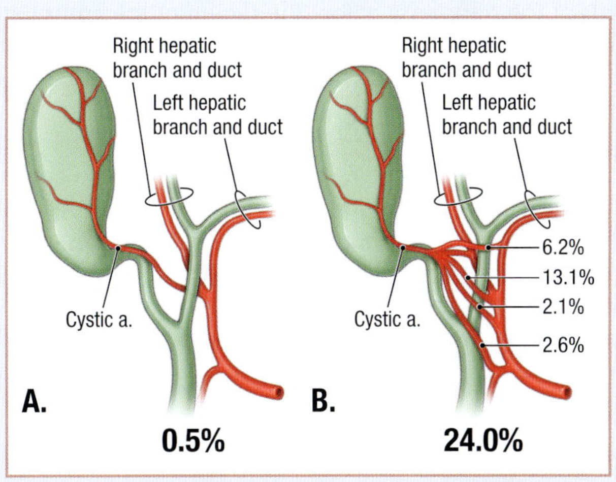

FIGURE B4.3 ● **A.** Cystic artery arising from hepatic artery proper at bifurcation. **B.** Alternate branching pattern percentages. Anterior views.

CLINICAL CORRELATION 4.6

Cystic Artery Variants

ATLAS 4.57A, 4.62

The cystic artery usually arises from the right hepatic artery, but other origins are possible. Typically, the cystic artery passes posterior to the common hepatic duct, although in about a quarter of individuals, it may pass anteriorly along various pathways as shown in FIGURE B4.3. Occasionally, the right hepatic artery may arise from the superior mesenteric artery, or an aberrant left hepatic artery may arise from the left gastric artery. During surgical removal of the stomach (gastrectomy), blood flow to an aberrant left hepatic artery could be interrupted, endangering the left lobe of the liver.

6. Use scissors to make a longitudinal cut through the wall of the gallbladder, beginning at the fundus and continuing through the neck into the **cystic duct**. If gallstones are present, remove them.
7. Look for the **spiral fold (valve)**, a fold in the mucosal lining of the neck continuing into the cystic duct allowing for bidirectional flow in and out of the organ.
8. The connection of the biliary system with the main pancreatic duct to drain into the second (descending) portion of the duodenum will be seen in the dissection of the duodenum and pancreas.

Dissection Follow-up

1. Correlate the location of each organ to the abdominal quadrant system.
2. Review the branches of the celiac trunk.
3. Describe the relationships of the structures in the hepatoduodenal ligament.
4. Review the boundaries of the omental foramen.
5. Review the parts of the organs dissected and their relationships to surrounding structures.
6. Return the gallbladder and other abdominal organs to their correct anatomical positions.
7. Use an embryology textbook to review the development of the embryonic foregut derivatives and their respective mesenteries.

MIDGUT AND HINDGUT DERIVATIVES

Dissection Overview

The small intestine consists of the duodenum, jejunum, and ileum and is the major site of digestion of food and absorption of nutrients. The small intestine has a rich blood supply and contains elaborate mucosal folds, which increase the surface area for absorption. The large intestine consists of the cecum, appendix, colon (ascending, transverse, descending, and sigmoid), rectum, and anal canal. The large intestine has a relatively smooth mucosal surface and functions primarily for water absorption and expelling fecal waste.

The superior mesenteric artery is responsible for blood supply to the small and large intestines up to the right two-thirds of the transverse colon, the region of the embryonic midgut. The superior mesenteric artery arises from the anterior surface of the abdominal aorta about 1 cm inferior to the celiac trunk at vertebral level L1. The superior mesenteric artery courses within the mesentery of the small intestine toward the terminal end of the ileum and cecum in the right lower abdominal quadrant.

The inferior mesenteric artery supplies the left third of the transverse colon, descending colon, sigmoid colon, and superior one-third of the rectum, the region of the embryonic hindgut. The inferior mesenteric artery arises from the anterior surface of the abdominal aorta at vertebral level L3. Except for the branches that pass through the sigmoid mesocolon to supply the sigmoid colon, the inferior mesenteric artery and its branches lie retroperitoneally.

The order of dissection will be as follows: The external features of the jejunum and ileum will be studied. The external features of the large intestine will be studied. The branches of the superior mesenteric artery will be dissected. The inferior mesenteric artery and its branches will be dissected. The origin and remainder of the field of supply of the superior mesenteric artery (to the duodenum and pancreas) will be dissected later.

Dissection Instructions

Midgut Derivatives

ATLAS 4.40, 4.41; VIDEO 4.6.2

Dissection Note: The jejunum and ileum will be studied together because the transition from one to the other is gradual.

1. Refer to FIGURE 4.29.
2. Reflect the **greater omentum** and **transverse colon** superiorly over the costal margin to expose the coils of the **jejunum** and **ileum** of the small intestine.
3. Identify the **mesentery proper**, the supportive peritoneal reflections suspending the intraperitoneal portions of the small intestine.

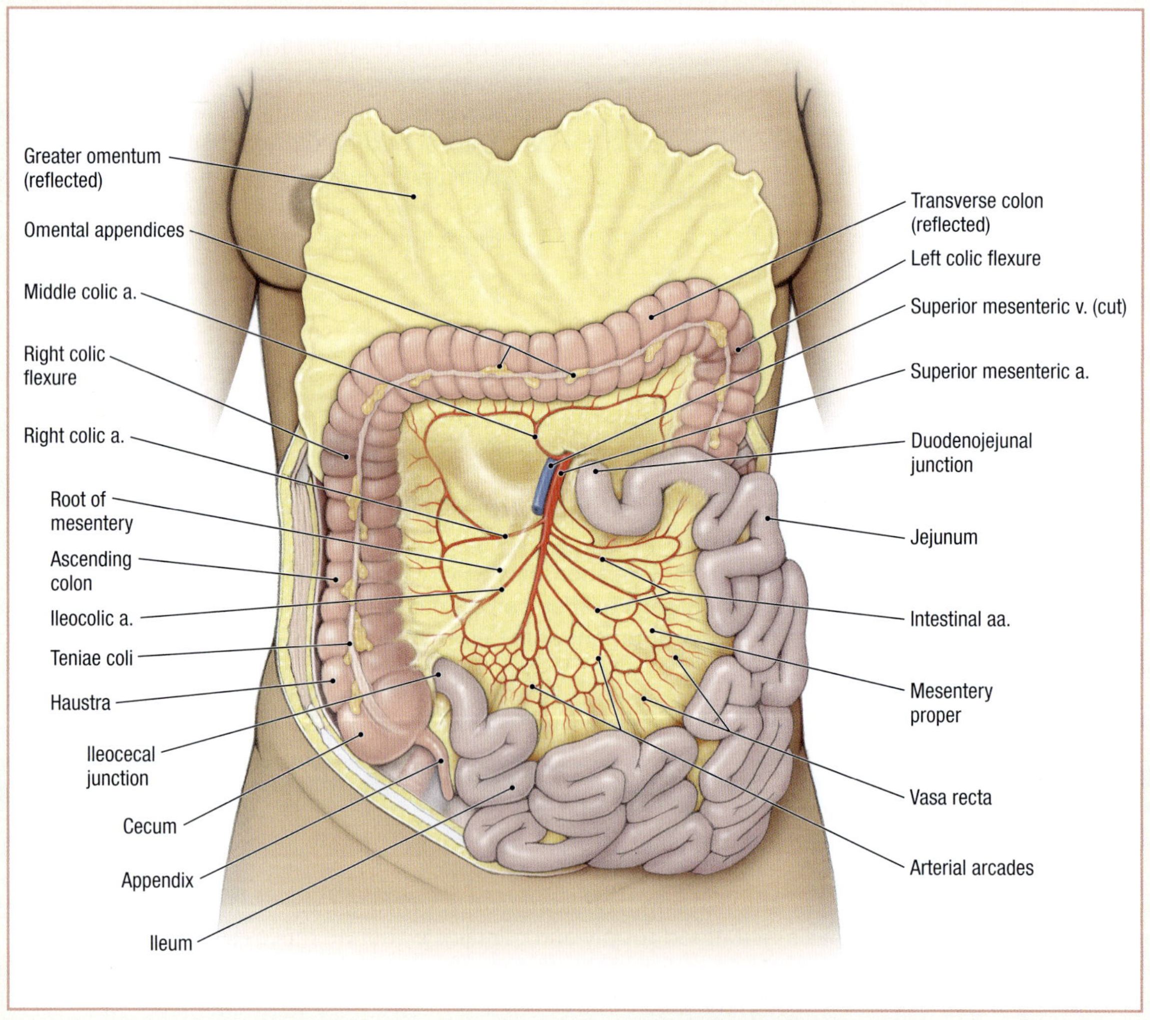

FIGURE 4.29 ● Midgut derivatives and branches of superior mesenteric artery. Anterior view.

4. Observe that the **root of the mesentery**, its point of origination, is attached to the posterior abdominal wall along an oblique line from the left upper quadrant to the right lower quadrant.
5. Move the intraperitoneal portion of the small intestine to the left side of the abdominal cavity and follow the jejunum proximally to find the **duodenojejunal junction**.
6. Gently pull the proximal jejunum away from the posterior abdominal wall and observe that the small intestine has limited mobility in this location as it is anchored at the duodenojejunal junction by the **suspensory ligament of the duodenum**, a fibromuscular band arising from the right crus of the diaphragm. *Note that the suspensory ligament passes posterior to the pancreas; thus, it cannot be seen at this time.*
7. Palpate the small intestine and observe that the wall of the jejunum is thicker than the wall of the ileum and that the overall diameter of the jejunum is larger.
8. Identify the termination of the ileum where it empties into the **cecum** at the **ileocecal junction**.
9. Verify that the root of the mesentery crosses the posterior abdominal wall from the duodenojejunal junction to the ileocecal junction. Observe that the mesentery is somewhat "fan-shaped," with the root about 15 cm long and its intestinal attachment nearly 6 m long.
10. In the right lower quadrant, identify the **cecum**, the first component of the **large intestine**.
11. Observe that the cecum is quite mobile and often almost completely invested by peritoneum, although it does not have a named mesentery. *Note that the cecum is classified as an intraperitoneal organ; however, the length of its mesentery and degree of its mobility varies considerably from individual to individual.*
12. Elevate the cecum slightly and observe the close relationship to the underlying **external iliac vessels** coursing toward the lower limb.
13. Identify the **appendix (vermiform appendix)** attached to the end of the cecum in one of several positions, although if present, most likely in a retrocecal position (see **Clinical Correlation 4.7**).

CLINICAL CORRELATION 4.7

Appendicitis

ATLAS 4.43

The appendix is a blind-ended intraperitoneal organ with limited known functionality, although with high clinical relevancy due to the common need to remove the organ when it becomes inflamed—appendicitis. In many individuals, the appendix lies in a retrocecal position posterior to the cecum; however, in some individuals, it may be found suspended inferior to the cecum, extend into the pelvic cavity, or in a low ratio of other orientations as shown in FIGURE B4.4. Verification of the orientation in the sick individual should be assessed prior to attempted removal in an appendectomy procedure.

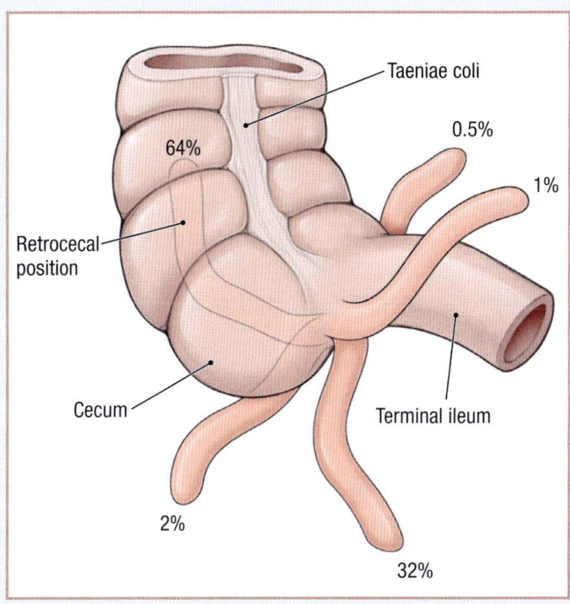

FIGURE B4.4 ● Variations in appendix orientations. Anterior view.

14. Observe that the appendix is suspended by a mesentery called the **mesoappendix**.
15. On the external surface of the large intestine, observe three features that distinguish it from the small intestine: **teniae coli**, the three narrow bands of longitudinal muscle running the length of the large intestine; **haustra (sacculations)**, the outpouchings of the wall of the colon; and **omental appendices (epiploic appendages)**, the small, fatty projections covered by peritoneum.
16. The teniae coli are named according to their location around the circumference of the large intestine with the **mesocolic tenia** along the attachment of the transverse and sigmoid mesocolons, the **omental tenia** where the omental appendices attach, and the **free tenia** where neither mesocolons nor omental appendices are attached.
17. Identify the **ascending colon** extending from the cecum to the **right colic flexure** and recall that it is a secondarily retroperitoneal organ.

18. Identify the **transverse colon** between the **right colic (hepatic) flexure** and **left colic (splenic) flexure** and observe that the transverse colon is suspended by the **transverse mesocolon** and freely mobile at this location.

Superior Mesenteric Artery and Vein

ATLAS 4.30, 4.31, 4.44; VIDEO 4.6.1

1. Refer to FIGURE 4.29.
2. Position the coils of the **jejunum** and **ileum** to the left side of the abdomen so the right side of the **mesentery proper** faces anteriorly.
3. Make a small incision through the peritoneum and use forceps to grasp it and slowly peel it away from the underlying blood vessels to expose branches of the superior mesenteric artery.
4. Remove the parietal peritoneum from the posterior abdominal wall on the right side of the root of the mesentery as far laterally as the ascending colon. *Note that all portions of the peritoneum on the surface of an organ are visceral, whether it is a retroperitoneal or an intraperitoneal organ.*
5. Identify the branches of the **superior mesenteric artery** coursing within the mesentery proper (see **Clinical Correlation 4.8**).

CLINICAL CORRELATION 4.8

Superior Mesenteric Artery Syndrome

ATLAS 4.68

The third part of the duodenum can become compressed between the superior mesenteric vessels and abdominal aorta, leading to a gastrovascular disorder known as superior mesenteric artery syndrome. Blockage of the duodenum results in blockage of the digestive tract and although rare may be life-threatening. The superior mesenteric artery may also compress the left renal vein against the abdominal aorta in "nutcracker syndrome," resulting in insufficient venous drainage of the left kidney, left adrenal gland, and left gonad.

6. Use blunt dissection to clean a short portion of the superior mesenteric artery, which is embedded in a variable amount of mesenteric fat. As you dissect, observe the **superior mesenteric plexus of nerves**, a dense autonomic nerve network surrounding the blood vessels.
7. Identify the **superior mesenteric vein** positioned along the right side of the superior mesenteric artery. *Note that the superior mesenteric vein is formed by tributaries that correspond in name and position to many of the branches of the superior mesenteric artery.*
8. Return to the mesentery proper and identify one or two **mesenteric lymph nodes**, if visible, along the branches of the superior mesenteric vessels. The mesentery may contain up to 200 lymph nodes, which drain into the **superior mesenteric lymph nodes** near the origin of the superior mesenteric artery from the abdominal aorta.
9. To facilitate identification of the intestinal arteries, the lymph nodes and autonomic nerves may be removed to clear the dissection field.
10. Observe that the superior mesenteric artery has 15 to 18 **intestinal arteries** originating from the left side of the superior mesenteric artery supplying the jejunum and ileum.
11. Observe that the intestinal arteries end in straight terminal branches called **vasa recta (straight arteries)**, which are interconnected by **arterial arcades**.
12. Identify the **middle colic artery** arising from the anterior surface of the superior mesenteric artery coursing through the transverse mesocolon to supply the transverse colon.
13. Clean the middle colic artery along a short distance and observe that it divides into a right and a left branch along the margin of the transverse colon.
14. Identify the **right colic artery** arising from the right side of the superior mesenteric artery passing to the right in a retroperitoneal position to supply the ascending colon.
15. Clean the right colic artery and observe that it often divides into a superior branch and an inferior branch.
16. Refer to FIGURE 4.30.
17. To the left of the superior mesenteric artery, identify the vast blood supply to the proximal jejunum.
18. Remove a portion of the peritoneum supporting the jejunum to clean and isolate the jejunal vasculature along a short portion of the organ's length.
19. Observe that only one or two **arcades** are found between adjacent **intestinal arteries**, resulting in relatively long **vasa recta** to the jejunum.
20. Remove a portion of the peritoneum supporting the ileum to clean and isolate a portion of the ileal vasculature along a short portion of the organ's length.
21. Examine the distal ileum's blood supply and observe that four or five **arcades** occur between adjacent **intestinal arteries**, resulting in relatively short **vasa recta**.
22. Refer to FIGURE 4.31.
23. Identify and clean the **ileocolic artery** arising from the distal extent of the superior mesenteric artery coursing toward the right lower quadrant in a retroperitoneal position to supply the cecum.
24. Identify the **anterior** and **posterior cecal arteries** arising from the **ileocolic artery** to provide blood supply to the cecum within the **cecal folds** surrounding the ileocecal junction.

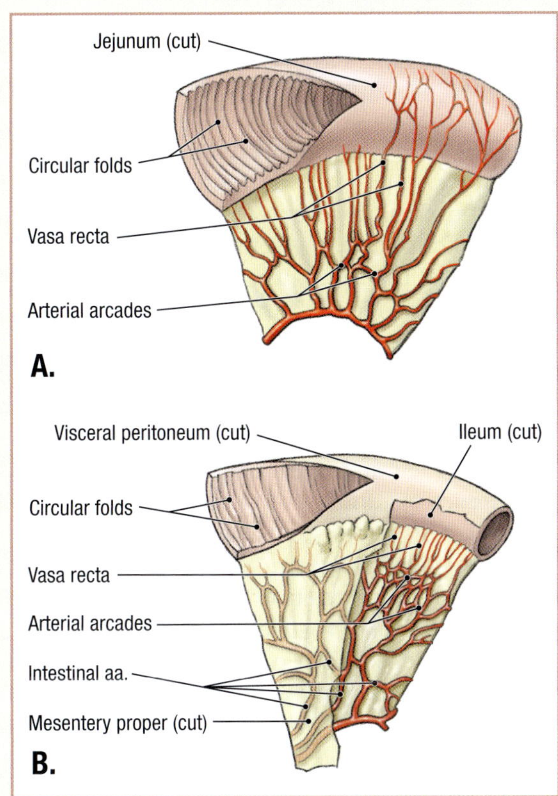

FIGURE 4.30 ● **A.** Arterial supply to jejunum. **B.** Arterial supply to ileum. Isolated views.

25. If the appendix has not been surgically removed in the cadaver, identify and clean the **appendicular artery**, a small vessel arising from the ileocolic artery within the mesoappendix, which anastomoses with intestinal branches and the right colic artery.

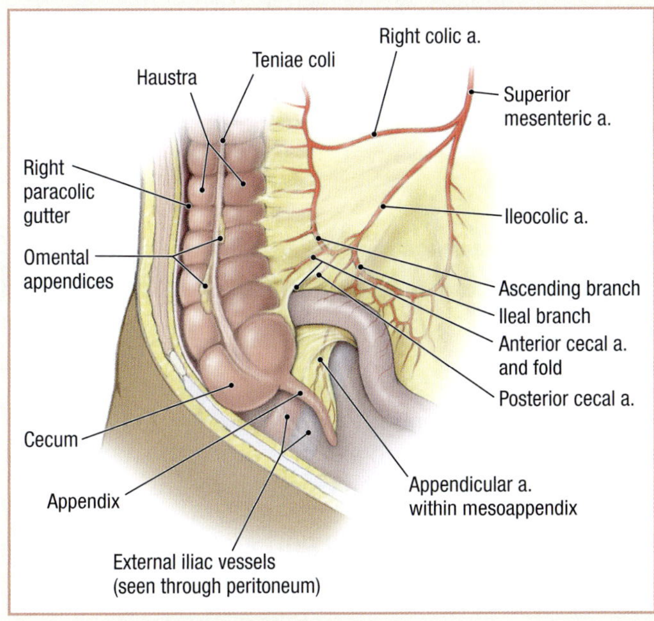

FIGURE 4.31 ● Branches of ileocolic artery. Anterior view.

Hindgut Derivatives

ATLAS 4.46, 4.48, 4.49; VIDEO 4.7.2

1. Refer to FIGURE 4.32.
2. Reflect the transverse colon and greater omentum superiorly over the costal margin to expose the posterior surface of the transverse mesocolon.
3. Move the small intestine to the right to expose the distal aspect of the large intestine.
4. Beginning in the left upper quadrant, verify that the **left colic flexure** lies at a more superior level than the right colic flexure due to the location of the liver.
5. Identify the **descending colon** from the left colic flexure to the left lower quadrant and recall that it is a secondarily retroperitoneal organ.
6. In the left lower quadrant, identify the **sigmoid colon** and its associated mesentery, the **sigmoid mesocolon**.
7. Observe that the sigmoid colon is a mobile intraperitoneal organ that ends in the pelvis at the level of the S3.
8. Follow the sigmoid colon inferiorly and identify the superior aspect of the **rectum** within the pelvic cavity inferior to the S3 vertebral level. *Note that the rectum and anal canal are contained entirely within the pelvic cavity and will be dissected with the pelvic viscera.*

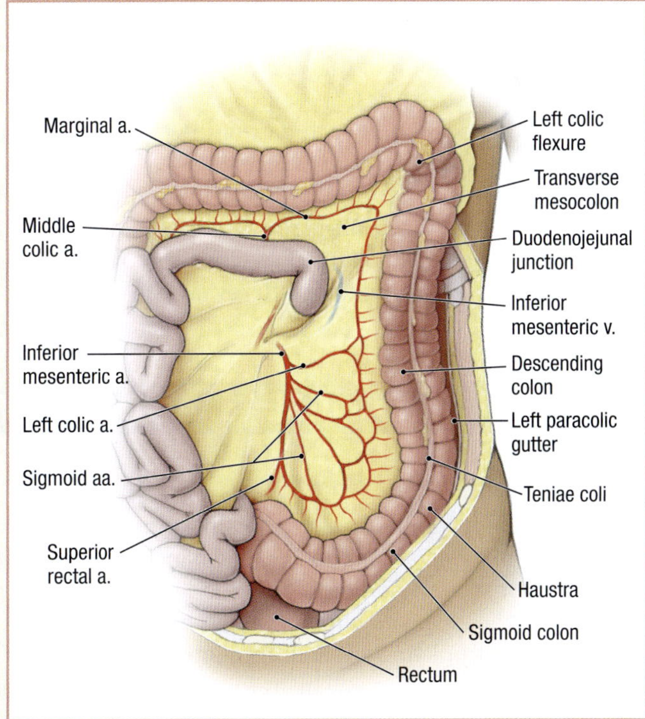

FIGURE 4.32 ● Hindgut derivatives and branches of inferior mesenteric artery. Anterior view.

Inferior Mesenteric Artery and Vein

ATLAS 4.31, 4.46; VIDEO 4.7.1

1. Refer to FIGURE 4.32.
2. Identify the **inferior mesenteric artery** where it arises from the abdominal aorta commonly posterior to the third part of the duodenum. If you have trouble finding the inferior mesenteric artery, locate one of its branches in the sigmoid mesocolon and trace that branch back to the main vessel and then proceed with the dissection of the peripheral branches.
3. Use a probe to clean the **branches of the inferior mesenteric artery** beginning with the **left colic artery** supplying the descending colon and left third of the transverse colon. *Note that the left colic artery anastomoses with the middle colic branch of the superior mesenteric artery and ascending branch of the first sigmoid artery.*
4. Identify three or four **sigmoid arteries** supplying the sigmoid colon. Observe that sigmoid arteries pass through the sigmoid mesocolon forming arcades like those of the intestinal arteries.
5. Identify the **superior rectal artery** descending into the pelvic cavity to supply the proximal part of the rectum. Make an effort to follow the superior rectal artery until it divides into a **right** and **left branch** on either side of the rectum.
6. Superior to the left colic artery, identify the **marginal artery of the colon** coursing along the inner circumference of the large intestine near the left colic flexure.
7. Observe that the marginal artery reaches the middle colic artery forming an anastomosis between the superior and inferior mesenteric arteries supplying the midgut and hindgut derivatives respectively.
8. Observe that the tributaries of the **inferior mesenteric vein** correspond to the branches of the inferior mesenteric artery.
9. Clean a portion of the inferior mesenteric vein and observe that it ascends on the left side of the inferior mesenteric artery.
10. Identify the left ureter just posterior to the inferior mesenteric vein and artery within the retroperitoneal space.
11. Lymph vessels that accompany the branches of the inferior mesenteric artery drain the descending colon and sigmoid colon. The lymphatic vessels drain into the **inferior mesenteric nodes** located around the origin of the inferior mesenteric artery from the abdominal aorta. *Note that in an embalmed specimen, it may be difficult to locate the lymphatic vessels; however, lymph nodes are generally identifiable in the mesentery.*
12. Return the small intestine and transverse colon to their correct anatomical positions.

Dissection Follow-up

1. Review the location of the jejunum and ileum relative to the abdominal quadrant system and their relationships to surrounding structures.
2. Review the location of each part of the large intestine relative to the abdominal quadrant system and the relationships to surrounding structures.
3. Review the branches of the superior mesenteric artery that supply the small intestine.
4. Review the branches of the superior mesenteric artery and inferior mesenteric artery that supply the large intestine.
5. Replace the small and large intestines and other displaced abdominal contents in their correct anatomical position.
6. Use an embryology textbook to review the embryonic midgut and hindgut derivatives.

DUODENUM, PANCREAS, AND HEPATIC PORTAL VEIN

Dissection Overview

The duodenum is the part of the small intestine between the stomach and jejunum and is the recipient of the ducts of the liver, gallbladder, and pancreas. The pancreas lies within the curve of the duodenum with its head directed at the descending or second portion of the duodenum. The pancreas is both an endocrine and exocrine organ. The duodenum and pancreas lie at the junction of the embryonic foregut and midgut and thus have a rich blood supply arising from both the celiac trunk and superior mesenteric artery.

The order of dissection will be as follows: The parts of the duodenum will be studied. The parts of the pancreas will be identified, and the main pancreatic duct will be dissected. The formation of the hepatic portal vein will be demonstrated.

Dissection Instructions

Duodenum

ATLAS 4.37, 4.38, 4.39, 4.59; VIDEO 4.8.1

1. Refer to FIGURE 4.33.
2. Reflect the transverse colon and greater omentum superiorly over the costal margin.
3. Use blunt dissection to separate and remove the remaining portion of the transverse mesocolon and connective tissue overlying the anterior surface of the duodenum and pancreas.
4. Identify the **four parts of the duodenum** beginning with the **superior (1st) part** at the L1 vertebral level, coursing in the transverse plane where it continues from the pylorus of the stomach.
5. Recall that the hepatoduodenal ligament, a portion of the lesser omentum, attaches to the first part of the duodenum. *Note that the first part is mostly intraperitoneal and has an expanded initial part called the ampulla which clinicians often call the duodenal cap or duodenal bulb.*
6. Identify the **descending (2nd) part** of the duodenum at the L2 vertebral level and observe that it is positioned to the right of midline and anterior to the hilum of the right kidney, right renal vessels, and inferior vena cava. *Note that the second part of the duodenum is retroperitoneal and will receive the bile duct and the pancreatic ducts.*
7. Identify the **horizontal (3rd) part** of the duodenum at the L3 vertebral level in a retroperitoneal location and observe that it is crossed anteriorly by the superior mesenteric vessels and posteriorly by the inferior vena cava, abdominal aorta, and inferior mesenteric artery. *Note that the inferior mesenteric vein is typically located to the left of the third part of the duodenum.*
8. Identify the **ascending (4th) part** of the duodenum at the L2 vertebral level. Observe that the ascending part of the duodenum is retroperitoneal throughout most of its length until it turns anteriorly to join the jejunum at the duodenojejunal junction.

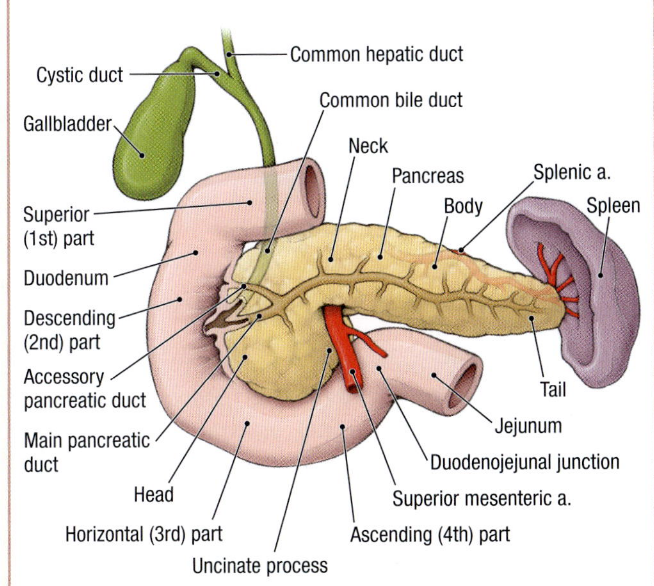

FIGURE 4.33 ● Pancreas and duodenum. Anterior view.

Pancreas

ATLAS 4.37, 4.38, 4.59B; VIDEO 4.8.2

1. Refer to FIGURE 4.33.
2. Identify the **pancreas** within the curvature of the duodenum posterior to the body of the stomach. *Note that the bulk of the pancreas is a secondarily retroperitoneal organ and lies across the midline against vertebral bodies L1–L3.*
3. Identify the **head of the pancreas** adjacent to the descending part of the duodenum anterior to the inferior vena cava.
4. Identify the **uncinate process** at the inferior margin of the head of the pancreas, a small projection that lies posterior to the superior mesenteric vessels.
5. Identify the **neck of the pancreas**, a short portion that lies anterior to the superior mesenteric vessels connecting the head and body of the pancreas.
6. Identify the **body of the pancreas** to the left of the mesenteric vessels posterior to the stomach, extending from right to left and slightly superiorly as it crosses the abdominal aorta.
7. Identify the **tail of the pancreas**, the narrow left end of the gland enclosed within the splenorenal ligament where it contacts the hilum of the spleen.
8. Use a probe to bluntly dissect into the anterior surface of the head of the pancreas and find the **main pancreatic duct**. *Note that main pancreatic duct often resembles a pale vein.*
9. Follow the main pancreatic duct through the neck and into the body and make an effort to identify the smaller **accessory pancreatic duct** draining into its superior side in the head of the pancreas.
10. Follow the common bile duct inferiorly posterior to the superior part of the duodenum and observe that it penetrates the deep aspect of the pancreatic tissue to join the main pancreatic duct near the left side of the descending part of the duodenum.
11. Refer to FIGURE 4.34.
12. Superior to the head of the pancreas, identify the **anterior and posterior superior pancreaticoduodenal arteries** arising from the superior pancreaticoduodenal artery, a branch of the gastroduodenal artery.
13. Inferior to the head of the pancreas, identify the **inferior pancreaticoduodenal artery** commonly

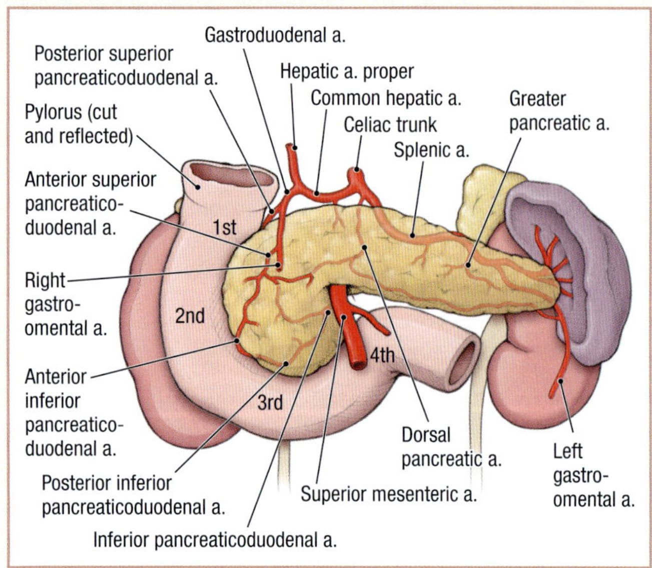

FIGURE 4.34 ● Blood supply of pancreas. Anterior view.

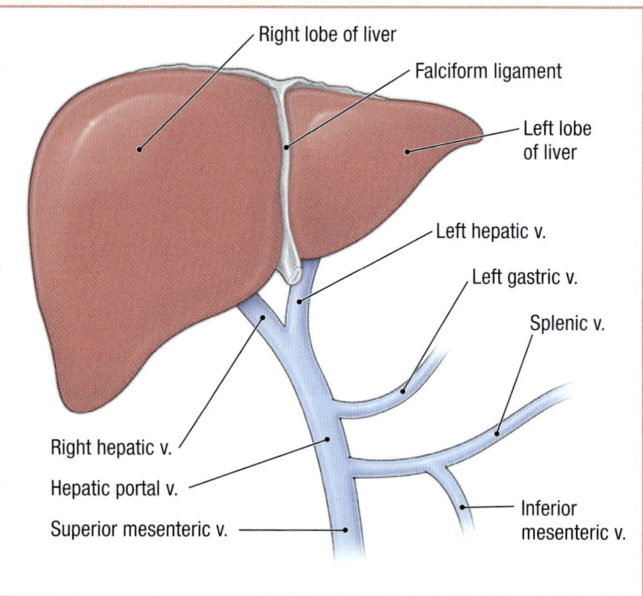

FIGURE 4.35 ● Hepatic portal vein. Anterior view.

arising as the most proximal branch of the superior mesenteric artery, although its origin is variable.

14. Return to the celiac trunk and follow the **splenic artery** as it passes to the left along the superior border of the pancreas where it may pass in and out of the glandular tissue.
15. Remove the remaining peritoneum over the anterior aspect of the pancreas and observe that up to 10 small branches of the splenic artery supply the body and tail of the pancreas, although only two will be named here: the **dorsal pancreatic artery**, entering the neck of the pancreas, and the **greater pancreatic (pancreatica magna) artery**, entering the pancreas about halfway between the neck and the tail. Recall that the splenic artery also gave rise to the short gastric arteries and left gastroomental artery.
16. Use blunt dissection to trace the superior mesenteric artery proximally toward its origin off the abdominal aorta and observe that it crosses anterior to the third part of the duodenum and posterior to the neck of the pancreas.

Hepatic Portal Vein

ATLAS 4.38, 4.65; VIDEO 4.8.3

1. Refer to FIGURE 4.35.
2. Identify the **splenic vein** where it courses posterior to the pancreas and inferior to the splenic artery.
3. Use blunt dissection to isolate the splenic vein posterior to the body of the pancreas and observe that it is typically flatter and straighter than the more tortuous thicker splenic artery.
4. Follow the splenic vein to the right where it is joined by the **superior mesenteric vein** to form the **hepatic portal vein**. Recall that the hepatic portal vein ascends in the hepatoduodenal ligament as part of the portal triad.
5. The veins of the pancreas correspond to the arteries and drain into the superior mesenteric and splenic veins and are ultimately tributaries to the hepatic portal vein.
6. Follow the hepatic portal vein superiorly until it branches into the **right** and **left hepatic veins** each directed at their respective lobe of the liver. *Note that the bifurcation of the hepatic portal vein into the individual hepatic veins may not be visible outside the liver.*
7. Identify the **left gastric vein** draining into the hepatic portal vein (see **Clinical Correlation 4.9**). *Note that this vessel may have been cut during dissection of the branches of the celiac trunk.*

CLINICAL CORRELATION 4.9

Portal Hypertension

ATLAS 4.66

The hepatic portal system of veins drains a significant portion of the intestinal tract and has no valves. When the hepatic portal vein becomes blocked, as can occur with cirrhosis of the liver, blood pressure increases in the hepatic portal system (portal hypertension) resulting in engorgement of the venous tributaries of the system. Gastroesophageal varices, enlargement of the gastric and esophageal veins, are a dangerous complication of portal hypertension as they may lead to internal bleeding if ruptured.

Four portal-systemic (portal-caval) anastomoses exist within the abdomen to allow for alternative routes of venous return in response to pressure changes: gastroesophageal (left gastric vein, esophageal veins, and azygos vein), anorectal (superior rectal vein and middle and inferior rectal veins), paraumbilical (paraumbilical veins and superficial epigastric veins), and retroperitoneal (colic veins and retroperitoneal veins).

8. Return to the field of distribution of the inferior mesenteric vein and follow it superiorly until it joins the portal system by draining into the superior mesenteric vein, splenic vein, or junction of the superior mesenteric and splenic veins.

Dissection Follow-up

1. Review the relationship of each part of the duodenum to the surrounding structures.
2. Review the branches of the celiac trunk and superior mesenteric artery.
3. Review the blood supply to the pancreas and duodenum.
4. Review the formation and field of drainage of the hepatic portal vein.
5. Trace a drop of blood from the small intestine to the inferior vena cava, naming all veins that are encountered along the way. Repeat this exercise beginning at the descending colon.
6. Replace the displaced abdominal contents in their correct anatomical position.
7. Use an embryology textbook to review the development of the pancreas and duodenum.

REMOVAL OF GASTROINTESTINAL TRACT

Dissection Overview

The digestive tract collectively serves to take in nourishment for the body and expel waste. The mechanical process of digestion begins in the oral cavity and descends via the esophagus to reach the stomach and duodenum where digestion continues. Absorption of the nutrients and chemical compounds occurs in the small intestine, primarily in the jejunum, whereas water reabsorption occurs in the large intestine, primarily in the ascending colon. The descending colon, sigmoid colon, and rectum store fecal matter prior to defecation via the anus.

The posterior features of the various parts of the gastrointestinal tract and the posterior abdominal wall are best dissected with the gastrointestinal tract removed from the abdominal cavity; however, many of the relationships may still be studied without complete removal. Two methods of intestinal removal will be described, and either may be followed depending on the needs of the course. If removal of the gastrointestinal tract is either not a part of your labs' dissection protocol, or time does not permit, you may follow the partial bloc removal instructions or orient the abdominal contents to one side or the other, leaving the tract in situ.

The order of dissection will be as follows: The stomach will be opened and reviewed. The small and large intestines will be opened regionally and reviewed. The gastrointestinal tract will then be removed either partially or en bloc and reviewed outside of the body. In the partial removal, only the small intestine and associated vessels will be removed. In full bloc removal, the rectum and esophagus will be cut using string ligatures to prevent spilling of their contents as well as transection of the arteries to the gastrointestinal tract (celiac trunk, superior mesenteric artery, and inferior mesenteric artery) allowing for full removal of the tract and associated organs.

Dissection Instructions

Opening the Stomach

ATLAS 4.32; VIDEO 4.9.1

1. Elevate the diaphragm and identify the opening of the **esophageal hiatus** allowing passage of the esophagus into the abdominal cavity.
2. Use blunt dissection to clean the anterior surface of the esophagus and cardia of the stomach.
3. Refer to FIGURE 4.36.
4. Use scissors to open the stomach along its anterior surface paralleling the curve of the lesser curvature (**Cut 1**).
5. Extend the cut through the fundus of the stomach horizontally toward the greater curvature of the stomach (**Cut 2**).
6. Open the stomach, and on its inner surface, identify the **rugae (gastric folds)**. If necessary, rinse and clean the mucosal surface to observe the internal structures. *Note that the rugae will flatten out with stomach expansion and are thus not always present.*
7. Observe the narrowing of the body of the stomach inferiorly at the **pyloric antrum** just prior to the **pyloric canal**.
8. Insert a probe into the pyloric canal and extend the cut through the anterior surface of the stomach into the pylorus following the path of the probe (**Cut 3**).
9. Create a short vertical incision at the end of the horizontal incision within the pylorus and open the pyloric region of the stomach (**Cut 4**).
10. At the end of the pyloric canal, identify the **pyloric sphincter**, a circular muscle which controls the passage of food into the **duodenum** via the **pyloric orifice**.

Opening the Small and Large Intestines

ATLAS 4.37, 4.40, 4.43; VIDEO 4.9.2

1. Extend the longitudinal cut from the pylorus of the stomach through the anterior wall of the duodenum following the shape of the duodenum through its second part (**Cut 5**).
2. Refer to FIGURE 4.37.
3. Spread open the second part of the duodenum and identify the **circular folds (plicae circulares)**. *Note that unlike the rugae of the stomach, the folds of the small intestine are transversely oriented and always present.*
4. Identify the **major (greater) duodenal papilla**, or ampulla of Vater, an elevation of mucosa on the posterior-medial wall of the second part of the duodenum which allows passage of the **hepatopancreatic duct**, the combined main pancreatic duct and common bile duct. *Note that the regulation of the opening is controlled by circular muscle in the wall of the papilla known as the hepatopancreatic sphincter (sphincter of Oddi).*
5. Identify the **minor (lesser) duodenal papilla**, the site of drainage of the accessory pancreatic duct, approximately 2 cm superior to the major duodenal papilla (if present).
6. Refer to FIGURE 4.38.
7. Use scissors to make one 5-cm longitudinal cut in the **proximal jejunum** and another in the **distal ileum**.
8. Rinse the mucosa within the two cut regions of the small intestine to compare the internal anatomy and observe that the **circular folds** are larger and closer together in the jejunum than they are in the ileum.

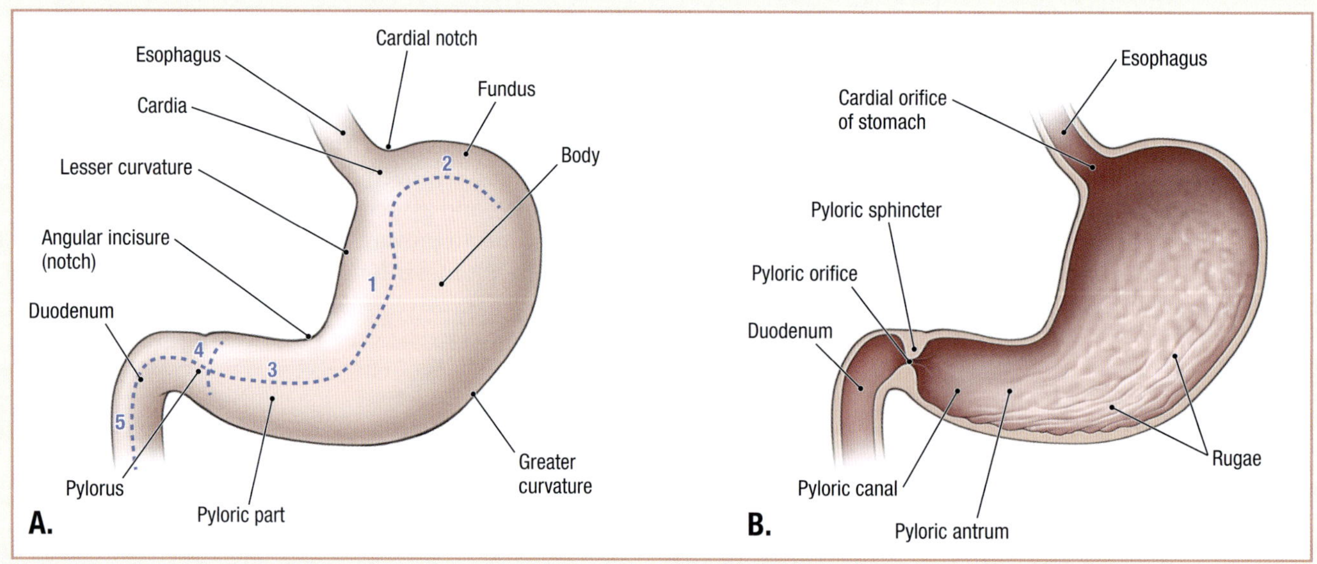

FIGURE 4.36 **A.** Cuts to open stomach. **B.** Internal features of stomach. Anterior views.

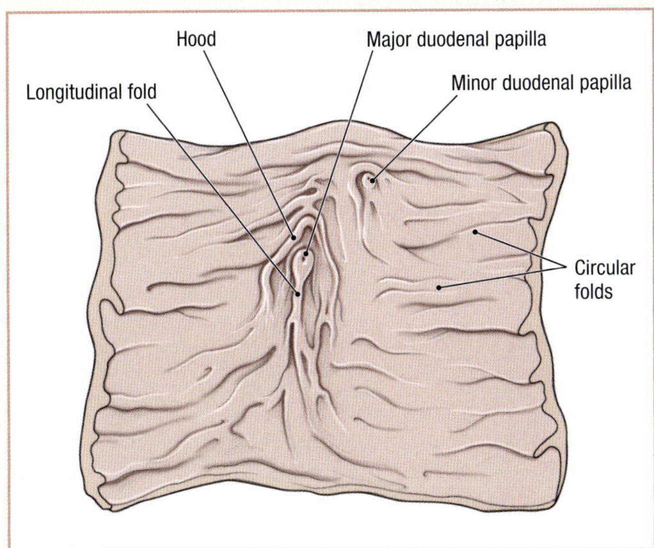

FIGURE 4.37 ● Mucosal features of descending duodenum. Isolated view.

9. Identify **solitary lymph nodes**, the small, raised bumps on the internal aspect of the ileum. *Note that the lymph nodules are present elsewhere in the digestive tract, although they are less visible. The prevalence of lymphatics within the ileum and cecal region is indicative of its role in assisting the immune system.*
10. Refer to FIGURE 4.39.
11. Use scissors to make a flap approximately 7.5 cm long in the anterior wall of the **cecum**.
12. Rinse the mucosa within the cecum and identify the **ileocecal orifice** located between the **superior and inferior lips of the ileocecal valve.**
13. Identify the **opening of the appendix** inside the cecum, using the appendix externally as a landmark for orientation.
14. On the inner surface of the cecum, observe the proximity of the opening of the appendix to the ileocecal orifice.
15. Observe that the inner surface of the colon consists of **semilunar folds (plicae semilunares)** between adjacent **haustra**, and its mucosa is relatively smooth compared to the other parts of the gastrointestinal tract.

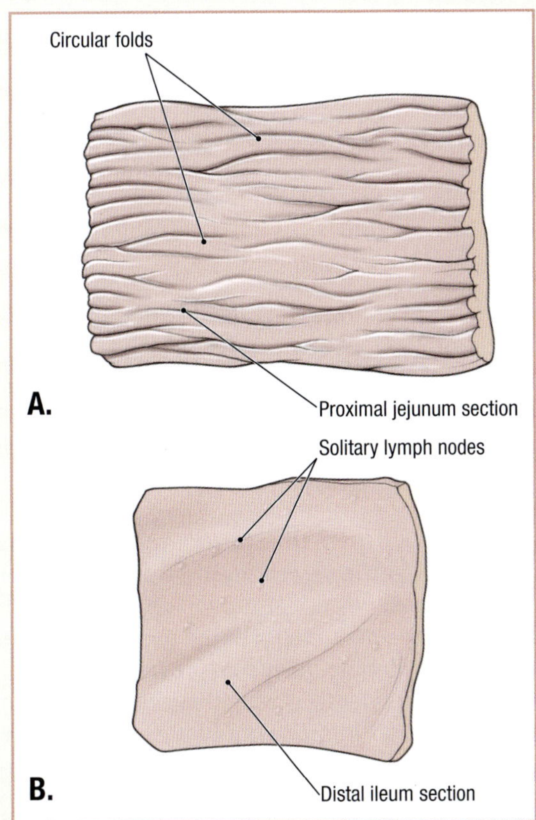

FIGURE 4.38 ● **A.** Mucosal features of proximal jejunum. **B.** Mucosal features of distal ileum. Isolated views.

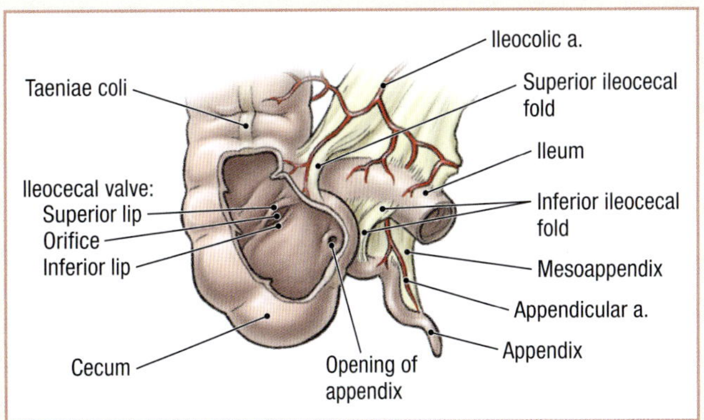

FIGURE 4.39 ● Ileocecal valve and blood supply to cecum and appendix. Anterior view.

Dissection Note: Select either the **Removal of Small Intestine** or **Removal of Gastrointestinal Tract** and disregard the dissection sequence for the other approach.

Removal of Small Intestine

ATLAS 4.25, 4.48, 4.49

Dissection Note: If your lab dissection protocol does not call for removal of the gastrointestinal tract, skip the following dissection protocol and perform the remaining abdominal dissections with the gastrointestinal tract *in situ*.

1. Refer to FIGURE 4.40A.
2. Locate the ascending (4th) part of the duodenum and the point of transition to the **duodenojejunal junction** to the left of the superior mesenteric artery and vein.
3. Transect the jejunum just below the duodenojejunal junction (**Cut 1**). *Note that it is not necessary to tie strings around the jejunum because typically it is void.*
4. Locate the distal part of the ileum and follow it to where it meets the cecum at the **ileocecal junction**.

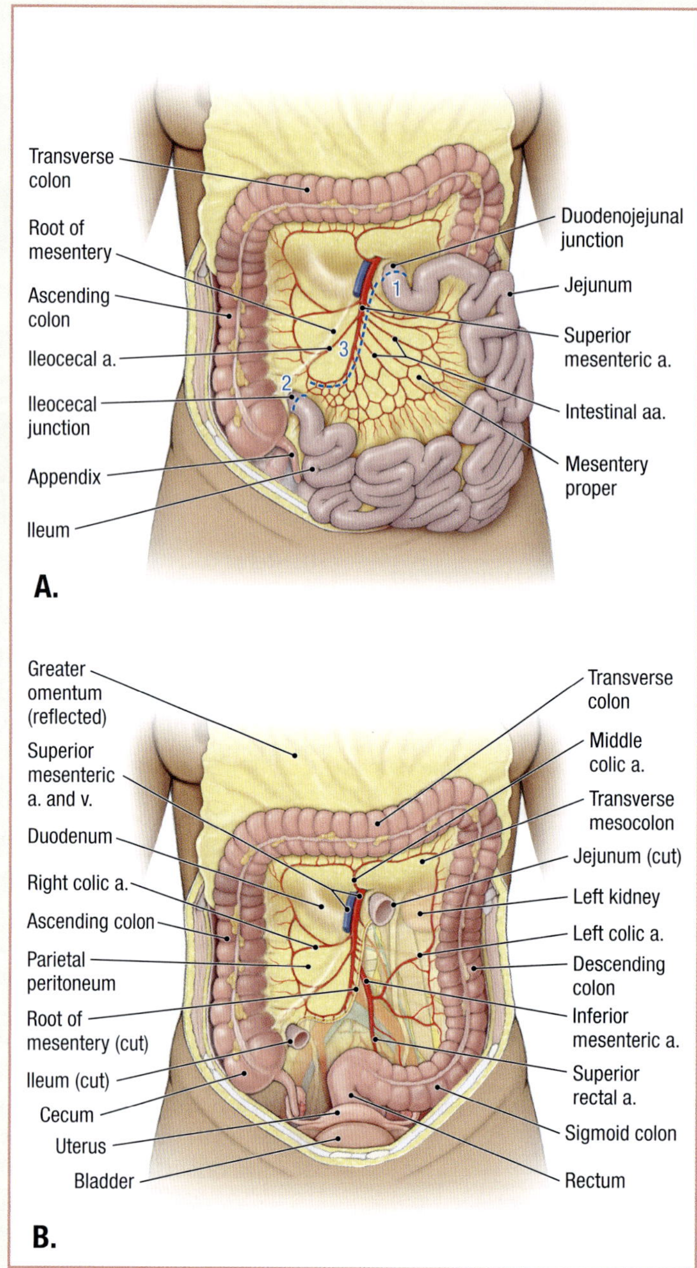

FIGURE 4.40 ■ **A.** Small intestine removal. **B.** Peritoneal reflections. Anterior views.

5. Transect the ileum just prior to the ileocecal junction (**Cut 2**). *Note that it is not necessary to tie strings around the ileum because typically it is void.*
6. Arrange the loops of the small intestine such that the path of the superior mesenteric artery, intestinal arteries, and ileocolic artery are visible.
7. Transect the jejunal and ileal intestinal arteries as they arise to the left of the superior mesenteric artery as well as the associated veins, lymphatics, and peritoneum from the level of the duodenojejunal junction to the ileocecal junction (**Cut 3**). The curved incision should spare the superior mesenteric artery itself as well as the vessels arising from it to supply the large intestine.
8. Ensure that the peritoneum of the mesentery proper and all associated neurovasculature has been completely cut, and gently elevate the jejunal and ileal portions of the small intestine out of the abdominal cavity.
9. Arrange the removed abdominal viscera on a dissecting table or large tray to study the parts from anterior and posterior views.
10. Refer to FIGURE 4.40B.

11. Return to the abdominal cavity to mobilize the abdominal organs for ease of dissection of the posterior abdominal viscera.
12. Free the stomach by cutting through any peritoneal attachments it may still have to the posterior abdominal wall and position it to the right side of the abdominal cavity to expose the vascular branches of the celiac trunk.
13. Grasp the spleen and gently pull it anteriorly and medially and carefully free the splenic vessels and body and tail of the pancreas from the posterior abdominal wall.
14. Insert your fingers posterior to the duodenum and free it and the head of the pancreas from the posterior abdominal wall. After mobilization, return the stomach, duodenum, pancreas, and spleen with their associated neurovasculature to anatomical position.
15. Cut the parietal peritoneum lateral to the ascending colon within the **right paracolic gutter** and free the ascending colon from the posterior abdominal wall.
16. Roll the ascending colon toward the midline and use your fingers to loosen its blood vessels from the posterior abdominal wall. After mobilization, return the ascending colon and associated neurovasculature to anatomical position.
17. Cut the parietal peritoneum lateral to the descending colon within the **left paracolic gutter** and use your fingers to free the descending colon from the posterior abdominal wall.
18. Roll the descending colon toward the midline and use your fingers to loosen its blood vessels from the posterior abdominal wall.
19. Use your fingers to separate the fascia and peritoneum surrounding the distal end of the sigmoid colon and rectum and gently pull them and the associated neurovasculature away from the sacrum and left ilium.
20. After mobilization, return the descending colon, sigmoid colon, rectum, and all associated neurovasculature to anatomical position.

Removal of Gastrointestinal Tract

ATLAS 4.25, 4.68; VIDEO 4.9.3

Dissection Note: If your lab dissection protocol does not call for removal of the gastrointestinal tract, skip the following dissection protocol and perform the remaining abdominal dissections with the gastrointestinal tract *in situ.*

1. Refer to FIGURE 4.40B and FIGURE 4.41.
2. Inferior to the thoracic diaphragm, identify the **esophagus** and cut the anterior and posterior vagal trunks just below where they pass through the diaphragm.
3. Tie a string around the esophagus just below the point where it emerges through the **esophageal hiatus** (**String 1 location**). When securing the knot, ensure to not pull the string so tightly as to sever the esophagus superior to the string. *Note that it is not necessary to tie two strings around the esophagus because typically it is void.*
4. Transect the esophagus inferior to the location of the tied string to ensure any contents within the esophagus remain enclosed within the lumen of the organ (**Cut 1**).
5. Free the stomach by cutting through any peritoneal attachments it may still have to the posterior abdominal wall and position it to the right side of the abdominal cavity to expose the vascular branches of the celiac trunk.
6. Transect the celiac trunk close to the abdominal aorta below the point of its trifurcation. Depending on the length of the celiac trunk, it may be possible to leave a very short stump.
7. Gently push the neck and body of the pancreas inferiorly and transect the superior mesenteric artery near the aorta, leaving a 1-cm stump.
8. Grasp the spleen and gently pull it anteriorly and medially and carefully free the splenic vessels, tail of the pancreas, and body of the pancreas from the posterior abdominal wall.
9. Insert your fingers posterior to the duodenum and free it and the head of the pancreas from the posterior abdominal wall.

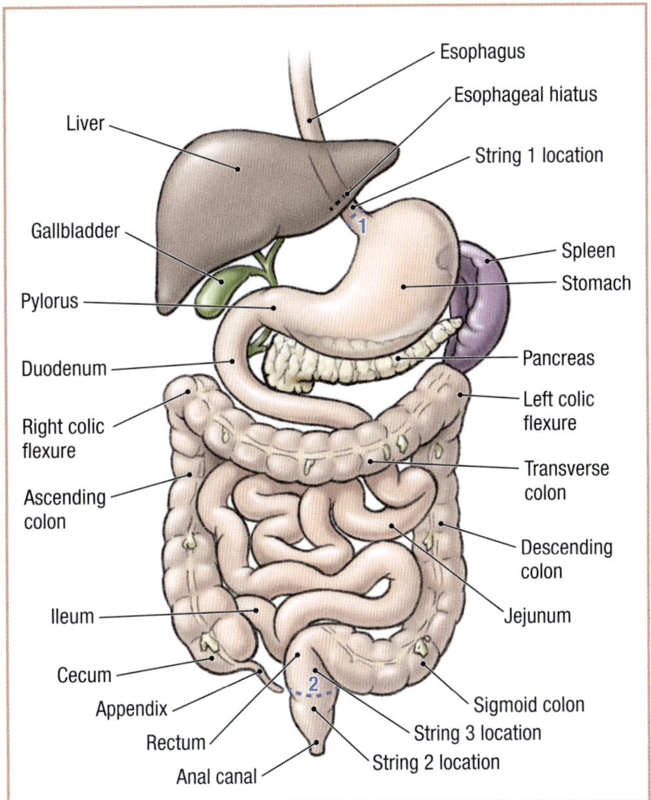

FIGURE 4.41 ● Gastrointestinal tract removal. Anterior view.

10. Cut the suspensory ligament of the duodenum close to the duodenojejunal junction.
11. Cut the parietal peritoneum lateral to the ascending colon within the **right paracolic gutter** and free the ascending colon from the posterior abdominal wall.
12. Roll the ascending colon toward the midline and use your fingers to loosen its blood vessels from the posterior abdominal wall.
13. Use scissors to cut the inferior mesenteric artery near the aorta, leaving a 1-cm stump.
14. Cut the parietal peritoneum lateral to the descending colon within the **left paracolic gutter** and use your fingers to free the descending colon from the posterior abdominal wall.
15. Roll the descending colon toward the midline and use your fingers to loosen its blood vessels from the posterior abdominal wall.
16. Use your fingers to separate the fascia and peritoneum surrounding the distal end of the sigmoid colon and rectum and gently pull them away from the sacrum and left ilium.
17. Gently squeeze the rectum as far inferiorly as possible to compress any remaining internal fecal matter contents and slowly work superiorly while squeezing to create a section of the internal lumen as void as possible distal to the sigmoid colon.
18. Tie a string as far inferiorly within the pelvic cavity as you can reach around the now somewhat void rectum (**String 2 location**) and another approximately 4 cm superior to this location (**String 3 location**). Make the knots tight to avoid slipping of the strings but do not tighten the string so much as to sever the colon.
19. Transect the rectum **between the strings** (**Cut 2**) to ensure as little remaining fecal matter as possible enters the dissection field.
20. Cut the superior rectal artery distally as well as any fascia preventing the rectum from being elevated out of the pelvic cavity.
21. Ensure that the gastrointestinal tract, liver, pancreas, and spleen are free of any peritoneal attachments and remove them from the abdominal cavity en bloc. Support the liver while removing the abdominal contents and be careful not to twist or tear the structures in the hepatoduodenal ligament.
22. Arrange the abdominal viscera on a dissecting table or large tray in anatomical position and study the parts from the anterior view.
23. Trace the branches of the celiac trunk, superior mesenteric artery, and inferior mesenteric artery to their areas of distribution.
24. Observe the formation and termination of the hepatic portal vein, noting the differences between the branching pattern of the arteries and the veins.
25. Turn the viscera and repeat the exercise of tracing the vessels from the posterior view.

Dissection Follow-up

1. Review the features of the gastrointestinal mucosa.
2. Compare the quantity and complexity of circular folds in the proximal and distal parts of the small intestine.
3. Compare this arrangement to the mucosal features seen in the stomach and large intestine and correlate your findings to the function of the organs dissected.
4. Recall the locations of valves in the gastrointestinal tract.
5. Store the removed abdominal viscera in a large plastic bag or return them to the abdominal cavity following your labs' dissection protocols. If a bag is used, wet the abdominal contents frequently with mold-inhibiting solution.

POSTERIOR ABDOMINAL VISCERA

Dissection Overview

The posterior abdominal viscera are in the retroperitoneal space between the parietal peritoneum and the muscles and bones of the posterior abdominal wall as shown in FIGURE 4.42. In addition to portions of the gastrointestinal tract, the retroperitoneal space contains the kidneys, ureters, suprarenal glands, aorta, inferior vena cava, and abdominal portions of the sympathetic trunks.

The kidneys play key roles in the proper elimination of waste and in maintaining homeostasis in a variety of ways including blood volume and pressure regulation. The kidneys are well protected by their position within the abdomen as well as by cushioning layers of fat, an outer pararenal layer and an inner perirenal layer separated by renal fascia.

The order of dissection will be as follows: The posterior abdominal viscera will be palpated, and the overlying parietal peritoneum removed. The renal fat and fascia will be removed, and the kidneys and suprarenal glands will be studied. The abdominal aorta and the inferior vena cava will be dissected. The muscles of the posterior abdominal wall will be studied. The lumbar plexus of nerves will be examined. The diaphragm and its openings will be studied.

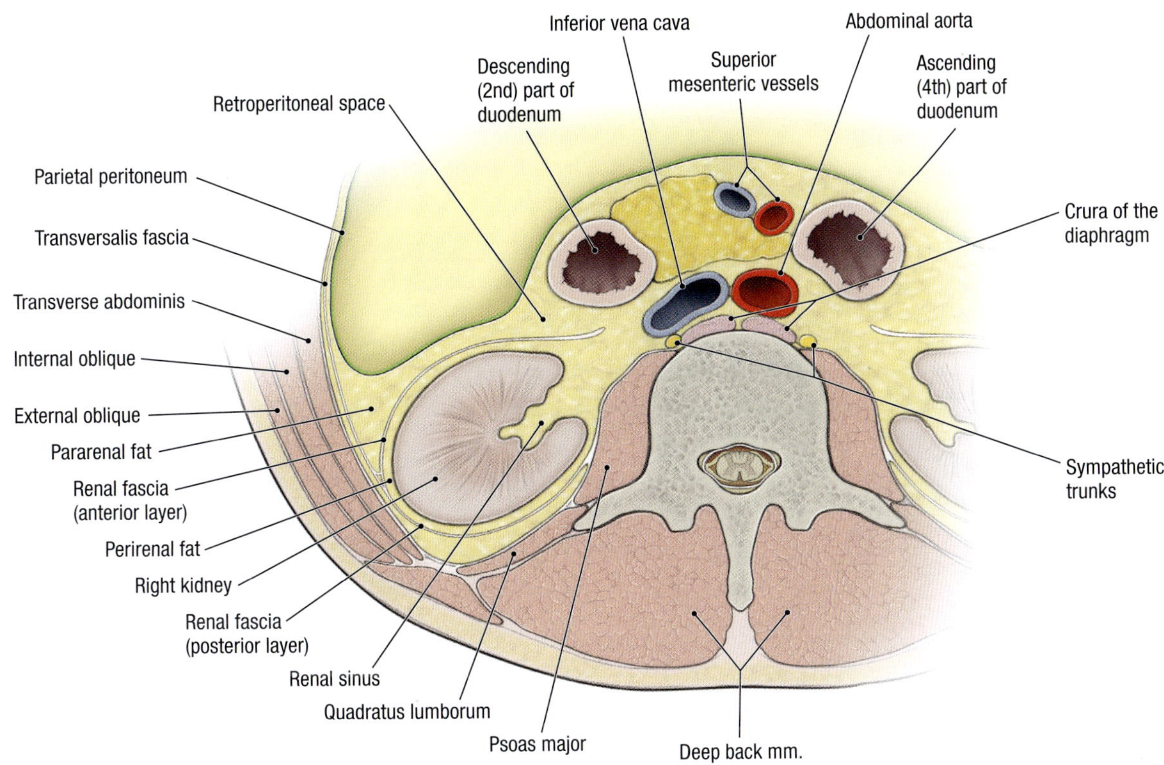

FIGURE 4.42 ■ Transverse section of posterior abdominal wall. Inferior view.

Dissection Instructions

Retroperitoneal Vasculature

ATLAS 4.25, 4.68, 4.69; VIDEO 4.10.1

Dissection Note: If the gastrointestinal track and associated organs were not removed from the abdominal cavity, or if only the small intestine was removed, it will be necessary to adjust the remaining viscera periodically throughout this dissection protocol. If necessary, use a sponge or paper towels to clean and dry the posterior abdominal wall in advance or during the session.

1. Refer to FIGURE 4.43.
2. Identify and palpate the **abdominal aorta** from its point of entrance to the abdominal cavity at the **aortic hiatus** of the diaphragm.
3. Clean the abdominal aorta inferiorly to demonstrate that it terminates at the level of L4 where it bifurcates into right and left **common iliac arteries**.
4. To the right of the abdominal aorta, identify and palpate the **inferior vena cava**. Observe that the inferior vena cava originates at the level of L5 where the right and left **common iliac veins** join.
5. Identify the **left renal vein** and use a probe to trace it from the left kidney across the midline to the inferior vena cava as it courses anterior to the renal arteries and aorta.
6. Identify and clean the **left suprarenal vein** draining into the superior aspect of left renal vein.
7. Identify the **left renal artery**, which lies posterior to the left renal vein. Follow the left renal artery to the hilum of the kidney and observe that it usually divides into several **segmental arteries** before entering the kidney. *Note that accessory renal arteries are common during development and an excellent example of anatomical variation.*

Dissecting Note: If dissecting a male cadaver, proceed to step 12.

8. In the **female cadaver**, identify and clean the **ovarian vessels**. Observe that the **ovarian arteries** branch directly from the anterolateral surface of the aorta at about vertebral level L2, inferior to the origin of the renal arteries.
9. Identify the **left ovarian vein** draining into the inferior aspect of the left renal vein.
10. Identify the **right ovarian vein** draining into the inferior vena cava.
11. Follow the ovarian vessels inferiorly toward the pelvic cavity until they cross the **external iliac vessels** but do not follow them into the pelvis at this time. Observe that the ovarian vessels cross anterior to the ureters along their descent.

Dissection Note: If you are dissecting a female cadaver, proceed to the dissection sequence for the **Kidneys**.

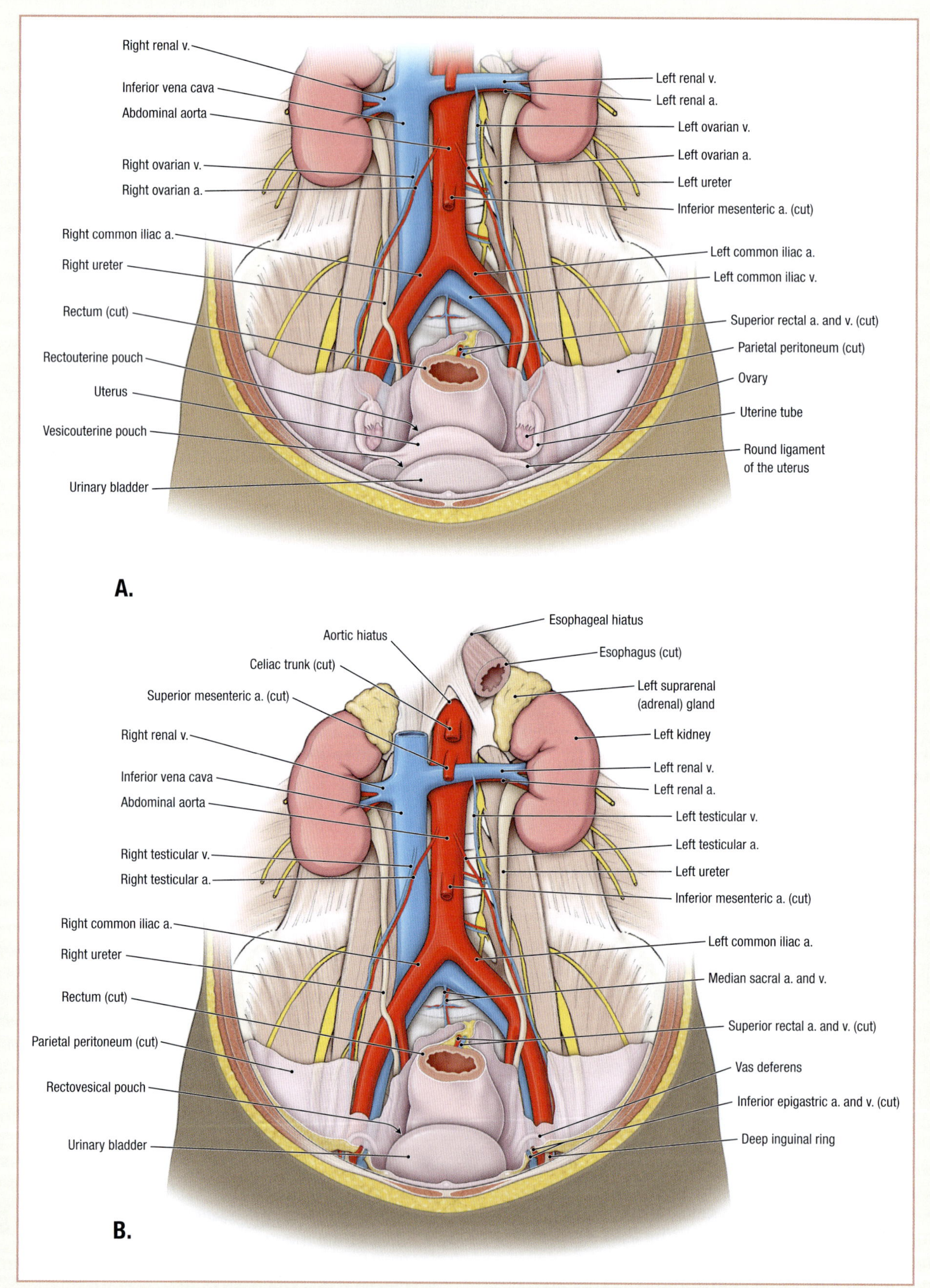

FIGURE 4.43 ■ **A.** Retroperitoneal vasculature and renal system in female. **B.** Retroperitoneal vasculature and renal system in male. Anterior views.

12. On a male cadaver, identify and clean the **testicular artery** and **vein** beginning at the deep inguinal ring and progressing superiorly.
13. Observe that the testicular vessels cross anterior to the ureter and are quite small and delicate. Make an effort not to damage the ureter while following the vessels.
14. The **right** and **left testicular arteries** branch directly from the anterolateral surface of the aorta at about vertebral level L2, inferior to the origin of the renal arteries.
15. Observe that the **left testicular vein** drains into the inferior aspect of the left renal vein, whereas the **right testicular vein** drains directly into the inferior vena cava (see **Clinical Correlation 4.10**).

CLINICAL CORRELATION 4.10

Testicular Varicocele

ATLAS 4.19, 4.68

Testicular varicocele occurs when the pampiniform plexus of veins becomes engorged with blood due to restriction of venous return from the testis. Testicular varicocele is more common on the left side because the left testicular vein drains into the left renal vein which is subject to compression where it passes posterior to the superior mesenteric artery.

Kidneys

ATLAS 4.67B, 4.68, 4.71; VIDEO 4.10.2

1. Refer to FIGURE 4.42 and FIGURE 4.43.
2. Palpate the **kidneys** and the **suprarenal (adrenal) glands** through the retroperitoneal fat between vertebral levels T12 and L3 where they lie lateral to the vertebral column.
3. Use blunt dissection to confirm that the kidneys are surrounded by an outer layer of **pararenal fat** and an inner layer of **perirenal fat** separated from one another by a thin layer of **renal fascia**.
4. Remove the outer layer of pararenal fat along with the renal fascia anterolaterally.
5. Carefully remove portions of the perirenal fat from the dissection field to increase visibility of the kidneys. Do not disrupt the fascia lining the posterior abdominal wall during the fat removal process.
6. Observe that the kidneys lie against the posterior abdominal wall and that the anterior surface of the kidneys face anterolaterally at an oblique angle following the curve of the vertebrae.
7. Observe that the **superior pole** of the kidney is separated from the suprarenal gland by a thin layer of renal fascia.
8. Use blunt dissection to identify the border between the kidney and the superiorly located suprarenal gland. Be careful not to remove the suprarenal gland with the fat.
9. Verify that the right kidney, through its peritoneal covering, is in contact with the right colic flexure, visceral surface of the liver, and second part of the duodenum.
10. Verify that the left kidney, through its peritoneal covering, is in contact with the tail of the pancreas, left colic flexure, stomach, and spleen.
11. Using the left renal artery as a hinge, turn the left kidney toward the right and observe the posterior surface of the left kidney.
12. Identify the **ureter**, the muscular duct that carries urine from the kidney to the urinary bladder.
13. Follow the ureter inferiorly to where it crosses the common iliac vessels and use blunt dissection to follow it into the pelvic cavity for a short distance.
14. Observe that the abdominal part of the ureter passes posterior to the gonadal (ovarian or testicular) vessels and crosses the anterior surface of the **psoas major**. *Note that if the gastrointestinal tract was removed, recall that the left ureter passed posterior to the branches of the inferior mesenteric artery and vein.*
15. Refer to FIGURE 4.44.
16. Follow the ureter superiorly and observe that it connects to the **renal pelvis** exiting the kidney at the **hilum**.
17. Observe that the hilum of the kidney faces anteromedially and that the lateral border faces posterolaterally.
18. Use a scalpel to divide the left kidney into anterior and posterior halves by splitting it longitudinally along its lateral border and open the two halves of the kidney like a book using the renal pelvis as the hinge.

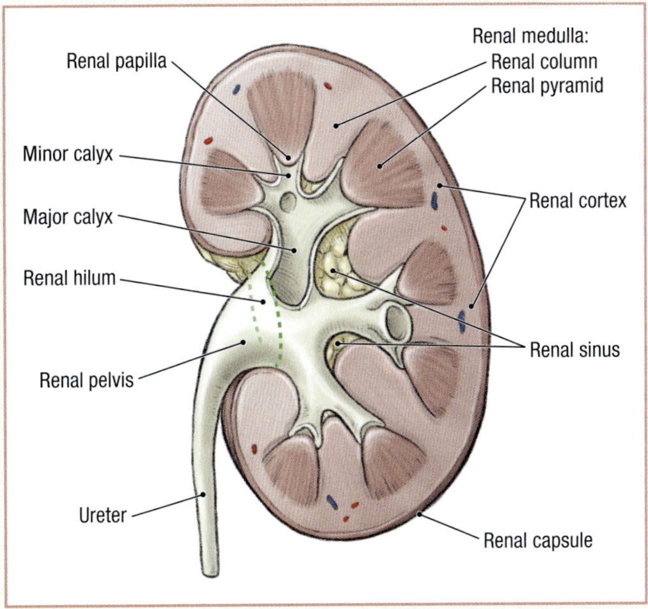

FIGURE 4.44 ● Coronal section of left kidney. Anterior view.

19. On the internal aspect of the kidney, identify the **renal cortex**, the outer zone of the kidney (about one-third of its depth).
20. Observe that the cortex is surrounded by the **renal capsule**, a thin fibrous capsule firmly attached to the surface of the kidney.
21. Deep to the renal cortex, identify the **renal medulla**, the inner zone of the kidney (about two-thirds of its depth). Observe that the renal medulla consists of **renal pyramids** separated by **renal columns**.
22. At the apex of a renal pyramid, identify a **renal papilla** projecting into a **minor calyx**. Observe that the **minor calyx** is a cup-like chamber and the beginning of the extrarenal duct system.
23. Observe that several minor calyces combine to form a **major calyx**, which drain into the **renal pelvis**, the funnel-like proximal end of the ureter that begins within the **renal sinus** and emerges from the renal hilum where it connects to the ureter at the **ureteropelvic junction** (see **Clinical Correlation 4.11**). *Note that the renal sinus is the space within the kidney occupied by the renal pelvis, calices, vessels, nerves, and fat.*

CLINICAL CORRELATION 4.11

Kidney Stones

ATLAS 4.72

Kidney stones (renal calculi) may form in the calyces and renal pelvis. Small kidney stones may spontaneously pass through the ureter into the bladder. Larger kidney stones may lodge at one of three natural constrictions of the ureter: (1) the ureteropelvic junction, where the renal pelvis becomes constricted to form the ureter, (2) where the ureter crosses the pelvic brim, and (3) at the entrance of the ureter into the urinary bladder. Kidney stones are often excruciatingly painful until they pass (naturally) or are treated (via invasive or noninvasive techniques).

24. Return the left kidney to its correct anatomical position.

Suprarenal Glands

ATLAS 4.69A, 4.70; VIDEO 4.10.3

Dissection Note: The suprarenal glands are fragile and may be easily torn or mistaken for adipose tissue, so care must be taken when dissecting them.

1. Refer to FIGURE 4.45.
2. Palpate the **suprarenal (adrenal) glands** within the remnants of the perirenal fat. *Note that often the boundaries of the glands are difficult to differentiate from the surrounding fat; therefore, use the vessels in the region to help delineate the border.*
3. Observe that the **right suprarenal gland** is commonly triangular and lies partially posterior to the inferior vena cava.
4. Observe that the **left suprarenal gland** is commonly semilunar and more exposed (see **Clinical Correlation 4.12**).

CLINICAL CORRELATION 4.12

Suprarenal Gland Development

ATLAS 4.70

The kidneys and suprarenal glands have different embryonic origins; thus, if the kidneys fail to ascend to their normal positions during development, the suprarenal glands still develop in a position lateral to the celiac trunk. In renal transplantation, the suprarenal glands may be separated from the deficient kidney at the relatively weak septum of renal fascia between the organs. As the natal kidney may still have minimal function and removal may damage the suprarenal glands, it may be left in place. To facilitate implantation, the donor kidney is typically placed in the iliac fossa with the new renal vessels connecting to the external iliac vessels.

5. Observe that each suprarenal gland receives multiple arteries from various sources and care must be taken to preserve these small delicate vessels.
6. Identify the **inferior suprarenal artery** arising from the renal artery by gently sliding a probe through the fat parallel to the expected direction of the vessels (inferior to superior).
7. Using a similar technique with the probe, carefully identify the **superior suprarenal artery** arising from the inferior phrenic artery (superior to inferior), and the **middle suprarenal artery** arising from the aorta near the celiac trunk (medial to lateral).
8. Observe that the left suprarenal vein empties into the superior aspect of the left renal vein, while the right suprarenal vein drains directly into the inferior vena cava.
9. Remove the remaining perirenal fat from the region, noting the presence of a vast collection of small nerve fibers paralleling the vessels. *Note that the suprarenal glands receive numerous sympathetic nerve fibers from the surrounding ganglia.*

Abdominal Aorta and Inferior Vena Cava

ATLAS 4.68, 4.80; VIDEO 4.10.4

1. Refer to FIGURE 4.45.
2. Identify the **abdominal aorta** and observe that it begins at vertebral level T12 as the continuation of the

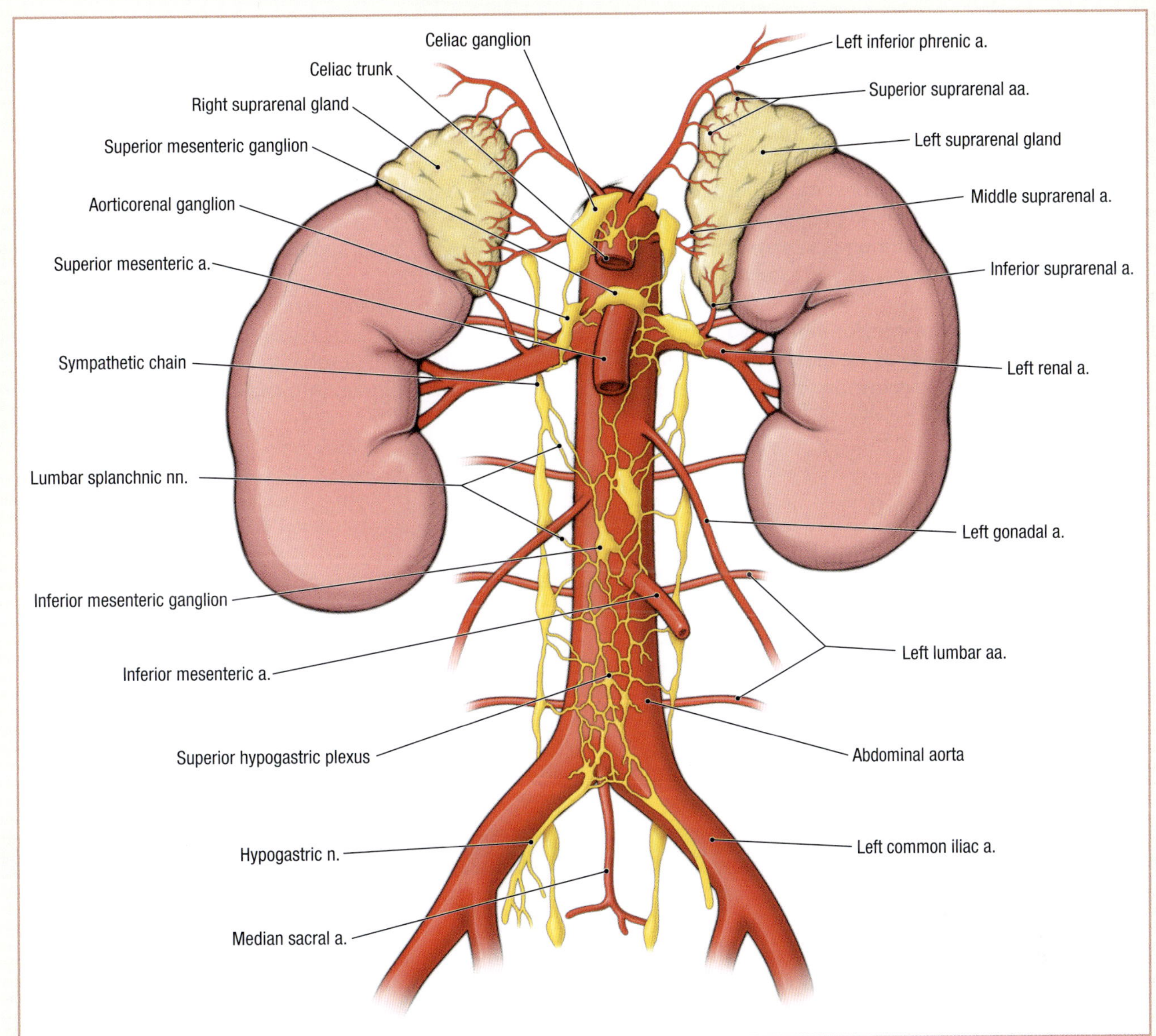

FIGURE 4.45 ● Paired and unpaired branches of abdominal aorta and autonomics of lumbar region. Anterior view.

thoracic aorta inferior to the diaphragm and ends by bifurcating at vertebral level L4 to form the **right** and **left common iliac arteries**.

3. Observe that the abdominal aorta has three types of branches: unpaired visceral, paired visceral, and paired somatic.
4. Identify the unpaired visceral arteries arising from the midline to the gastrointestinal tract: **celiac trunk**, **superior mesenteric artery**, and **inferior mesenteric artery**.
5. Identify the paired visceral arteries coursing to the three paired abdominal organs: **middle suprarenal arteries**, **renal arteries**, and **gonadal** (ovarian or testicular) **arteries**.
6. Identify the paired somatic arteries to the abdominal wall: **inferior phrenic arteries** and **lumbar arteries**.
7. Identify at least one of four pairs of **lumbar arteries** and observe that the right lumbar arteries cross the lumbar vertebral bodies to pass posterior to the inferior vena cava. *Note that on both sides, the lumbar arteries pass deep to the psoas major.*
8. On the inferior surface of the diaphragm, clean the **inferior phrenic arteries** and trace them back to their point of origin from the aorta near the aortic hiatus. Recall that these arteries give rise to superior suprarenal arteries.
9. At the termination of the abdominal aorta, identify and clean the proximal portion of the **common iliac arteries** near vertebral level L4. *Note that the common iliac arteries supply blood to the pelvis and lower limbs and will be dissected in more detail with the pelvis.*

10. Observe that **preaortic (prevertebral) ganglia** surround the abdominal aorta and its visceral branches forming a complex network of autonomic nerves.
11. Identify the **celiac, superior mesenteric, aorticorenal**, and **inferior mesenteric ganglia.**
12. Observe that connections from the preaortic ganglia extend along the lateral aspect of the aorta inferiorly to the **superior hypogastric plexus** and **hypogastric nerves**, which carry autonomic information to and from the pelvis.
13. Refer back to FIGURE 4.43.
14. Identify and clean the **inferior vena cava** beginning at the L5 vertebral level as well as its major tributaries, the **right** and **left common iliac veins.** Recall that the inferior vena cava ends at the T8 vertebral level by passing through the diaphragm to empty into the right atrium of the heart.
15. Observe that the inferior vena cava receives venous drainage from the paired abdominal organs (**renal, suprarenal**, and **gonadal veins**) either directly (right side) or indirectly (left side). *Note that the inferior vena cava has no unpaired visceral branches because the hepatic portal system collects all the blood from the gastrointestinal tract, which after filtration in the liver drains to the inferior vena cava via the hepatic veins.*
16. Identify and clean the paired somatic veins from the abdominal wall (lumbar veins and inferior phrenic veins), which drain into the inferior vena cava.

Dissection Follow-up

1. Review the relationships of each kidney to the surrounding structures.
2. Trace the path taken by a drop of urine from the renal papilla through the ureter to the level of the pelvic brim, noting the points of possible constriction.
3. Review the shape, position, relationships, arterial supply, and venous drainage of each suprarenal gland.
4. Review the branches of the abdominal aorta (paired and unpaired visceral and somatic).
5. Review the location of the autonomic ganglia in the lumbar region.
6. Review the tributaries of the inferior vena cava.
7. Replace the kidneys and other abdominal contents in their correct anatomical positions.

POSTERIOR ABDOMINAL WALL

Dissection Overview

The posterior abdominal wall is composed of the vertebral column, muscles that move the vertebral column, muscles that move the lower limbs, and the diaphragm. The nerves of the posterior abdominal wall arise from the anterior rami of spinal nerves T12–L4. The lumbar plexus (L1–L4) is formed within the psoas major, and its branches can be seen as they emerge from the lateral border of the muscle. Nerves of the lumbar plexus that innervate the abdominal wall and aspects of the lower limb will be dissected with the posterior abdominal wall.

The order of dissection will be as follows: Muscles that form the posterior abdominal wall will be identified. The branches of the lumbar plexus will be studied and isolated. The abdominal part of the sympathetic trunk will be studied.

Dissection Instructions

Muscles of Posterior Abdominal Wall

ATLAS 4.77, 4.88; VIDEO 4.11.1

Dissection Note: While identifying the muscles of the posterior abdominal wall, *do not* yet remove the overlying fascia or clean the muscles as nerves in the region may be damaged.

1. Refer to FIGURE 4.46.
2. Move each respective kidney, suprarenal gland, and remaining abdominal viscera toward the contralateral side to perform the following steps on each side of the body.
3. Remove any remaining renal fat and fascia from the posterior abdominal wall on each side of the abdominal cavity, ensuring you do not cut the associated neurovasculature of the organs.
4. Identify the **psoas major** on the lateral aspects of the lumbar vertebrae.
5. Look for the **psoas minor** and observe that it has a long flat tendon passing down the anterior surface of the psoas major. *Note that the psoas minor is absent in some individuals or may be present on only one side of the body in others.*
6. Identify the **iliacus** lateral to the psoas major in the depression of the iliac fossa. *Note that the iliacus*

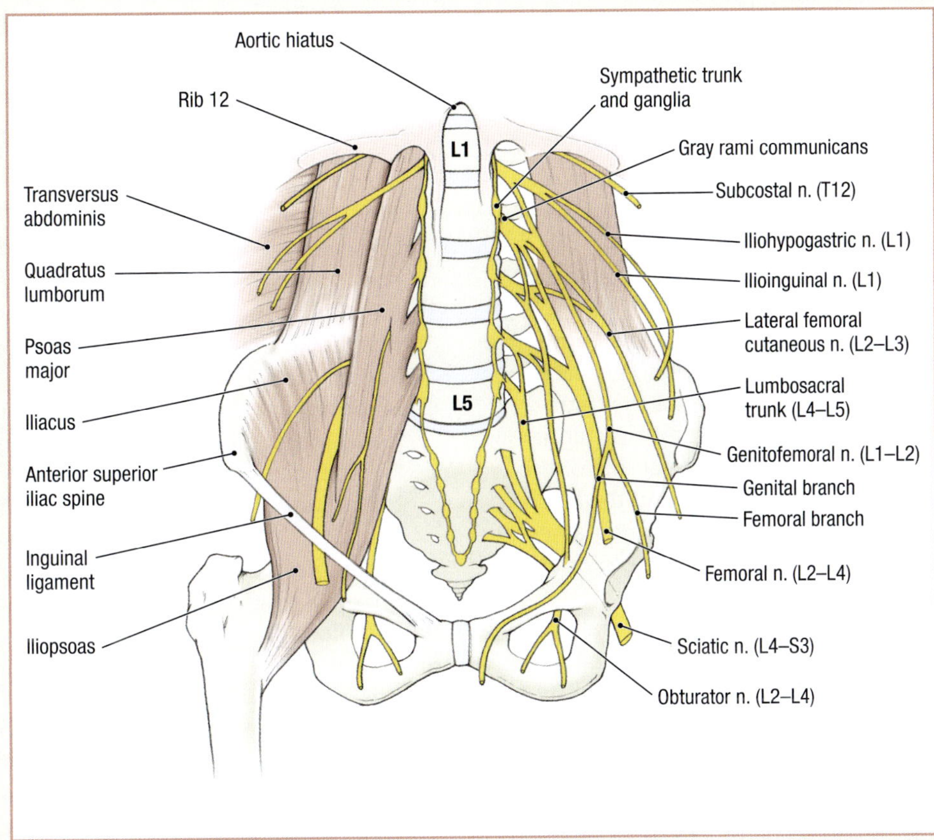

FIGURE 4.46 ● Lumbar plexus and muscles of posterior abdominal wall. Anterior view.

and psoas major merge deep to the inguinal ligament to form a functional unit collectively called the ***iliopsoas***.

7. Identify the **quadratus lumborum** lateral to the psoas major but superior to the iliac crest.
8. Review the attachments, actions, and innervations of the psoas major, psoas minor, iliacus, and quadratus lumborum (see **TABLE 4.2**).
9. Identify the **transversus abdominis**, one of the anterolateral abdominal wall muscles, and observe that it lies posterior to the quadratus lumborum.
10. Verify that the posterior surface of each kidney is related, through the renal fat and fascia, to the diaphragm, psoas major, quadratus lumborum, and transversus abdominis.
11. Observe that the superior pole of the right kidney is near the 12th rib and that the superior pole of the left kidney is slightly higher, near the 11th rib.

Lumbar Plexus

ATLAS 4.77, 4.78; VIDEO 4.11.2

Dissection Note: The branching pattern of the nerves of the lumbar plexus varies somewhat between individuals. Use the peripheral relationships of the nerves (their region of distribution or a point of exit from the abdominal cavity) for positive identification.

1. Refer to FIGURE 4.46.
2. Identify the **genitofemoral nerve** on the anterior surface of the psoas major. Observe that the genitofemoral nerve divides into **genital** and **femoral branches** superior to the inguinal ligament.
3. Identify the **genital branch of the genitofemoral nerve** and observe that it passes through the deep inguinal ring to enter the inguinal canal. *Note that the genital branch is the motor nerve to the cremaster, the thin muscle responsible for elevation of the testis in the male.*
4. Identify the **femoral branch of the genitofemoral nerve** and observe that it passes deep to the inguinal ligament on the anterior surface of the external iliac artery. *Note that the femoral branch supplies a small area of skin inferior and medial to the inguinal ligament.*
5. Use blunt dissection to remove the extraperitoneal fascia from the posterior abdominal wall lateral to the psoas major. The branches of the lumbar plexus are embedded in the extraperitoneal fascia and care must be taken not to damage them.
6. Palpate rib 12 and identify the **subcostal nerve** about 1 cm inferior and parallel to it.

7. Find the **iliohypogastric** and **ilioinguinal nerves**, which descend steeply across the anterior surface of the quadratus lumborum. *Note that frequently, these two nerves arise from a common L1 trunk with the iliohypogastric nerve located more superiorly and do not separate until they reach the lateral abdominal wall.*
8. To positively identify the ilioinguinal nerve, follow it through the anterolateral abdominal wall into the inguinal canal where it then exits via the superficial inguinal ring.
9. Identify the **lateral cutaneous nerve of the thigh** where it passes deep to the inguinal ligament near the ASIS. The lateral cutaneous nerve of the thigh supplies the skin on the lateral aspect of the thigh.
10. Identify the **femoral nerve** on the lateral side of the psoas major in the groove between it and the iliacus. The femoral nerve innervates the iliacus and passes deep to the inguinal ligament to provide motor and sensory branches to the anterior thigh.
11. Identify the **obturator nerve** medial and parallel to the psoas major within the lateral aspect of the pelvic cavity deep to the common iliac vessels. The obturator nerve supplies motor and sensory innervation to the medial thigh.
12. Identify the **lumbosacral trunk** medial to the obturator nerve. Observe that the lumbosacral trunk is a large nerve formed by contributions from the anterior ramus of L4 and the anterior ramus of L5. The lumbosacral trunk passes into the pelvis to join the sacral plexus and should be followed only a short distance at this time.
13. On the left side of the abdominal cavity, follow each nerve of the lumbar plexus proximally into the psoas major and observe that each branch of the lumbar plexus passes through the muscle at a different depth.
14. Clean the posterior abdominal wall to clearly display each nerve of the lumbar plexus as well as the superior extent of each muscle passing deep to the diaphragm.

Abdominal Part of Sympathetic Trunk

ATLAS 4.78, 4.81, 4.82A; VIDEO 4.11.3

1. Refer to FIGURE 4.46.
2. On the left side of the posterior abdominal wall, identify and clean the **sympathetic trunk**. Observe that the sympathetic trunk lies on the lumbar vertebral bodies between the crus of the diaphragm and the psoas major.
3. Identify **lumbar splanchnic nerves** that pass anteriorly from the lumbar sympathetic ganglia to the aortic autonomic nerve plexus.
4. Beginning at the genitofemoral nerve, remove the psoas major piece by piece, on one side only, to fully expose the lumbar plexus. Pay attention not to damage the lumbar vessels or the sympathetic trunk.
5. Cut and remove the psoas major to a point just proximal to its passage deep to the inguinal ligament and place its pieces in the tissue container.
6. With the psoas major removed, examine the point of exit of each spinal nerve from its intervertebral foramen and verify the spinal level contributions to each named nerve (e.g., femoral nerve—L2, L3, L4).
7. Identify rami communicantes that pass posteriorly from the sympathetic ganglia to the lumbar anterior rami. *Note that the gray rami of the lower lumbar region are the longest in the body because the sympathetic trunk crosses the anterolateral surface of the lumbar vertebral bodies.*
8. Observe that the rami communicantes lie against the lateral surface of the vertebral bodies. To assist finding the rami communicantes, clean and follow the lumbar arteries from their origin off the abdominal aorta and observe the relationship of the arteries, veins, and nerves in the lumbar region.
9. Review the autonomic nerve supply of the abdominal viscera.

Dissection Follow-up

1. Review the proximal and distal attachments as well as the action of each of the muscles of the posterior abdominal wall in **TABLE 4.2**.
2. Review the three muscles that form the anterolateral abdominal wall (external oblique, internal oblique, and transversus abdominis).
3. Follow each branch of the lumbar plexus peripherally and review the region of innervation of each of these nerves.
4. Review the abdominal part of the sympathetic trunk, lumbar splanchnic nerves, and rami communicantes (both gray and white).
5. Replace the abdominal contents in their correct anatomical positions.

TABLE 4.2 Muscles of Posterior Abdominal Wall

Muscle	*Proximal Attachments*	*Distal Attachments*	*Actions*	*Innervation*
Psoas major	Lumbar vertebrae (bodies, intervertebral discs, and transverse processes)	Lesser trochanter of the femur	Flexes the thigh and extends the vertebral column	L1–L4 (anterior rami)
Psoas minor	Lateral surface of T12 and L1	Iliopubic eminence and arcuate line of the ilium	Tilts pelvis posteriorly	L1–L2 (anterior rami)
Iliacus	Iliac fossa	Lesser trochanter of the femur	Flexes the thigh	Femoral n.
Quadratus lumborum	12th rib and lumbar transverse processes	Iliolumbar ligament and iliac crest	Flexes vertebral column laterally and anchors the rib cage during respiration	T12–L4 (anterior rami)

Abbreviation: n., nerve.

DIAPHRAGM

Dissection Overview

The diaphragm forms the superior boundary of the abdominal cavity and the inferior boundary of the thoracic cavity. The diaphragm is the principal muscle of respiration and has a right half and a left half (hemidiaphragms). Openings through the diaphragm allow passage of structures between the thoracic and abdominal cavities while maintaining respiratory function. From superior and anterior to inferior and posterior, these openings are the caval foramen, esophageal hiatus, and aortic hiatus.

The order of dissection will be as follows: The parts of the diaphragm will be identified. The openings of the diaphragm and their associated contents will be studied. The phrenic nerve will be reviewed. The greater splanchnic nerves that pass through the diaphragm will be studied.

Dissection Instructions

Diaphragm

ATLAS 3.75, 4.77, 4.79A, 4.88; VIDEO 4.12.1

Dissection Note: If the ribs were previously cut, separate them to either side to increase visibility and ease of access to the diaphragm. If the ribs were not yet cut, consider separating them now following the dissection sequence entitled **Reflection of Diaphragm** before proceeding.

1. Refer to FIGURE 4.47.
2. Use blunt dissection to remove the parietal peritoneum and connective tissue off the abdominal surface of the diaphragm, sparing the inferior phrenic vessels.
3. Identify the **central tendon of the diaphragm**, the aponeurotic center of the diaphragm and distal attachment of all of its muscular parts. Recall that the pericardial sac fused with the superior aspect of the central tendon.
4. The muscular portion of the diaphragm can be subdivided into sternal, costal, and lumbar parts. Identify the **sternal part** of the diaphragm, two small bundles of muscle fibers attaching to the posterior surface of the xiphoid process.
5. Identify the **costal part** of the diaphragm, the location where muscle fibers attach to the inferior six ribs and their costal cartilages.
6. Identify the **lumbar part** of the diaphragm formed by the two crura (right and left) and the muscle fibers arising from the medial and lateral arcuate ligaments.
7. Identify the **right crus** of the diaphragm and observe that it has attachments to the bodies of vertebrae

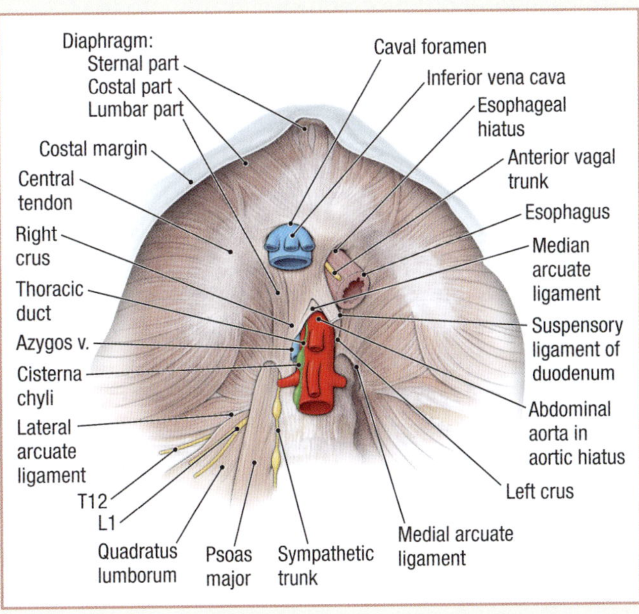

FIGURE 4.47 ■ Respiratory diaphragm. Inferior view.

L1–L3 and wraps around the esophagus to form the **esophageal hiatus**.

8. Identify the remnants of the **suspensory ligament of the diaphragm** arising from the right crus of the diaphragm.
9. Identify the **left crus** of the diaphragm and observe that it has attachments to the bodies of vertebrae L1 and L2.
10. Identify the **arcuate ligaments** that serve as inferior attachments for some of the muscle fibers of the diaphragm.
11. Identify the **lateral arcuate ligament** bridging the anterior surface of the quadratus lumborum, the **medial arcuate ligament** bridging the anterior surface of the psoas major, and the **median arcuate ligament** (unpaired) bridging the anterior surface of the aorta at the aortic hiatus.
12. Identify the **caval (vena caval) foramen** passing through the central tendon at vertebral level T8 allowing passage of the **inferior vena cava** through the diaphragm.
13. Identify the **esophageal hiatus** passing through the right crus at vertebral level T10 and observe that the **esophagus** and vagal trunks pass through this opening (see **Clinical Correlation 4.13**).

CLINICAL CORRELATION 4.13

Diaphragmatic Hernias and Paralysis

ATLAS 4.79

Herniation of either abdominal or thoracic contents may occur through or around the diaphragm due to cavity pressure changes, trauma, or developmental anomalies. A hiatal hernia allows passage of the stomach through the esophageal hiatus into the thoracic cavity and, although a congenital malformation, may occur posterior to or through the diaphragm, a possibly life-threatening condition.

Pain from the diaphragm is carried by the phrenic nerves (C3–C5) and referred to the region of the shoulder supplied by the supraclavicular cutaneous nerves arising from the same vertebral levels. The diaphragm can be paralyzed in cases of midcervical spinal cord injuries but is spared in low-cervical spinal cord injuries. A paralyzed hemidiaphragm cannot contract (descend); so, it will be positioned higher than normal in the thorax on a chest radiograph.

14. Identify the **aortic hiatus** passing posterior to the diaphragm at vertebral level T12 and observe that the **aorta**, **azygos** and **hemiazygos veins**, and **thoracic duct** pass through this opening.
15. Observe that the **sympathetic trunk** passes posterior to the diaphragm between its muscle fibers and the posterior abdominal wall musculature.
16. Within the thorax, identify the right and left phrenic nerves and recall that they provide motor innervation to the right and left hemidiaphragms, sensory innervation to the diaphragmatic parietal pleura, mediastinal parietal pleura, fibrous pericardium, parietal layer of serous pericardium, and the parietal peritoneum on the inferior aspect of the diaphragm. *Note that the pleural and peritoneal coverings of the peripheral part of the diaphragm receive sensory fibers from the lower intercostal nerves (T5–T11) and subcostal nerve.*
17. To increase mobility of the diaphragm, cut the right phrenic nerve 4 cm proximal to the superior surface of the diaphragm and push the right hemidiaphragm inferiorly.
18. Clean and follow the azygos vein and the thoracic duct inferiorly toward where they pass through the aortic hiatus. To verify the opening in the diaphragm that the azygos vein and thoracic duct pass through, gently push a probe through the aortic hiatus parallel to the aorta and observe the proximity of these structures.
19. Identify the greater splanchnic nerve in the right thorax and observe that it arises from vertebral levels T5–T9. Follow the greater splanchnic nerve inferiorly and verify that it penetrates the crus of the diaphragm to enter the abdominal cavity. *Note that the main portion of the greater splanchnic nerve distributes to the celiac ganglion where its sympathetic axons will synapse.*
20. Inferior to the greater splanchnic nerve, make an effort to identify and clean the lesser splanchnic nerve arising from vertebral levels T10–T11. *Note that the least splanchnic nerve is difficult to identify as it arises from vertebral level T12 deep to the posterior attachments of the diaphragm.*
21. Find the celiac ganglion if not previously removed near the celiac trunk and observe its connection with the thoracic splanchnic nerves.
22. Near the celiac ganglion, locate the **cisterna chyli (chyle cistern)**, a thin-walled lymphatic structure at the inferior end of the thoracic duct.

Dissection Follow-up

1. Review the attachments of the diaphragm to the skeleton of the thoracic wall.
2. Trace the course of the thoracic aorta as it passes through the aortic hiatus to become the abdominal aorta.
3. Review the course of the esophagus and vagal trunks through the esophageal hiatus.
4. Recall the position of the heart on the superior surface of the diaphragm and review the course of the inferior vena cava to the right atrium through the liver and diaphragm.
5. Observe that the thoracic duct passes through the aortic hiatus and that the splanchnic nerves (greater, lesser, and least) penetrate the crura.
6. Replace the abdominal contents in their correct anatomical positions.

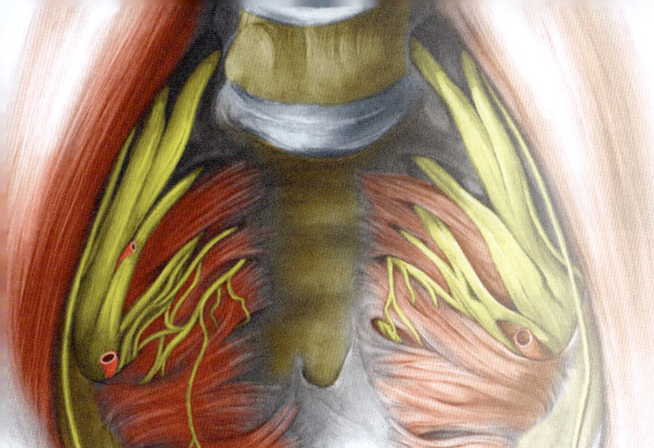

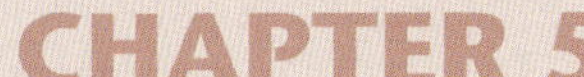

CHAPTER 5

Pelvis and Perineum

REFERENCES

ATLAS = *Grant's Atlas of Anatomy*, 16th ed., figure number

VIDEO = *Grant's Dissection Videos*, video sequence number

The pelvis is the most inferior aspect of the trunk and area of transition to the lower limbs. The bony pelvis provides support and protection for lower abdominal and pelvic organs, acts as a strong support for the vertebral column, and is the site of attachment for muscles acting on the trunk and lower limb. The pelvic cavity may be subdivided into a greater (false) pelvis, the superior portion continuous with the abdominal cavity, and a lesser (true) pelvis, the inferior portion encircled by the pelvic bones, with the transition occurring at the plane of the pelvic inlet as shown in FIGURE 5.1.

The pelvic cavity contains the rectum, urinary bladder, and internal genitalia. The perineum is the region of the trunk located between the thighs and separated from the pelvic cavity by the pelvic diaphragm. The perineum contains the anal canal, urethra, and external genitalia (vulva in the female and penis and scrotum in the male).

This chapter begins with the dissection of structures in the anal triangle common to both sexes (see **Clinical Correlation 5.1: Sex and Gender**). Dissection of internal and external genitalia is divided into two sections: one for female cadavers and one for male cadavers. Students are expected to learn the anatomy of both the female and male pelvis and perineum; therefore, each dissection team should partner with another team dissecting a cadaver of the opposite sex.

CLINICAL CORRELATIONS

During your dissection protocol, you may encounter anatomical variations, clinical conditions, disease processes, or medical devices in your cadaveric donor. The following select clinical correlations will be described in more detail throughout this chapter.

Pelvis and Perineum

5.1. Sex and Gender, see the **Bony Pelvis** sequence. ATLAS 4.17
5.2. Lymphatic Drainage of Labia Majora, see the **Labia Majora** sequence. ATLAS 5.30C, 5.30D
5.3. Obstetric Considerations, see the **Female Superficial Perineal Pouch** sequence. ATLAS 5.32, 5.49, 5.50
5.4. Uterine Orientation and Life Changes, see the **Female Pelvic Peritoneum** sequence. ATLAS 5.21, 5.22, 5.27A, 5.27B
5.5. Hemorrhoids, see the **Female Rectum and Anal Canal** sequence. ATLAS 5.16D, 5.18D
5.6. Hysterectomy, see the **Female Pelvic Blood Vessels** sequence. ATLAS 5.28, 5.33C, 5.35A
5.7. Vasectomy, see the **Spermatic Cord** sequence. ATLAS 5.37
5.8. Lymphatic Drainage of Scrotum and Testis, see the **Testis** sequence. ATLAS 4.20C, 5.43
5.9. Rupture of Male Urethra, see the **Male Superficial Perineal Pouch** sequence. ATLAS 5.60
5.10. Circumcision, see the **Penis** sequence. ATLAS 5.61
5.11. Cystotomy, see the **Male Pelvic Peritoneum** sequence. ATLAS 5.48B, 5.48E, 5.48F, 5.63
5.12. Benign Prostatic Hyperplasia and Digital Rectal Examination, see the **Male Rectum and Anal Canal** sequence. ATLAS 5.37, 5.40
5.13. Hypogastric Nerve Damage, see the **Male Pelvic Nerves** sequence. ATLAS 5.44

ANAL TRIANGLE

Dissection Overview

The perineum is a diamond-shaped area inferior to the pelvic diaphragm between the thighs. The perineum is commonly divided into two triangles for descriptive purposes: the urogenital triangle anteriorly and the anal triangle posteriorly. At the outset of dissection, it is important to understand that these two triangles are not in the same plane but an angle to one another and that the pelvic diaphragm separates the pelvic cavity from the perineum.

The ischioanal (ischiorectal) fossa is a wedge-shaped area on either side of the anus within the anal triangle. The apex of the wedge is directed superiorly toward the coccyx, and the base is beneath the skin. The ischioanal fossa is filled with loose fat to accommodate physical changes within the pelvis such as distension of the anal canal during the passage of feces or movement of the fetus during childbirth.

The order of dissection will be as follows: The skeleton of the female and male pelvis will be reviewed. The skin of the gluteal region will be removed and the gluteus maximus retracted. The nerves and vessels of the ischioanal fossa will be dissected. The fat will be removed from the ischioanal fossa to reveal the inferior surface of the pelvic diaphragm.

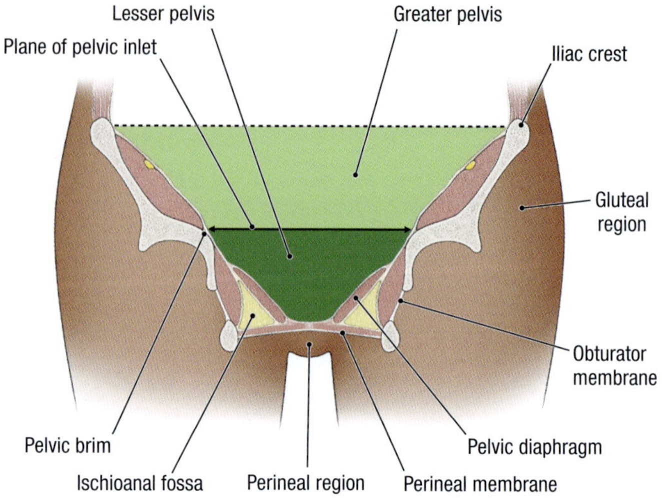

FIGURE 5.1 ● Coronal section through pelvis. Anterior view.

Skeletal Anatomy

Refer to an articulated bony pelvis and identify the following skeletal features.

Bony Pelvis

ATLAS 5.3, 5.8B

1. Refer to FIGURE 5.2.
2. Observe that the bony **pelvis** is formed by the **hip bones (os coxae), sacrum,** and **coccyx**.
3. Inferior to the sacrum, identify the fused coccygeal vertebrae making up the **coccyx** and observe that they do not articulate with the hip bones.
4. Identify the roughened area of the **ischial tuberosity** on the most inferior aspect of the bony pelvis. The ischial tuberosity is the area of attachment for the hamstrings and **sacrotuberous ligament**.
5. Identify the **iliac crest** of the ilium, the most superior aspect of the bony pelvis.
6. Follow the iliac crest posteriorly and identify the **posterior superior iliac spine (PSIS)**.
7. Compare a female and male pelvis and observe that the distance between the ischial tuberosities is commonly greater in the female than the male (see **Clinical Correlation 5.1**).

CLINICAL CORRELATION 5.1

Sex and Gender

ATLAS 4.17

The sex of an individual occurs on a spectrum rather than binarized categories. Sex refers to the gonadal development of ovaries or testes as determined by chromosomal patterning (i.e., xx female, xy male, and xxy or xyy intersex). Gonads produce hormones responsible for phenotypic (visual characteristics) expression at birth of the external genitalia and secondary sex characteristics. For educational purposes in this text, a simplified binary of female or male is used to refer to the congenital- or birth-assigned sex and the associated physical characteristics correlating to each. As such, the female gonad is the ovary, whereas the male gonad is the testis.

The gender of an individual also occurs on a spectrum; is not binarized; and cannot be determined, categorized, or defined by anatomy but only by the individual themselves. Identity terms may include but are not limited to female, male, nonbinary, third gender, androgynous, gender fluid, genderqueer, or transgender.

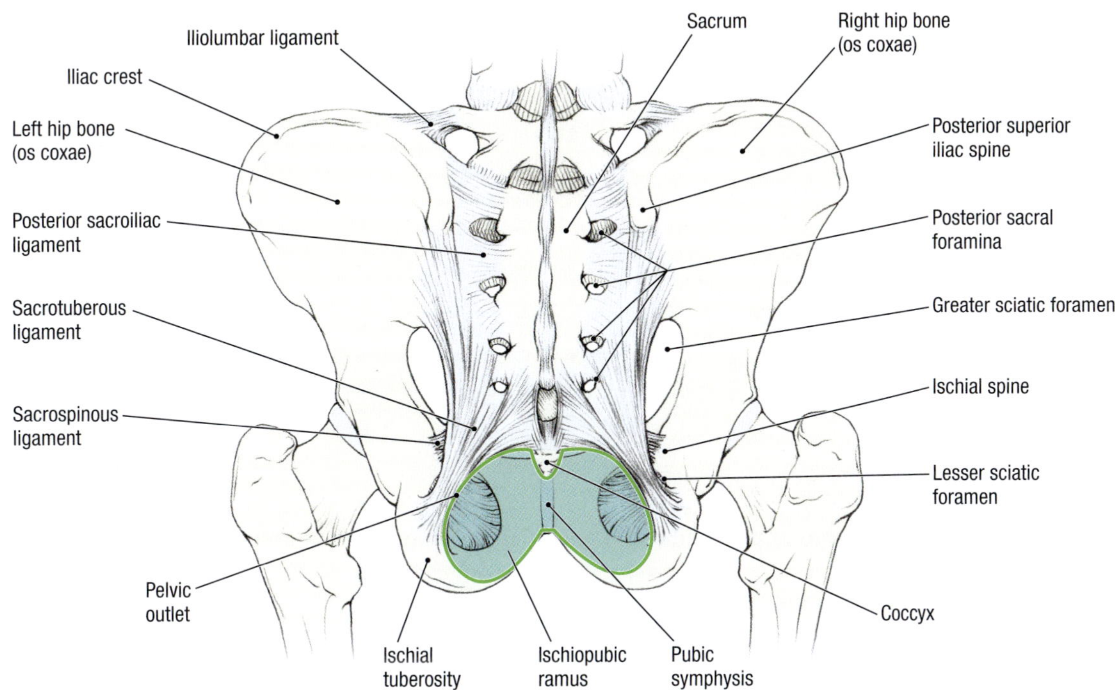

FIGURE 5.2 ● Bones and ligaments of pelvis. Posterior view.

8. From a posterior perspective, identify the **ischial spine** of the ischium and observe that this bony projection is directed toward the sacrum.
9. Observe that the ischial spine separates the **greater sciatic notch** from the **lesser sciatic notch** and serves as a point of attachment for the **sacrospinous ligament**.
10. Compare a female and male pelvis and observe that the distance between the ischial spines is commonly greater in the female than the male.
11. On the sacrum, identify the **posterior sacral foramina** and observe that they connect to the **sacral canal** and are continuous with the **anterior sacral foramina**.
12. On an articulated pelvis, observe that the **sacroiliac articulation** is strengthened by both a **posterior sacroiliac ligament** and an **anterior sacroiliac ligament**. *Note that the sacroiliac articulation is a synovial joint between the auricular surface of the sacrum and the ilium.*
13. On an articulated pelvis, observe that the **iliolumbar ligament** strengthens the articulation at the **lumbosacral joint** and that the **supraspinous ligament** courses along the spinous processes of the lumbar vertebrae to the **median sacral crest**.
14. Identify the **pelvic outlet** and observe that it is bound anteriorly by the **inferior margin of the pubic symphysis**; posteriorly by the **tip of the coccyx**; and laterally by the **ischiopubic rami**, **ischial tuberosities**, and **sacrotuberous ligaments**.
15. Compare a female and male pelvis and observe that the pelvic outlet is commonly larger and more rounded in the female than the male.

Surface Anatomy

The surface anatomy of the pelvis and perineum may be studied on a cadaver, although fixation of tissue during embalming may make it difficult to distinguish bone from well-preserved soft tissues in some specimens.

Urogenital and Anal Triangles

ATLAS 5.45, 5.46, 5.53B

1. Refer to FIGURE 5.3.
2. With the cadaver lying in the prone position, palpate the tip of the **coccyx** in the midline posteriorly.
3. On the lateral aspects of the perineum bilaterally, palpate the **ischial tuberosities**, the lateral boundary points of both the anal and urogenital triangles.

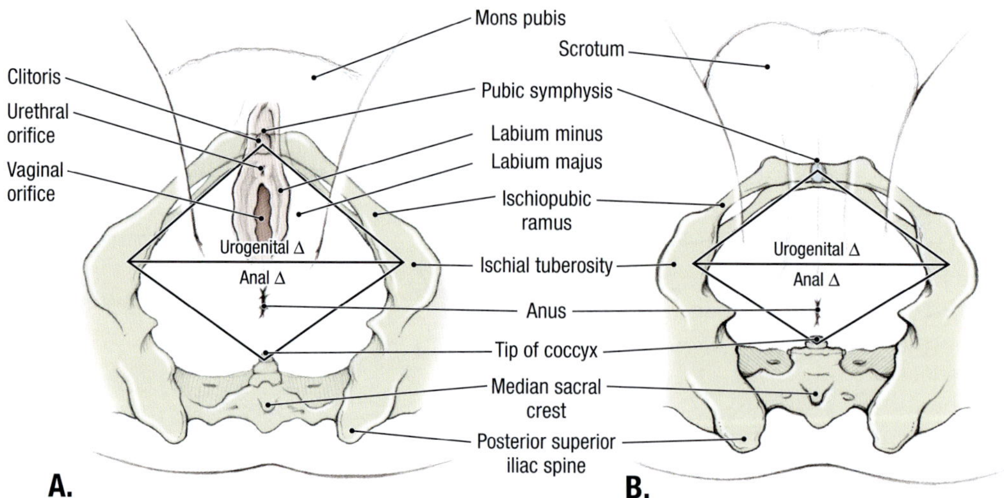

FIGURE 5.3 Boundaries of urogenital and anal triangles in female (**A**) and male (**B**) in supine positions. Inferior views.

4. Identify the **anal triangle**, the posterior part of the perineum containing the **anus**.
5. Retract the gluteal folds away from the midline and identify the **opening of the anal canal.**
6. Identify the **urogenital triangle**, the anterior part of the perineum containing the **urethra** and **external genitalia.**
7. Observe that the urogenital triangle in the female contains the **vulva,** the female external genitalia that includes the **labia (majora** and **minora), clitoris,** and **vaginal** and **urethral orifices** in the space of the **vestibule.**
8. Observe that the urogenital triangle in the male contains the **penis** and **scrotum.**

Dissection Instructions

Skin Incisions of Gluteal Region

ATLAS 5.49A, 5.57; VIDEO 5.1.1

Dissection Note: Prior to commencing with skin incisions, decide to either perform a full- or partial-thickness approach and to either reflect or remove the skin from the dissection field. See **Removing Skin** in the **Introduction Chapter** for descriptions.

If the lower limb has been dissected previously, reflect the gluteus maximus laterally and move ahead to the **ischioanal fossa** dissection sequence.

1. Refer to FIGURE 5.4.
2. With the cadaver in the prone position, make an incision from the tip of the coccyx (S), superiorly along the lateral border of the sacrum and the iliac crest, to the midaxillary line (T). *Note that if the back has been skinned, this incision has been made previously.*
3. Make a midline skin incision from the median sacral crest and tip of the coccyx (S) to a point near the posterior edge of the anus.
4. Make an incision encircling the anus.

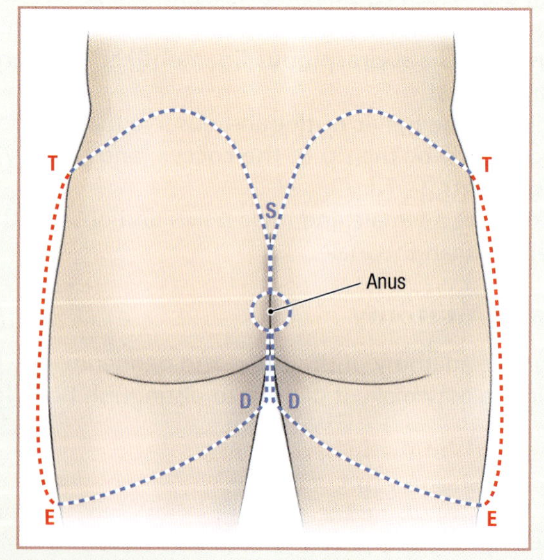

FIGURE 5.4 Skin incisions of gluteal region. Posterior view.

5. Make an incision from the anterior edge of the anus down the medial surface of the thigh (D) for approximately 7.5 cm.
6. Make a skin incision from the medial surface of the thigh (D) obliquely to the lateral surface of the thigh (E) approximately 30 cm inferior to the iliac crest.
7. If reflecting the skin, use the uncut sections of skin laterally as hinge points between the iliac crest (T) and the lateral surface of the thigh (E) to leave the skin attached along the peripheral aspect of the gluteal region. Reflect the skin only as far laterally as the midaxillary line.
8. If removing the skin, make a vertical skin incision from the iliac crest (T) along the midaxillary line to the lateral aspect of the thigh (E).
9. If using a partial-thickness skin removal method, remove the skin, but not the subcutaneous tissue, from medial to lateral using either a pair of locking forceps or the buttonhole technique. At any point, the portions of skin may be cut into smaller segments to facilitate removal.
10. If using a full-thickness skin removal method, remove the subcutaneous tissue from the surface of the gluteus maximus along with the skin, taking care to not cut too deeply. *Do not yet remove the subcutaneous tissue within the ischioanal fossa.*
11. If the skin is to be removed, detach the skin along the periphery and place it in the tissue container.

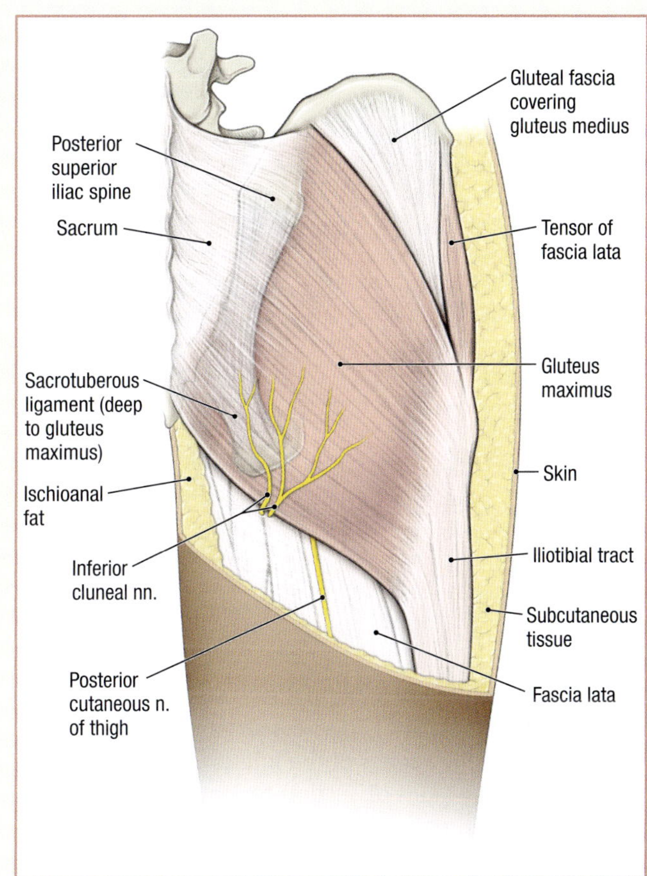

FIGURE 5.5 ● Fascia of gluteal region. Posterior view.

Subcutaneous Tissue of Gluteal Region

ATLAS 5.50A, 5.54, 5.58; VIDEO 5.1.2

Dissection Note: The loose ischioanal fat is part of the subcutaneous tissue of this region but is a different texture than the dense fat overlying the ischial tuberosities. Despite the relatively large amounts of fat, proceed slowly within the ischioanal fossa to avoid tearing the delicate neurovascular structures of the region.

1. Refer to FIGURE 5.5.
2. If you have not already done so with the skin removal, remove the subcutaneous tissue from the surface of the **gluteus maximus** superiorly and place it in the tissue container.
3. Observe that the large gluteus maximus attaches along its lateral aspect to the **iliotibial tract (IT band)**, the condensation of the thick **fascia lata** of the thigh.
4. Along the inferior aspect of the gluteus maximus within the subcutaneous tissue, identify one or two of the **inferior cluneal nerves**, the cutaneous nerve branches in the region.
5. Clean and define the inferior border of the **gluteus maximus** by removing the remaining subcutaneous tissue and separate it from the ischioanal fat and deep gluteal connective tissue. *Note that it is not necessary to save the inferior cluneal nerves but take care not to cut the fascia lata of the posterior thigh.*
6. Deep to the inferior border of the gluteus maximus, palpate the **sacrotuberous ligament**. *Note that the gluteus maximus is attached to the sacrotuberous ligament and sacrum medially.*
7. Retract the gluteus maximus superiorly to broaden the dissection field and expose the **ischioanal fat**.
8. Along the superior border of the gluteus maximus, identify the **gluteus medius** but do not yet remove the overlying **gluteal fascia**.

Ischioanal Fossa

ATLAS 5.54, 5.58; VIDEO 5.1.2

1. Refer to FIGURE 5.6.
2. Lateral to the anus, use scissors to create an incision directed toward the gluteus maximus within the ischioanal fat to a depth of approximately 3 cm (**Cut 1**).
3. Using the scissor technique, or your preferred method of blunt dissection, push and separate the fat with the blunt outer edge of the scissors or probe to enlarge the opening in the ischioanal fat.

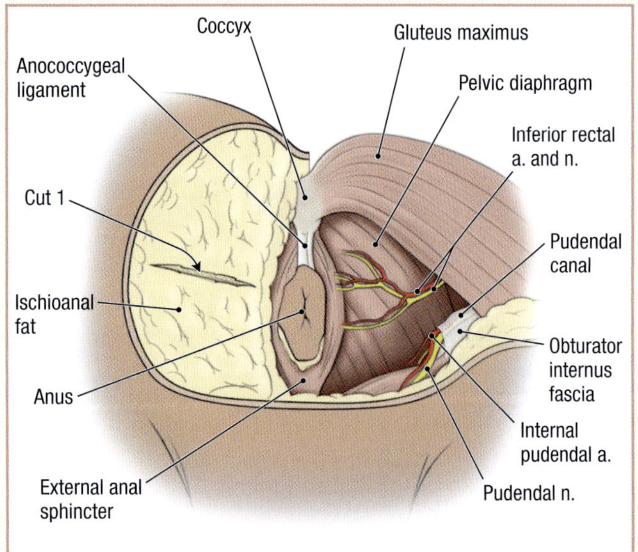

FIGURE 5.6 ● Ischioanal fossa superficial (*left*) and deep (*right*) dissections. Inferior view.

4. Within the ischioanal fat, palpate and identify the **inferior rectal (anal) nerve** and **vessels.**
5. Preserve the branches of the inferior rectal nerve and vessels using blunt dissection to remove the surrounding fat, drying the area with paper towels if necessary. *Note that the inferior rectal nerve innervates the external anal sphincter and skin around the anus.*
6. Use blunt dissection to clean the **external anal sphincter** surrounding the anus medially, part of the medial boundary of the ischioanal fossa. *Note that the external anal sphincter has three parts: a subcutaneous portion encircling the anus, a superficial portion anchoring the anus to the perineal body and coccyx, and a deep portion forming a ring of muscle fused with the pelvic diaphragm.*
7. Use blunt dissection to clean the inferior surface of the **pelvic diaphragm**, the medial and superior boundaries of the ischioanal fossa. *Note that the inferior boundary of the ischioanal fossa is the skin of the region.*
8. Use blunt dissection to expose the **fascia of the obturator internus**, the lateral boundary of the ischioanal fossa.
9. Laterally, observe that the inferior rectal nerve and vessels are surrounded by the fascia of the obturator internus in a space known as the **pudendal canal.**
10. Place gentle traction on the inferior rectal vessels and nerve and observe that a ridge is raised in the obturator internus fascia demarcating the path of the pudendal canal.
11. Gently place a probe within the pudendal canal to verify the path of the canal and carefully cut the overlying obturator fascia, taking care to not cut the underlying nerves and vessels.
12. Observe that the inferior rectal vessels and nerve exit the inferior aspect of the pudendal canal to enter the ischioanal fossa. *Note that the superior aspect of the canal communicates with the lesser sciatic foramen.*
13. Use blunt dissection to elevate and clean the contents of the pudendal canal, the **pudendal nerve** and **internal pudendal artery** and **vein.**

Dissection Follow-up

1. Review the boundaries of the true pelvis and confirm that the pelvic diaphragm separates the pelvic cavity from the perineum.
2. Use the dissected specimen to review the boundaries of the ischioanal fossa.
3. Review the location of the external anal sphincter, its blood supply, and its pattern of innervation as a skeletal muscle under voluntary control.
4. If a full- or partial-thickness skin reflection was performed, replace the reflected portions of skin back to anatomical position.

FEMALE EXTERNAL GENITALIA, UROGENITAL TRIANGLE, AND PERINEUM

Dissection Overview

If you are dissecting a male cadaver, refer to the **Scrotum, Spermatic Cord, and Testis** section and use this section for review with a female cadaver.

In the embryo, the female and male external genitalia have similar origins and remain morphologically similar until a certain stage in development. Thus, many of the structures of the external genitalia have a homologous counterpart in the opposite sex such as the labia majora in the female and scrotum in the male, or the clitoris in the female and penis in the male.

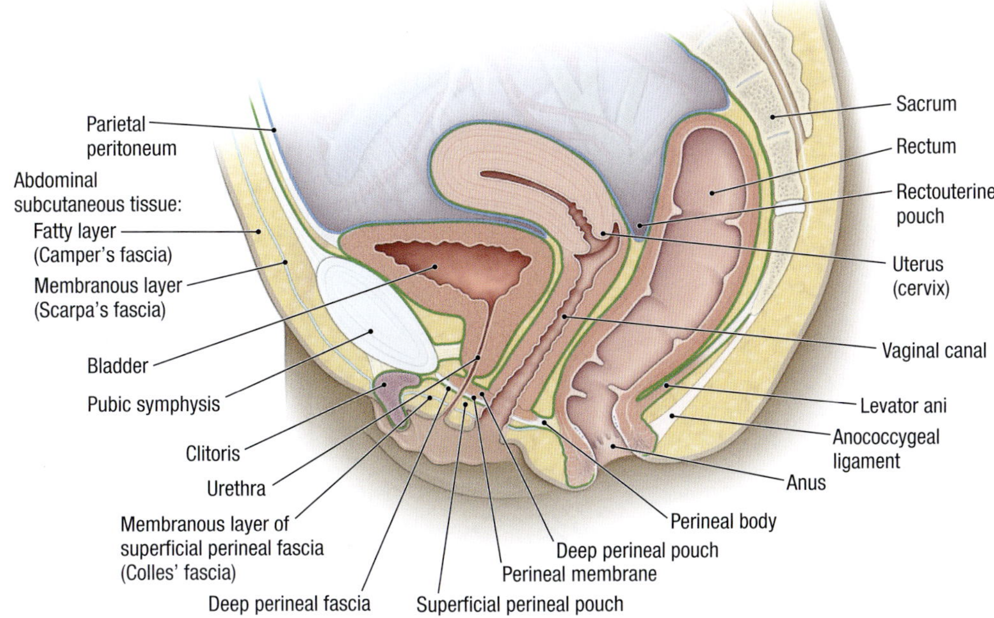

FIGURE 5.7 Fasciae of female perineum. Midsagittal view.

In all individuals, the superficial perineal fascia has a superficial fatty layer and a deep membranous layer. In the female, the superficial fatty layer provides the shape of the labia majora and is continuous with the fat of the lower abdominal wall (Camper's fascia), ischioanal fossa, and thigh as shown in FIGURE 5.7. The membranous layer of superficial perineal fascia (Colles' fascia) is continuous with the membranous layer of superficial fascia of the lower abdominal wall (Scarpa's fascia). The membranous layer of the superficial perineal fascia is attached to the ischiopubic ramus as far posteriorly as the ischial tuberosity and to the posterior edge of the perineal membrane and forms the superficial boundary of the superficial perineal pouch (space).

The order of dissection of the female urogenital triangle will be as follows: The round ligament of the uterus will be followed from the superficial inguinal ring for a short distance into the superior part of the labia majora. The external genitalia will be examined. The skin will be removed from the labia majora. The superficial perineal fascia will be removed, and the contents of the superficial perineal pouch will be identified. The contents of the deep perineal pouch will be described but only minimally dissected.

Skeletal Anatomy

Refer to an articulated bony pelvis and identify the following skeletal features.

Female Bony Pelvis

ATLAS 5.5, 5.8

1. Refer to FIGURE 5.8.
2. Identify the three bones comprising the hip bone: **ilium**, **ischium**, and **pubis**.
3. Orient the bony pelvis in anatomical position (erect posture) and observe that the **anterior superior iliac spine** and anterior aspect of the pubis at the **pubic tubercle** align in a coronal plane.
4. On the anterior surface of the ilium, identify the **iliac fossa**. Observe that the iliac fossae are directed toward one another and form the lateral boundaries of the **false (greater) pelvis**, the portion of the bony pelvis superior to the **pelvic inlet (brim)**.
5. Observe that the pelvic inlet is formed by the **sacral promontory** and **anterior border of the ala (wing) of the sacrum** posteriorly; arcuate line of the ilium laterally; and pecten pubis, pubic crest of the pubic bones, and **pubic symphysis** anteriorly.
6. Observe that in anatomical position, the plane of the pelvic inlet forms an angle of approximately 55° to the horizontal.
7. Observe that the lesser pelvis is located inferior to the pelvic inlet and surrounded by bone. *Note that the inferior boundary of the lesser pelvis is the pelvic diaphragm.*
8. Identify the **obturator foramen**, the large opening on the anterior aspect of the bony pelvis.

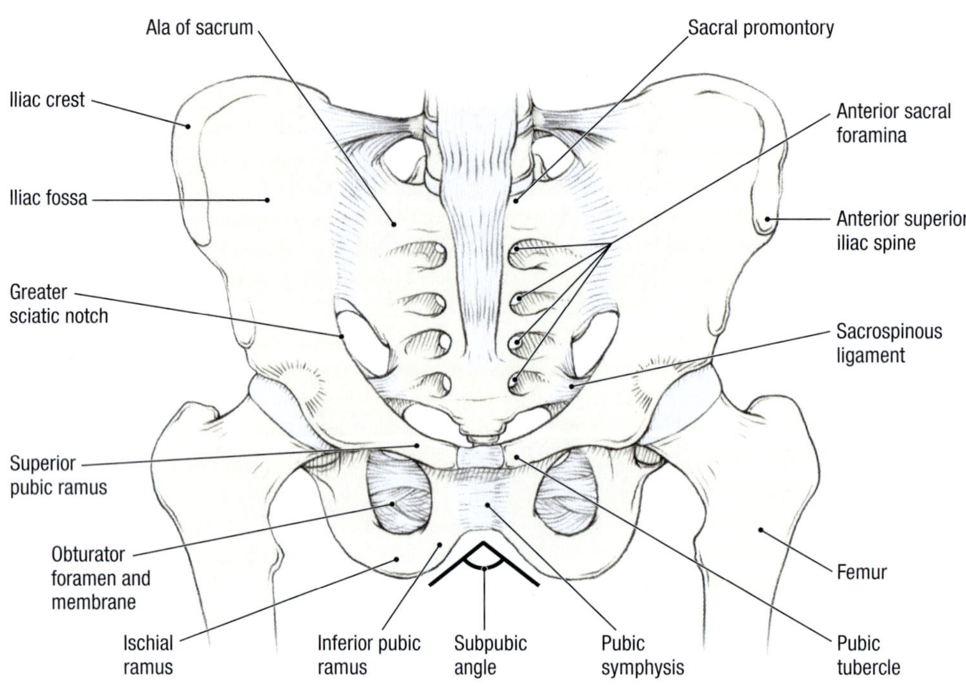

FIGURE 5.8 ● Female bony pelvis. Anterior view.

9. Observe that in anatomical position, the obturator foramen faces inferiorly and is bound by the **superior pubic ramus** anteriorly, **ischiopubic ramus** medially, and body of the **ischium** laterally.
10. Observe that the ischiopubic ramus is formed by the **ischial ramus** and **inferior pubic ramus**, often not easily delineated.
11. Compare a female and male bony pelvis and observe that the **subpubic angle** (angle of the pubic arch) is commonly wider, the distance between the ischial spines is greater, the pelvic inlet is more oval, and that the greater pelvis is often wider and shorter in females.

Surface Anatomy

The surface anatomy of the perineum may be studied on a cadaver; however, fixation of tissue during embalming may make it difficult during palpation to distinguish bone from well-preserved soft tissues in some specimens.

Female External Genitalia

ATLAS 5.1A, 5.45; VIDEO 5.8.1

1. Refer to FIGURE 5.9.
2. With the cadaver in a supine position, stretch the thighs widely apart and brace them.
3. Examine the **vulva**, the female external genitalia.
4. Observe that the **mons pubis** is the region of the female external genitalia anterior to the pubic symphysis filled with fat and covered with pubic hair.
5. Identify the **labia majora** (sing. **labium majus**), the paired cutaneous swellings extending from the mons pubis superiorly to the perineum inferiorly (see **Clinical Correlation 5.2**). Locate where the right and left sides of the labia majora meet anteriorly at the **anterior labial commissure** and posteriorly at the **posterior labial commissure**.
6. Identify the **clitoris** just posterior to the anterior labial commissure.
7. Observe that the **glans** of the clitoris is covered by the **prepuce** on its dorsal surface, whereas the **frenulum of the clitoris** curves posteriorly for a short distance along the ventral surface. *Note that the glans, prepuce, and frenulum of the clitoris are homologous to the male counterparts on the penis except that they do not contain the urethra.*
8. Medial to the labia majora, identify the **labia minora** (sing. **labium minus**) and observe that unlike the labia majora, these folds are not covered with hair. *Note that the labia minora have numerous sebaceous glands and overlie the bulbs of the vestibule.*
9. Identify the **frenulum of labia minora** just anterior to the posterior labial commissure.
10. Identify the region of the **vestibule of the vagina** between the labia minora.

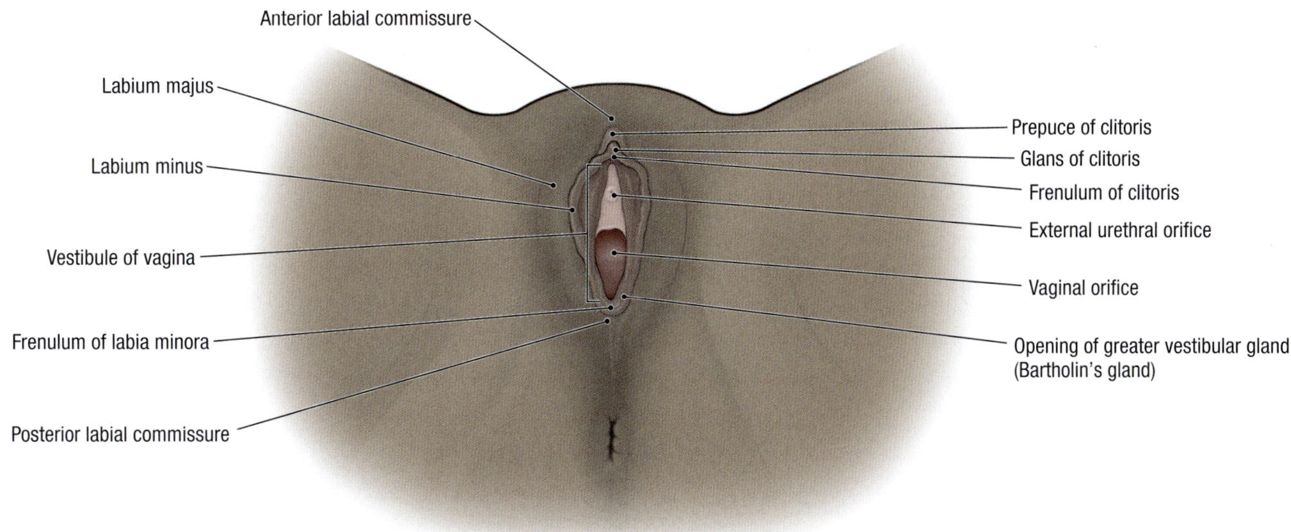

FIGURE 5.9 ■ Surface anatomy of female external genitalia. Inferior view.

11. Within the vestibule, identify the smaller anteriorly located **external urethral orifice** and the larger posteriorly located **vaginal orifice**. *Note that within the vestibule, the openings of the paraurethral ducts are present on each side of the external urethral orifice, although it is unlikely that they will be visible in the cadaveric specimen.*

Dissection Instructions

Labia Majora

ATLAS 5.45, 5.49A; VIDEO 5.8.2

Dissection Note: The dissection of the labia majora corresponds to the dissection of the scrotum in male cadavers. Partner with a dissection team that has a male cadaver for the dissection of the external genitalia. You are expected to observe and learn the anatomy for both sexes.

1. Refer back to FIGURE 4.8C.
2. At the **superficial inguinal ring**, identify the **round ligament of the uterus**.
3. Use blunt dissection to demonstrate that the round ligament of the uterus emerges from the superficial inguinal ring and spreads out into the subcutaneous tissue of the **labia majora** (see **Clinical Correlation 5.2**). *Note that the round ligament is a delicate structure that can be demonstrated for only 1 to 2 cm distal to the superficial inguinal ring.*

CLINICAL CORRELATION 5.2

Lymphatic Drainage of Labia Majora

ATLAS 5.30C, 5.30D

Lymphatics from the labia majora drain to the superficial inguinal lymph nodes. Inflammation of the labia majora may cause tender, enlarged superficial inguinal lymph nodes.

Skin Incisions of Female Urogenital Triangle

ATLAS 5.49A, 5.50A, 5.54; VIDEO 5.8.3

Dissection Note: It is recommended to perform a partial-thickness skin removal technique leaving the subcutaneous tissue intact because cutting too deeply may easily damage many of the structures in the region. To facilitate dissection, position yourself between the lower limbs with the trunk of the cadaver pulled toward the end of the dissection table.

1. Refer to FIGURE 5.10.
2. With the cadaver in the supine position, stretch the thighs widely apart and brace them.
3. Make a transverse incision from the anterior aspect of the right thigh (N) across the mons pubis to the anterior aspect of the left thigh (N). *Note that if the abdomen was previously dissected, a portion of this incision was already made.*
4. Make a skin incision connecting from the anterior aspect of each thigh (N) posteriorly to a point in the posterior thigh (M) in line with the horizontal incision bifurcating the anterior margin of the anus (J).
5. Make a skin incision from the midline of the mons pubis (E) to the anterior labial commissure (R).
6. Make a skin incision in the midline from posterior labial commissure (K) to the anterior margin of the anus (J).

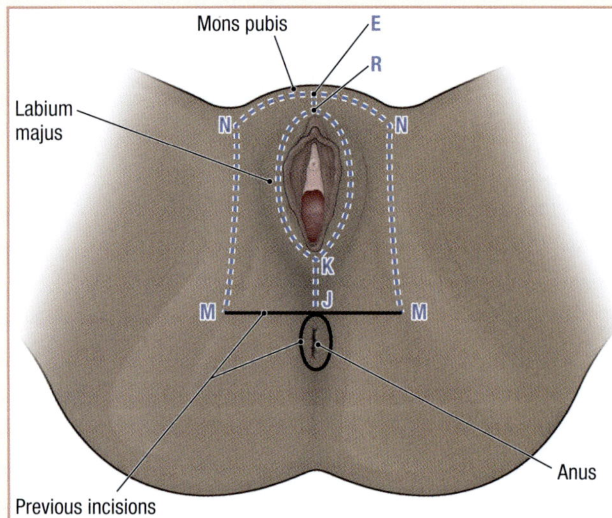

FIGURE 5.10 ● Skin incisions of female perineum. Inferior view.

7. Make a skin incision that follows the medial surface of the labia majora beginning at the anterior labial commissure (R) to the posterior labial commissure (K) just lateral to the labia minora on each side.
8. Remove the skin from the labia majora from medial to lateral.
9. Detach each skin flap along the medial surface of the thigh and place it in the tissue container.
10. Remove the mass of fat contained in the labia majora and place it in the tissue container.
11. If the cadaver has a large amount of fat in the subcutaneous tissue of the medial thighs, carefully remove a portion of the fat corresponding to the areas of removed skin.

Female Superficial Perineal Pouch

ATLAS 5.49A, 5.50A, 5.51, 5.53; VIDEO 5.8.4

1. Refer to FIGURE 5.11.
2. In the female, three muscles occupy the superficial pouch on each side: ischiocavernosus, bulbospongiosus, and superficial transverse perineal. The pairs of muscles overlay the erectile tissue of the region and contribute to the contents of the superficial perineal pouch with their accompanying neurovascular structures.
3. Beginning posteriorly in the ischioanal fossa, identify the **posterior labial nerve** and **vessels** and observe that they are terminal branches of the **superficial branch of the perineal artery and nerve**, which supply the posterior part of the labia majora. *Note that the superficial branch of the perineal artery and nerve enter the urogenital triangle by passing lateral to the external anal sphincter.*
4. Use blunt dissection to remove the fat and superficial perineal fascia about 2 cm lateral to the labium minus and identify the **membranous layer of the superficial perineal fascia (Colles' fascia)**.

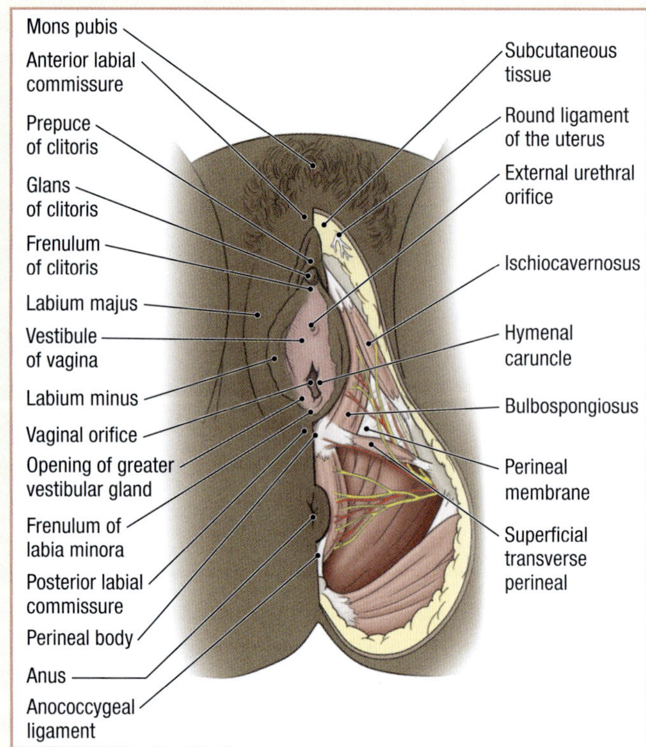

FIGURE 5.11 ● Contents of female superficial perineal pouch. Inferior view.

5. Review the attachments of the Colles' fascia by palpating the **ischiopubic ramus** and **ischial tuberosity** as well as the posterior edge of the **perineal membrane**. *Note that the Colles' fascia forms the superficial boundary of the* ***superficial perineal pouch*** *(space).*
6. Use blunt dissection to find the **bulbospongiosus** deep to the labium minus overlying the **bulb of the vestibule**. *Note that the bulbospongiosus in the female does not join the contralateral muscle across the midline as it does in the male.*
7. Review the attachments and actions of the **bulbospongiosus** (see **TABLE 5.1**).
8. Lateral to the bulbospongiosus, use blunt dissection to clean the surface of the **ischiocavernosus** overlying the superficial surface of the **crus of the clitoris** along the ischiopubic ramus.
9. Use blunt dissection to find the **superficial transverse perineal** at the posterior border of the urogenital triangle.
10. Observe that the superficial transverse perineal helps to support the **perineal body**, a fibromuscular mass located anterior to the anal canal and near the posterior edge of the bulbospongiosus (see **Clinical Correlation 5.3**). *Note that the superficial transverse perineal may be delicate and difficult to find. Limit the time you spend looking for it.*

CLINICAL CORRELATION 5.3

Obstetric Considerations

ATLAS 5.32, 5.49, 5.50

To alleviate the pain of childbirth, multiple nerve blocks may be performed. A spinal block at the L3/L4 vertebral level will introduce anesthesia from the waist down, including the perineum, pelvic floor, and birth canal. Alternatively, a caudal epidural block will anesthetize most of the perineal region, the entire birth canal, and pelvic floor without affecting the lower limbs. A pudendal nerve block is the most localized and only blocks the portion of the perineum innervated by the pudendal nerve in the perineum, thus sparing the upper portion of the birth canal and uterus so the mother can still feel uterine contractions.

As the head of the baby passes through the vaginal canal during childbirth, the anus is forced posteriorly toward the sacrum and coccyx, the urethra is forced anteriorly toward the pubic symphysis, and considerable pressure is exerted on the levator ani. Perineal lacerations during childbirth are common, and it may be necessary to surgically widen the vaginal orifice (episiotomy). If the perineal body is lacerated, it must be repaired to prevent weakness of the pelvic floor; otherwise, it could result in prolapse of the urinary bladder, uterus, or rectum.

11. Refer to FIGURE 5.12.
12. Use blunt dissection to clean between the three muscles of the superficial perineal pouch until a small triangular opening is created.
13. Within the triangular opening, identify the **perineal membrane**, the deep boundary of the superficial perineal pouch.
14. On the left side of the cadaver, remove the bulbospongiosus and identify the **bulb of the vestibule**, an elongated mass of erectile tissue lateral to the vaginal orifice.
15. Identify the **greater vestibular gland** in the superficial perineal pouch immediately posterior to the bulb of the vestibule. *Note that in the cadaver, the greater vestibular gland is difficult to find.*
16. Anteriorly, the bulbs of the two sides are joined at the **commissure of the bulbs** which is continuous with the **glans clitoris.** Do not attempt to find the commissure of the bulbs.
17. On the left side of the cadaver, remove the ischiocavernosus overlying the **crus of the clitoris**. Observe that the crus of the clitoris attaches to the ischiopubic ramus and is continuous with the corpus cavernosum clitoris.

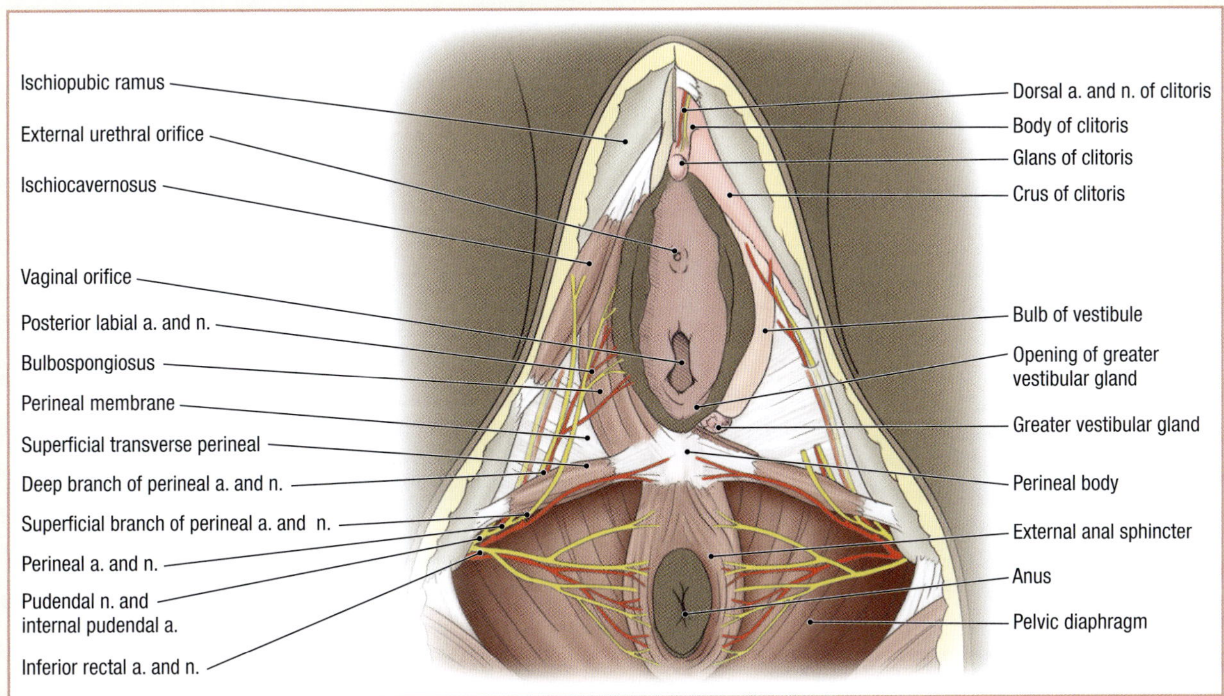

FIGURE 5.12 ● Contents of female superficial perineal pouch in superficial (*right*) and deep (*left*) dissections. Inferior view.

Clitoris

ATLAS 5.52, 5.53; VIDEO 5.8.4

1. Refer to FIGURE 5.13A.
2. Follow the crura of the clitoris anteriorly and identify the **body of the clitoris** and the **glans of the clitoris**, the most distal aspect of the erectile tissue.
3. On the dorsal aspect of the clitoris, remove the overlying connective tissue and identify the **dorsal vein of the clitoris** in the midline.
4. To either side of the dorsal vein, identify the smaller **dorsal artery of the clitoris.**
5. Continue dissecting lateral to the dorsal artery and identify the **dorsal nerve of the clitoris.** *Note that despite the comparatively smaller mass of the clitoris, the dorsal nerve is approximately the same size with as many nerve endings as the homologous dorsal nerve of the penis in the male.*
6. Make a transverse cut through the body of the clitoris just proximal to the glans of the clitoris (**Cut 1**).
7. Refer to FIGURE 5.13B.
8. Study the erectile bodies of the clitoris and observe that the corpora cavernosa are oval shaped and surrounded by the **tunica albuginea**, a layer of connective tissue, which fuse to form a midline septum.
9. Within the erectile tissue of a cut corpora cavernosa, make an effort to identify the **deep artery of the clitoris** near the midline septum on each side.

Female Deep Perineal Pouch

ATLAS 5.52A, 5.53A

Dissection Note: The deep perineal pouch lies superior (deep) to the perineal membrane and will be minimally dissected as few of the structures are easily identifiable.

1. Refer to FIGURE 5.13A to study the **contents of the deep perineal pouch in the female.**
2. Identify the **urethra** in the midsagittal plane and observe that it pierces the **perineal membrane.** The female urethra extends from the internal urethral orifice in the urinary bladder to the external urethral orifice in the vestibule of the vagina (about 4 cm).
3. Observe that the **external urethral sphincter (sphincter urethrae)** surrounds the membranous urethra. The external urethral sphincter is voluntary and when contracted compresses the membranous urethra and stops the flow of urine.
4. Posterior to the opening of the **urethra**, identify the **vaginal opening.**
5. Identify the **smooth muscle** along the posterior margin of the deep perineal pouch. Collectively, the muscles within the deep perineal pouch plus the perineal membrane are known as the **urogenital diaphragm.** *Note that the fiber direction and function of the smooth muscle align with those of the superficial transverse perineal in the superficial perineal pouch.*
6. Review the attachments and actions of the **external urethral sphincter** (see **TABLE 5.1**).
7. Coursing anterior along the lateral margin of the deep perineal pouch, identify the **branches of the internal pudendal artery and vein** (most notably, the **dorsal artery of the clitoris**) and the **branches of the pudendal nerve** (most notably, the **dorsal nerve of the clitoris**), which supply the external urethral sphincter, smooth muscle of the region, and clitoris.

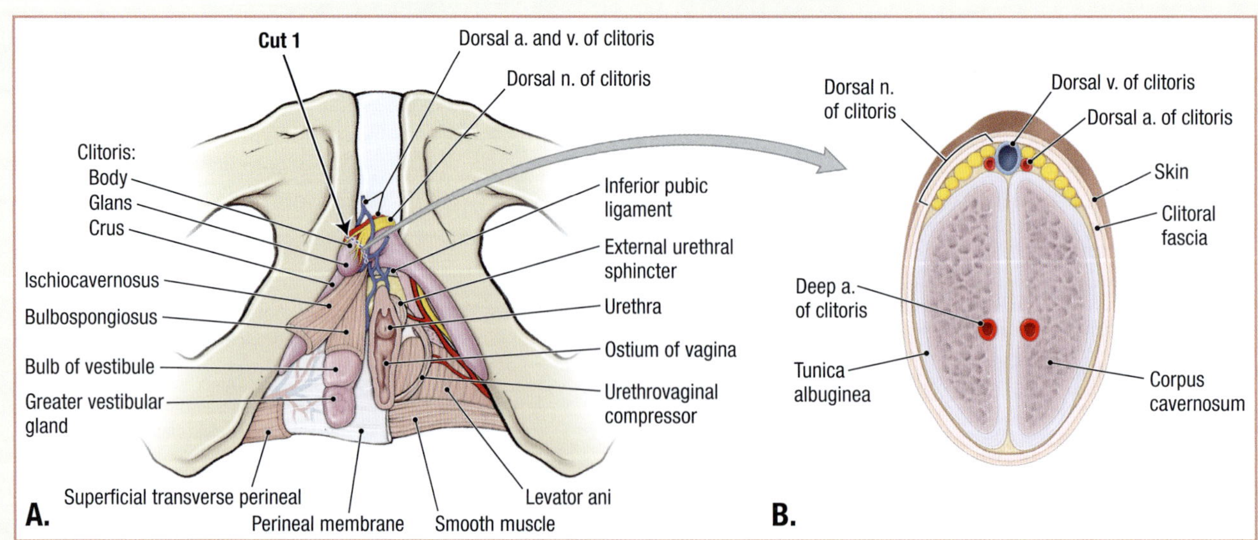

FIGURE 5.13 ■ **A.** Contents of female deep perineal pouch (*left*). Inferior view. **B.** Transverse section of clitoris.

Dissection Follow-up

1. Review the muscles of the female superficial perineal pouch in **TABLE 5.1**.
2. Replace the muscles of the urogenital triangle in their correct anatomical positions.
3. Review the contents of the female superficial perineal pouch. Visit a dissection table with a male cadaver and view the contents of the superficial perineal pouch.
4. Review the course of the internal pudendal artery from its origin in the pelvis.
5. Review the course and branches of the pudendal nerve.
6. Review the path of the female urethra and note its course from the urinary bladder to the perineum as compared to the male urethra.
7. Return the reflected portions of tissue back to anatomical position.

TABLE 5.1 Female Superficial and Deep Perineal Pouches

SUPERFICIAL GROUP OF MUSCLES				
Muscle	*Anterior Attachments*	*Posterior Attachments*	*Actions*	*Innervation*
Bulbospongiosus	Corpus cavernosum clitoris	Perineal body	Compresses the bulb of the clitoris	Deep branch of the perineal n. (branch of pudendal n.)
Ischiocavernosus	Crus of the clitoris	Ischial tuberosity and ischiopubic ramus	Forces blood from the crus of the clitoris into the distal part of the corpus cavernosum clitoris	
Superficial transverse perineal	Perineal body (medial attachment)	Ischial tuberosity (lateral attachment)	Provides support to the perineal body	Perineal n. (branch of pudendal n.)
DEEP GROUP OF MUSCLES				
Muscle	*Anterior Attachments*	*Posterior Attachments*	*Actions*	*Innervation*
Deep transverse perineal	Perineal body (medial attachment)	Ischial tuberosity (lateral attachment)	Provides support to the perineal body	Perineal n. (branch of pudendal n.)
External urethral sphincter	Attaches to itself around the urethra		Compresses the membranous urethra and stops the flow of urine	Deep branch of the perineal n. (branch of pudendal n.)

Abbreviation: n., nerve.

FEMALE PELVIC CAVITY

Dissection Overview

The female pelvic cavity contains the urinary bladder, female internal genitalia, and rectum. The term *adnexa* refers to the ovaries, uterine tubes, and ligaments of the uterus. If the uterus or adnexa have been surgically removed (hysterectomy) or are otherwise not present in your cadaver, examine these structures in other cadavers.

The order of dissection will be as follows: The peritoneum will be studied in the female pelvic cavity. The pelvis will be sectioned in the midline, and the cut surface of the sectioned pelvis will be studied. The uterus and vagina will be studied. The uterine tube will be traced from the uterus to the ovary. The ovary will be studied.

Dissection Instructions

Female Pelvic Peritoneum

ATLAS 5.14, 5.21D; VIDEO 5.9.1

1. Refer to FIGURE 5.14.
2. Identify the peritoneum on the posterior aspect of the anterior abdominal wall superior to the pubis (**1**).
3. Observe that the peritoneum reflects from the anterior abdominal wall inferiorly across the apex of the urinary bladder (**2**).
4. Observe that the peritoneum courses along the superior surface of the urinary bladder (**3**) but not its posterior surface.
5. Identify the **paravesical fossa** (paired), the shallow depressions in the peritoneal cavity on the lateral sides of the urinary bladder.

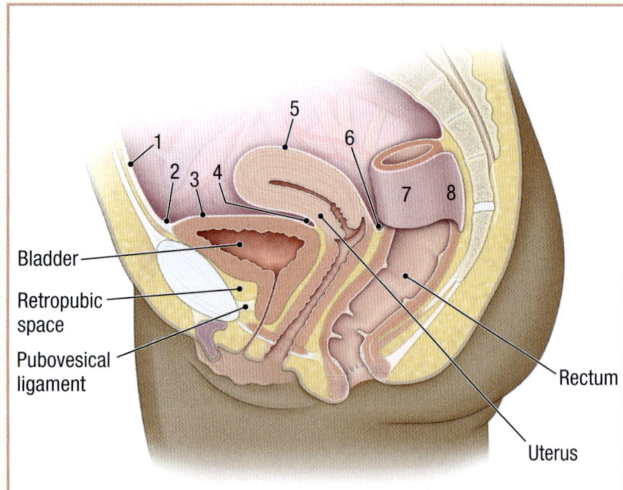

FIGURE 5.14 ● Female pelvic peritoneum. Midsagittal view.

6. Follow the lining of the peritoneum posteriorly and observe that it passes from the superior surface of the urinary bladder to the uterus to form the **vesicouterine pouch** (**4**).
7. Observe that the peritoneum in the female additionally covers the fundus and body of the uterus (**5**) and contacts the wall of the posterior part of the vaginal fornix (see **Clinical Correlation 5.4**).

CLINICAL CORRELATION 5.4

Uterine Orientation and Life Changes

ATLAS 5.21, 5.22, 5.27A, 5.27B

The adult uterus is typically anteverted (tilted anteriorly) and anteflexed (bent anteriorly) over the surface of the urinary bladder. The orientation and position of the uterus allows for expansion into the abdominal cavity during pregnancy, although simultaneously, it compresses the urinary bladder preventing filling, thus increasing the need and frequency of urination.

The uterus grows throughout childhood and adolescence and will gain a thicker muscular wall following single or multiple pregnancies. Following parturition, the uterus will regress to a smaller size and substantially decrease in volume and thickness following menopause.

8. Observe that the peritoneum covers a depression between the uterus and the rectum, the **rectouterine pouch** (the pouch of Douglas) (**6**), the lowest point in the female abdominopelvic cavity.
9. Follow the peritoneum superiorly along the posterior aspect of the pelvic cavity on the anterior surface of the rectum (**7**) and observe that it is continuous with the sigmoid mesocolon at the level of the third sacral vertebra.
10. Identify the **pararectal fossa** (paired), the shallow depressions in the peritoneal cavity on the lateral sides of the rectum (**8**).

Broad Ligament

ATLAS 5.21D, 5.24, 5.35; VIDEO 5.9.2

1. Refer to FIGURE 5.15.
2. Identify the **broad ligament of the uterus**, layers of peritoneum extending bilaterally from the sides of the uterus to the pelvic wall. *Note that the connective tissue enclosed between the two layers of the broad ligament is called **parametrium**.*
3. Observe that the **uterine tube** is contained within the **mesosalpinx**, the superior margin of the broad ligament.
4. Identify the **mesovarium**, the portion of the broad ligament suspending the ovaries, and the **mesometrium**, the portion of the broad ligament adjacent to the body of the uterus.
5. Identify the **round ligament of the uterus** (paired), visible through the anterior layer of the broad ligament.
6. Observe that the round ligament of the uterus passes over the pelvic brim and exits the abdominal cavity by passing through the deep inguinal ring lateral to the inferior epigastric vessels. *Note that the round ligament of the uterus passes through the inguinal canal to end in the labium majus.*
7. Identify the **ovarian ligament** (paired), a fibrous cord within the broad ligament connecting the ovary to the uterus.
8. Identify the **suspensory ligament of the ovary** (paired), a peritoneal fold covering the ovarian vessels between the posterior abdominal wall and true pelvis.
9. Observe that the **endopelvic fascia (extraperitoneal fascia)** includes distinct condensations of tissue to support the uterus: the **uterosacral (sacrogenital) ligament** (paired), extending from the cervix to the sacrum underlying the **uterosacral fold**; the **transverse cervical ligament (cardinal ligament)** (paired), extending from the cervix to the pelvic wall; and the **pubocervical (pubovesical)** (paired) ligament, extending from the pubis to the cervix.

Sectioning of Female Pelvis

ATLAS 5.14; VIDEO 5.9.3

Dissection Note: The pelvis will be divided in the midline up to vertebral level L3 with a saw. Subsequently, the left side of the body will be transected at vertebral level L3, enabling removal of the left lower limb and left hemi pelvis. The right lower limb and right side of the pelvis will remain attached to the trunk.

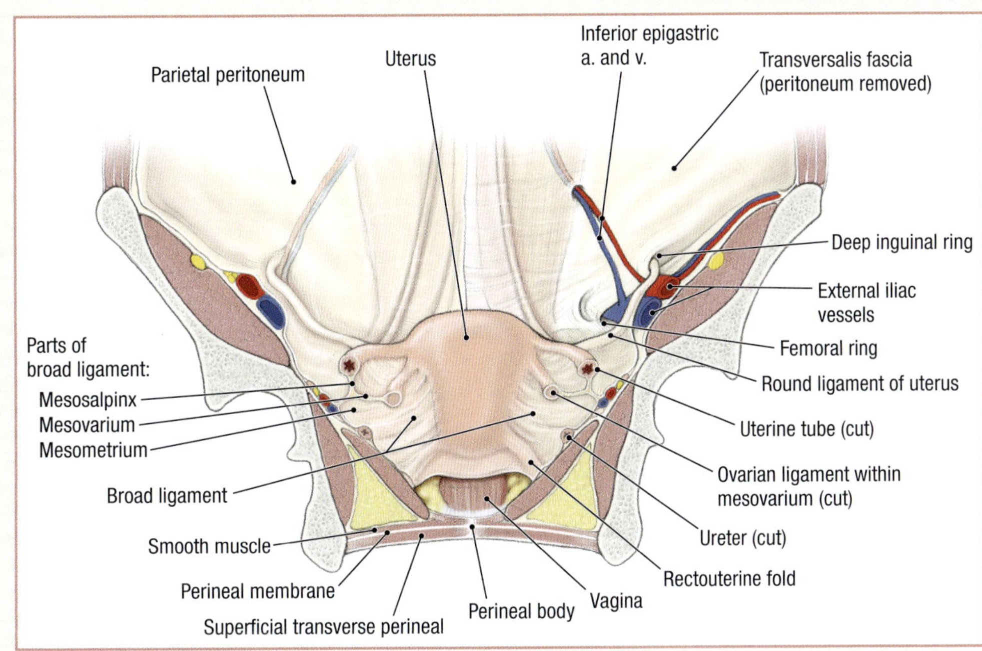

FIGURE 5.15 ● Uterus, broad ligament, and female internal genitalia with removed peritoneum (*right*). Posterior view.

1. Refer to FIGURE 5.16A.
2. In the female pelvic cavity, make a midline cut beginning posterior to the pubic symphysis through the superior surface of the urinary bladder (**Cut 1**). Spread open the bladder and sponge the interior if necessary.
3. If present, position the uterus in the midline and use a scalpel to divide the uterus in *its* median plane, which may or may not align with the midline of the pelvis (**Cut 2**).
4. Extend the cut through the midline of the cervix into the vaginal canal inferiorly.
5. Extend the midline cut in the posterior direction, cutting through the anterior and posterior walls of the rectum and distal part of the sigmoid colon (**Cut 3**).
6. Clean the internal aspect of the rectum and anal canal. *Use caution when cleaning and moving fecal matter. Refer to your instructor for proper safety techniques.*
7. Use a scalpel to cut the left common iliac vein, left common iliac artery, left ovarian vessels, and left ureter about 1 cm distal to their respective points of origin (**Cuts 4**).
8. Cut through the left lumbar arteries at vertebral levels L4 and L5 and reflect the abdominal aorta to the right side of the abdominal cavity.
9. Use a scalpel to make an incision from the midaxillary line to the vertebral column through the muscles of the lateral abdominal wall about 2 cm superior to the iliac crest (**Cut 5**).
10. Cut through the nerves of the left lumbar plexus where they cross the horizontal incision and any remaining fibers of the left psoas major and quadratus lumborum at vertebral level L3.
11. Refer to FIGURE 5.16B.
12. Identify the internal urethral orifice in the bladder and insert a probe into it. Using the probe as a guide, cut through the inferior part of the bladder, dividing the urethra.
13. In the perineum, insert the tip of a probe into the external urethral orifice. Use the probe as a guide to make a midline cut through the clitoris, dividing it into right and left sides. Extend this cut posteriorly, dividing the urethra and vagina into right and left sides (**Cut 6**).
14. In the midline, extend the cut to the tip of the coccyx cutting through the perineal membrane, perineal body, and anal canal (**Cut 7**).
15. Refer to FIGURE 5.16C.
16. With the cadaver in the supine position, use a saw to cut through the pubic symphysis in the midline from anterior to posterior, stopping at the inferior border of the pubic symphysis (**Cut 8**).
17. Turn the cadaver 90° to the right, so it is lying on its right side. Prop the cadaver or have your lab partners hold the body so it does not fall or rotate.
18. Have your lab partners abduct the left lower limb to facilitate sectioning of the sacrum.
19. Cut through the sacrum from posterior to anterior (**Cut 9**). Make an effort to not allow the saw to contact the soft tissue structures that were cut with the scalpel. Retract the soft tissue structures out of the path of the blade if necessary.
20. Forcibly spread apart the lower limbs to expand the opening division of the sacrum and extend the midline cut as far superiorly as the body of the third lumbar vertebra.

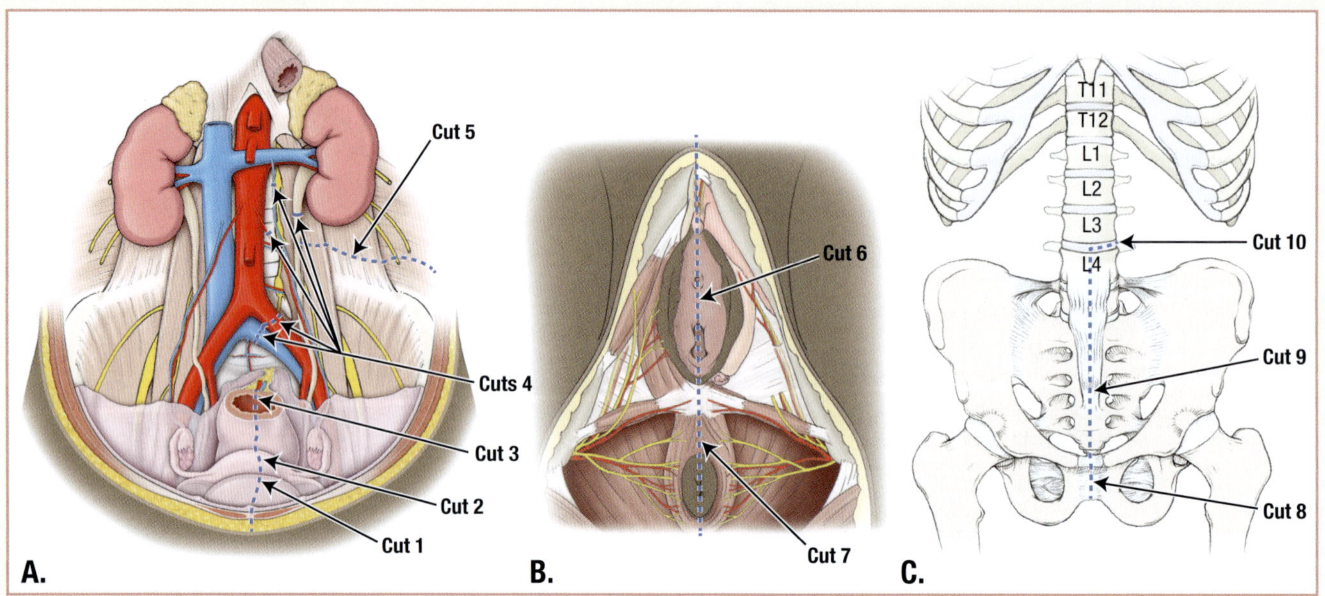

FIGURE 5.16 ■ **A.** Soft tissue cuts for female pelvic bisection. Anterior view. **B.** Perineal cuts for female pelvic bisection. Inferior view. **C.** Skeletal cuts for female pelvic bisection and left lower limb and pelvis detachment. Anterior view.

21. Adduct the left lower limb and use the saw to cut horizontally through the left half of the intervertebral disc between L3 and L4 (**Cut 10**), sparing the inferior aspect of the abdominal aorta.
22. Once the horizontal and vertical cuts are connected, return the cadaver to the supine position.
23. Cut any remaining pieces of tissue preventing the left lower limb from being removed and pull the left lower limb away from the rest of the cadaver.
24. Clean the rectum and anal canal on both sides of the bisected pelvic specimen.

Female Internal Genitalia

ATLAS 5.21A, 5.33A; VIDEO 5.9.4

1. Refer to FIGURE 5.17.
2. Trace the sectioned urethra from the urinary bladder to the **external urethral orifice** and identify the

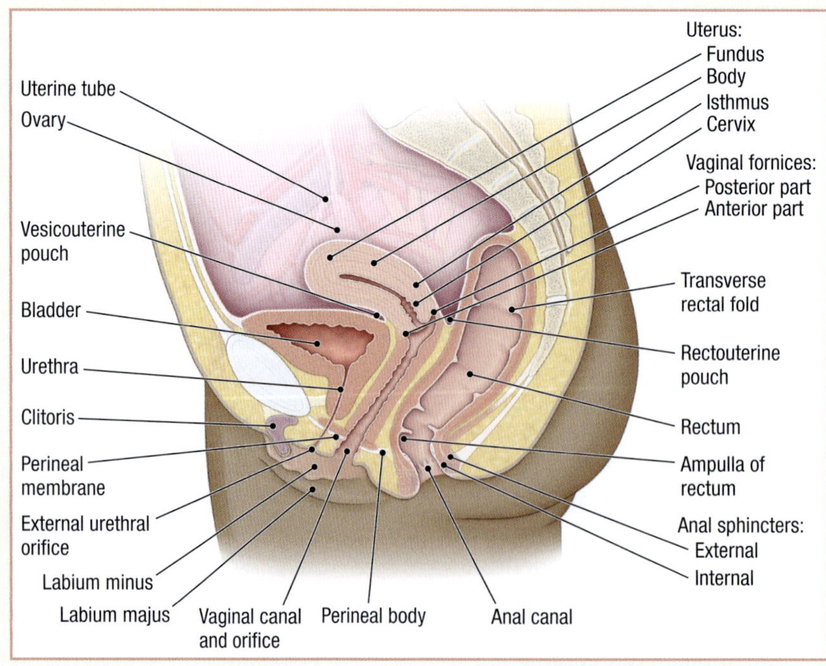

FIGURE 5.17 ■ Midline section of female pelvis. Midsagittal view.

external urethral sphincter. *Note that the external urethral sphincter may be difficult to see.*

3. In the sectioned specimen, identify the **vagina** and observe that the anterior vaginal wall is shorter than the posterior vaginal wall.
4. Within the vaginal canal, identify the **vaginal fornix** surrounding the inferior most aspect of the uterus, the **cervix**. Observe that the vaginal fornix has **anterior**, **posterior**, and **lateral** (paired: right and left) **parts**.
5. Observe that the posterior wall of the vagina (near the posterior part of the vaginal fornix) is in contact with the peritoneum lining the rectouterine pouch.
6. Study the **uterus** and observe that it is tilted approximately 90° anterior to the axis of the vagina (anteverted). *Note that the position of the uterus changes as the bladder fills and during pregnancy.*
7. Identify the **fundus of the uterus**, the rounded portion superior to the attachments of the uterine tubes.
8. Inferior to the fundus, identify the **body of the uterus** with its **vesical surface** facing the vesicouterine pouch and its **intestinal surface** facing the rectouterine pouch. *Note that the broad ligament is attached to the lateral surface of the body of the uterus.*
9. Identify the **isthmus of the uterus**, the narrowed portion of the body superior to the cervix.
10. Refer to FIGURE 5.18.
11. Identify the **uterine cavity** and observe that in a sagittal section, it appears as a slit, whereas in a coronal section, it is triangular in appearance.
12. Observe that the uterine wall contains three distinct layers: the **myometrium**, the thick muscular wall forming the bulk of the wall; the **endometrium**, the innermost aspect of the uterine wall formed by uterine mucosa; and the **perimetrium**, the peritoneal layer covering the external surface of the uterus. *Note that the tissues within the broad ligament are called parametrium.*
13. Identify the **uterine (fallopian) tube**. Use your fingers to follow the uterine tube as it passes laterally within the mesosalpinx beginning at the **isthmus**, the narrow medial one-third of the uterine tube.
14. Continue to palpate laterally along the length of the uterine tube and identify the **ampulla**, the widest and longest part of the uterine tube and most common site of fertilization and ectopic pregnancy.
15. Identify the **infundibulum**, the funnel-like end of the uterine tube, and the **fimbriae**, the fingerlike processes surrounding its distal margin.
16. Identify the **ovary**, the female gonad responsible for production of the oocyte and the reproductive hormones of estrogen and progesterone.
17. Observe that the ovary is ovoid, or almond shaped, with a **tubal (distal) extremity** where the ovarian vessels enter the ovary, and a **uterine (proximal) extremity** attached to the ovarian ligament.
18. Observe that the ovary sits in the **ovarian fossa**, a shallow depression in the lateral pelvic wall bounded by the ureter, external iliac vein, and uterine tube.

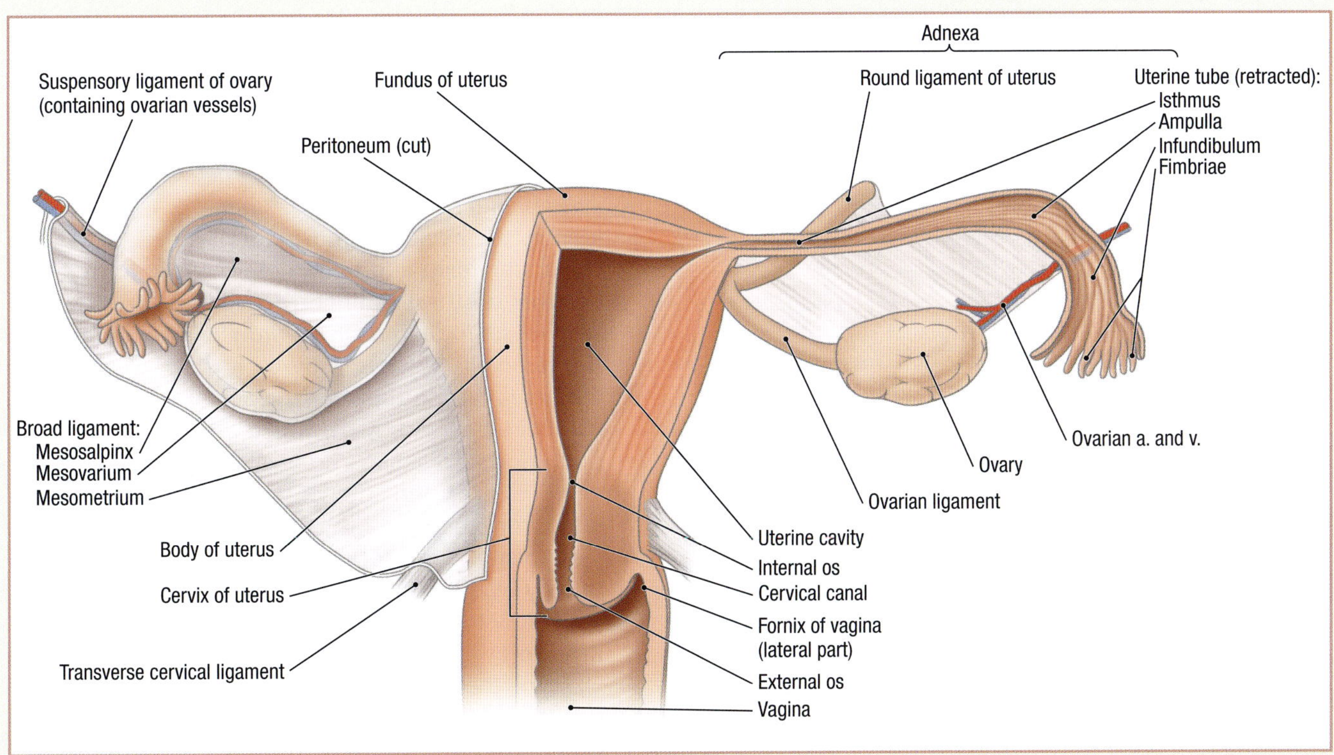

FIGURE 5.18 ● Broad ligament and female internal genitalia. Posterior view.

Dissection Follow-up

1. Review the position of the female pelvic viscera within the pelvic cavity.
2. Visit a dissection table with a male cadaver and observe the position of the male pelvic viscera.
3. Review the peritoneum in the female pelvic cavity. Visit a dissection table with a male cadaver and compare differences in the female and male peritoneum.
4. Trace the round ligament of the uterus from the superficial inguinal ring to the uterus.
5. Compare the pelvic course of the ductus deferens with the pelvic course of the round ligament of the uterus.
6. Review the parts of the broad ligament and review the function of the endopelvic fascia in passive support of the uterus.
7. Review the abdominal origin and course of the ovarian vessels through the suspensory ligament of the ovary.
8. Return the reflected tissue back to anatomical position.

FEMALE URINARY BLADDER, RECTUM, AND ANAL CANAL

Dissection Overview

The urinary bladder is a reservoir for urine which when empty is located within the pelvic cavity and when filled extends into the abdominal cavity. The urinary bladder is a retroperitoneal organ surrounded by endopelvic fascia. Between the pubic symphysis and the urinary bladder, there is a potential space called the retropubic space (prevesical space). The retropubic space is filled with fat and loose connective tissue to accommodate expansion of the urinary bladder. The pubovesical ligament is a condensation of fascia that ties the neck of the urinary bladder to the pubis defining the inferior limit of the retropubic space. The lower two-thirds of the rectum is surrounded by endopelvic fascia. The upper one-third of the rectum is partially covered by peritoneum.

The order of dissection will be as follows: The parts of the urinary bladder will be studied. The interior of the urinary bladder will be studied. The interior of the rectum and anal canal will be studied.

Dissection Instructions

Female Urinary Bladder

ATLAS 5.21A, 5.22A, 5.56A, 5.56B; VIDEO 5.10.1

1. Refer to FIGURE 5.19.
2. Identify the **apex of the urinary bladder**, the pointed part directed toward the anterior abdominal wall attaching to the urachus.

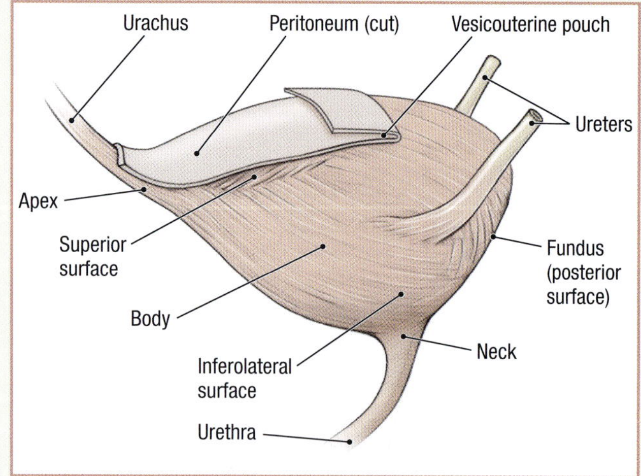

FIGURE 5.19 ● Parts of female urinary bladder. Lateral view.

3. Observe that the **body of the urinary bladder** is located between the apex and the **fundus (base) of the urinary bladder**, the inferior part of the posterior wall.
4. Observe the proximity of the fundus of the bladder to the vagina and uterus. *Note that in the male, the fundus is related to the ductus deferens, seminal vesicles, and rectum.*
5. Identify the **neck of the urinary bladder**, where the urethra exits and the wall thickens to form the **internal urethral sphincter**. *Note that the internal urethral sphincter is an involuntary muscle controlled by the autonomic nervous system.*
6. Observe that the **superior surface** of the urinary bladder is covered by peritoneum, whereas the **posterior surface** lies immediately adjacent to the anterior cervix and anterior wall of the vagina, separated from them by a thin layer of endopelvic fascia.
7. Verify that the **inferolateral** (paired) **surface** of the urinary bladder is covered by endopelvic fascia and lies below the reflection point of the peritoneum.
8. Refer to FIGURE 5.20.
9. Examine the wall of the urinary bladder noting its thickness and observe that it consists of bundles of smooth muscle called **detrusor**. *Note that the mucous membrane lining most of the inner surface of*

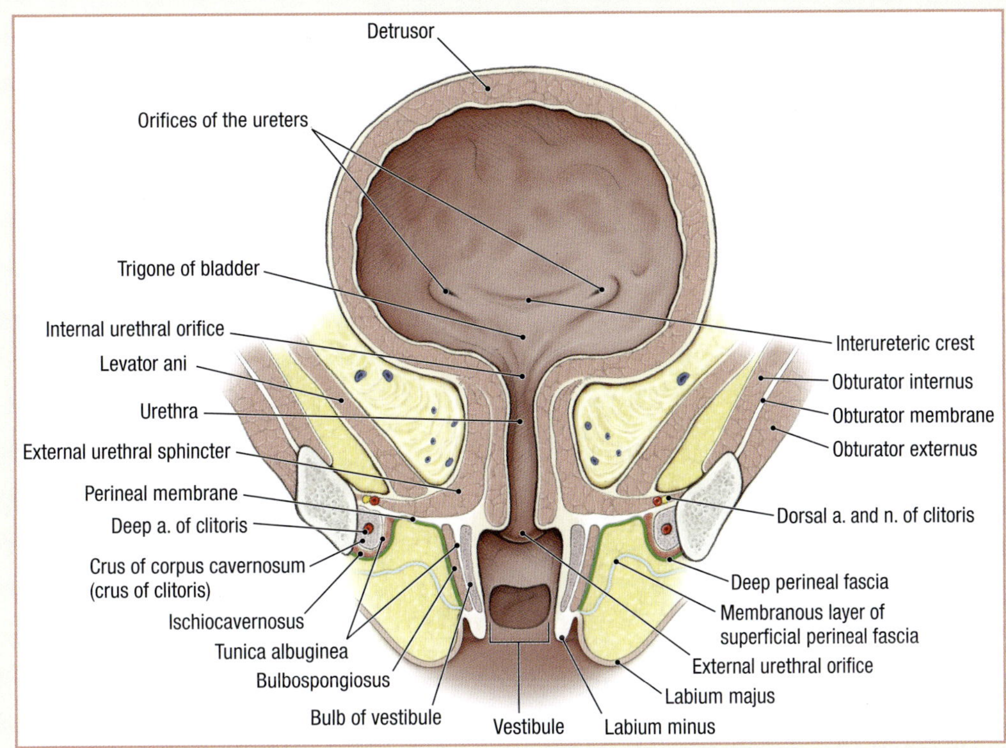

FIGURE 5.20 ● Coronal section of female urinary bladder and vestibule. Anterior view.

the urinary bladder lies in folds when the bladder is empty but flatten to accommodate expansion when the bladder is full.

10. Study the inner surface of the fundus and identify the **trigone of the urinary bladder (urinary trigone)**, a smooth, triangular region of mucous membrane defined by lines between the **internal urethral orifice** and the two **ureteric orifices**. *Note that the urinary trigone has now been bisected.*
11. Observe that the **internal urethral orifice** is located at the most inferior point in the urinary bladder at the inferior aspect of the trigone.
12. Identify the **interureteric crest**, a visible ridge extending between the orifices of the ureters.
13. Insert the tip of a probe into the orifice of the ureter to confirm that the ureter passes through the muscular wall of the urinary bladder in an oblique direction. *Note that when the urinary bladder is full (distended), the pressure of the accumulated urine flattens the part of the ureter within the wall of the bladder, thus preventing reflux of urine back into the ureter.*
14. Locate the point where the ureter crosses the external iliac artery or the bifurcation of the common iliac artery.
15. Use blunt dissection to follow the ureter to the fundus of the urinary bladder, observing that it crosses inferior to the **uterine artery** and superior to the **vaginal artery** along its course.

Female Rectum and Anal Canal

ATLAS 5.14, 5.16C, 5.16D, 5.17; VIDEO 5.10.2

1. Refer to FIGURE 5.21.
2. Identify the **rectum** at its point of origin at the level of the third sacral vertebra and observe that it follows the curvature of the sacrum and coccyx.
3. Identify the **ampulla of the rectum**, the dilated portion of the rectum proximal to the point where the rectum bends approximately 80° posteriorly at the **anorectal flexure**.
4. Examine the inner surface of the rectum and observe that the mucous membrane is smooth except for the presence of **transverse rectal folds**, one on the right and two on the left. *Note that the transverse rectal folds may be difficult to identify in some cadavers.*
5. Identify the **anal canal** inferior to the anorectal flexure and observe it is only 2.5 to 3.5 cm in length and passes out of the pelvic cavity into the anal triangle of the perineum.
6. Examine the inner surface of the anal canal proximally and identify the **anal columns**, 5 to 10 longitudinal ridges of mucosa containing branches of the **superior rectal artery** and **vein** (see **Clinical Correlation 5.5**). *Note that the mucosal features of the anal canal may be difficult to identify.*

CLINICAL CORRELATION 5.5

Hemorrhoids

ATLAS 5.16D, 5.18D

Hemorrhoids, or piles, are dilations of the veins around the anal canal and commonly occur in adults with or without underlying pathology. Hemorrhoids can result from conditions that increase intraabdominal pressure (such as obesity and pregnancy), or portal hypertension, which may be a consequence of cirrhosis of the liver. Increases in blood pressure and engorgement of the veins contained in the anal columns result in internal hemorrhoids. Internal hemorrhoids are covered by mucous membrane and are relatively insensitive to painful stimuli because the mucous membrane is innervated by autonomic nerves. External hemorrhoids are enlargements of the tributaries of the inferior rectal veins, are covered by skin, and are very sensitive to painful stimuli because they are innervated by somatic nerves (inferior rectal nerves).

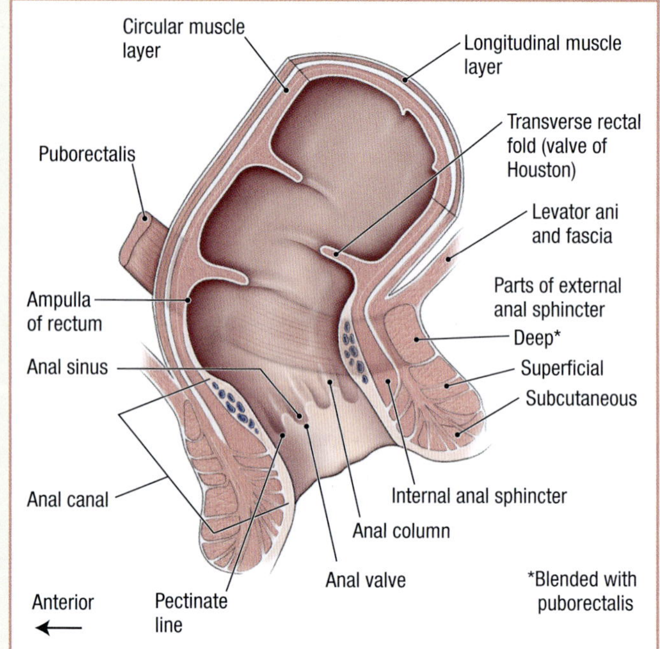

FIGURE 5.21 • Distal rectum, anal sphincters, and anal canal. Midsagittal view.

7. Identify the semilunar folds of mucosa forming the **anal valves**, which unite the distal ends of the anal columns. Between the anal valve and the wall of the anal canal is a small pocket called an **anal sinus**.
8. Identify the **pectinate line**, the irregular line formed by the contour of the collective anal valves.
9. Identify the **external anal sphincter** in the sectioned specimen surrounding the anal canal. *Note that the external anal sphincter is composed of skeletal muscle and is under voluntary control.*
10. Identify the **internal anal sphincter** in the sectioned specimen surrounding the anal canal. *Note that the internal anal sphincter is composed of smooth muscle and is under involuntary control.*
11. Observe that the longitudinal muscle of the anal canal separates the two sphincter muscles. If you have difficulty identifying the anal sphincters, use a scalpel to cut another section through the wall of the anal canal to improve the clarity of the dissection.

Dissection Follow-up

1. Use the dissected specimen to review the features of the urinary bladder, rectum, and anal canal.
2. Review the relationships of the uterus, vagina, and ureters to the rectum and fundus of the urinary bladder.
3. Visit a dissection table with a male cadaver and review the relationships of the seminal vesicles, ampulla of the ductus deferens, and ureters to the rectum and fundus of the urinary bladder.
4. Review the pelvic course of the ureter and function of the urinary bladder.
5. Review the female urethra. Visit a table with a male cadaver and review the parts of the male urethra.
6. Compare muscle type and innervation of the external and internal anal sphincters.
7. Return all reflected tissue back to anatomical position.

FEMALE INTERNAL ILIAC ARTERY AND SACRAL PLEXUS

Dissection Overview

Anterior to the sacroiliac articulation, the common iliac artery divides to form the external and internal iliac arteries. The external iliac artery distributes to the lower limb, and the internal iliac artery distributes to the pelvis, gluteal region, and perineum. The internal iliac artery commonly divides into anterior and posterior divisions, although arterial variation frequently occurs. Branches arising from the anterior division are mainly visceral and supply the urinary bladder, internal genitalia, external genitalia, rectum, and gluteal region. Branches arising from the posterior division are parietal and supply the pelvic walls and gluteal region.

The somatic nerve plexuses of the pelvic cavity, sacral and coccygeal, are located between the pelvic viscera and lateral pelvic wall in the endopelvic fascia and formed by contributions from anterior rami of spinal nerves L4–Co1. The primary visceral nerve plexus of the pelvic cavity is the inferior hypogastric plexus (pelvic plexus), formed by contributions from the hypogastric nerves, sacral splanchnic nerves (sympathetic), and pelvic splanchnic nerves (parasympathetic).

The order of dissection will be as follows: The branches of the posterior division of the internal iliac artery will be identified. The branches of the anterior division of the internal iliac artery will be identified. The nerves of the sacral plexus will be dissected. The pelvic portion of the sympathetic trunk will be dissected.

Dissection Instructions

Female Pelvic Blood Vessels

ATLAS 5.17, 5.29; VIDEO 5.11.1

Dissection Note: The internal iliac artery has one of the most variable branching patterns of any artery, and it is worth noting at the outset of this dissection that you must use the target distribution of the branches to identify them, not their pattern of branching or point of origin. The dissection of the pelvic vasculature may be performed on both the right and left sides of the hemisected pelvis; however, it is recommended to focus the dissection on just the right side because a deeper dissection will be performed on the left side with the detached lower limb.

1. Refer to FIGURE 5.22.
2. Identify the **internal iliac vein** and observe that its tributaries largely parallel the nearby arteries but are plexiform in nature. To clear the dissection field, remove all tributaries to the internal iliac vein as each correlating artery is identified and cleaned.
3. Identify the locations of the **vesical venous plexus**, **uterine venous plexus**, **vaginal venous plexus**, and **rectal venous plexus**, all of which drain into the internal iliac vein.
4. Identify and clean the **common iliac artery** and follow it distally until it bifurcates into the **external iliac artery** and **internal iliac artery**.
5. Use blunt dissection to follow the internal iliac artery into the pelvis and identify its **anterior** and **posterior divisions**.
6. Begin identification of the branches of the posterior division of the internal iliac artery by finding the most posterior and superior branch, the **iliolumbar artery**.

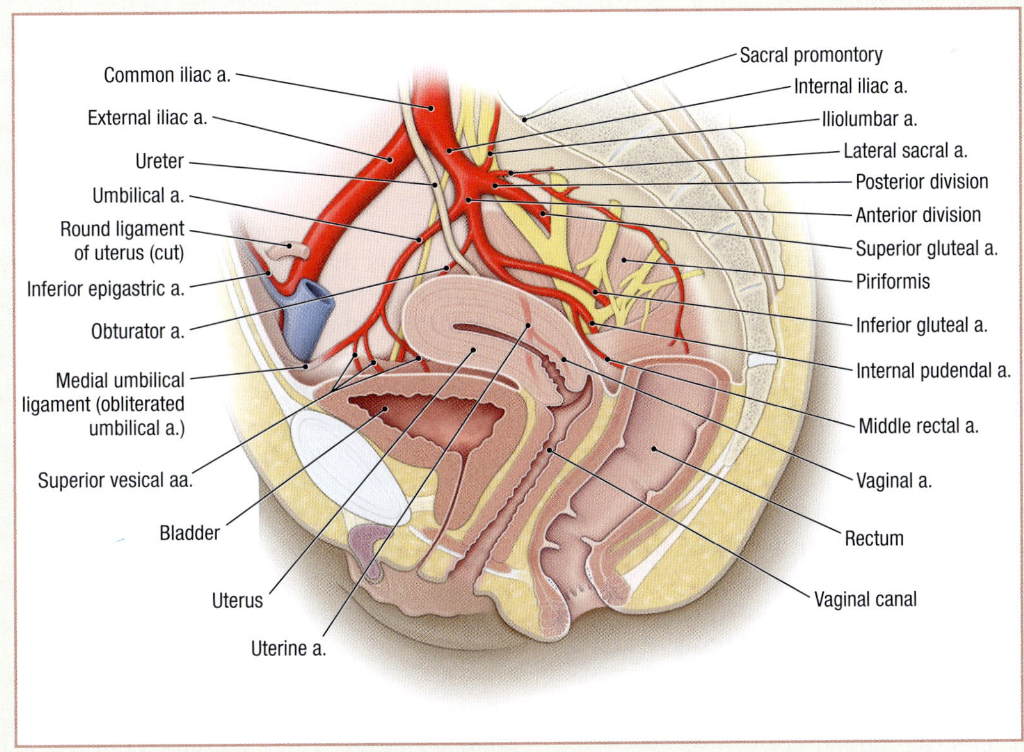

FIGURE 5.22 ■ Branches of female internal iliac artery. Midsagittal view.

7. Observe that the **iliolumbar artery** branches posteriorly from the posterior division and then ascends lateral to the **sacral promontory**, lumbar vertebrae, lumbosacral trunk, and obturator nerve.
8. Identify the **lateral sacral artery**, which frequently gives rise to a superior branch and an inferior branch. Observe that the inferior branch passes anterior to the sacral ventral rami. *Note that the lateral sacral artery may arise from a common trunk with the iliolumbar artery.*
9. Identify the last and typically largest branch of the posterior division, the **superior gluteal artery**, which exits the pelvic cavity through the greater sciatic foramen superior to the piriformis.
10. Identify the branches of the **anterior division of the internal iliac artery** beginning with the **umbilical artery**.
11. In the medial umbilical fold, identify the **medial umbilical ligament** (the remnant of the umbilical artery) and use blunt dissection to trace it posteriorly to the umbilical artery.
12. Identify and clean several **superior vesical arteries** arising from the inferior surface of the umbilical artery which descend to the superolateral part of the urinary bladder.
13. Inferior to the umbilical artery, identify the **obturator artery** passing into the obturator canal with the **obturator nerve**. It may help to find the obturator artery where it enters the obturator canal in the lateral wall of the pelvis and then follow it posteriorly to its origin. *Note that the obturator artery arises from the external iliac or inferior epigastric arteries in about a quarter of individuals as the aberrant obturator artery, which crosses the pelvic brim to enter the obturator canal. The aberrant obturator artery is particularly at risk for injury during surgical repair of a femoral hernia.*
14. Follow the anterior division of the internal iliac artery toward the pelvic floor and identify the **inferior gluteal artery**.
15. Observe that the inferior gluteal artery commonly passes out of the pelvic cavity into the gluteal region through the greater sciatic foramen inferior to the piriformis. *Note that the inferior gluteal artery may share a common trunk with the internal pudendal artery, or less commonly, with the superior gluteal artery.*
16. Identify the **uterine artery** coursing along the inferior attachment of the broad ligament.
17. Use blunt dissection to trace the uterine artery to the lateral aspect of the uterus and observe that it passes superior to the ureter (see **Clinical Correlation 5.6**). Commonly, the uterine artery divides into a large superior branch to the body and fundus of the uterus and a smaller branch to the cervix and vagina.

CLINICAL CORRELATION 5.6

Hysterectomy

ATLAS 5.28, 5.33C, 5.35A

A hysterectomy, surgical removal of the uterus, may be performed in cases of uterine disease such as uterine fibroids, endometrioses, uterine prolapse, or uterine or cervical cancer, although incidence rates for non-cancerous reasons has declined. Hysterectomies may be performed trans-abdominally, or trans-vaginally, in open, laparoscopic, or robotic-assisted approach. Depending on the severity of the pathology, a portion of the uterus (subtotal), the entire uterus (total), or the uterus and ovaries (radical) may be removed. Ligation of the uterine artery will occur distal to the origin of the vaginal branches to facilitate healing.

The proximity of the ureter to the uterine artery near the lateral fornix of the vagina is of clinical importance during a hysterectomy when the uterine artery is tied off and cut. The ureter may be unintentionally clamped, tied off, and cut where it crosses the uterine artery, resulting in serious consequences for the corresponding kidney. To recall this relationship, use the mnemonic device "water under the bridge." The "water" is the urine within the ureter, and the "bridge" is the uterine artery.

18. Observe the close relationship of the lateral part of the vaginal fornix to the uterine artery. *Note that in a living person, pulsations of the uterine artery may be palpated through the lateral part of the vaginal fornix.*
19. Identify the **vaginal artery** and observe that it passes across the floor of the pelvis inferior to the ureter to supply the vagina and urinary bladder. *Note that the male cadaver does not have a vaginal or uterine artery but rather an inferior vesical artery.*
20. Identify the ureter and observe that it passes between the vaginal artery and the uterine artery.
21. Identify the **internal pudendal artery** anterior to the inferior gluteal artery. Observe that the internal pudendal artery exits the pelvic cavity through the greater sciatic foramen medial to the inferior gluteal artery as it will enter the lesser sciatic foramen to reach the perineum. *Note that the internal pudendal artery often arises from a common trunk with the inferior gluteal artery.*

Female Pelvic Nerves

ATLAS 5.13, 5.29A, 5.31; VIDEO 5.11.2

Dissection Note: The dissection of the pelvic nerves may be performed on both the right and left sides of the hemisected pelvis; however, it is recommended to focus the dissection on just the right side because a deeper

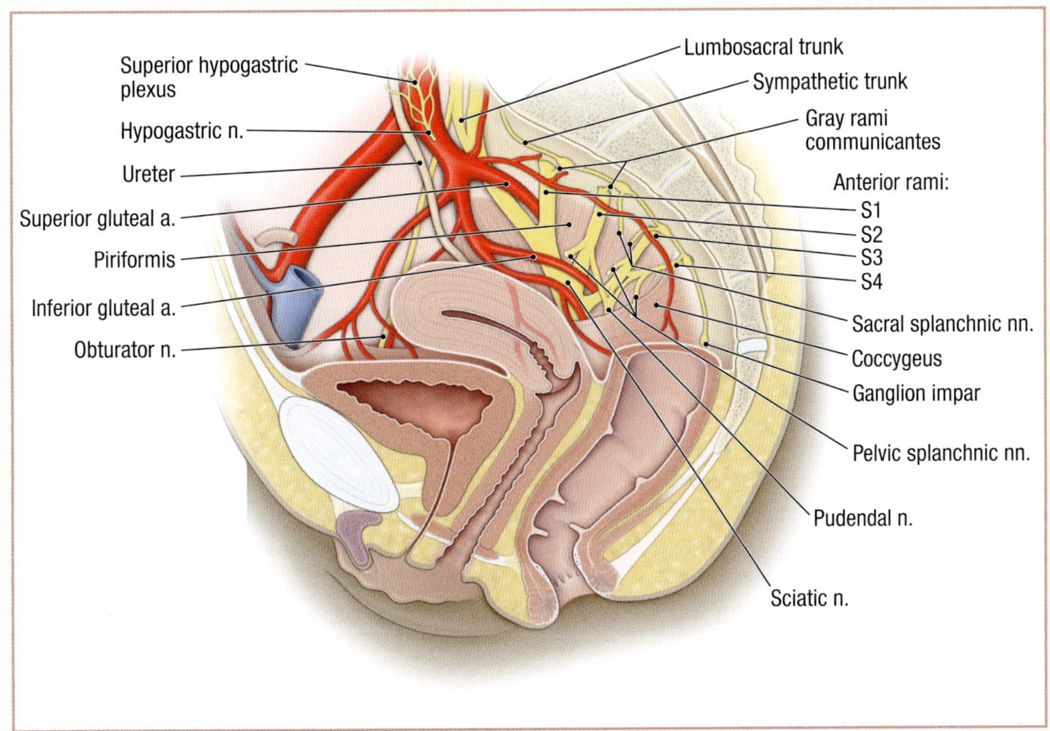

FIGURE 5.23 ● Sacral and autonomic nerve plexuses in female pelvis. Midsagittal view.

dissection will be performed on the left side with the detached lower limb.

1. Refer to FIGURE 5.23.
2. Use blunt dissection to free the rectum from the anterior surface of the sacrum and coccyx.
3. Retract the rectum medially and identify the **sacral plexus** of nerves on the anterior surface of the piriformis.
4. Just lateral to the sacral promontory, identify and clean the **lumbosacral trunk** (anterior rami of L4 and L5) and verify that it joins the sacral plexus.
5. Inferior to the lumbosacral trunk, identify the anterior rami of S2 and S3 which emerge between the proximal attachments of the piriformis.
6. Identify the **sciatic nerve** and observe that it is formed by the anterior rami of spinal nerves L4–S3. The sciatic nerve exits the pelvis by passing through the greater sciatic foramen to enter the gluteal region inferior to the piriformis, although variations are common.
7. Observe that the **superior gluteal artery** usually passes between the **lumbosacral trunk** and the **anterior ramus of spinal nerve S1** and exits the pelvis through the greater sciatic foramen superior to the piriformis.
8. Observe that the **inferior gluteal artery** usually passes between the anterior rami of spinal nerves S2 and S3, but may pass between the anterior rami of spinal nerves S1 and S2, to exit the pelvis through the greater sciatic foramen inferior to the piriformis.
9. Identify the **pudendal nerve** and observe that it is formed by contributions from the anterior rami of spinal nerves S2, S3, and S4. *Note that the pudendal nerve exits the pelvis through the greater sciatic foramen inferior to the piriformis where it then enters the perineum by passing through the lesser sciatic foramen.*
10. Identify the **pelvic splanchnic nerves (nervi erigentes)**. Observe that pelvic splanchnic nerves are branches of the anterior rami of spinal nerves S2, S3, and S4. *Note that pelvic splanchnic nerves carry presynaptic parasympathetic axons for innervation of pelvic organs and the embryonic hindgut.*
11. Identify the **sacral portion of the sympathetic trunk** on the anterior surface of the sacrum medial to the ventral sacral foramina. Observe that the sympathetic trunk continues from the abdominal region into the pelvis and that the two sides join in the midline near the level of the coccyx to form the **ganglion impar**.
12. Identify the **gray rami communicantes**, which connect the sympathetic ganglia to the sacral anterior rami. *Note that each gray ramus communicans carries postsynaptic sympathetic fibers to an anterior ramus for distribution to the lower extremity and perineum.*
13. Identify the **sacral splanchnic nerves** arising from two or three of the sacral sympathetic ganglia and observe that they pass directly to the **inferior hypogastric plexus**. *Note that sacral splanchnic nerves carry sympathetic fibers that distribute to the pelvic viscera.*
14. On the right side of the pelvic cavity, follow the inferior hypogastric plexus superiorly toward the condensation of the plexus into the **right hypogastric nerve**. Use an illustration to identify the **superior hypogastric plexus** and review the origins of the autonomics in both the superior and inferior hypogastric plexuses.

Dissection Follow-up

1. Review the location of the terminal branches of the abdominal aorta.
2. Use the dissected specimen to review the branches of the internal iliac artery and the region supplied by each.
3. Review the relationship of the uterine and vaginal arteries to the ureter.
4. Review the branches of the sacral plexus.
5. Review the course of the pudendal nerve from the pelvic cavity to the urogenital triangle.
6. Return the reflected tissue back to anatomical position.

FEMALE PELVIC DIAPHRAGM

Dissection Overview

The pelvic diaphragm is the muscular floor of the pelvic cavity formed by the levator ani and coccygeus as well as their surrounding fasciae. The pelvic diaphragm extends from the pubic symphysis anteriorly to the coccyx posteriorly. Laterally, the pelvic diaphragm is attached to the fascia covering the obturator internus. Openings in the midline of the pelvic diaphragm, the urogenital hiatus and anal hiatus, allow passage of the urethra, vagina, and anal canal.

The order of dissection will be as follows: The pelvic viscera will be retracted medially. The obturator internus, tendinous arch of the levator ani, and levator ani will be identified. The urethra, vaginal canal, and anal canal will be cut, and the pelvic viscera reflected.

Dissection Instructions

Female Pelvic Diaphragm

ATLAS 5.9, 5.11, 5.12; VIDEO 5.12.1

Dissection Note: Perform the following dissection sequence on only one side of the cadaver. If the left lower limb was removed during the bisection of the pelvis, it is recommended that the deep dissection be performed on the left side to preserve the continuity of the vasculature into the abdominal cavity on the right side.

1. Refer to FIGURE 5.24A.
2. Retract the rectum, vagina, uterus, and urinary bladder medially and identify the **pelvic diaphragm**.
3. Use blunt dissection to remove any remaining fat and connective tissue from the superior surface of the pelvic diaphragm.
4. Locate the **obturator canal** piercing the obturator internus by identifying and following the obturator artery and nerve.
5. Palpate the medial surface of the ischial spine through the levator ani and identify the **tendinous arch of the levator ani**. Observe that the tendinous arch lies just inferior to a line connecting the ischial spine and the obturator canal. *Note that the tendinous arch is a thickening in the obturator fascia and the origin of part of the levator ani.*

Dissection Note: Identify the three components of the **levator ani** by their anterolateral attachments. Learn, but do not dissect, their posterior attachments.

6. Refer to FIGURE 5.24B.
7. Identify the **puborectalis** (paired) attaching anteriorly to the body of the pubis and posteriorly to the puborectalis of the opposite side (in a midline raphe). The puborectalis form the margin of the urogenital hiatus and a "puborectal sling," which maintains the **anorectal flexure** of the rectum. *Note that during defecation, the puborectalis relaxes, the anorectal flexure straightens, and the elimination of fecal matter is facilitated.*
8. Identify the **pubococcygeus** (paired) attaching from the body of the pubis anteriorly to the coccyx and **anococcygeal raphe (ligament)** posteriorly.
9. Identify the **iliococcygeus** (paired) attaching from the tendinous arch anterolaterally to the coccyx and anococcygeal raphe posteriorly. *Note that the levator ani supports the pelvic viscera and resists increases in intraabdominal pressure.*
10. Identify the **coccygeus** (paired) attaching from the ischial spine anteriorly to the lateral border of the coccyx and lowest part of the sacrum posteriorly.
11. Place the fingers of one hand in the ischioanal fossa inferior to the pelvic diaphragm and the fingers of the other hand on the superior surface of the pelvic diaphragm to palpate the thickness of the pelvic diaphragm.
12. Turn the left lower limb and observe that the **obturator internus** forms the lateral wall of the ischioanal fossa and perineum inferior to the pelvic diaphragm, and the lateral wall of the pelvic cavity superior to the pelvic diaphragm.

Dissection Note: The medial attachment of the obturator internus is the margin of the obturator foramen

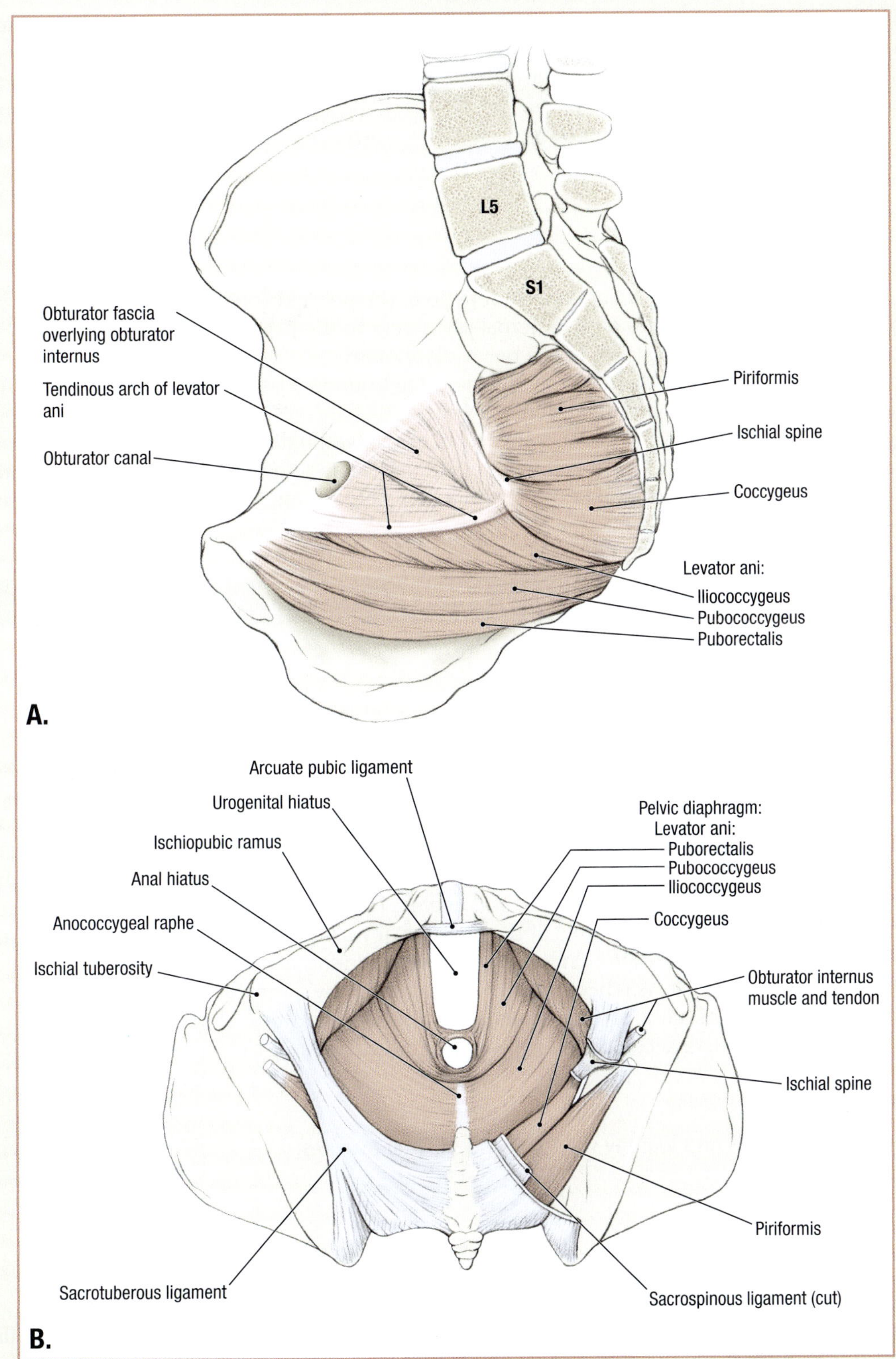

FIGURE 5.24 ● Female pelvic diaphragm. **A.** Midsagittal view. **B.** Inferior view.

and inner surface of the obturator membrane, and its lateral attachment is the greater trochanter of the femur. The obturator internus will be studied further when the gluteal region is dissected.

13. Observe that the urethra and vagina pass through the **urogenital hiatus** of the pelvic diaphragm.
14. Observe that the anal canal passes through the **anal hiatus** of the pelvic diaphragm.

15. If the muscles forming the pelvic diaphragm remain difficult to see, make an incision through the inferior aspect of the urinary bladder, vaginal canal, and anal canal and detach the viscera from the pelvic floor. Leave the viscera attached to the neurovascular structures so the relationships are maintained for later review.
16. Review the general pattern of lymphatic drainage of the pelvis and the location of the **common iliac**, **external iliac**, **internal iliac**, **sacral**, and **lumbar nodes**.

Dissection Follow-up

1. Review the proximal attachment and action of each muscle of the pelvic diaphragm.
2. Review the relationship of the branches of the internal iliac artery to the pelvic diaphragm.
3. Review the relationship of the sacral plexus to the pelvic diaphragm.
4. Review the role played by the pelvic diaphragm in forming the boundary between the pelvic cavity and the perineum and in supporting the pelvic and abdominal viscera.
5. Compare the lymphatic drainage of the perineal structures to the lymphatic drainage of the ovary.
6. Review the formation of the thoracic duct to complete your understanding of the lymph drainage from this region.
7. Visit a dissection table with a male cadaver and perform a complete review of the dissected male pelvis.

SCROTUM, SPERMATIC CORD, AND TESTIS

Dissection Overview

If you dissected a female cadaver, use the remainder of this chapter for review with a male cadaver.

The female and male gonads, ovaries and testes, respectively, develop from common embryonic tissue. While the ovary remains within the pelvis during development, the testis will descend to a location outside the abdominopelvic cavity within the scrotum. In the embryo, the scrotum forms as an outpouching of the anterior abdominal wall during the descent of the testis; therefore, most layers of the abdominal wall are represented in the scrotum. The superficial fascia of the scrotum is represented by dartos fascia containing smooth muscle fibers and no fat.

The spermatic cord contains the structures connecting between the testis and the abdominopelvic cavity: the ductus deferens, testicular vessels, lymphatics, smooth muscle, and nerves. The contents of the spermatic cord are surrounded by three spermatic fascial layers derived from layers of the abdominal wall. Each layer was added to the spermatic cord as the testis and associated structures passed through the inguinal canal during development.

The order of dissection will be as follows: The scrotum will be opened by a vertical cut along its anterior surface. The spermatic cord will be followed from the superficial inguinal ring into the scrotum. The testis will be removed from the scrotum. The spermatic cord will be dissected. The testis will be studied.

Skeletal Anatomy

Refer to an articulated bony pelvis and identify the following skeletal features.

Male Bony Pelvis

ATLAS 5.3A, 5.6, 5.8

1. Refer to FIGURE 5.25.
2. Identify the three bones comprising the hip bone: **ilium**, **ischium**, and **pubis**.
3. Orient the bony pelvis in anatomical position (erect posture) and observe that the **anterior superior iliac spine** and anterior aspect of the pubis at the **pubic tubercle** align in a coronal plane.
4. On the anterior surface of the ilium, identify the **iliac fossa**. Observe that the iliac fossae are directed toward one another and form the lateral boundaries of the **false (greater) pelvis**, the portion of the bony pelvis superior to the **pelvic inlet (brim)**.
5. Observe that the pelvic inlet is formed by the **sacral promontory** and **anterior border of the ala (wing) of the sacrum** posteriorly; arcuate line of the ilium laterally; and pecten pubis, pubic crest of the pubic bones, and **pubic symphysis** anteriorly.
6. Observe that in anatomical position, the pelvic inlet forms an angle of approximately 55° from the horizontal plane.
7. Observe that the lesser pelvis is located inferior to the pelvic inlet and surrounded by bone. *Note that the inferior boundary of the lesser pelvis is the pelvic diaphragm.*

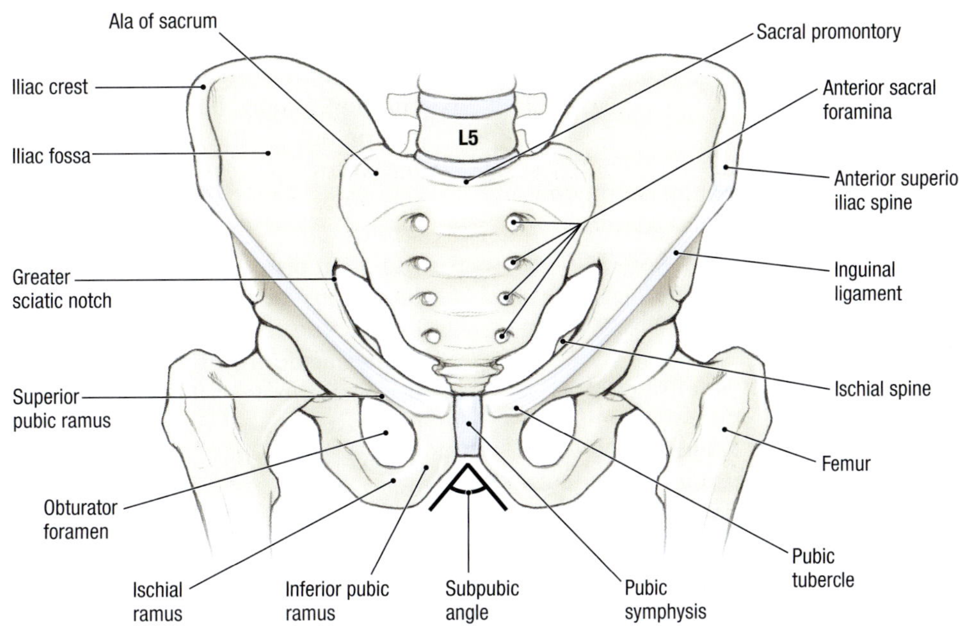

FIGURE 5.25 Male bony pelvis. Anterior view.

8. Identify the **obturator foramen**, the large opening on the anterior aspect of the bony pelvis.
9. Observe that in anatomical position, the obturator foramen faces inferiorly and is bound by the **superior pubic ramus** anteriorly, **ischiopubic ramus** medially, and body of the **ischium** laterally.
10. Observe that the ischiopubic ramus is formed by the **ischial ramus** and **inferior pubic ramus**, often not easily delineated.
11. Compare a male and female bony pelvis and observe that the **subpubic angle** (angle of the pubic arch) is commonly narrower, the distance between the ischial spines is less, the pelvic inlet is more heart shaped, and the greater pelvis is often narrower and taller in males.

Surface Anatomy

The surface anatomy of the perineum may be studied on a cadaver; however, note that fixation of tissue during embalming may make it difficult to distinguish bone from well-preserved soft tissues in some specimens.

Male External Genitalia

ATLAS 5.2, 5.46

1. Refer to FIGURE 5.26.
2. Place the body in a supine position. Stretch the thighs widely apart and brace them.
3. Identify the **shaft of the penis**, the pendant male reproductive organ located in the midline.
4. Observe that the shaft of the penis connects to the trunk in the pubic region at the **root of the penis**.
5. If the abdominal wall has been dissected, identify the **suspensory ligament of the penis** coursing through the subcutaneous tissue providing additional fibrous support to the penis.
6. Identify the **glans of the penis** at the distal end of the shaft of the penis, demarcated from the shaft by the ridge of tissue forming the **corona**. *Note that in an uncircumcised penis, the glans is either partially or fully covered by the prepuce, or foreskin, which will need to be reflected to view the corona.*
7. Identify the **external urethral orifice**, the terminal distal end of the male penile urethra.
8. Posterior to the penis, identify the **scrotum**, the extension of skin surrounding the bilaterally located testes.

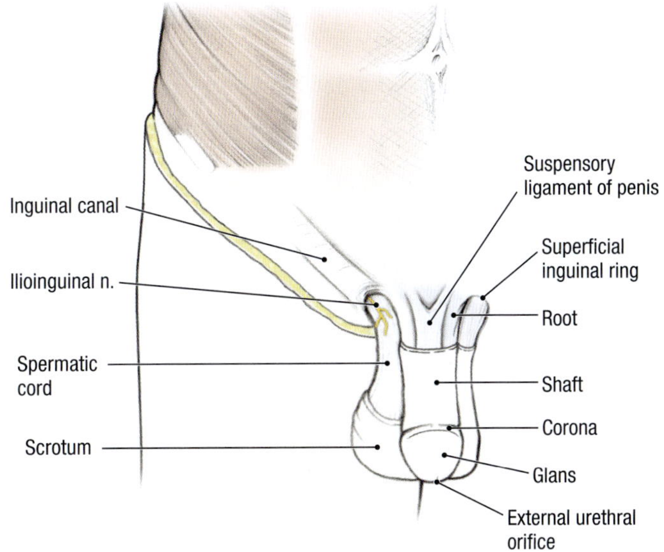

FIGURE 5.26 Surface anatomy of male external genitalia. Anterior view.

Dissection Instructions

Scrotum

ATLAS 4.16, 5.46, 5.48F; VIDEO 5.2.1

Dissection Note: The dissection of the scrotum corresponds to the dissection of the labia majora in female cadavers. Partner with a dissection team that has a female cadaver for the dissection of the external genitalia because you are expected to observe and learn the anatomy for both sexes.

1. Refer to FIGURE 5.26.
2. Identify the **spermatic cord** emerging from the **superficial inguinal ring.**
3. Beginning inferior to the superficial inguinal ring, push your finger or a blunt instrument into to the subcutaneous tissue of the inguinal region to separate the spermatic cord and fascia from the surrounding fat.
4. Use blunt dissection to follow the spermatic cord down into the scrotum by creating a space encircling the spermatic cord along its path of descent. *Note that minimal force is typically needed to separate the spermatic cord from the surrounding tissue.*
5. Refer to FIGURE 5.27.

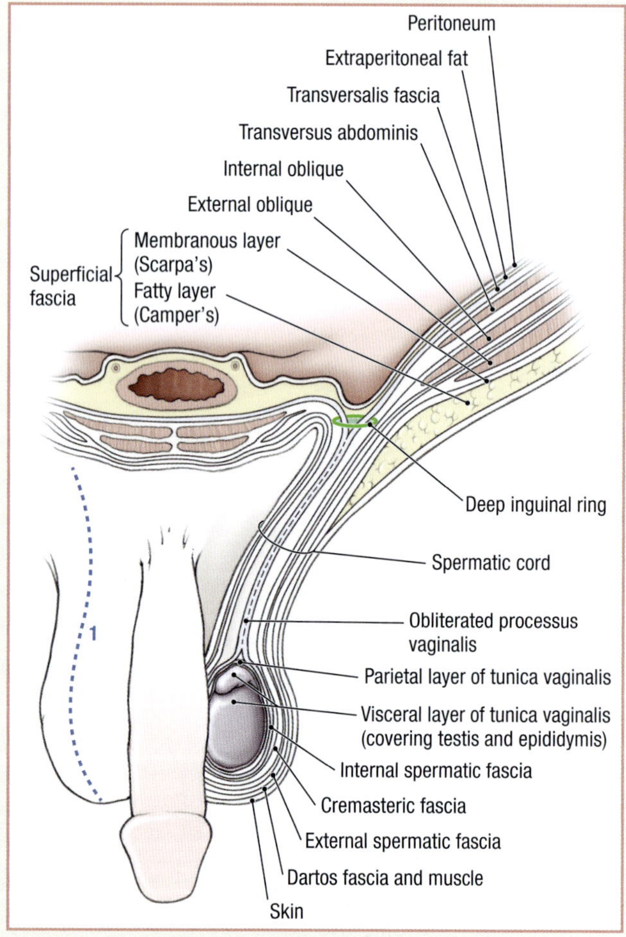

FIGURE 5.27 ● Contributions of anterior abdominal wall to spermatic fascia. Anterior view.

6. Make a vertical incision down the anterior surface of the scrotum along the path of the enlarged space cutting through the skin and dartos fascia, ensuring you do not cut the spermatic cord (**Cut 1**). *Note that the dartos fascia contains the smooth muscle fibers of the dartos, which is responsible for the wrinkling of the scrotal skin.*
7. Use blunt dissection to free the spermatic cord and testis from the surrounding scrotal tissue.
8. Identify the **scrotal ligament** (the remnant of the **gubernaculum testis**), a band of tissue anchoring the inferior pole of the testis to the scrotum.
9. Use scissors to cut the scrotal ligament and reflect the spermatic cord and attached testis laterally from the scrotum.
10. Observe that the **scrotal septum** divides the scrotum into two compartments.

Spermatic Cord

ATLAS 4.16, 4.19, 4.20A; VIDEO 5.2.2

Dissection Note: Perform the following dissection sequence on only one side.

1. Refer to FIGURE 5.27 and FIGURE 5.28.
2. Palpate the spermatic cord and identify the location of the **ductus deferens (vas deferens)** within the surrounding fascia by feeling for the hardest and most "cord-like" structure in the spermatic cord.
3. Carefully make a vertical incision through the **external spermatic fascia,** the outermost covering of the spermatic cord derived from the external oblique aponeurosis (**Cut 1**).

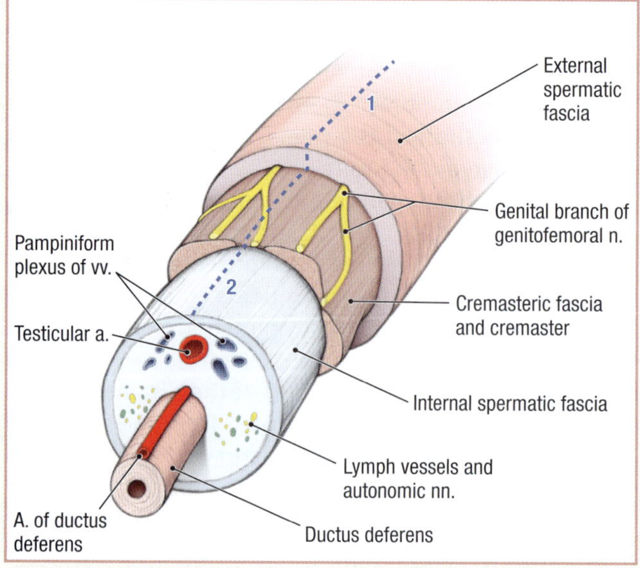

FIGURE 5.28 ● Transverse sections through spermatic cord. Oblique view.

4. Gently spread apart the external spermatic fascia and identify the **cremasteric muscle** and **fascia** derived from the internal oblique. *Note that the cremaster is innervated by the genital branch of the genitofemoral nerve and responsible for elevation of the testis.*
5. Make a vertical incision through the cremasteric layer and the **internal spermatic fascia**, the deepest of the three spermatic cord coverings derived from the transversalis fascia (**Cut 2**).
6. Identify the now exposed **ductus (vas) deferens** and use blunt dissection to separate it from the surrounding **pampiniform plexus of veins** (see **Clinical Correlation 5.7**).

CLINICAL CORRELATION 5.7

Vasectomy

ATLAS 5.37

The ductus deferens can be surgically interrupted through ligation or excision in the superior part of the scrotum, a procedure known as a vasectomy or deferentectomy. Sperm production in the testis continues, but the spermatozoa cannot reach the urethra; thus, following a vasectomy, ejaculated fluid will no longer contain sperm, rendering the individual sterile.

7. Within the plexus of vein, identify the **artery of the ductus deferens**, a small artery located on the surface of the ductus deferens.
8. Follow the ductus deferens superiorly through the inguinal canal toward the deep inguinal ring and confirm that it passes through the deep inguinal ring lateral to the inferior epigastric vessels.
9. Identify the **testicular artery** and use blunt dissection to separate it from the pampiniform plexus of veins. Observe that the testicular artery can be distinguished from the veins by its slightly thicker wall and tortuous course. *Note that sensory nerve fibers, autonomic nerve fibers, and lymphatic vessels accompany the blood vessels in the spermatic cord but are likely too small to differentiate.*

Testis

ATLAS 4.16, 4.19B, 4.20; VIDEO 5.2.3

Dissection Note: Perform the following dissection sequence on only one side.

1. Refer to FIGURE 5.29.
2. Observe that the testis is covered by the layers of spermatic fascia as well as the **tunica vaginalis**, a serous sac derived from peritoneum with parietal and visceral layers (see **Clinical Correlation 5.8**). The testes are the male gonad responsible for production of sperm and the reproductive hormone testosterone.

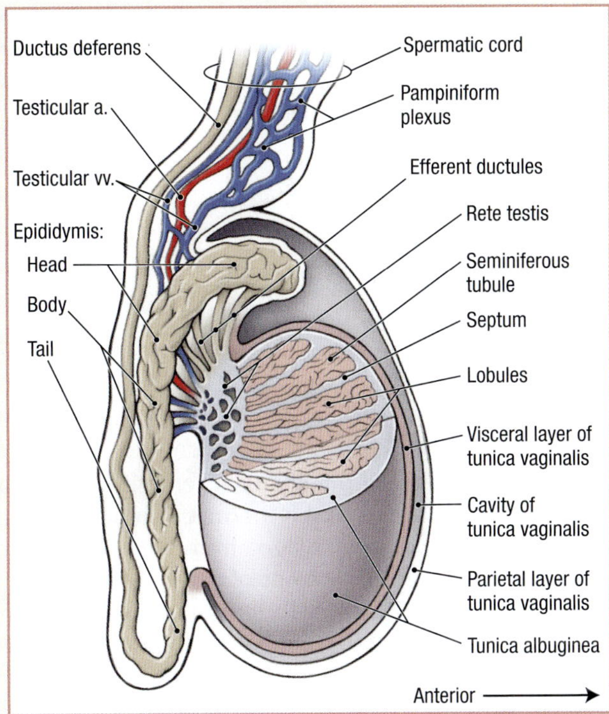

FIGURE 5.29 ● Parts of right testis and epididymis. Lateral view.

CLINICAL CORRELATION 5.8

Lymphatic Drainage of Scrotum and Testis

ATLAS 4.20C, 5.43

Lymphatics from the scrotum drain to the superficial inguinal lymph nodes. Inflammation of the scrotum may cause tender, enlarged superficial inguinal lymph nodes. In contrast, lymphatics from the testis follow the testicular vessels through the inguinal canal into the abdominal cavity where they drain into lumbar (lateral aortic) and preaortic lymph nodes. Testicular tumors may metastasize to lumbar and preaortic lymph nodes, not to superficial inguinal lymph nodes.

3. Use scissors to cut the outer **parietal layer of the tunica vaginalis** along its anterior surface and open it widely.
4. Observe that the **visceral layer of the tunica vaginalis** covers the anterior, medial, and lateral surfaces of the **testis** but not its posterior surface. *Note that the cavity of the tunica vaginalis is a potential space containing a very small amount of serous fluid.*
5. Use blunt dissection to follow the ductus deferens inferiorly until it joins the **tail of the epididymis**, the inferior part of the epididymis that turns superiorly to follow the curve of the testis.

6. Follow the epididymis superiorly to identify the **body of the epididymis**, the middle part that is slightly narrower in diameter, and the **head of the epididymis**, the superior expanded part that receives the efferent ductules.
7. Use a scalpel to carefully section the testis along its anterior surface longitudinally from its superior pole to its inferior pole.
8. Use the epididymis as a hinge and open the halves of the testis as you would open a book.
9. Identify the **tunica albuginea**, the thick fibrous capsule of the testis now visible from the cross-sectional view.
10. Identify the multiple **septa** dividing the interior of the testis into **lobules**.
11. Use a fine-tipped probe or small forceps to tease some of the **seminiferous tubules** out of one lobule and observe their convoluted appearance and tight organization. *Note that the seminiferous tubules are the site of sperm production, although maturation occurs in the epididymis prior to ejaculation.*

Dissection Follow-up

1. Review the course of the ductus deferens from the abdominal wall to the testis.
2. Review the coverings of the spermatic cord and layers of the abdominal wall from which they are derived.
3. Trace the route of spermatozoa from their origin in the seminiferous tubule to the ejaculatory duct.
4. Replace the reflected portions of tissue back to anatomical position.
5. Visit a dissection table with a female cadaver and complete the **Dissection Follow-up** for the **Female External Genitalia, Urogenital Triangle, and Perineum** dissection.

MALE UROGENITAL TRIANGLE, PENIS, AND PERINEUM

Dissection Overview

The subcutaneous tissue of the male perineum has a superficial fatty layer and a deep membranous layer like the subcutaneous tissue of the lower anterior abdomen. The Camper's fascia, the superficial fatty layer of the anterior abdominal wall, thins out with relatively little to no fat along the shaft of the penis or scrotum. The membranous layer of the fascia of the anterior abdominal wall (Scarpa's fascia) continues as the superficial perineal fascia (Colles' fascia) and the dartos fascia of the penis and scrotum as shown in FIGURE 5.30.

The order of dissection of the male urogenital triangle will be as follows: The skin will be removed from the urogenital triangle. The superficial perineal fascia will be removed, and the contents of the superficial perineal pouch will be identified. The skin will be removed from the penis, and its parts will be studied. The contents of the deep perineal pouch will be described but not dissected.

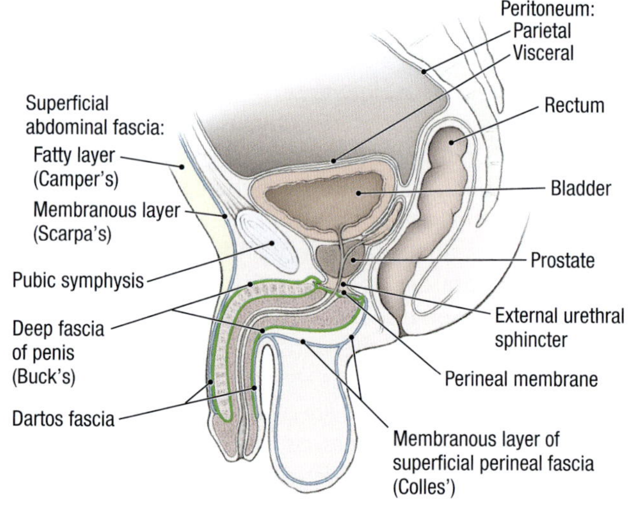

FIGURE 5.30 ● Fasciae of male perineum. Midsagittal view.

Dissection Instructions

Skin Incisions of Male Urogenital Triangle

ATLAS 5.57, 5.58; VIDEO 5.3.1

Dissection Note: Partner with a dissection team that has a female cadaver for the dissection of the urogenital triangle to compare the two sexes. It is recommended to perform a partial-thickness skin removal technique, leaving the subcutaneous tissue intact because cutting too deeply may easily damage many of the structures in the region. To facilitate dissection, position yourself between the lower limbs with the trunk of the cadaver pulled toward the end of the dissection table.

1. Refer to FIGURE 5.31.
2. With the cadaver in the supine position, stretch the thighs widely apart and brace them.
3. Retract the spermatic cord and testis bilaterally away from the penis.

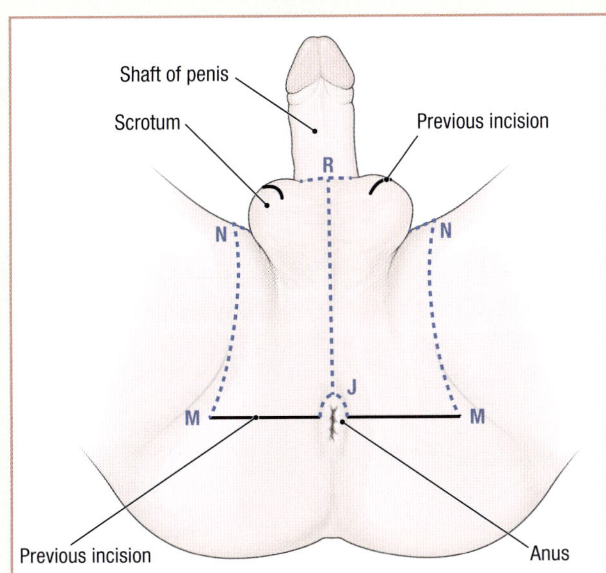

FIGURE 5.31 ● Skin incisions for male perineum. Inferior view.

4. Make a skin incision that encircles the proximal end of the penis (R), making sure to not cut too deeply as the skin is very thin in this region.
5. Make a midline skin incision posterior to the proximal end of the penis (R) that splits the scrotum along the scrotal septum to the anterior margin of the anus (J).
6. Make an incision in the midline superior to the penis to the point where the skin of the abdomen was removed previously.
7. Make a transverse incision from the anterior aspect of the right thigh (N) across the midline superior to the penis to the anterior aspect of the left thigh (N). *Note that if the abdomen was previously dissected, a portion of this incision was already made.*
8. Make a skin incision connecting from the anterior aspect of each thigh (N) posteriorly to a point in the posterior thigh (M) in line with the horizontal incision bifurcating the anterior margin of the anus (J).
9. Reflect the skin flaps from medial to lateral.
10. Detach the scrotum and skin flaps along the medial surface of the thigh and place them in the tissue container.
11. If the cadaver has a large amount of fat in the subcutaneous tissue of the medial thighs, remove a portion of the fat corresponding to the areas of removed skin.

Male Superficial Perineal Pouch

ATLAS 5.57, 5.58; VIDEO 5.3.2

1. Refer to FIGURE 5.32A.
2. In the male, three muscles occupy the superficial pouch on each side: ischiocavernosus, bulbospongiosus, and superficial transverse perineal.

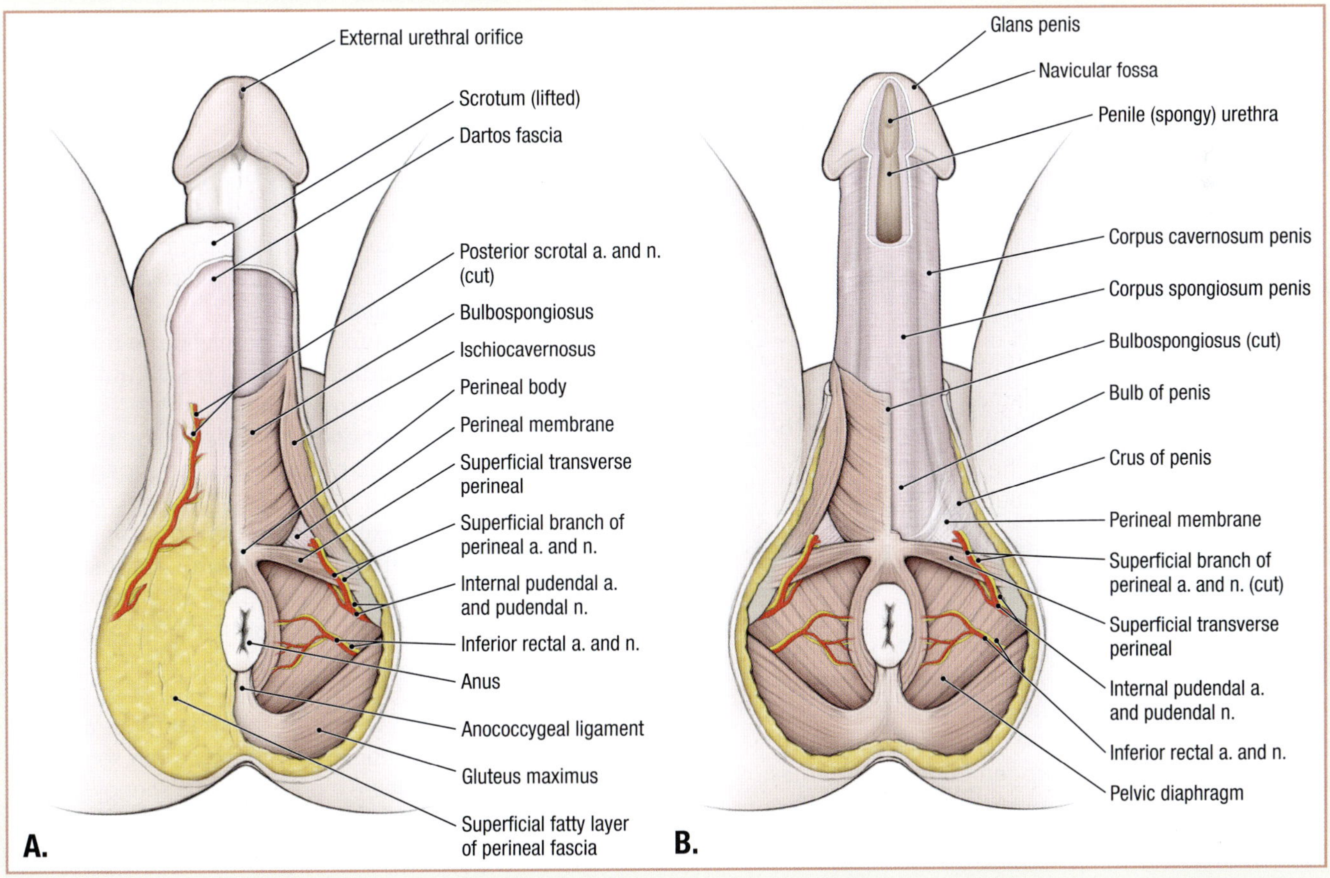

FIGURE 5.32 ● Contents of male superficial perineal pouch in superficial (**A**) and deep (**B**) dissections. Inferior views.

The pairs of muscles overlay the erectile tissue of the region and contribute to the contents of the superficial perineal pouch with their accompanying neurovascular structures.

3. Beginning posteriorly in the ischioanal fossa, identify the **posterior scrotal nerve and vessels** and observe that they are terminal branches of the **superficial branch of the perineal artery and nerve** and supply the posterior part of the scrotum. *Note that the superficial branch of the perineal artery and nerve enter the urogenital triangle by passing lateral to the external anal sphincter.*
4. Use blunt dissection to remove the fat and superficial perineal fascia of the urogenital triangle and identify the **membranous layer of the superficial perineal fascia (Colles' fascia)**.
5. Review the attachments of the Colles' fascia by palpating the **ischiopubic ramus** and **ischial tuberosity** as well as the posterior edge of the **perineal membrane**. *Note that the Colles' fascia forms the superficial boundary of the **superficial perineal pouch** (space).*
6. Use blunt dissection to find the **bulbospongiosus** centrally in the urogenital triangle with the right and left halves fusing at a midline raphe.
7. Observe that the bulbospongiosus covers the surface of the **bulb of the penis**, the central tube of erectile tissue containing the urethra (see **Clinical Correlation 5.9**).

CLINICAL CORRELATION 5.9

Rupture of Male Urethra

ATLAS 5.60

If the penile or spongy urethra is injured in the perineum, urine may escape into the superficial perineal pouch. The urine may spread into the shaft of the penis if the deep (Buck's) fascia is not compromised or into the scrotum, penis, and upward into the lower abdominal wall if the deep fascia is ruptured (see FIGURE B5.1). The fluid would extend into the space between the membranous layer of the abdominal superficial (Scarpa's) fascia and the deep (investing) fascia covering the aponeurosis of the external oblique.

If the membranous or intermediate urethra is ruptured by comparison, extravasation of urine and blood occurs into the deep perineal pouch or compartment. Fluid in the deep perineal pouch may pass through the urogenital hiatus to enter the pelvic cavity and spread around the prostate or bladder internally.

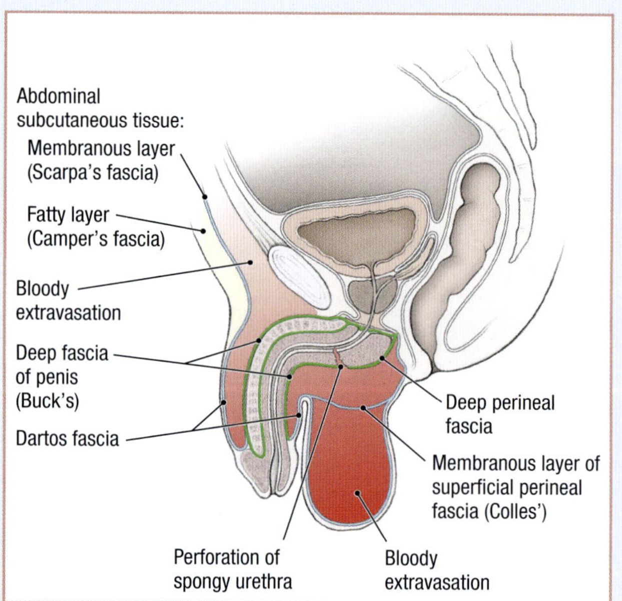

FIGURE B5.1 ● Rupture of penile urethra in perineum with extravasated urine and blood in superficial perineal pouch and lower abdomen wall. Midsagittal view.

8. Review the attachments and actions of the **bulbospongiosus** (see **TABLE 5.2**).
9. Lateral to the bulbospongiosus, use blunt dissection to clean the surface of the **ischiocavernosus** overlying the superficial surface of the **crus of the penis**.
10. Use blunt dissection to find the **superficial transverse perineal** at the posterior border of the urogenital triangle.
11. Observe that the superficial transverse perineal helps to support the **perineal body**, a fibromuscular mass located anterior to the anal canal and posterior to the bulbospongiosus. *Note that the superficial transverse perineal may be delicate and difficult to find. Limit the time you spend looking for it.*
12. Use blunt dissection to clean between the three muscles of the superficial perineal pouch until a small triangular opening is created.
13. Within the triangular opening, identify the **perineal membrane**, the deep boundary of the superficial perineal pouch.
14. Use a scalpel to make a shallow incision along the midline raphe of the bulbospongiosus and remove it on the left side of the cadaver. Take care because this is a thin muscle and effort must be made to not cut too deeply.
15. Refer to FIGURE 5.32B.
16. Identify the **bulb of the penis** and use an illustration to observe that it is continuous with the corpus spongiosum penis and contains a portion of the spongy urethra.
17. On the left side of the cadaver, remove the ischiocavernosus overlying the **crus of the penis**.

18. Verify that the crus of the penis attaches to the ischiopubic ramus and is continuous with the corpus cavernosum penis.

Penis

ATLAS 5.59, 5.61, 5.62; VIDEO 5.3.3

Dissection Note: In anatomical position, the penis is erect, thus making the surface of the penis closest to the anterior abdominal wall, the dorsal surface of the penis. The superficial fascia of the penis (dartos fascia) has no fat and contains the superficial dorsal vein of the penis, which may be easily cut if the skin incisions are made too deep.

1. Refer to FIGURE 5.32.
2. Identify the **root of the penis**, the part of the penis attached to the ischiopubic rami (bulb and crura).
3. Identify the **body (shaft) of the penis**, the part of the penis that is pendant containing the corpora cavernosa and corpus spongiosum penis.
4. Identify the **glans penis** at the distal end of the penis, the continuation of the corpus spongiosum penis containing the penile urethra, which terminates at the **external urethral orifice**.
5. Around the circumference of the glans, identify the **corona of the glans**. In an uncircumcised specimen, identify the **prepuce** (foreskin), which must be retracted to expose the corona.
6. Observe the midline location of the **frenulum** on the ventral surface of the glans connecting along the distal shaft of the penis.
7. Use a scalpel to make a shallow midline skin incision through the skin along the ventral surface of the penis.
8. Use a probe or forceps to gently elevate the skin from around the shaft of the penis and detach it along with the prepuce, if present, by cutting the skin just proximal to the corona of the glans (see **Clinical Correlation 5.10**). Do not attempt to remove the skin of the glans.

CLINICAL CORRELATION 5.10

Circumcision

ATLAS 5.61

Circumcision is the removal of the foreskin or prepuce of the penis. An uncircumcised prepuce covers all or part of the glans, whereas a circumcised prepuce would leave the glans either fully or partially exposed. Smegma, or accumulations of secretions, may accumulate within the preputial sac, the space between the glans and the prepuce in an uncircumcised penis, leading to irritation and sensitivity. Occasionally, the prepuce is not elastic enough to fully retract over the glans during an erection or intercourse, a condition known as phimosis, which may need surgical correction.

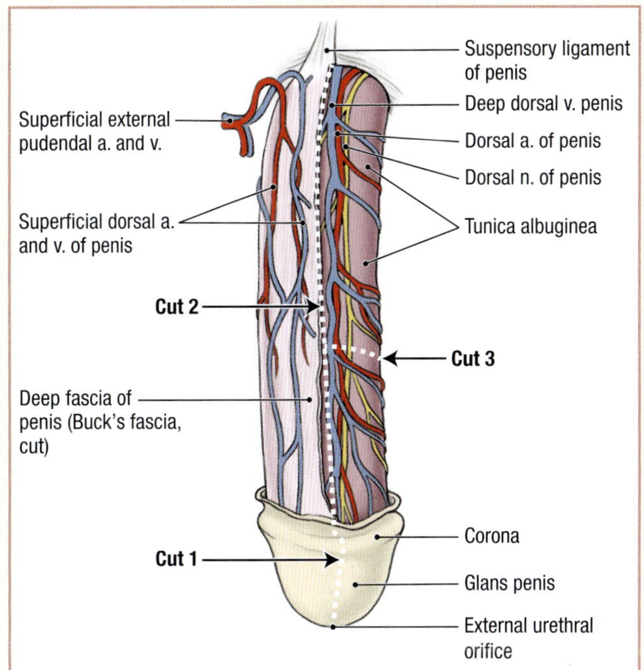

FIGURE 5.33 ● Exposed arteries and nerves of penis with skin (*left*) and superficial fascia (*right*) removed. Dorsal view.

9. Refer to FIGURE 5.33.
10. On the dorsal surface of the penis, identify and clean the **superficial dorsal vein**. The superficial dorsal vein of the penis drains into the **superficial external pudendal vein**, which then drains into the great saphenous vein to return to the femoral vein.
11. On the dorsum of the penis, use blunt dissection to dissect through the **deep fascia of the penis** and identify the **deep dorsal vein of the penis** (unpaired) in the midline. *Note that most of the blood from the penis drains through the deep dorsal vein into the* ***prostatic venous plexus****.*
12. Identify and clean the **dorsal artery of the penis** (paired) on each side of the deep dorsal vein. The dorsal artery of the penis is a terminal branch of the internal pudendal artery.
13. Identify and clean the **dorsal nerve of the penis** (paired) on each side of the midline lateral to the deep dorsal artery. *Note that the dorsal nerve of the penis is a branch of the pudendal nerve.*
14. Use blunt dissection to trace the dorsal artery and nerve of the penis proximally.
15. Observe that the dorsal artery and nerve of the penis course deep to the perineal membrane before they emerge onto the dorsum of the penis. The deep dorsal vein passes between the pubic arch and the anterior edge of the perineal membrane to enter the pelvis. *Note that the deep dorsal vein does not accompany the deep dorsal artery and dorsal nerve proximal to the body of the penis.*

Spongy (Penile) Urethra

ATLAS 5.61D, 5.63, 5.64; VIDEO 5.3.4

Dissection Note: The male urethra is described as having four regions: preprostatic, prostatic, membranous, and spongy (penile). The spongy urethra is the portion located within the corpus spongiosum penis. To examine the internal features of the spongy urethra, the glans and shaft of the penis will be cut longitudinally along the midline and one haft transected axially.

1. Refer to FIGURE 5.33.
2. Identify the **external urethral orifice** at the tip of the glans penis.
3. Gently insert a probe into the external urethral orifice and use a scalpel to cut down to the probe from both the dorsal and ventral surfaces of the penis in the median plane of the penis (**Cut 1**). *Note that the pathway of the spongy urethra may not be a straight line or may be slightly off center.*
4. Advance the probe proximally and continue to divide the penis until you reach a point inferior to the pubic symphysis where the two corpora cavernosa separate from the bulb of the penis (**Cut 2**). Dorsal to the probe, the cut should pass between the corpora cavernosa and split the deep dorsal vein longitudinally. Ventral to the probe, the cut should divide the corpus spongiosum into equal halves.
5. Carefully continue the cut through the bulb of the penis along the path of the urethra but do not cut through the perineal membrane. *Note that the urethra bends at a sharp angle and passes through the perineal membrane.*
6. Observe the sagittal section of the penis and identify the **glans penis**, the distal expansion of the corpus spongiosum. *Note that the glans penis caps the two corpora cavernosa at the distal extent of the penis.*
7. Identify the penile (spongy) urethra within the erectile tissue of the corpus spongiosum and observe that it terminates by passing through the glans to the external urethral orifice.
8. Examine the interior of the spongy urethra at the glans penis and identify the **navicular fossa**, a widening of the urethra.
9. In the proximal part of the spongy urethra in the bulb of the penis, look for the openings of the ducts of the bulbourethral glands. *Note that the opening of the ducts may be too small to see.*
10. On the left side of the penis, make a transverse cut through the body of the penis about midway down its length (**Cut 3**).
11. Refer to FIGURE 5.34.
12. Observe that the deep fascia of the penis (Buck's fascia) is an investing fascia surrounding the corpus spongiosum (unpaired), corpus cavernosum (paired), deep dorsal vein (unpaired), dorsal artery (paired), and dorsal nerve of the penis (paired).

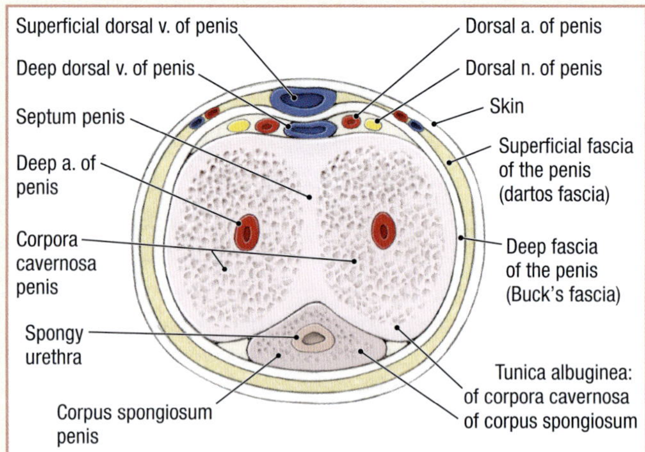

FIGURE 5.34 ■ Transverse section through midshaft of penis. Inferior view.

13. On the dorsal aspect of the transversely cut surface, identify the **corpus cavernosum** and observe that it is surrounded by the thick fascia of the **tunica albuginea of the corpus cavernosum**. *Note that the bisection of the penis likely cut through the septum penis, separating the corpora cavernosa.*
14. On the ventral aspect of the transversely cut surface, identify the **corpus spongiosum** and observe that it is surrounded by the **tunica albuginea of the corpus spongiosum**.
15. Study the erectile tissue within the corpus cavernosum penis and identify the **deep artery of the penis** near the center of the tubular erectile tissue. *Note that the origin of the deep artery of the penis is the internal pudendal artery.*

Male Deep Perineal Pouch

ATLAS 5.59, 5.60A

Dissection Note: The deep perineal pouch lies superior (deep) to the perineal membrane and will be minimally dissected, as few of the structures are easily identifiable.

1. Refer to FIGURE 5.35.
2. Identify the **membranous (intermediate) urethra** in the midsagittal plane where it pierces the **perineal membrane**. The membranous urethra extends from the perineal membrane to the prostate gland and is the shortest (about 1 cm), thinnest, narrowest, and least distensible part of the urethra.
3. Surrounding the membranous urethra, identify the **external urethral sphincter (sphincter urethrae)** and the obliquely oriented fibers of the **compressor urethrae**. *Note that the external urethral sphincter is a voluntary muscle, while the compressor urethrae is an involuntary muscle; both muscles, however, act to compress the membranous urethra and stop the flow of urine.*

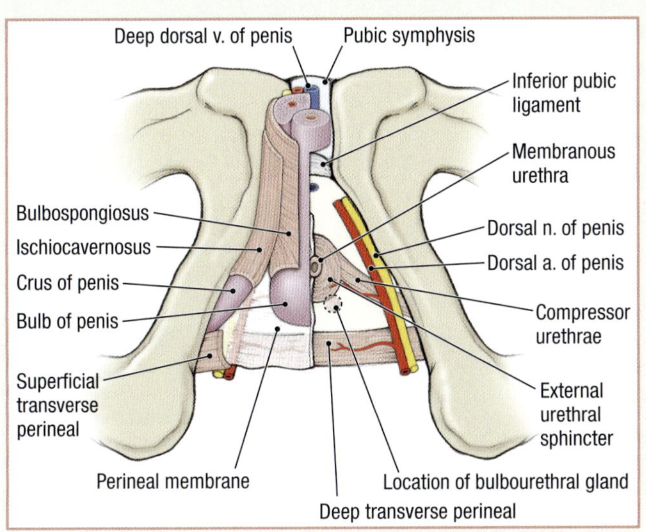

FIGURE 5.35 ● Contents of the male superficial (*left*) and deep (*right*) perineal pouches. Inferior view.

4. Posterolateral to the urethra, identify the location of the **bulbourethral gland**. The bulbourethral glands are located in the deep perineal pouch bilaterally, but their ducts pass through the perineal membrane to drain into the proximal portion of the spongy urethra in the superficial perineal pouch.
5. Identify the **deep transverse perineal** (paired) along the posterior margin of the deep perineal pouch. Collectively, the muscles within the deep perineal pouch plus the perineal membrane are known as the **urogenital diaphragm.** *Note that the deep transverse perineal fiber direction and function are identical to those of the superficial transverse perineal in the superficial perineal pouch.*
6. Review the attachments and actions of the **external urethral sphincter** and the **deep transverse perineal** (see **TABLE 5.2**).
7. Coursing anteriorly along the lateral margin of the deep perineal pouch, identify the **branches of the internal pudendal artery and vein** (most notably, the dorsal artery of the penis) and the **branches of the pudendal nerve** (most notably, the dorsal nerve of the penis). *Note that the pudendal neurovascular structures supply the external urethral sphincter, deep transverse perineal, and penis.*

Dissection Follow-up

1. Review the muscles of the male superficial perineal pouch in **TABLE 5.2**.
2. Review the course of the internal pudendal artery from its origin in the pelvis.
3. Review the course and branches of the pudendal nerve.
4. Review the course of the deep dorsal vein of the penis into the pelvis to join the prostatic venous plexus.
5. Review the parts of the male urethra.
6. Return the muscles of the urogenital triangle and reflected portions of tissue to their correct anatomical positions.
7. Visit a dissection table with a female cadaver and view the contents of the superficial perineal pouch.

TABLE 5.2 Male Superficial and Deep Perineal Pouches

Muscle	*Anterior Attachments*	*Posterior Attachments*	*Actions*	*Innervation*
SUPERFICIAL GROUP OF MUSCLES				
Bulbospongiosus	Contralateral bulbospongiosus muscle at the midline raphe	Perineal body	Compress the bulb of the penis to expel urine or semen	Deep branch of the perineal n. (branch of pudendal n.)
Ischiocavernosus	Crus of the penis	Ischial tuberosity and ischiopubic ramus	Forces blood from the crus of the penis into the distal part of the corpus cavernosum penis	Deep branch of the perineal n. (branch of pudendal n.)
Superficial transverse perineal	Perineal body (medial attachment)	Ischial tuberosity (lateral attachment)	Provides support to the perineal body	Perineal n. (branch of pudendal n.)
DEEP GROUP OF MUSCLES				
Muscle	*Anterior Attachments*	*Posterior Attachments*	*Actions*	*Innervation*
Deep transverse perineal	Perineal body (medial attachment)	Ischial tuberosity (lateral attachment)	Provides support to the perineal body	Perineal n. (branch of pudendal n.)
External urethral sphincter	Attaches to itself around the urethra		Compresses the membranous urethra and stops the flow of urine	Deep branch of the perineal n. (branch of pudendal n.)

Abbreviation: n., nerve.

MALE PELVIC CAVITY

Dissection Overview

The male pelvic cavity contains the urinary bladder, male internal genitalia, and rectum as shown in FIGURE 5.36. The organs within the true pelvis are often classified as infraperitoneal because they are located inferior to the peritoneum. Recall that the pelvic structures are located superior to the pelvic diaphragm and perineal membrane.

The order of dissection will be as follows: The peritoneum will be studied in the male pelvic cavity. The pelvis will be sectioned in the midline, and the cut surface of the sectioned pelvis will be studied. The ductus deferens will be traced from the anterior abdominal wall to the region between the urinary bladder and rectum. The seminal vesicles and prostate gland will be studied.

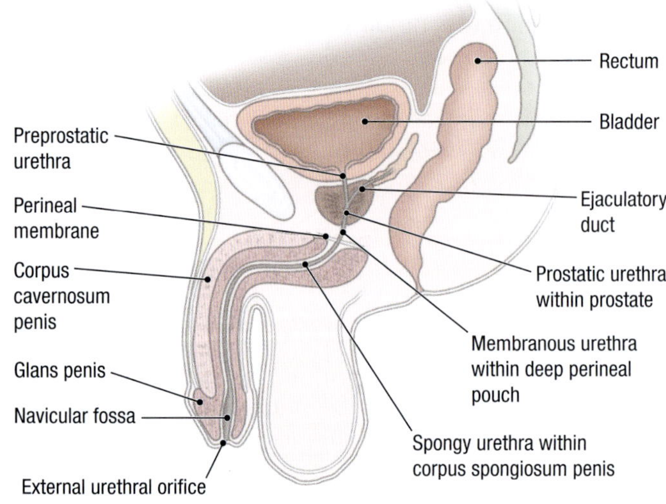

FIGURE 5.36 ● Parts of male urethra. Midsagittal view.

Dissection Instructions

Male Pelvic Peritoneum

ATLAS 5.15, 5.36; VIDEO 5.4.1

1. Refer to FIGURE 5.37.
2. Identify the peritoneum on the posterior aspect of the anterior abdominal wall superior to the pubis (**1**).
3. Observe that the peritoneum reflects from the anterior abdominal wall inferiorly across the apex of the urinary bladder (**2**) (see **Clinical Correlation 5.11**).

CLINICAL CORRELATION 5.11

Cystotomy

ATLAS 5.48B, 5.48E, 5.48F, 5.63

Cystotomy is a surgical incision made into the urinary bladder, often as a method of treatment to alleviate urethral blockages caused by small tumors, foreign bodies, or urinary calculi due to urinary tract infections. A needle inserted just superior to the pubis (suprapubic access) can penetrate a filled urinary bladder without entering the peritoneal cavity. As the urinary bladder fills, the peritoneal reflection from the anterior body wall to the urinary bladder is elevated above the level of the pubis, and the depth and breadth of the paravesical fossa and the rectovesical fossa will increase. Sampling urine through direct collection in the bladder allows a physician to obtain a less contaminated sample for analysis than a transurethral sample obtained through catheterization.

4. Observe that the peritoneum courses along the superior surface of the urinary bladder (**3**) and its posterior surface superiorly (**4**).
5. Identify the **paravesical fossa** (paired), the shallow depressions in the peritoneal cavity on the lateral sides of the urinary bladder.
6. Observe that the peritoneum descends posterior to the bladder in proximity to the superior ends of the seminal vesicles (**5**).
7. Follow the peritoneum posterior to the bladder and identify the **rectovesical pouch** (**6**), the reflection between the urinary bladder and the rectum. *Note that the rectovesical pouch is the lowest point in the male abdominopelvic cavity.*

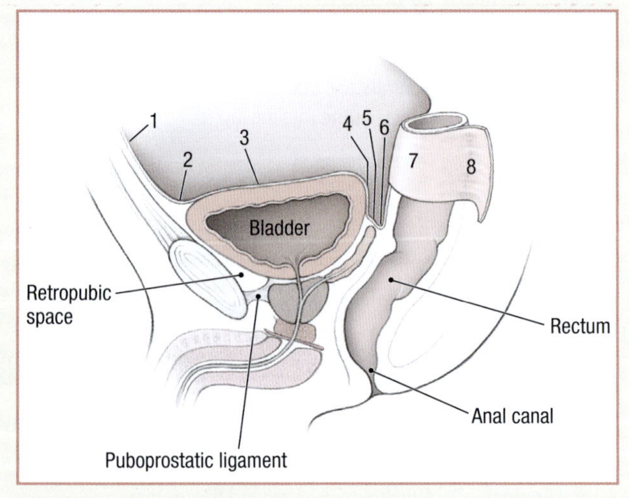

FIGURE 5.37 ● Male pelvic peritoneum. Midsagittal view.

8. Follow the peritoneum superiorly along the posterior aspect of the pelvic cavity on the anterior surface of the rectum (**7**) and observe that it is continuous with the sigmoid mesocolon at the level of the third sacral vertebra.
9. Identify the **pararectal fossa** (paired), the shallow depressions in the peritoneal cavity on the lateral sides of the rectum (**8**).

Sectioning of Male Pelvis

ATLAS 5.15, 5.16A, 5.48B; VIDEO 5.4.2

Dissection Note: The pelvis will be divided in the midline up to vertebral level L3 with a saw. Subsequently, the left side of the body will be transected at vertebral level L3, enabling removal of the left lower limb and the left hemi pelvis. The right lower limb and right side of the pelvis will remain attached to the trunk.

1. Refer to FIGURE 5.38A.
2. In the male pelvic cavity, make a midline cut beginning posterior to the pubic symphysis through the superior surface of the urinary bladder (**Cut 1**). Spread open the bladder and sponge the interior if necessary.
3. Identify the internal urethral orifice in the bladder and insert a probe into it. Use the probe as a guide to continue the midline cut inferior to the urinary bladder to divide the prostatic urethra and prostate gland.
4. Extend the midline cut in the posterior direction, cutting through the anterior and posterior walls of the rectum and the distal part of the sigmoid colon (**Cut 2**).
5. Clean the internal aspect of the rectum and anal canal. *Use caution when cleaning and moving fecal matter. Refer to your instructor for proper safety techniques.*
6. Use a scalpel to cut the left common iliac vein, left common iliac artery, left testicular vessels, and left ureter about 1 cm distal to their respective points of origin (**Cuts 3**).
7. Cut through the left lumbar arteries at vertebral levels L4 and L5 and reflect the abdominal aorta to the right side of the abdominal cavity.
8. Use a scalpel to make an incision from the midaxillary line to the vertebral column through the muscles of the lateral abdominal wall about 2 cm superior to the iliac crest (**Cut 4**).
9. Cut through the nerves of the left lumbar plexus where they cross the horizontal incision and any remaining fibers of the left psoas major and quadratus lumborum at vertebral level L3.
10. Refer to FIGURE 5.38B.
11. In the perineum, use a scalpel blade to make a cut in the midline between the halves of the bulb of the penis from the pubic symphysis to the coccyx passing through the perineal membrane, perineal body, and anal canal (**Cut 5**).
12. Refer to FIGURE 5.38C.
13. With the cadaver in the supine position, use a saw to cut through the pubic symphysis in the midline from anterior to posterior (**Cut 6**), stopping at the inferior border of the pubic symphysis.
14. Turn the cadaver 90° to the right, so it is lying on its right side and prop the cadaver, or have your lab partners hold the body, so it does not fall or rotate.
15. Have your lab partners abduct the left lower limb to facilitate the sectioning of the sacrum.
16. Cut through the sacrum from posterior to anterior (**Cut 7**). Make an effort not to allow the saw to pass

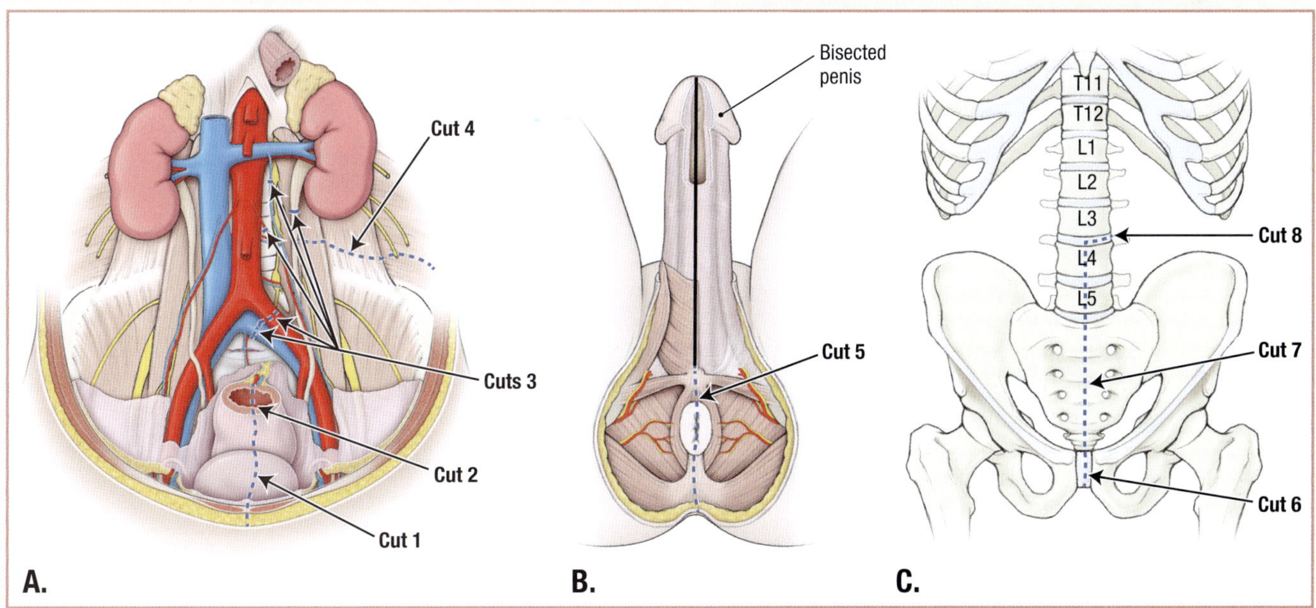

FIGURE 5.38 ■ **A.** Soft tissue cuts for male pelvic bisection. Anterior view. **B.** Perineal cuts for male pelvic bisection. Inferior view. **C.** Skeletal cuts for male pelvic bisection and left lower limb and pelvis detachment. Anterior view.

between the soft tissue structures that were cut with the scalpel, retracting them out of the path of the blade if necessary.

17. Forcibly spread apart the lower limbs to expand the opening division of the sacrum and extend the midline cut as far superiorly as the body of the third lumbar vertebra.
18. Adduct the left lower limb and use the saw to cut horizontally through the left half of the intervertebral disc between L3 and L4 (**Cut 8**), sparing the inferior aspect of the abdominal aorta.
19. Once the horizontal and vertical cuts are connected, return the cadaver to the supine position.
20. Cut any remaining pieces of tissue preventing the left lower limb from being removed and pull the left lower limb away from the rest of the cadaver.
21. Clean the rectum and anal canal on both sides of the bisected pelvic specimen.

Male Internal Genitalia

ATLAS 5.15, 5.16A, 5.37; VIDEO 5.4.3

1. Refer to FIGURE 5.39.
2. Identify the **perineal membrane** deep to the bulb of the penis. *Note that the perineal membrane can be identified as a thin line at the deep edge of the bulb of the penis.*
3. Superior (deep) to the perineal membrane, identify the **external urethral sphincter** surrounding the **membranous urethra**. *Note that the external urethral sphincter may be difficult to see in the sectioned specimen.*
4. On the sectioned pelvis, identify the four parts of the urethra: **(1) preprostatic**, **(2) prostatic**, **(3) membranous (intermediate)**, and **(4) spongy (penile)**.
5. Examine the interior of the **prostatic urethra** and observe that it is about 3 cm in length and passes through the prostate gland.
6. Refer to FIGURE 5.40.
7. Identify the longitudinal ridge of the **urethral crest** on the posterior wall of the prostatic urethra in the midline.
8. Identify the **seminal colliculus**, an enlargement of the urethral crest, and observe the presence of the **prostatic sinuses** on either side.
9. On the surface of the seminal colliculus, identify the **prostatic utricle**, the small opening in the midline.
10. On either side of the prostatic utricle, identify the **openings of the ejaculatory ducts**.
11. Refer to FIGURE 5.41.
12. Locate the **ductus deferens** near the inner surface of the anterior abdominal wall where it passes through the **deep inguinal ring** lateral to the **inferior epigastric vessels**.
13. Use blunt dissection to peel the peritoneum off the lateral wall of the pelvic cavity near the deep inguinal ring.
14. Detach the peritoneum at the point of reflection between the rectum and urinary bladder and place it in the tissue container.
15. Identify the **femoral ring** medial to the **external iliac vessels** passing inferior (deep) to the inguinal ligament.
16. Use blunt dissection to trace the ductus deferens from the deep inguinal ring toward the midline of the pelvis and observe that the ductus deferens passes superior and then medial to the branches of the internal iliac artery and superior to the ureter.

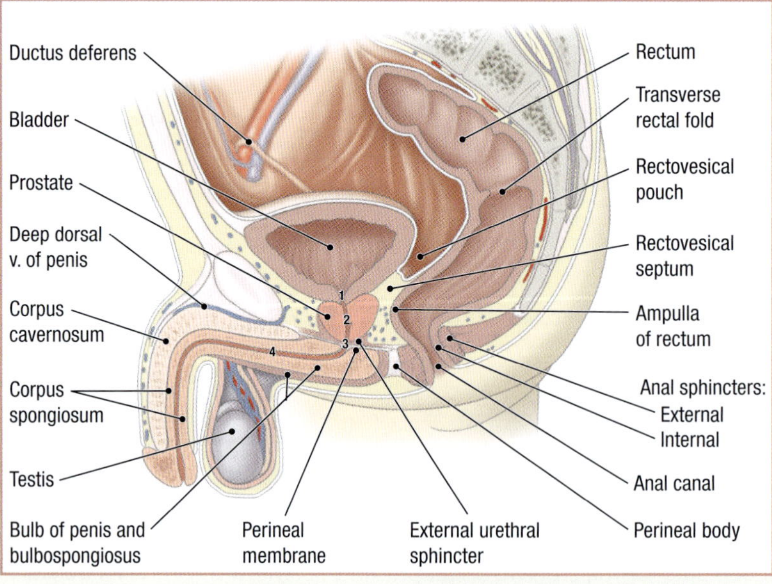

FIGURE 5.39 ● Midline section of male pelvis. Midsagittal view.

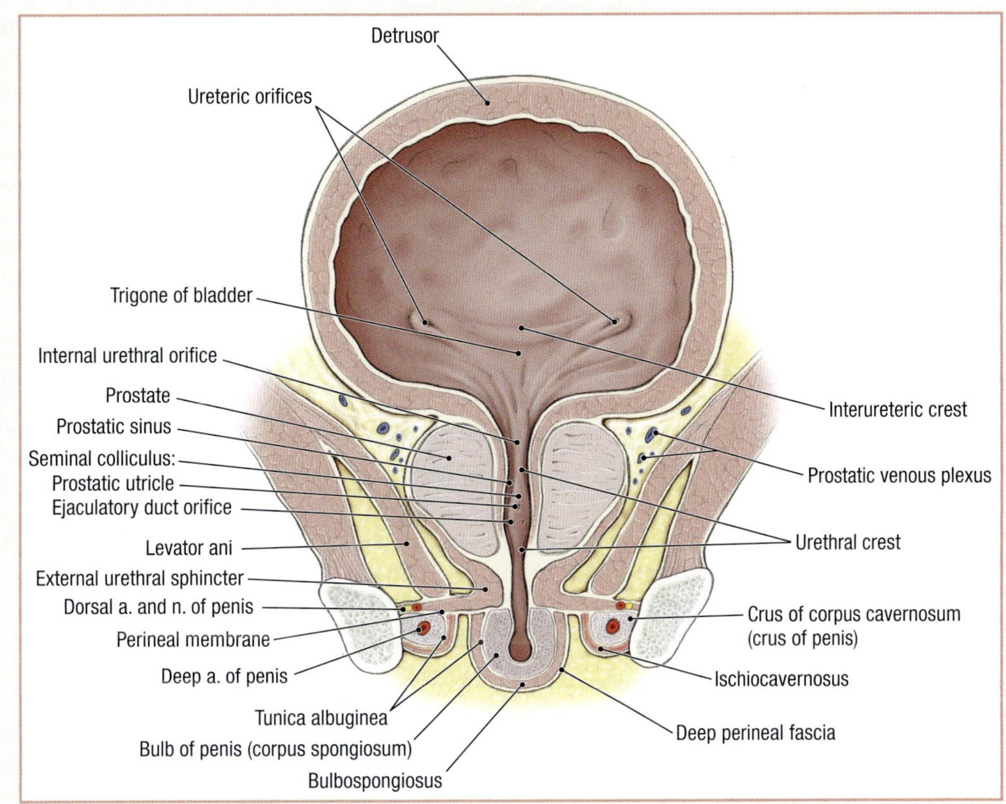

FIGURE 5.40 ■ Coronal section of male urinary bladder and proximal urethra. Anterior view.

17. Trace the ductus deferens into the rectovesical septum, the endopelvic fascia between the rectum and urinary bladder, and observe that the ductus deferens is in contact with the fundus (posterior surface) of the **urinary bladder**.
18. Identify the **ampulla of the ductus deferens**, the enlarged portion just before its termination.
19. Identify the **seminal vesicle** located inferolateral to the ampulla of the ductus deferens. *Note that the duct of the seminal vesicle joins the ductus*

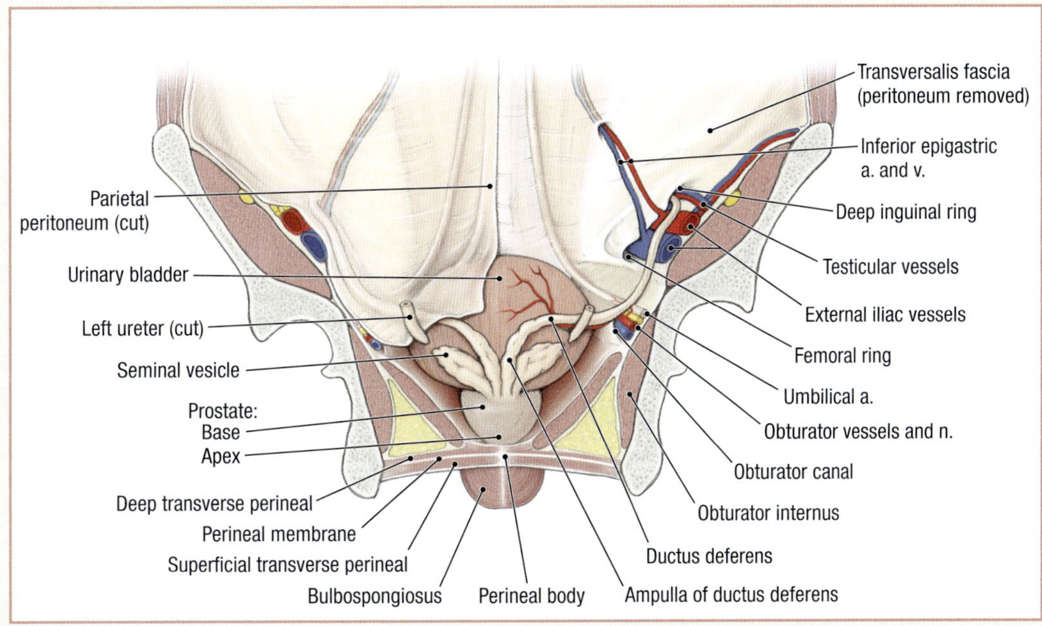

FIGURE 5.41 ■ Male urinary bladder and internal genitalia with removed peritoneum (*right*). Posterior view.

deferens to form the ejaculatory duct close to the prostate.

20. Use blunt dissection to release the seminal vesicle from the rectovesical septum. Pay attention because the **ejaculatory duct** is delicate and easily torn where it enters the prostate. *Note that the ejaculatory ducts empty into the prostatic urethra from their openings on the seminal colliculus.*
21. Identify the **prostate** inferior to the urinary bladder.
22. Observe that the **apex** of the prostate is directed inferiorly and that the **base** of the prostate is located superiorly against the neck of the urinary bladder.

Dissection Follow-up

1. Review the position of the male pelvic viscera within the lesser pelvis and compare it to the position of the viscera in the female pelvis.
2. Describe the differences in the male and female peritoneum.
3. Follow the ductus deferens from the epididymis to the ejaculatory duct, recalling its relationships to vessels, nerves, the ureter, and the seminal vesicle along this path.
4. Visit a dissection table with a female cadaver and follow the round ligament of the uterus from the labium majus to the uterus and compare this route to the course of the ductus deferens in the male pelvis.
5. Return the reflected tissue in the right hemipelvis back to anatomical position.
6. Return left lower limb and hemisected pelvis back to anatomical position.

MALE URINARY BLADDER, RECTUM, AND ANAL CANAL

Dissection Overview

The urinary bladder is a reservoir for urine which when empty is located within the pelvic cavity and when filled extends into the abdominal cavity. Organs located inferior to the peritoneum are classified as subperitoneal organs and are surrounded by endopelvic fascia. The urinary bladder and lower two-thirds of the rectum are subperitoneal, whereas the upper third of the rectum is partially covered by peritoneum.

Between the pubic symphysis and the urinary bladder is a potential space called the retropubic space (prevesical space). The retropubic space is filled with fat and loose connective tissue to accommodate the expansion of the urinary bladder. The inferior limit of the retropubic space is defined by the puboprostatic ligament, a condensation of fascia that ties the prostate to the inner surface of the pubis.

The order of dissection will be as follows: The parts of the urinary bladder will be studied. The interior of the urinary bladder will be studied. The interior of the rectum and anal canal will be studied.

Dissection Instructions

Male Urinary Bladder

ATLAS 5.37A, 5.38, 5.41A; VIDEO 5.5.1

1. Refer to FIGURE 5.42.
2. Identify the **apex of the urinary bladder,** the pointed part directed toward the anterior abdominal wall attaching to the urachus.
3. Observe that the **body of the urinary bladder** is located between the apex and the **fundus (base) of the urinary bladder**, the inferior part of the posterior wall.
4. Observe the proximity of the fundus to the ductus deferens, seminal vesicles, and rectum.

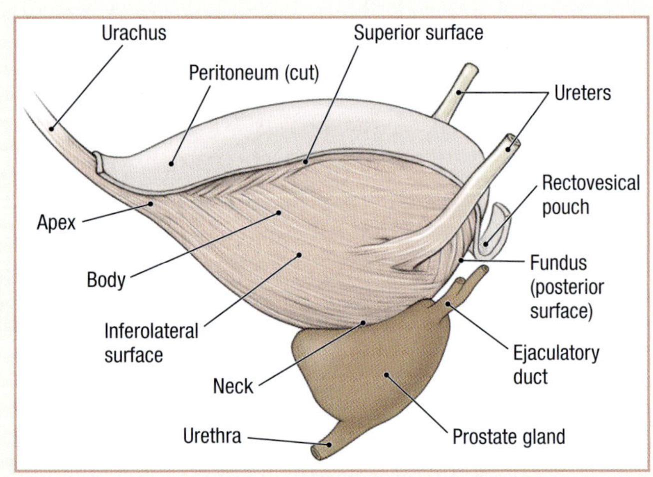

FIGURE 5.42 ● Parts of male urinary bladder. Lateral view.

5. Identify the **neck of the urinary bladder**, where the urethra exits and the wall thickens to form the **internal urethral sphincter**. *Note that the internal urethral sphincter is an involuntary muscle controlled by the autonomic nervous system.*
6. Observe that the **superior surface** of the urinary bladder is covered by peritoneum, whereas the **posterior surface** lies immediately adjacent to the rectum.
7. Verify that the **inferolateral** (paired) surface of the urinary bladder is covered by endopelvic fascia and lies below the reflection point of the peritoneum.
8. Refer back to FIGURE 5.40.
9. Examine the **wall of the urinary bladder**, noting its thickness and observe that it consists of bundles of smooth muscle called **detrusor**. *Note that the mucous membrane lining most of the inner surface of the urinary bladder lies in folds when the bladder is empty but flattens out to accommodate expansion when the bladder is full.*
10. Study the inner surface of the fundus and identify the **trigone of the urinary bladder (urinary trigone)**, a smooth, triangular region of mucous membrane defined by lines between the **internal urethral orifice** and the two **ureteric orifices**. *Note that the urinary trigone has now been bisected.*
11. Observe that the internal urethral orifice is located at the most inferior point in the urinary bladder at the inferior aspect of the trigone.
12. Identify the **interureteric crest**, a visible horizontal ridge extending between the orifices of the ureters.
13. Insert the tip of a probe into the orifice of the ureter to confirm that the ureter passes through the muscular wall of the urinary bladder in an oblique direction. *Note that when the urinary bladder is full (distended), the pressure of the accumulated urine flattens the part of the ureter within the wall of the bladder, thus preventing reflux of urine back into the ureter.*
14. Locate the point where the ureter crosses the external iliac artery or the bifurcation of the common iliac artery.
15. Use blunt dissection to follow the ureter to the fundus of the urinary bladder, observing that it crosses inferior to the **vas deferens** along its course.

Male Rectum and Anal Canal

ATLAS 5.15, 5.16, 5.18; VIDEO 5.5.2

1. Refer back to FIGURE 5.39 and FIGURE 5.43.
2. Identify the **rectum** at its point of origin at the level of the third sacral vertebra and observe that it follows the curvature of the sacrum and coccyx.
3. Identify the **ampulla of the rectum**, the dilated portion of the rectum proximal to the point where the rectum bends approximately 80° posteriorly at the **anorectal flexure** (see **Clinical Correlation 5.12**).

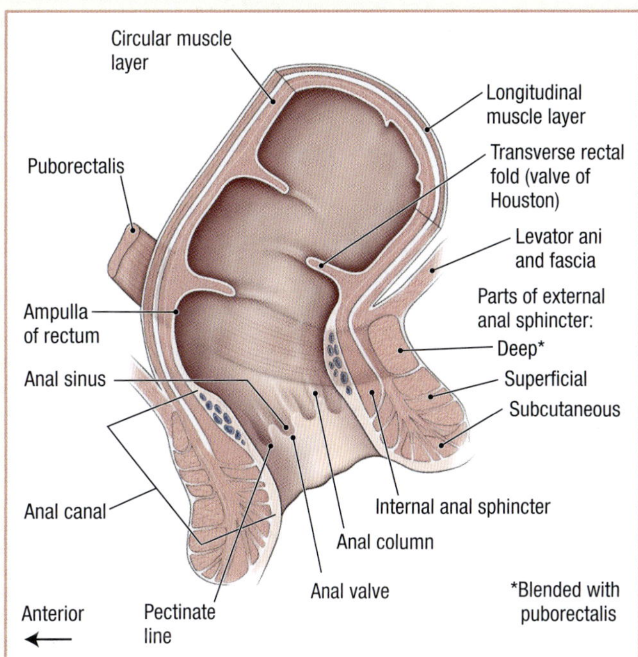

FIGURE 5.43 ● Distal rectum, anal sphincters, and anal canal. Midsagittal view.

CLINICAL CORRELATION 5.12

Benign Prostatic Hyperplasia and Digital Rectal Examination

ATLAS 5.37, 5.40

The prostate continues to grow throughout life in a condition known as benign prostatic hyperplasia (BPH). BPH can cause partial or total obstruction of the urethral orifice or the prostatic urethra and lead to urgency (a sudden desire to urinate), nocturia (needing to void during the night), and dysuria (difficult or painful urination). BPH may also cause infections, enlargement of the urinary bladder or kidneys, or result in erectile dysfunction. The size and consistency of the prostate, in particular, the posterior lobe (the most common location of prostate cancer), can be assessed by palpation through the anterior wall of the rectum by a digital rectal examination (DRE).

4. Observe that the prostate gland and seminal vesicles are located adjacent to the anterior wall of the rectum.
5. Examine the inner surface of the rectum and observe that the mucous membrane is smooth except for the presence of **transverse rectal folds**, one on the right and two on the left. *Note that the transverse rectal folds may be difficult to identify in some cadavers.*
6. Identify the **anal canal** inferior to the anorectal flexure and observe that it is only 2.5 to 3.5 cm in length and passes out of the pelvic cavity into the anal triangle of the perineum.

7. Examine the inner surface of the anal canal proximally and identify the **anal columns**, 5 to 10 longitudinal ridges of mucosa containing branches of the **superior rectal artery** and **vein**. *Note that the mucosal features of the anal canal may be difficult to identify.*
8. Identify the semilunar folds of mucosa forming the **anal valves**, which unite the distal ends of the anal columns. Between the anal valve and the wall of the anal canal is a small pocket called an **anal sinus**.
9. Identify the **pectinate line**, the irregular line formed by the contour of the collective anal valves.
10. Identify the **external anal sphincter** in the sectioned specimen surrounding the anal canal. *Note that the external anal sphincter is composed of skeletal muscle and is under voluntary control.*
11. Identify the **internal anal sphincter** in the sectioned specimen surrounding the anal canal. *Note that the internal anal sphincter is composed of smooth muscle and is under involuntary control.*
12. Observe that the longitudinal muscle of the anal canal separates the two sphincter muscles. If you have difficulty identifying the anal sphincters, use a scalpel to cut another section through the wall of the anal canal to improve the clarity of the dissection.

Dissection Follow-up

1. Use the dissected specimen to review the features of the urinary bladder, rectum, and anal canal.
2. Review the relationships of the seminal vesicles, ampulla of the ductus deferens, and ureters to the rectum and fundus of the urinary bladder.
3. Visit a dissection table with a female cadaver and review the relationships of the uterus, vagina, and ureters to the rectum and fundus of the urinary bladder.
4. Review the pelvic course of the ureter and function of the urinary bladder.
5. Review the male urethra and compare it with the female urethra.
6. Review all parts of the large intestine and recall its function in absorption of water and in compaction and elimination of fecal material.
7. Compare muscle type and innervation of the external and internal anal sphincters.
8. Return all reflected tissue back to anatomical position.

MALE INTERNAL ILIAC ARTERY AND SACRAL PLEXUS

Dissection Overview

Anterior to the sacroiliac articulation, the common iliac artery divides to form the external and internal iliac arteries. The external iliac artery distributes to the lower limb, and the internal iliac artery distributes to the pelvis, gluteal region, and perineum. The internal iliac artery commonly divides into anterior and posterior divisions, although arterial variation frequently occurs. Branches arising from the anterior division are mainly visceral and supply the urinary bladder, internal genitalia, external genitalia, rectum, and gluteal region. Branches arising from the posterior division are parietal and supply the pelvic walls and gluteal region.

The somatic nerve plexuses of the pelvic cavity, sacral and coccygeal, are located between the pelvic viscera and lateral pelvic wall in the endopelvic fascia and formed by contributions from anterior rami of spinal nerves L4–Co1. The primary visceral nerve plexus of the pelvic cavity is the inferior hypogastric plexus (pelvic plexus), formed by contributions from the hypogastric nerves, sacral splanchnic nerves (sympathetic), and pelvic splanchnic nerves (parasympathetic).

The order of dissection will be as follows: The branches of the posterior division of the internal iliac artery will be identified. The branches of the anterior division of the internal iliac artery will be identified. The nerves of the sacral plexus will be dissected. Subsequently, the pelvic portion of the sympathetic trunk will be dissected.

Dissection Instructions

Male Pelvic Blood Vessels

ATLAS 5.41, 5.42; VIDEO 5.6.1

Dissection Note: The internal iliac artery has one of the most variable branching patterns of any artery, and it is worth noting at the outset of this dissection that you must use the target distribution of the branches to identify them, not their pattern of branching or point of origin.

The dissection of the pelvic vasculature may be performed on both the right and left sides of the hemisected pelvis; however, it is recommended to focus the dissection on just the right side because a deeper dissection will be performed on the left side with the detached lower limb.

1. Refer to FIGURE 5.44.
2. Identify the **internal iliac vein** and observe that its tributaries largely parallel the nearby arteries but are plexiform in nature. To clear the dissection field, remove all tributaries to the internal iliac vein as each correlating artery is identified and cleaned.
3. Identify the locations of the **prostatic venous plexus, vesical venous plexus,** and **rectal venous plexus,** all of which drain into the internal iliac vein.
4. Identify the **deep dorsal vein of the penis** just inferior to the pubic symphysis and verify that it empties into the prostatic venous plexus.
5. Identify and clean the **common iliac artery** and follow it distally until it bifurcates into the **external iliac artery** and **internal iliac artery.**
6. Use blunt dissection to follow the internal iliac artery into the pelvis and identify its **anterior** and **posterior divisions.**
7. Begin identification of the branches of the posterior division of the internal iliac artery by finding the most posterior and superior branch, the **iliolumbar artery.**
8. Observe that the **iliolumbar artery** passes posteriorly from the posterior division and then ascends lateral to the **sacral promontory,** lumbar vertebrae, lumbosacral trunk, and obturator nerve.
9. Identify the **lateral sacral artery,** which frequently gives rise to a superior branch and an inferior branch. Observe that the inferior branch passes anterior to the sacral ventral rami. *Note that the lateral sacral artery may arise from a common trunk with the iliolumbar artery.*
10. Identify the branches of the **anterior division of the internal iliac artery** beginning with the **umbilical artery.**
11. In the medial umbilical fold, identify the **medial umbilical ligament** (the remnant of the umbilical artery) and use blunt dissection to trace it posteriorly to the umbilical artery.
12. Identify and clean several **superior vesical arteries** arising from the inferior surface of the umbilical artery which descend to the superolateral part of the urinary bladder.
13. Inferior to the umbilical artery, identify the **obturator artery** passing into the obturator canal with the **obturator nerve.** It may help to find the obturator artery where it enters the obturator canal in the lateral wall of the pelvis and then follow it posteriorly to its origin. *Note that the obturator artery arises from the external iliac or inferior epigastric arteries in about a quarter of individuals as the aberrant obturator artery, which crosses the pelvic brim to enter the obturator canal. The aberrant obturator artery is particularly at risk for injury during surgical repair of a femoral hernia.*

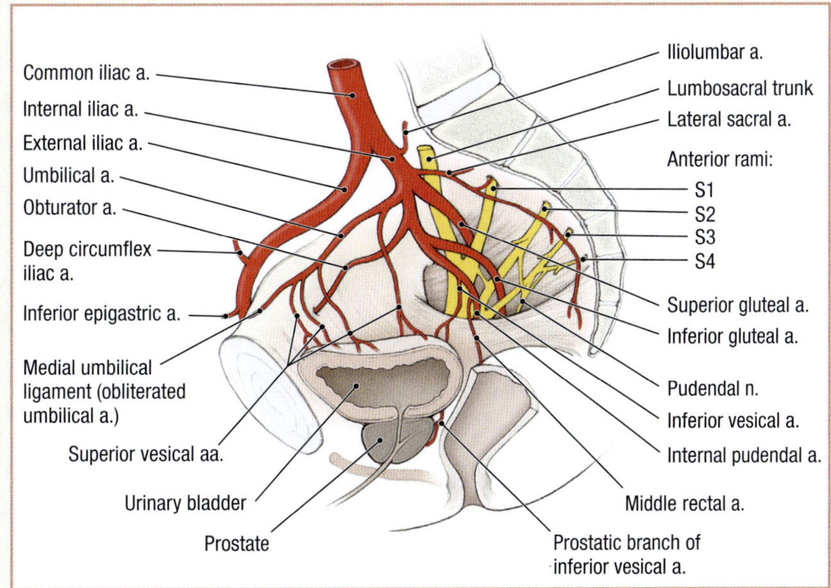

FIGURE 5.44 ● Branches of male internal iliac artery. Midsagittal view.

14. Follow the anterior division of the internal iliac artery toward the pelvic floor and identify the **inferior gluteal artery**.
15. Observe that the inferior gluteal artery commonly passes out of the pelvic cavity into the gluteal region through the greater sciatic foramen inferior to the piriformis. *Note that the inferior gluteal artery may share a common trunk with the internal pudendal artery or, less commonly, with the superior gluteal artery.*
16. Identify the **inferior vesical artery** off the anterior aspect of the anterior division of the internal iliac artery. Observe that the inferior vesical artery courses toward the fundus of the urinary bladder to supply the bladder, seminal vesicle, and prostate. *Note that the inferior vesical artery is a named branch only in the male; in the female, it is an unnamed branch of the vaginal artery.*
17. Identify the **middle rectal artery** coursing medially toward the rectum. The middle rectal artery often arises from a common trunk with the inferior vesical artery, making positive identification difficult. *Note that the middle rectal artery, like the inferior vesical artery, sends branches to the seminal vesicle and prostate.*
18. Identify the **internal pudendal artery** anterior to the inferior gluteal artery. Observe that the internal pudendal artery exits the pelvic cavity through the greater sciatic foramen medial to the inferior gluteal artery as it will enter the lesser sciatic foramen to reach the perineum. *Note that the internal pudendal artery often arises from a common trunk with the inferior gluteal artery.*

Male Pelvic Nerves

ATLAS 5.12A, 5.13, 5.44; VIDEO 5.6.2

Dissection Note: The dissection of the pelvic nerves may be performed on both the right and left sides of the hemisected pelvis; however, it is recommended to focus the dissection on just the right side because a deeper dissection will be performed on the left side with the detached lower limb.

1. Refer to FIGURE 5.45.
2. Use blunt dissection to free the rectum from the anterior surface of the sacrum and coccyx.
3. Retract the rectum medially and identify the **sacral plexus** of nerves on the anterior surface of the piriformis.
4. Just lateral to the sacral promontory, identify and clean the **lumbosacral trunk** (anterior rami of L4 and L5) and verify that it joins the sacral plexus.
5. Inferior to the lumbosacral trunk, identify the anterior rami of S2 and S3, which emerge between the proximal attachments of the piriformis.
6. Identify the **sciatic nerve** and observe that it is formed by the anterior rami of spinal nerves L4–S3. The sciatic nerve exits the pelvis by passing through the greater sciatic foramen to enter the gluteal region, usually inferior to the piriformis, although variations are common.
7. Observe that the **superior gluteal artery** usually passes between the **lumbosacral trunk** and the **anterior ramus of spinal nerve S1** and exits the pelvis through the greater sciatic foramen superior to the piriformis.

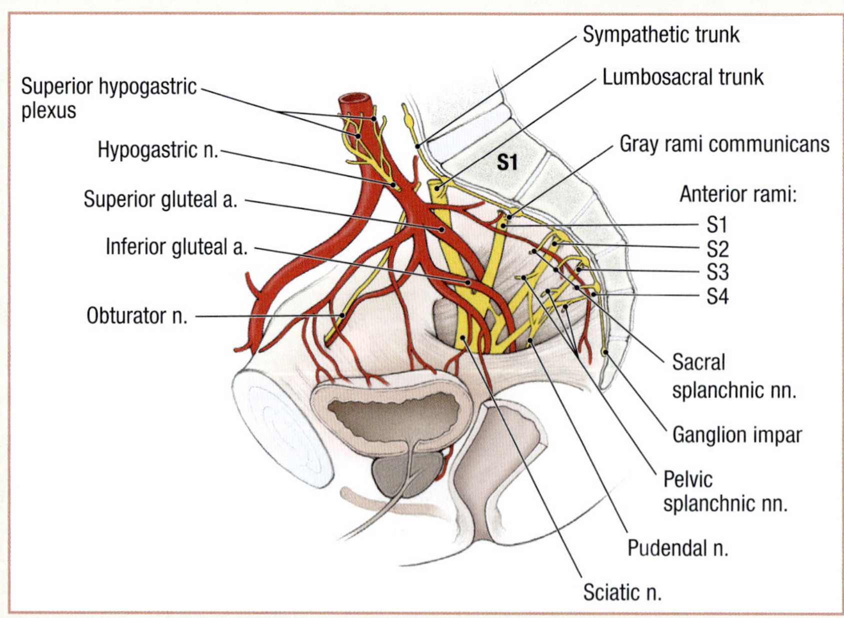

FIGURE 5.45 ● Sacral and autonomic nerve plexuses in male pelvis. Midsagittal view.

8. Observe that the **inferior gluteal artery** usually passes between the anterior rami of spinal nerves S2 and S3, but may pass between the anterior rami of spinal nerves S1 and S2, to exit the pelvis through the greater sciatic foramen inferior to the piriformis.
9. Identify the **pudendal nerve** and observe that it is formed by contributions from the anterior rami of spinal nerves S2, S3, and S4. *Note that the pudendal nerve exits the pelvis through the greater sciatic foramen inferior to the piriformis where it then enters the perineum by passing through the lesser sciatic foramen.*
10. Identify the **pelvic splanchnic nerves (nervi erigentes)**. Observe that pelvic splanchnic nerves arise from the anterior rami of spinal nerves S2, S3, and S4. *Note that pelvic splanchnic nerves carry presynaptic parasympathetic axons for innervation of pelvic organs and the embryonic hindgut.*
11. Identify the **sacral portion of the sympathetic trunk** located on the anterior surface of the sacrum medial to the ventral sacral foramina. Observe that the sympathetic trunk continues from the abdominal region into the pelvis and that the two sides join in the midline near the level of the coccyx to form the **ganglion impar**.
12. Identify the **gray rami communicantes**, which connect the sympathetic ganglia to the sacral anterior rami. *Note that each gray ramus communicans carries postsynaptic sympathetic fibers to an anterior ramus for distribution to the lower extremity and perineum.*
13. Identify the **sacral splanchnic nerves** arising from two or three of the sacral sympathetic ganglia and observe that they pass directly to the **inferior hypogastric plexus** (see **Clinical Correlation 5.13**). *Note that sacral splanchnic nerves carry sympathetic fibers that distribute to the pelvic viscera.*

CLINICAL CORRELATION 5.13

Hypogastric Nerve Damage

ATLAS 5.44

The inferior hypogastric plexus is in the endopelvic fascia lateral to the rectum, bladder, seminal vesicles, and prostate. The inferior hypogastric plexus, as well as its superior contribution of the hypogastric nerve, could be injured during pelvic surgery. Damage to the autonomic plexus could cause loss of bladder control and erectile dysfunction.

14. On the right side of the pelvic cavity, follow the inferior hypogastric plexus superiorly toward the condensation of the plexus into the **right hypogastric nerve**. Use an illustration to identify the **superior hypogastric plexus** and review the origins of the autonomics in both the superior and inferior hypogastric plexuses.

Dissection Follow-up

1. Review the location of the terminal branches of the abdominal aorta.
2. Use the dissected specimen to review the branches of the internal iliac artery and the region supplied by each.
3. Review the relationship of the ureter to the vas deferens.
4. Review the formation of the sacral plexus.
5. Review the course of the pudendal nerve from the pelvic cavity to the urogenital triangle.
6. Return all reflected tissue back to anatomical position.

MALE PELVIC DIAPHRAGM

Dissection Overview

The pelvic diaphragm is the muscular floor of the pelvic cavity formed by the levator ani and coccygeus as well as their surrounding fasciae. The pelvic diaphragm extends from the pubic symphysis anteriorly to the coccyx posteriorly. Laterally, the pelvic diaphragm is attached to the fascia covering the obturator internus. Openings in the midline of the pelvic diaphragm, the urogenital hiatus and anal hiatus, allow passage of the urethra and anal canal.

The order of dissection will be as follows: The pelvic viscera will be retracted medially. The obturator internus, tendinous arch of the levator ani, and the levator ani will be identified. The vas deferens, prostate, and anal canal will be cut, and the pelvic viscera reflected.

Dissection Instructions

Dissection Note: Perform the following dissection sequence on only one side of the cadaver. If the left lower limb was removed during the bisection of the pelvis, it is recommended that this dissection be performed on the left side to preserve the continuity of the vasculature into the abdominal cavity on the right side.

Male Pelvic Diaphragm

ATLAS 5.10, 5.11, 5.12; VIDEO 5.7.1

1. Refer to FIGURE 5.46A.
2. Retract the rectum, urinary bladder, prostate, and seminal vesicles medially and identify the **pelvic diaphragm**.
3. Use blunt dissection to remove any remaining fat and connective tissue from the superior surface of the pelvic diaphragm.
4. Locate the **obturator canal** piercing the obturator internus by identifying and following the obturator artery and nerve.
5. Palpate the medial surface of the ischial spine through the levator ani and identify the **tendinous arch of the levator ani**. Observe that the tendinous arch lies just inferior to a line connecting the ischial spine and the obturator canal. *Note that the tendinous arch is a thickening in the obturator fascia and the origin of part of the levator ani.*

Dissection Note: Identify the three components of the **levator ani** by their anterolateral attachments. Learn, but do not dissect, their posterior attachments.

6. Refer to FIGURE 5.46B.
7. Identify the **puborectalis** (paired) attaching anteriorly to the body of the pubis and posteriorly to the puborectalis of the opposite side (in a midline raphe). The puborectalis form the margin of the urogenital hiatus, and a "puborectal sling," which maintains the **anorectal flexure** of the rectum. *Note that during defecation, the puborectalis relaxes, the anorectal flexure straightens, and the elimination of fecal matter is facilitated.*
8. Identify the **pubococcygeus** (paired) attaching from the body of the pubis anteriorly to the coccyx and the **anococcygeal raphe (ligament)** posteriorly.
9. Identify the **iliococcygeus** (paired) attaching from the tendinous arch anterolaterally to the coccyx and the anococcygeal raphe posteriorly. *Note that the levator ani supports the pelvic viscera and resists increases in intraabdominal pressure.*
10. Identify the **coccygeus** (paired) attaching from the ischial spine anteriorly to the lateral border of the coccyx and lowest part of the sacrum posteriorly.
11. Place the fingers of one hand in the ischioanal fossa inferior to the pelvic diaphragm and the fingers of the other hand on the superior surface of the pelvic diaphragm to palpate the thickness of the pelvic diaphragm.
12. Turn the left lower limb and observe that the **obturator internus** forms the lateral wall of the ischioanal fossa and perineum inferior to the pelvic diaphragm, and the lateral wall of the pelvic cavity superior to the pelvic diaphragm.

Dissection Note: The medial attachment of the obturator internus is the margin of the obturator foramen and inner surface of the obturator membrane, and its lateral attachment is the greater trochanter of the femur. The obturator internus will be studied further when the gluteal region is dissected.

13. Observe that the urethra and anal canal pass through midline openings in the pelvic diaphragm called the **urogenital hiatus** and **anal hiatus**, respectively.
14. To increase the visibility of the pelvic diaphragm, cut the **vas deferens** a few centimeters away from the deep inguinal ring and reflect it along with the pelvic viscera medially.
15. If the muscles forming the pelvic diaphragm remain difficult to see, make an incision through the inferior aspect of the prostate and anal canal and detach the viscera from the pelvic floor. Leave the viscera attached to the neurovascular structures, so the relationships are maintained for later review.
16. Review the general pattern of lymphatic drainage of the pelvis and the location of the **common iliac**, **external iliac**, **internal iliac**, **sacral**, and **lumbar nodes**.

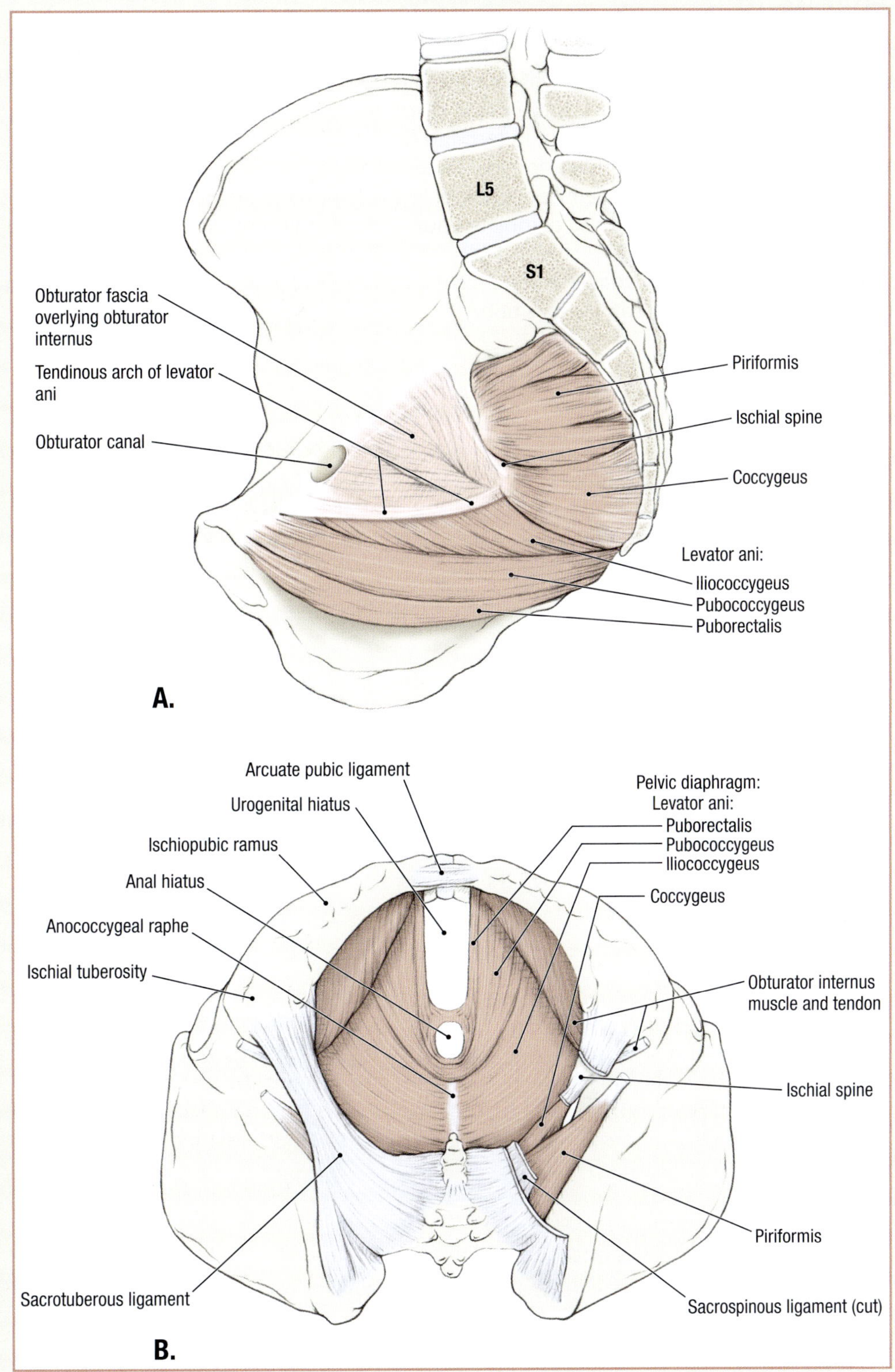

FIGURE 5.46 ■ Male pelvic diaphragm. **A.** Midsagittal view. **B.** Inferior view.

Dissection Follow-up

1. Review the proximal attachment and action of each muscle of the pelvic diaphragm.
2. Review the relationship of the branches of the internal iliac artery to the pelvic diaphragm.
3. Review the relationship of the sacral plexus to the pelvic diaphragm.
4. Review the role played by the pelvic diaphragm in forming the boundary between the pelvic cavity and the perineum and in supporting the pelvic and abdominal viscera.
5. Compare the lymphatic drainage of the perineal contents to the lymphatic drainage of the testis.
6. Review the formation of the thoracic duct to complete your understanding of the lymphatic drainage from this region.
7. Visit a dissection table with a female cadaver and perform a complete review of the dissected female pelvis.
8. Return all reflected tissue back to anatomical position.

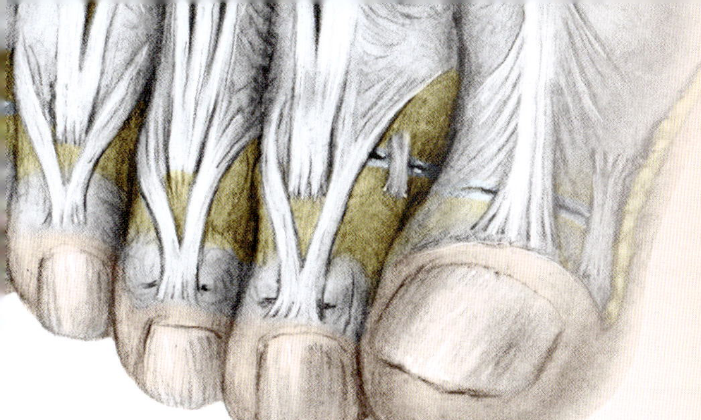

CHAPTER 6
Lower Limb

REFERENCES

ATLAS = *Grant's Atlas of Anatomy*, 16th ed., figure number

VIDEO = *Grant's Dissection Videos*, video sequence number

The lower limb extends from the hip to the tips of the toes and is divided into four regions: the gluteal region, thigh, leg, and foot. It is worth noting that the term *leg* refers only to the portion of the lower limb between the knee and ankle, not to the entire lower limb. The functional requirements of the lower limb are weight bearing, locomotion, and maintenance of equilibrium. Although the upper and lower limbs develop with a similar pattern of organization, the lower limb rotates such that the equivalent surface of the palm corresponds to the sole of the foot, with the thumb being lateral in the hand and the great toe medial in the foot. The developmental rotation of the lower limb is constructed for strength at the cost of mobility. Some of the muscles that control the lower limb are intrinsic (originate and terminate within the lower limb) and some are extrinsic (originate in the pelvis or gluteal region and terminate within the lower limb).

CLINICAL CORRELATIONS

During your dissection protocol, you may encounter anatomical variations, clinical conditions, disease processes, or medical devices in your cadaveric donor. The following select clinical correlations will be described in more detail throughout this chapter.

Lower Limb

6.1. Varicose Veins and Saphenous Cut Down, see the **Subcutaneous Tissue of Anterior Lower Limb** sequence. ATLAS 6.14A, 6.15B
6.2. Femoral Triangle and Femoral Hernia, see the **Femoral Triangle** sequence. ATLAS 6.21
6.3. Patellar Tendon (Quadriceps) Reflex, see the **Quadriceps Femoris** sequence. ATLAS 6.10B, 6.48
6.4. Intragluteal Injections, see the **External Rotators of Hip** sequence. ATLAS 6.34
6.5. Sciatic Nerve Injury, see the **Posterior Compartment of Thigh** sequence. ATLAS 6.31C, 6.36A, 6.36B
6.6. Common Fibular Nerve Injury, see the **Anterior Compartment of Leg** sequence. ATLAS 6.62C, 6.65B
6.7. Neck of Femur Fracture, see the **Hip Joint** sequence. ATLAS 6.43
6.8. Knee Injuries, see the **Knee Joint Posterior Approach** sequence. ATLAS 6.50, 6.51
6.9. Ankle Injuries, see the **Ankle Joint** sequence. ATLAS 6.85

SUBCUTANEOUS TISSUE OF LOWER LIMB

Dissection Overview

The subcutaneous tissue of the lower limb contains fat, superficial fascia, lymphatics, superficial veins, and cutaneous nerves. In the living body, the superficial veins of the lower limb may be visible through the skin and used for venipuncture or cannulation. In the cadaver, the superficial veins are not conspicuous.

The order of dissection will be as follows: The entire lower limb will be skinned except the sole of the foot. The superficial veins and cutaneous nerves will be dissected. The subcutaneous tissue and fat will be removed, leaving select superficial veins and cutaneous nerves intact. The deep fascia of the thigh will be studied.

Skeletal Anatomy

Refer to an articulated skeleton or disarticulated lower limb skeleton to identify the following skeletal features.

Anterior Hip

ATLAS 6.2A, 6.30A

1. Refer to FIGURE 6.1.
2. Identify the three bones comprising the hip bone from an anterior view: **ilium**, **ischium**, and **pubis**.
3. Observe that the three bones of the hip fuse within the **acetabulum**, the cuplike depression forming the socket of the hip joint. *Note that the point of fusion of the three bones in the acetabulum is referred to as the triradiate cartilage in youth and adolescents, typically not visible in the adult after skeletal fusion.*
4. On the anterior aspect of the pelvis, identify the **anterior superior iliac spine (ASIS)** and **anterior inferior iliac spine (AIIS)** of the ilium.
5. Follow the curve of the pelvic inlet along the **pecten pubis** to the **pubic tubercle**.
6. Align the pelvis in anatomical position and verify that the pubic tubercle and ASIS are aligned in a coronal plane.
7. Identify the **obturator foramen** and observe that it is bounded superiorly by the **superior pubic ramus** and inferomedially by the ischiopubic ramus, composed of the **inferior pubic ramus** and **ischial ramus**.

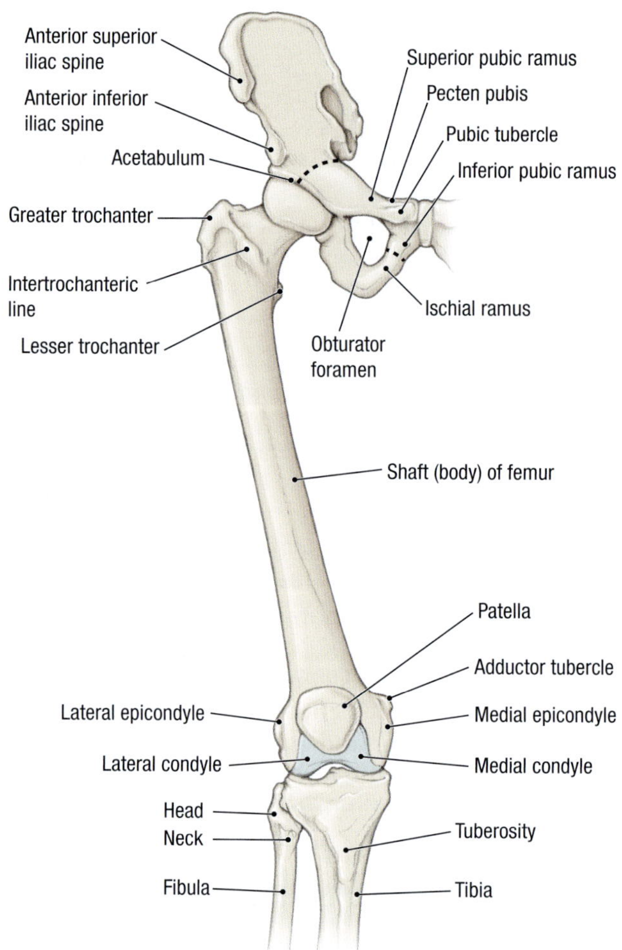

FIGURE 6.1 ● Skeleton of right hip, thigh, and knee. Anterior view.

Anterior Femur

ATLAS 6.2A, 6.30A

1. Refer to FIGURE 6.1.
2. On the superolateral aspect of the proximal femur, identify the **greater trochanter**.
3. On the anterior aspect of the proximal femur, follow the **intertrochanteric line** inferomedially from the greater trochanter to the **lesser trochanter**.
4. On the distal femur laterally, identify the **lateral epicondyle** superior to the **lateral condyle**.
5. On the distal femur medially, identify the **adductor tubercle** on the **medial epicondyle** superior to the **medial condyle**.

Anterior Proximal Tibia, Fibula, and Patella

ATLAS 6.2A

1. Refer to FIGURE 6.1.
2. On the proximal tibia, identify the **medial** and **lateral condyles**.
3. Observe that the **fibular head** articulates with the tibia inferior to the lateral condyle but does not articulate with the femur.
4. On the anterior surface of the proximal tibia, identify the **tibial tuberosity**.
5. On the **patella**, identify the anterior surface and the articular surface (posterior).

Surface Anatomy

The surface anatomy of the lower limb may be studied on a living subject or on a cadaver. On the cadaver, note that fixation of tissue during embalming may make it difficult to distinguish bone from well-preserved soft tissues in some specimens.

Lower Limb

ATLAS 6.1A

1. Refer to FIGURE 6.2.
2. Place the cadaver in the supine position.
3. Beginning on the lateral aspect of the hip, palpate the **iliac crest**.
4. Follow the path of the iliac crest anteriorly and identify the **ASIS** on the anterior aspect of the hip. *Note that the ASIS should be palpable even in larger cadavers because little Camper's fascia develops at this location.*
5. Move your fingers inferomedially from the ASIS to the pubic region following the path of the inguinal ligament and palpate the **pubic tubercle**.
6. In the midline of the lower limb, between the thigh and leg, palpate the **patella** or "kneecap" on the anterior aspect of the knee.
7. Observe that the patella has a relatively small degree of mobility in the fixed tissue of the embalmed cadaver compared to a living individual.
8. At the knee, palpate the **medial femoral epicondyle** and **lateral femoral epicondyle** on the medial and lateral aspects of the knee, respectively.
9. On the anterior aspect of the leg beginning just below the knee, palpate the **tibial tuberosity** and then, continuing inferiorly toward the ankle, palpate the **anterior border of the tibia**.
10. At the ankle, palpate the **medial malleolus** and **lateral malleolus** on the medial and lateral aspects of the ankle, respectively.

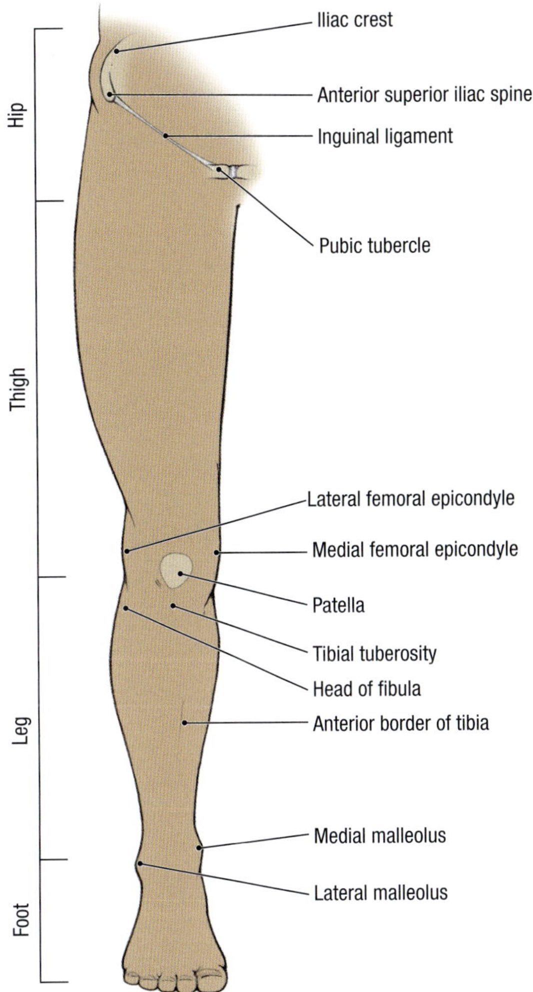

FIGURE 6.2 Surface anatomy of right lower limb. Anterior view.

Dissection Instructions

Dissection Note: Prior to commencing with skin incisions, note that the superficial veins and cutaneous nerves are easily damaged in the lower limb if skin incisions are made too deeply. It is thus recommended that along the medial and anterior surface of the limb, a partial-thickness skinning technique be implemented. If you are not studying the superficial veins or nerves, perform a full-thickness approach and either reflect or remove the skin from the dissection field. See **Removing Skin** in the **Introduction Chapter** for descriptions.

Skin Incisions of Lower Limb

VIDEO 6.1.1

1. Refer to FIGURE 6.3.
2. Place the cadaver in the supine position.
3. Make an incision from the ASIS (F) along the inguinal ligament (Q) to the pubic tubercle. *Note that if the abdomen has previously been dissected, this incision has been made.*
4. Extend the cut from the pubic tubercle inferiorly along the medial side of the thigh (D). *Note that if the perineum has previously been dissected, this incision has been made.*
5. Elevate the skin overlying the inguinal ligament (Q) to verify the depth of the skin and subcutaneous tissue of the region.
6. Make a vertical incision from the midpoint of the inguinal ligament (Q) inferiorly through the thigh, bisecting the skin overlying the patella until you reach the tibial tuberosity (R) in the leg.

Dissection Note: While making the skin incision along the thigh, preserve the underlying superficial veins and pay attention to not cut too deeply through the thin skin overlying the knee to avoid damaging the underlying tendons.

7. Extend the vertical incision from the tibial tuberosity (R) following the path of the anterior border of the tibia to a point just superior to the ankle (S).
8. Continue the vertical incision from the leg along the dorsum of the foot until a point just proximal to the toes (G).
9. Carefully make a shallow transverse incision across the dorsum of the foot just proximal to the webs of

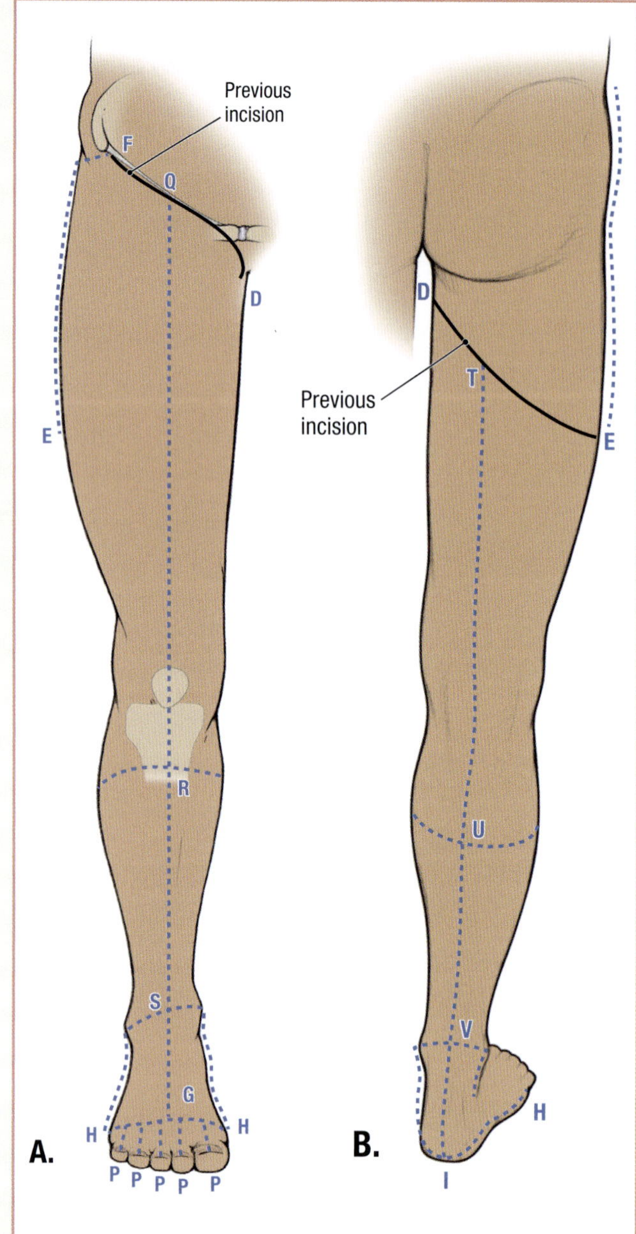

FIGURE 6.3 ● Skin incisions of right lower limb. **A.** Anterior view. **B.** Posterior view.

the toes (H to H). *Note that the skin is very thin on the dorsum of the foot, and care must be taken to not cut too deeply.*

10. Make a transverse skin incision from the anterior aspect of the leg (S) medially to the medial malleolus and laterally to the lateral malleolus.
11. Make a transverse skin incision from the tibial tuberosity (R) around the anterior aspect of the leg both medially and laterally to the periphery of the limb.
12. Reflect the skin from the lower limb beginning at the vertical incision at the midline of the inguinal ligament (Q) to the dorsum of the foot (G) medially and laterally as far as possible from the supine position.
13. Make additional transverse skin incisions as needed to speed up the skinning process by dividing the skinned regions into smaller portions.
14. Detach the skin from the dorsum of the foot peripherally along the medial and lateral aspects of the foot (I to H) while leaving the thick skin of the sole of the foot intact.
15. If the toes will be dissected, make a cut along the dorsal midline of each toe from the horizontal line across the webbing of the toes (H to H) to the proximal end of the nail (P) and remove the skin from the dorsal surface of each digit.
16. Place the cadaver in the prone position.
17. If the skin of the gluteal region has not previously been removed, work from medial to lateral and detach the skin from the gluteal region and lateral side of the hip (F to E).
18. Make an incision along the posterior midline of the thigh beginning at a point inferior to the gluteal folds (T) to a point inferior to the knee (U).
19. Continue the vertical incision from just below the knee (U) to a point posterior to the ankle overlying the calcaneal tendon (V).
20. Carefully extend the vertical incision from the posterior aspect of the ankle (V) along the path of the calcaneal tendon, paying attention to not cut too deeply until you reach the inferior aspect of the heel (I).
21. Extend the transverse skin incisions begun around the anterior surface of the limb at both the knee and ankle to join the vertical incision along the posterior aspect of the limb (T to I).
22. Beginning at the vertical incision (T to I), reflect large portions of the skin medially and laterally to the peripheral aspects of the lower limb.
23. Remove the skin from the thigh and leg and place it in the tissue container. Do not yet remove the skin from the sole of the foot.

Dissection Note: Reflecting the skin with portions still attached will block views of the underlying anatomy; thus, it is recommended to completely remove the skin. If the skin is removed in large portions, it may, however, be used later to wrap the lower limb postdissection to prevent desiccation.

Subcutaneous Tissue of Posterior Lower Limb

ATLAS 6.9B, 6.18; VIDEO 6.1.2

1. Refer to FIGURE 6.4B.
2. With the cadaver in the prone position, examine the structures contained in the **subcutaneous tissue** of the posterior lower limb.
3. Identify and clean the **small (lesser) saphenous vein** where it passes posterior to the lateral malleolus at the ankle and observe that it arises from the lateral end of the **dorsal venous arch of the foot.**

4. Use blunt dissection to follow the small saphenous vein superiorly and observe that it pierces the deep fascia overlying the **popliteal fossa** to drain into the popliteal vein. Do not follow the small saphenous vein into the popliteal fossa at this time.

5. Identify the **sural nerve** on the posterior aspect of the leg. Observe that the sural nerve pierces the deep fascia halfway down the posterior aspect of the leg and courses parallel to the small saphenous vein. *Note that the sural nerve innervates the skin of the lateral aspect of the ankle and foot.*

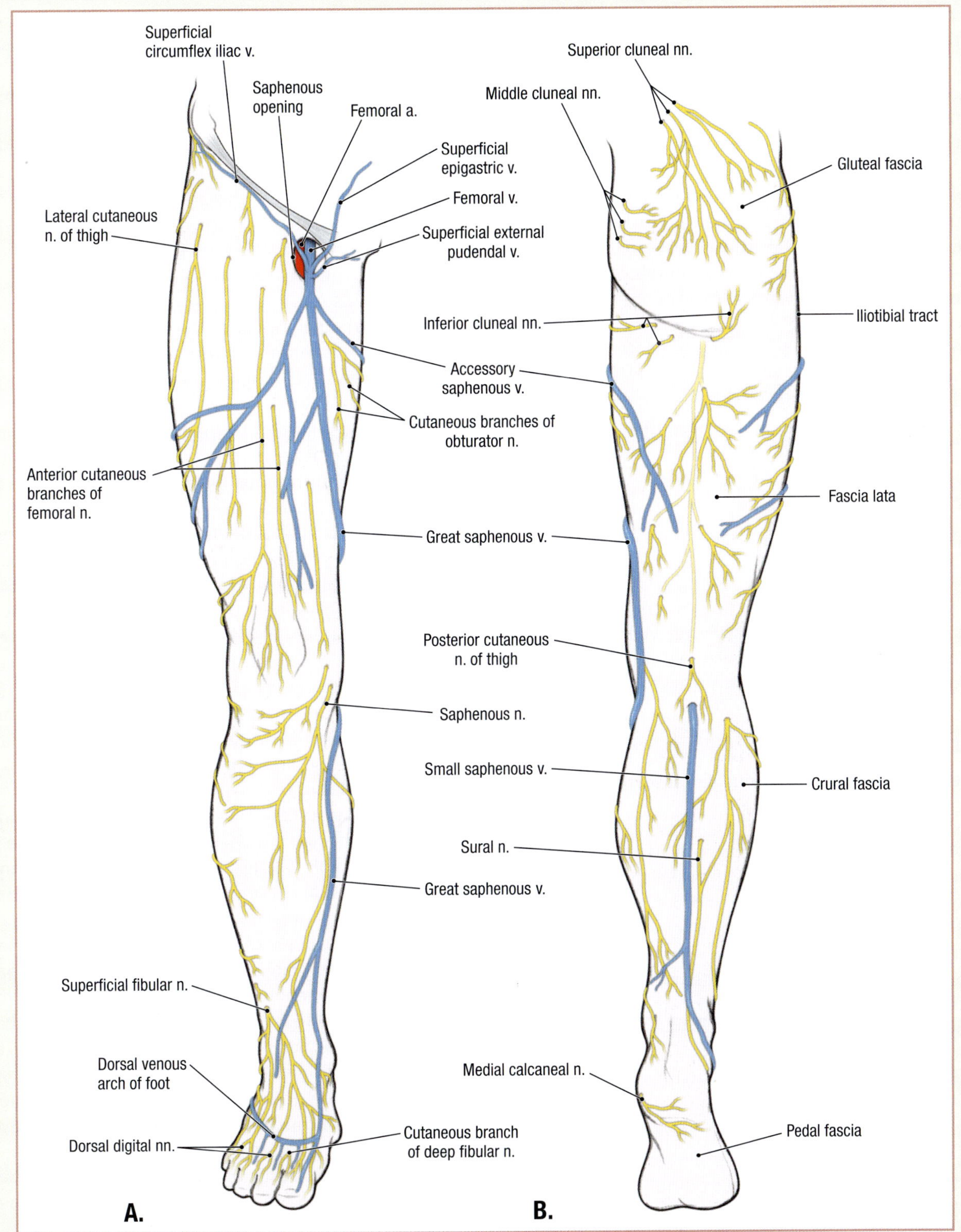

FIGURE 6.4 Cutaneous nerves, superficial veins, and deep fascia of right lower limb. **A.** Anterior view. **B.** Posterior view.

6. Identify the **posterior cutaneous nerve of the thigh** overlying the posterior aspect of the popliteal fossa. The posterior cutaneous nerve of the thigh is difficult to follow superiorly because it lies deep to the deep fascia. *Note that branches of this nerve pierce the deep fascia to supply the skin on the posterior surface of the thigh and popliteal fossa.*
7. Identify the **cluneal nerves**, which innervate the skin of the gluteal region if they have not already been cut or removed.
8. Observe that the **superior cluneal nerves** (posterior rami of L1–L3) and **middle cluneal nerves** (posterior rami of S1–S3) innervate the upper and middle parts of the buttock.
9. Observe that the **inferior cluneal nerves** (posterior rami of S2–S3) and branches of the **posterior cutaneous nerve of the thigh** (posterior rami of S1–S3) wrap around the inferior border of the gluteus maximus and innervate the skin over the lower part of the buttock.
10. Remove all remnants of subcutaneous tissue from the posterior aspect of the gluteal region, thigh, and leg while preserving the deep fascia, cutaneous nerves, and superficial veins that have been dissected.

Subcutaneous Tissue of Anterior Lower Limb

ATLAS 6.9A, 6.14A, 6.18; VIDEO 6.1.3

1. Refer to FIGURE 6.4A.
2. Turn the cadaver to the supine position.
3. Identify and clean the **great saphenous vein** where it courses anterior to the medial malleolus at the ankle (see **Clinical Correlation 6.1**).

CLINICAL CORRELATION 6.1

Varicose Veins and Saphenous Cut Down

ATLAS 6.14A, 6.15B

Superficial and perforating veins contain valves that prevent the backflow of blood. If the valves become incompetent, the veins distend and become tortuous, a condition known as varicose veins.

Clinically, the great saphenous vein may be used as a point of entrance for cannulation to provide a patient with prolonged administration of drugs, blood, or electrolytes. The great saphenous vein is accessed by making a small incision anterior to the medial malleolus, a procedure known as saphenous cut down. Portions of the great saphenous vein may also be removed and used as graft vessels in coronary bypass surgery, although the vessel direction would need to be reversed so the valves do not prevent arterial blood flow.

4. Follow the great saphenous vein into the foot and observe that it arises from the medial end of the **dorsal venous arch of the foot.**
5. Use blunt dissection to follow the great saphenous vein toward the knee and observe that it passes posterior to the medial epicondyle of the femur. *Note that the location of the great saphenous vein posterior to the knee reduces tension on the vessel when the knee is flexed and may usually be found about a hand's span posterior to the patella.*
6. Continue to follow the great saphenous vein into the thigh and observe that beginning at the level of the knee, it courses anterolaterally to eventually lie on the anterior surface of the proximal thigh.
7. Along the course of the great saphenous vein, identify the many unnamed superficial veins, which drain into it, as well as the **perforating veins**, which connect the great saphenous vein to the deep venous system.
8. On the medial aspect of the thigh, identify the **accessory saphenous vein**, a named tributary that drains the subcutaneous tissue and skin of the medial side of the thigh.
9. About 4 cm inferior to the inguinal ligament, observe that the great saphenous vein pierces the **saphenous opening (saphenous hiatus)** to drain into the femoral vein.

Dissection Note: The saphenous opening, a thinning in the deep fascia of the thigh (fascia lata), will be dissected later. Do not disrupt the saphenous opening at this time.

10. Observe that at the saphenous opening, the **superficial external pudendal vein**, the **superficial epigastric vein**, and the **superficial circumflex iliac vein** join the great saphenous vein.
11. In the proximal thigh, identify the **lateral femoral cutaneous nerve** where it passes deep to the lateral end of the inguinal ligament to innervate the skin of the lateral thigh.
12. Identify the **anterior cutaneous branches of the femoral nerve**, which innervate the skin of the anterior thigh. Observe that the cutaneous branches of the femoral nerve enter the subcutaneous tissue lateral to the great saphenous vein.
13. On the medial side of the knee, identify the **saphenous nerve** where it pierces the deep fascia to accompany the great saphenous vein into the leg. *Note that the saphenous nerve is a branch of the femoral nerve that innervates the skin on the anterior and medial sides of the leg and medial side of the ankle and foot.*
14. Medial to the great saphenous vein, identify the **cutaneous branches of the obturator nerve**, which innervate the skin of the medial thigh.
15. Identify the **superficial fibular nerve** in the distal third of the leg where it pierces the deep fascia of the leg superior to the lateral malleolus.

16. Follow the superficial fibular nerve onto the dorsum of the foot. *Note that the superficial fibular nerve innervates the dorsum of the foot and sends dorsal digital nerves to the skin of the toes.*
17. On the dorsum of the foot, identify the **dorsal digital branches of the deep fibular nerve** between the 1st (great) and 2nd toes. *Note that the innervation pattern between the toes is used for the assessment of deep fibular nerve function.*
18. Refer to FIGURE 6.5.
19. In the proximal thigh, identify the location of the **horizontal group of superficial inguinal lymph nodes** located about 2 cm inferior to the inguinal ligament.
20. Identify the **vertical group of superficial inguinal lymph nodes** encircling the proximal end of the **great saphenous vein**. *Note that the superficial inguinal lymph nodes collect lymphatic drainage from the lower limb, inferior part of the anterior abdominal wall, gluteal region, perineum, and external genitalia.*
21. Identify the **deep inguinal lymph nodes** through the fascia overlying the **saphenous opening** but do not yet dissect them. *Note that the deep inguinal lymph nodes collect lymphatic drainage from the superficial nodes and drain through the femoral canal into the abdomen deep to the inguinal ligament.*
22. Remove the remnants of subcutaneous tissue from the anterior thigh, leg, and foot while preserving the superficial veins, cutaneous nerves, and deep fascia.
23. Refer back to FIGURE 6.4.
24. Examine the deep fascia of the lower limb beginning with the **gluteal fascia** overlying the gluteal muscles.

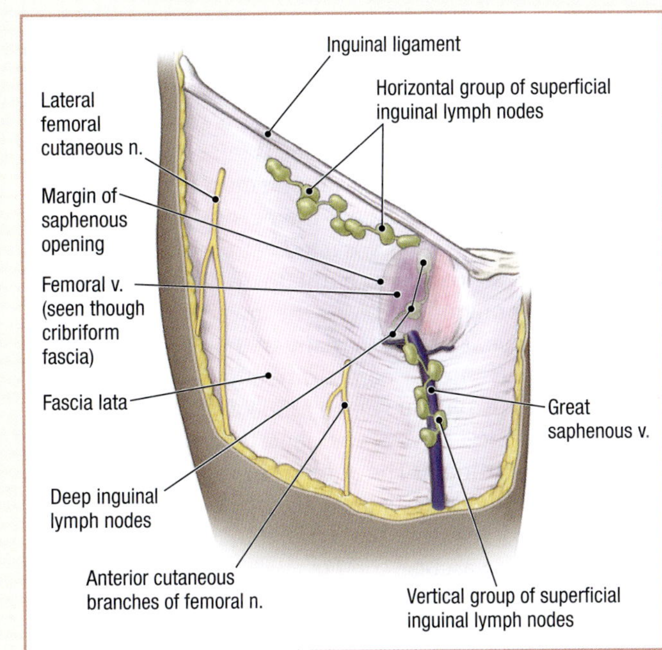

FIGURE 6.5 ● Saphenous opening and superficial inguinal lymph nodes. Anterior view.

25. Progress inferiorly and identify the **fascia lata** in the thigh, which thickens laterally to form the **iliotibial tract (IT band)**.
26. Identify the **crural fascia**, the deep fascia of the leg, and observe how tight and thick it is compared to the fascia lata.
27. Identify the **pedal fascia**, the deep fascia of the foot.

Dissection Follow-up

1. Trace the course of the superficial veins from distal to proximal and note where perforating veins drain deeply.
2. Review the location and pattern of distribution of the cutaneous nerves of the lower limb.
3. Review the location and attachments of the deep fascia of the lower limb.
4. Review the lymphatic drainage of the lower limb.

ANTERIOR COMPARTMENT OF THIGH

Dissection Overview

The fascia lata is connected to the femur by intermuscular septa to form the three fascial compartments of the thigh: anterior (extensor), medial (adductor), and posterior (flexor) compartments as shown in FIGURE 6.6. The muscles found within each compartment receive motor innervation primarily through a single nerve. Thus, the anterior compartment is related to the femoral nerve, the medial compartment to the obturator nerve, and the posterior compartment to branches of the sciatic nerve. The muscles located on the borders of two compartments receive dual innervation and thus are often categorized differently in various texts.

The anterior compartment of the thigh contains the iliopsoas, sartorius, and quadriceps femoris (rectus femoris, vastus lateralis, vastus intermedius, and vastus medialis). For ease of dissection, the pectineus and tensor of fascia lata will be dissected with the muscles of the anterior compartment of the thigh. The femoral artery, the major blood supply to the lower limb, and the femoral nerve, along with many of their branches, pass through the anterior compartment of the thigh.

The order of dissection will be as follows: The fascia lata of the thigh will be reviewed, and the saphenous opening will be studied. The anterior surface of the superior part of the fascia lata will be opened to expose the femoral triangle. The femoral triangle will be dissected, and its vascular contents will be followed distally. The sartorius will be identified, and the adductor canal will be dissected. The anterior surface of the inferior part of the fascia lata will be opened, and the remaining anterior thigh muscles will be studied.

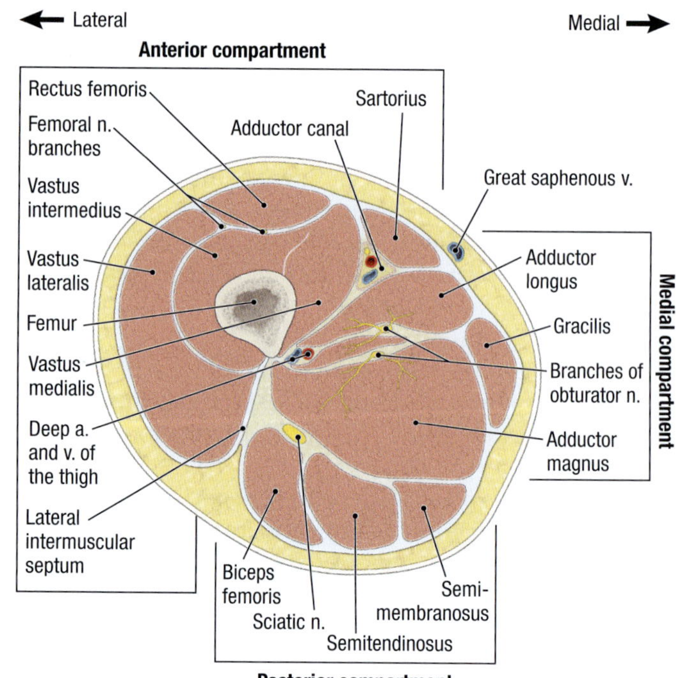

FIGURE 6.6 ● Axial section through right thigh. Inferior view.

Dissection Instructions

Saphenous Opening

ATLAS 6.19, 6.20; VIDEO 6.2.1

1. Refer to FIGURE 6.7.
2. Remove any remnants of subcutaneous tissue on the anterior surface of the fascia lata.

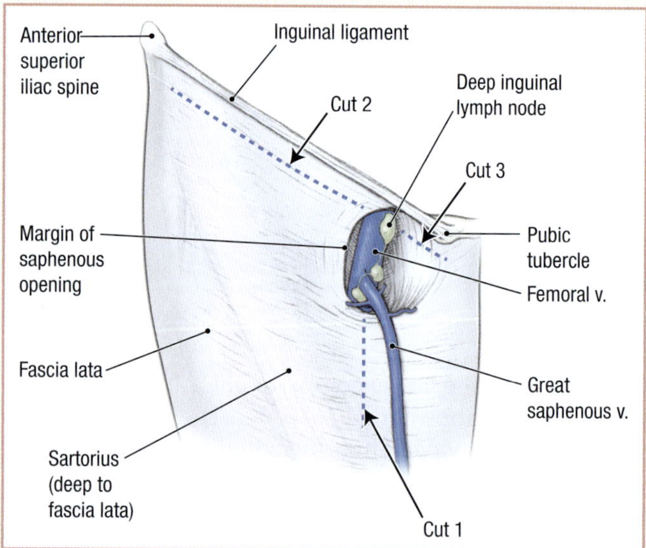

FIGURE 6.7 ● Opening fascia lata over right femoral triangle. Anterior view.

3. Remove the superficial inguinal lymph nodes around the saphenous opening while preserving the great saphenous vein.
4. Follow the great saphenous vein superiorly and observe that it passes through the **saphenous opening** approximately 4 cm inferior to the inguinal ligament.
5. Use blunt dissection to remove the connective tissue around the great saphenous vein where it penetrates the fascia lata and define the margin of the **saphenous opening**.
6. Observe that the saphenous opening is a natural weak point in the fascia lata covered with a relatively thin layer of fascia.
7. Trace the great saphenous vein through the saphenous opening and observe that it drains into the anterior aspect of the **femoral vein**.
8. Identify the path of the sartorius coursing deep to the fascia lata.
9. Use scissors to make a vertical incision through the fascia lata from the saphenous opening to the **sartorius** (**Cut 1**).
10. Use scissors to make a horizontal cut through the fascia lata laterally from the superior margin of the saphenous opening to a point directly inferior to the **ASIS** (**Cut 2**) paralleling the inguinal ligament.
11. Use scissors to make a second horizontal cut through the fascia lata medially from the superior margin of the saphenous opening to a point directly inferior to the **pubic tubercle** (**Cut 3**).

12. Use blunt dissection to elevate and separate the fascia lata from the underlying deeper structures.

Femoral Triangle

ATLAS 6.20B, 6.21; VIDEO 6.2.2

1. Refer to FIGURE 6.8.
2. Reflect the flaps of fascia lata medially and laterally to open the superficial boundary or "roof" of the **femoral triangle**.
3. Use scissors to remove the flaps of fascia lata overlying the femoral triangle and the anterior surface of the proximal thigh.
4. Observe that the base of the triangle (**superior border**) is formed by the **inguinal ligament** and its apex is directed inferiorly at the point where the sartorius crosses the adductor longus.
5. Identify and clean the proximal portion of the **sartorius**, which forms the **lateral boundary of the femoral triangle**.
6. Identify and clean the proximal portion of the **adductor longus**, which forms the **medial boundary of the femoral triangle**.
7. From lateral to medial, the major **contents of the femoral triangle** are the **femoral nerve**, **femoral artery**, and **femoral vein**. *Note that the femoral triangle also contains fat, fascia, lymphatics, branches of the femoral artery and nerve, and tributaries of the vein including the great saphenous vein.*
8. Retract the femoral artery, vein, and nerve and identify the two muscles forming the **floor of the femoral triangle**, the **iliopsoas** laterally and the **pectineus** medially. *Note that the iliacus and psoas major collectively are named the iliopsoas inferior to the inguinal ligament.*

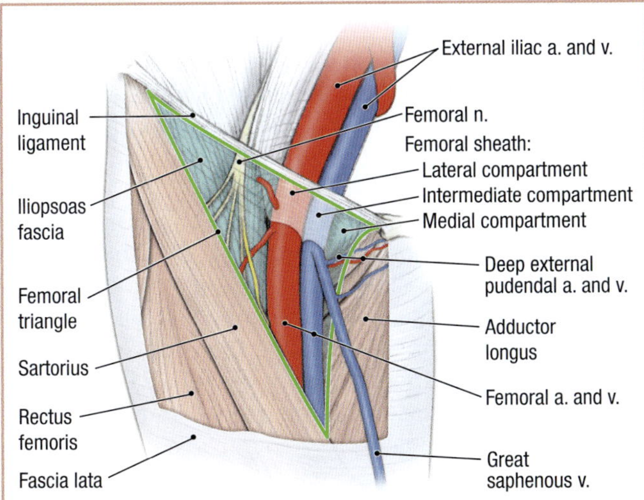

FIGURE 6.8 ● Boundaries and contents of right femoral triangle. Anterior view.

9. Identify the **femoral sheath**, an extension of transversalis fascia descending into the thigh from the abdominal cavity around the femoral vessels. The femoral sheath is divided into three compartments by fascial extensions.
10. Identify the femoral artery in the **lateral compartment** and the femoral vein in the **intermediate compartment** of the femoral sheath. Observe that the femoral vessels are the continuation of the external iliac vessels, with the name changing at the inguinal ligament.
11. The medial compartment of the femoral sheath is also called the **femoral canal**, and its proximal opening into the abdominal cavity is the **femoral ring** (see **Clinical Correlation 6.2**). *Note that the femoral canal contains lymphatic vessels and lymph nodes and is more readily seen from the abdominal side of the inguinal ligament.*

CLINICAL CORRELATION 6.2

Femoral Triangle and Femoral Hernia

ATLAS 6.21

Within the femoral triangle, the pulse of the femoral artery can be palpated about 3 cm inferior to the midpoint of the inguinal ligament. The femoral vein lies immediately medial to the femoral artery and lateral to the space of the femoral ring. A catheter introduced into the femoral artery can be advanced superiorly into the aorta and its branches. A catheter introduced into the femoral vein can be advanced superiorly into the inferior vena cava and the right atrium of the heart.

The femoral ring is a site of potential femoral herniation, a protrusion of abdominal viscera through the femoral ring into the femoral canal. Contents within the femoral hernia may become incarcerated or strangulated due to the inflexibility of the surrounding structures.

12. Observe that the lateral-to-medial arrangement of structures passing deep to the inguinal ligament (including the contents of the femoral sheath) can be identified by use of the mnemonic device **NAVL** (pronounced navel): femoral **N**erve, femoral **A**rtery, femoral **V**ein, and **L**ymphatics.
13. Identify the **femoral nerve** lateral to the femoral artery and observe that it lies on the floor of the femoral triangle external to the femoral sheath.
14. Follow the femoral nerve inferiorly and observe that it divides into numerous branches to innervate the muscles and skin of the anterior thigh.
15. Verify that the **anterior cutaneous branches of the femoral nerve** enter the subcutaneous tissue by penetrating the fascia lata along the anterior surface of the sartorius.

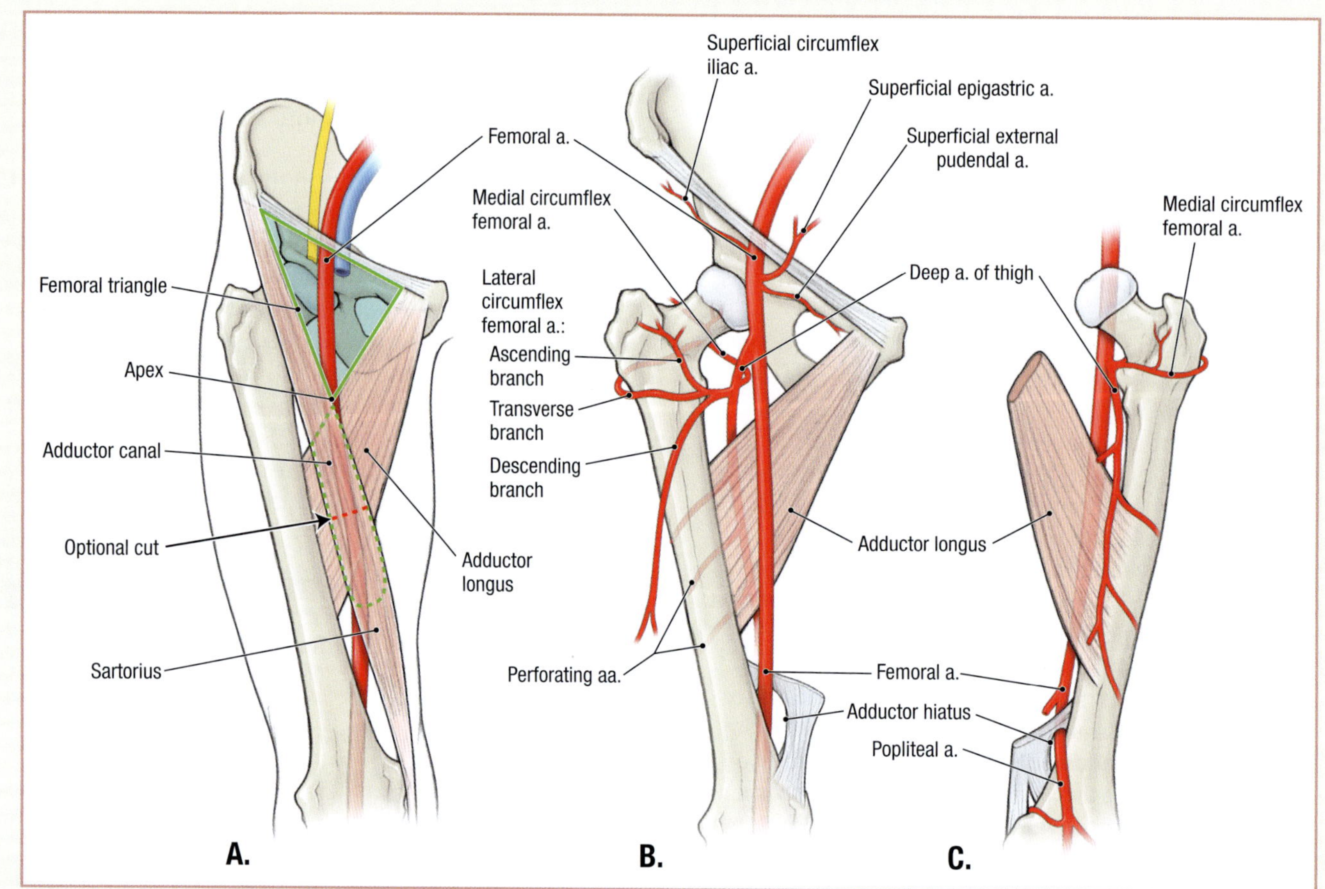

FIGURE 6.9 ■ **A.** Femoral triangle and adductor canal. Anterior view. **B.** Branches of femoral artery. Anterior view. **C.** Deep artery of thigh and medial circumflex femoral artery. Posterior view.

16. Use blunt dissection to clean the **femoral artery** and **femoral vein** within the femoral triangle.
17. Refer to FIGURE 6.9A.
18. Observe that inferior to the apex of the femoral triangle, the **femoral artery and vein** course between the sartorius and the adductor longus and enter a space known as the **adductor canal**. Do not yet dissect the adductor canal because this will be done later.
19. Refer to FIGURE 6.9B.
20. Inferior to the inguinal ligament, identify and clean the **superficial epigastric artery** coursing superiorly and superficially from the femoral artery.
21. Coursing more deeply from the femoral artery, identify and clean the laterally oriented **superficial circumflex iliac artery** and the medially oriented **superficial external pudendal artery**.
22. Gently retract the femoral artery medially and identify the **deep artery of the thigh (profunda femoris)** coursing parallel to the femoral artery but *posterior* to the adductor longus. *Note that the deep artery of the thigh supplies the medial and posterior compartments of the thigh.*
23. Identify and clean the **lateral circumflex femoral artery** arising from the deep artery of the thigh. *Note that the lateral circumflex femoral artery may arise from the deep artery of the thigh or directly from the femoral artery.*
24. Follow the lateral circumflex femoral artery laterally deep to the superior end of the rectus femoris and observe that it supplies the muscles and soft tissues of the lateral part of the thigh by three main branches: ascending, transverse, and descending.
25. Identify the **ascending branch**, which passes superiorly deep to the tensor of the fascia lata to anastomose with the superior gluteal and deep circumflex iliac arteries.
26. Identify the **transverse branch**, which passes deep to the rectus femoris to anastomose with the medial circumflex femoral artery.
27. Identify the **descending branch**, which also passes deep to the rectus femoris and then courses inferiorly on the anterior surface of the vastus intermedius to anastomose with the genicular arteries at the knee.
28. Refer to FIGURE 6.9C.
29. Identify the **medial circumflex femoral artery** arising from the deep artery of the thigh. *Note that the medial circumflex femoral artery may arise from the*

deep artery of the thigh or directly from the femoral artery.

30. Follow the medial circumflex femoral artery posteriorly between the pectineus and iliopsoas. *Note that in addition to supplying the soft tissues of the region, the medial circumflex femoral artery provides an important blood supply to the neck of the femur.*
31. Carefully retract the femoral vessels to clean the surface of the iliopsoas and pectineus forming the floor of the femoral triangle.
32. Review the attachments and actions of the iliopsoas and pectineus (see **TABLE 6.1**).

Adductor Canal and Sartorius

ATLAS 6.22, 6.28; VIDEO 6.2.3

1. Refer to FIGURE 6.9A and FIGURE 6.10.
2. Identify the **adductor canal**, a fascial compartment located deep to the sartorius containing the femoral artery, vein, and nerve branches.
3. Observe that the adductor canal begins at the **apex of the femoral triangle** and ends at the **adductor hiatus** near the knee. *Note that the adductor hiatus demarcates the transition point of femoral vessels within the adductor canal and popliteal vessels within the popliteal fossa.*
4. Use scissors to cut the fascia lata along the superficial surface of the sartorius from the ASIS to the medial epicondyle of the femur.
5. Use blunt dissection to separate the **sartorius** from the deep fascia enclosing it and observe that the sartorius crosses both the hip and knee joints.
6. Retract the sartorius so its superior and inferior attachments can be defined and its blood and nerve supplies can be identified.
7. Review the attachments and actions of the sartorius (see **TABLE 6.1**).
8. Gently pull the sartorius laterally and observe a sheath of dense connective tissue encloses the femoral vessels within the **adductor canal**.
9. Use scissors to open the adductor canal along its anterior aspect and observe that inferiorly the **femoral vein** lies posterior to the **femoral artery**. Recall that in the femoral triangle, the femoral vessels were side by side with the vein positioned medial to the artery.
10. Use blunt dissection to follow the femoral artery distally through the **adductor hiatus**, where its name changes to **popliteal artery**.
11. Within the adductor canal, identify two named branches of the femoral nerve, the **nerve to vastus medialis** and the **saphenous nerve**. *Note that the nerve to vastus medialis provides motor innervation to the vastus medialis and that the saphenous nerve is a cutaneous nerve innervating the skin on the medial side of the leg, ankle, and foot.*
12. If visibility of the contents within the adductor canal is limited, on one side of the cadaver, cut the sartorius at its midpoint and reflect the muscle halves superiorly and inferiorly (**Optional cut**).

Quadriceps Femoris

ATLAS 6.5, 6.24, 6.25; VIDEO 6.2.4

1. Refer to FIGURE 6.10.
2. Use scissors to make a vertical cut through the fascia lata from the apex of the femoral triangle superiorly to the superior border of the patella inferiorly.

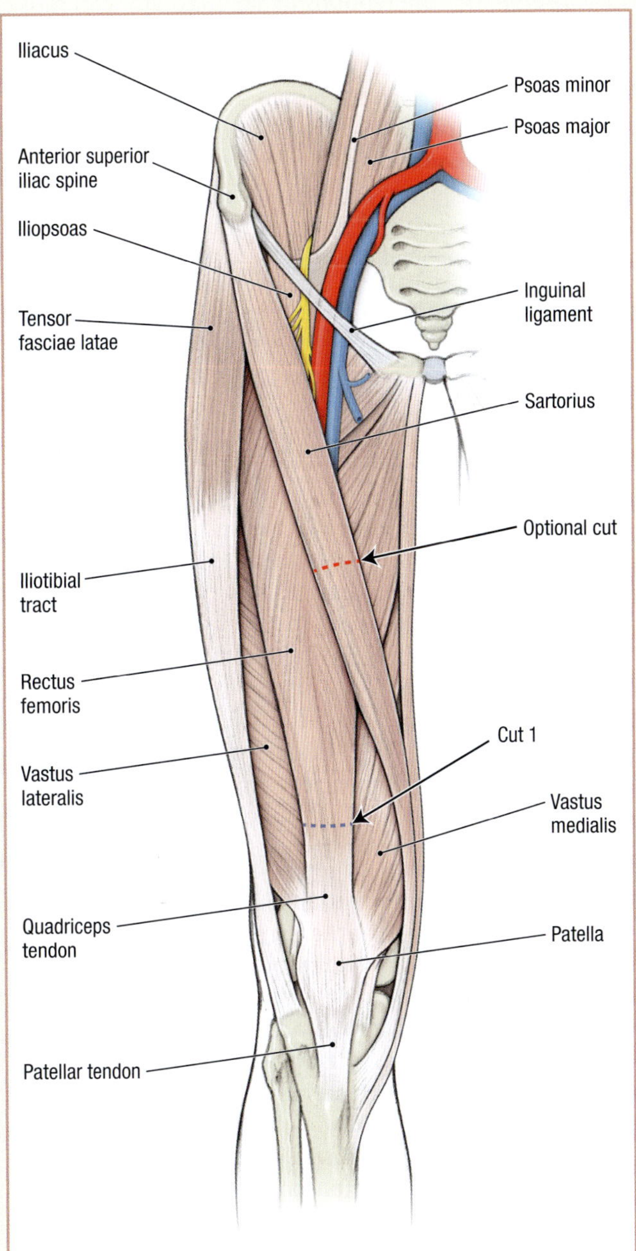

FIGURE 6.10 ■ Anterior compartment of right thigh. Anterior view.

3. Make a transverse incision in the fascia lata superior to the patella extending from the medial femoral epicondyle to the lateral femoral epicondyle.
4. Use blunt dissection to open the fascia lata widely and follow the inner surface laterally to verify that it is attached to the **lateral intermuscular septum**. *Note that the lateral intermuscular septum is attached to the linea aspera on the posterior aspect of the femur.*
5. Identify the **quadriceps femoris** (rectus femoris, vastus lateralis, vastus intermedius, and vastus medialis) and observe that it occupies most of the anterior compartment of the thigh.
6. Observe that the tendons of all four quadricep muscles unite to form the **quadriceps femoris tendon** superior to the patella.
7. Inferior to the patella, identify the **patellar (tendon) ligament** attaching to the tibial tuberosity (see **Clinical Correlation 6.3**). *Note that the patella is a sesamoid bone formed within a tendon; therefore, the inferior attachment of the quadriceps femoris is ultimately on the tibial tuberosity.*

CLINICAL CORRELATION 6.3

Patellar Tendon (Quadriceps) Reflex

ATLAS 6.10B, 6.48

Tapping the patellar tendon stimulates the patellar reflex (quadriceps reflex; knee jerk) and tests the function of the femoral nerve and spinal cord. Tapping the tendon activates muscle spindles in the quadriceps femoris, sending afferent impulses in the femoral nerve to spinal cord segments L2–L4. Within the spinal cord, an interneuron rapidly sends the incoming sensory information from the posterior horn to the motor cell bodies in the anterior horn of gray matter. Efferent impulses are then carried by the femoral nerve to the quadriceps femoris, resulting in a brief muscular contraction under normal function.

8. Identify and clean the surface of the **rectus femoris** in the midline of the anterior thigh and observe that it crosses the hip and knee joints and thus will assist movement at both joints.
9. Identify and clean the surface of the **vastus lateralis** on the lateral side of the anterior thigh.
10. Identify and clean the surface of the **vastus medialis** on the medial side of the anterior thigh.
11. On one side of the cadaver, transect the rectus femoris (**Cut 1**) and reflect its component parts superiorly and inferiorly.
12. Deep to the reflected rectus femoris, identify the **vastus intermedius** between the vastus lateralis and vastus medialis.

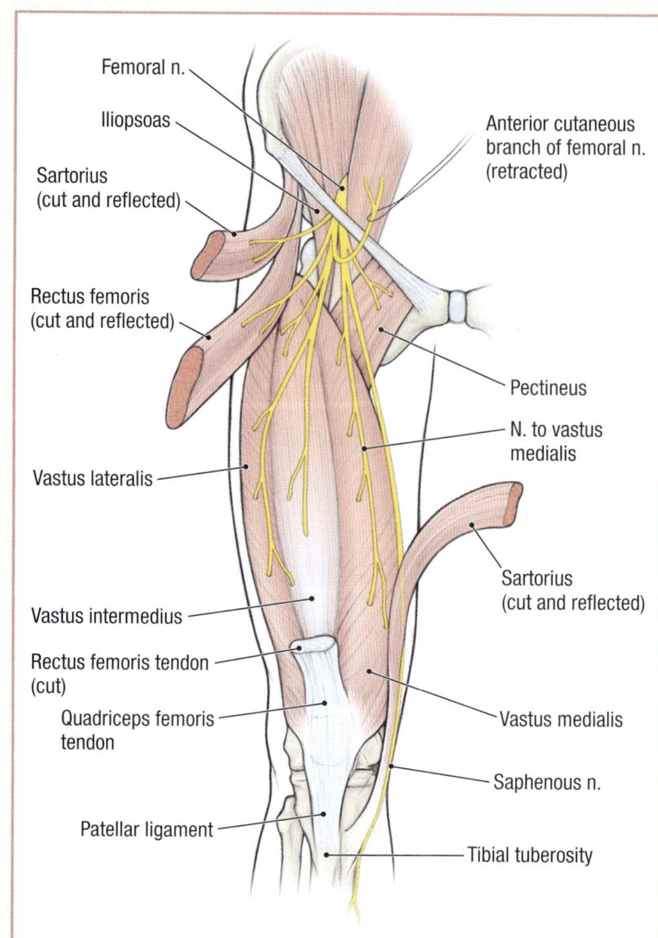

FIGURE 6.11 Branches of right femoral nerve. Anterior view.

13. Review the attachments and actions of the quadriceps (see **TABLE 6.1**).
14. Refer to FIGURE 6.11.
15. Observe that the descending branch of the lateral circumflex femoral artery can be seen on the anterior surface of the vastus intermedius deep to the rectus femoris.
16. Identify the **motor branches of the femoral nerve** to the anterior thigh muscles. *Note that the femoral nerve innervates the sartorius and pectineus in addition to innervating the quadriceps femoris.*
17. Locate the nerve to vastus medialis within the adductor canal and follow its branches to the vastus medialis.

Tensor of Fascia Lata

ATLAS 6.24A, 6.29; VIDEO 6.2.5

1. Refer back to FIGURE 6.10.
2. Identify the **IT band** on the lateral aspect of the thigh.

3. Elevate the remaining fascia lata from the anterior aspect of the thigh and cut through the fascia along a line from the ASIS superiorly to a point just lateral to the lateral femoral condyle inferiorly. Leave most of the fascia undisturbed along the lateral aspect of the thigh and just define the anterior edge of the IT tract at this time.
4. Within the IT band proximally, identify the **tensor fasciae latae (tensor of the fascia lata, TFL)**. *Note that the TFL is often categorized with the gluteal muscles despite its location on the anterior aspect of the hip due to its motor innervation by the superior gluteal nerve.*
5. Observe that the TFL is enclosed within the fascia lata inferior to the ASIS and connects to the IT tract distally. The IT tract serves to strengthen the lateral aspect of the knee and is an insertion point for the TFL and gluteus maximus.
6. Make a short incision through the fascia lata paralleling the anterior aspect of the TFL.
7. Use blunt dissection to separate the medial and lateral surfaces of the TFL from the surrounding fascia lata.
8. Remove a small portion of the fascia lata to expose the anterior and lateral surfaces of the TFL but do not disrupt the IT tract or the attachments of the muscle.
9. Review the attachments and actions of the TFL (see **TABLE 6.1**).

Dissection Follow-up

1. Use the dissected specimen to review the boundaries and contents of the femoral triangle.
2. Review the origin and course of the femoral artery and its branches in the thigh.
3. Review the attachments and actions of the muscles of the anterior compartment of the thigh as shown in **TABLE 6.1**.
4. Review the pattern of motor innervation to the muscles in the anterior compartment of the thigh, noting the muscles receiving dual innervation.
5. Replace the muscles of the anterior compartment of the thigh back to anatomical position.

TABLE 6.1 Muscles of Anterior Thigh

<table>
<tr><td colspan="5">ANTERIOR THIGH</td></tr>
<tr><td>Muscle</td><td>Proximal Attachments</td><td>Distal Attachments</td><td>Actions</td><td>Innervation</td></tr>
<tr><td>Pectineus</td><td>Pecten pubis and superior ramus of the pubis</td><td>Pectineal line of the femur</td><td>Adducts and flexes the thigh</td><td>Femoral n. and obturator n.</td></tr>
<tr><td>Iliopsoas</td><td>Iliac fossa (iliacus) and TP and bodies of vertebrae T12–L5 (psoas major)</td><td>Lesser trochanter of the femur</td><td>Flexes the thigh</td><td rowspan="2">Femoral n.</td></tr>
<tr><td>Sartorius</td><td>Anterior superior iliac spine</td><td>Medial surface of the proximal tibia</td><td>Flexes and laterally rotates the thigh; flexes and medially rotates the leg</td></tr>
<tr><td>Tensor fasciae latae</td><td>Anterior superior iliac spine</td><td>Iliotibial tract</td><td>Abducts, medially rotates, and flexes the thigh</td><td>Superior gluteal n.</td></tr>
<tr><td colspan="5">QUADRICEPS</td></tr>
<tr><td>Muscle</td><td>Proximal Attachments</td><td>Distal Attachments</td><td>Actions</td><td>Innervation</td></tr>
<tr><td>Rectus femoris</td><td>Anterior inferior iliac spine</td><td rowspan="4">Tibial tuberosity</td><td>Flexes the thigh and extends the leg</td><td rowspan="4">Femoral n.</td></tr>
<tr><td>Vastus medialis</td><td>Medial lip of the linea aspera and intertrochanteric line</td><td rowspan="3">Extends the leg</td></tr>
<tr><td>Vastus lateralis</td><td>Lateral lip of the linea aspera and greater trochanter</td></tr>
<tr><td>Vastus intermedius</td><td>Anterior and lateral surfaces of the femur</td></tr>
</table>

Abbreviations: L, lumbar vertebrae; n., nerve; T, thoracic vertebrae; TP, transverse process.

MEDIAL COMPARTMENT OF THIGH

Dissection Overview

The medial compartment of the thigh contains six muscles: gracilis, adductor longus, adductor brevis, pectineus, adductor magnus, and obturator externus. The muscles of the medial compartment are organized loosely into layers separated by the deep artery of the thigh and obturator nerve, the nerve responsible for providing motor innervation to the muscles. The shared function of the medial compartment of the thigh is to adduct the thigh; thus, this group of muscles is also known as the adductors.

The order of dissection will be as follows: The fascia lata will be removed from the medial thigh. The gracilis will be studied. The adductors will be separated from each other by following the medial circumflex femoral artery, the deep artery of the thigh, and the branches of the obturator nerve.

Dissection Instructions

Medial Compartment of Thigh

ATLAS 6.27, 6.28; VIDEO 6.3.1

1. Refer to FIGURE 6.12.
2. Use blunt dissection to elevate the fascia lata on the medial aspect of the thigh and identify the **gracilis**, the most medial muscle of the thigh.

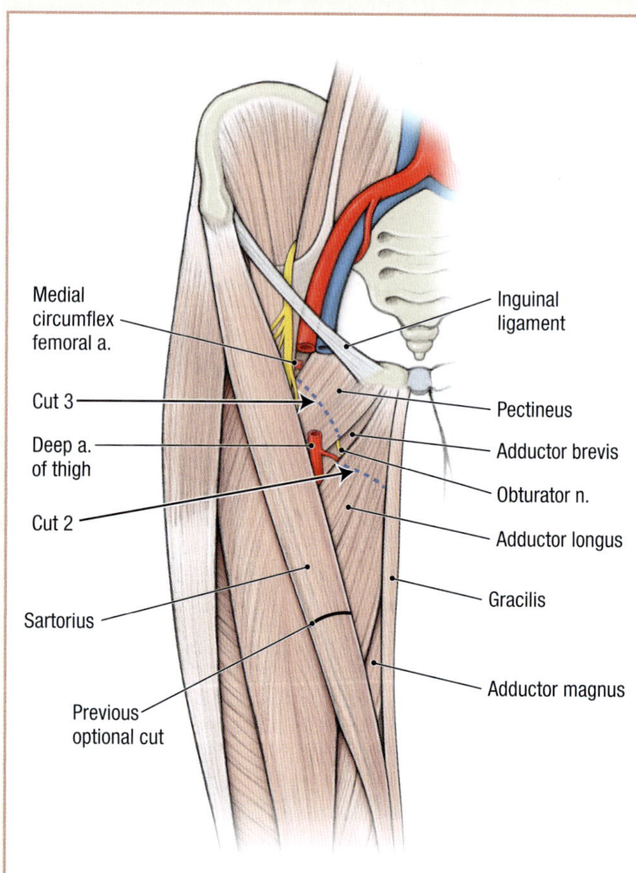

FIGURE 6.12 ■ Contents of medial compartment of right thigh. Anterior view.

3. Use scissors to cut the fascia lata from its attachments to the pelvis superiorly and along the medial intermuscular septum, paying attention not to remove the gracilis in the process.
4. Remove the cut portion of the fascia lata and place it in the tissue container.
5. Use blunt dissection to define the borders of the gracilis and observe that it crosses the hip and knee joints and thus will assist movement at both joints.
6. Review the attachments, actions, and innervation of the gracilis (see **TABLE 6.2**).
7. Lateral to the gracilis, identify the **adductor longus**, the medial boundary of the femoral triangle.
8. Lateral to the adductor longus, identify the **pectineus**, part of the floor of the femoral triangle.
9. Verify through palpation that the superior attachments of the gracilis, pectineus, and adductor longus are on the pubic bone.
10. Review the attachments, actions, and innervation of the adductor longus and pectineus (see **TABLE 6.2**).
11. Gently pull the adductor longus medially and the pectineus laterally to identify the location of the more deeply located **adductor brevis**.
12. Gently elevate the inferior edge of the adductor longus and identify the **adductor magnus**.
13. Observe that the adductor magnus lies deep to the adductor longus immediately lateral to the gracilis. *Note that the adductor magnus has both an adductor (pubofemoral) and a hamstring (ischiocondylar) portion and thus shares actions and innervations with the muscles in the medial and posterior compartments of the thigh.*
14. Review the attachments, actions, and innervation of the adductor brevis and adductor magnus (see **TABLE 6.2**).

Neurovasculature of Medial Thigh

ATLAS 6.6, 6.27, 6.28; VIDEO 6.3.1

1. Refer to FIGURE 6.12.
2. Within the femoral triangle, identify the **deep artery of the thigh** where it branches from the femoral artery.

3. Follow the deep artery of the thigh inferiorly and observe that it passes anterior to the pectineus and posterior to the adductor longus.
4. Use blunt dissection to define the borders of the pectineus and adductor longus while preserving the deep artery of the thigh.
5. Follow the deep artery of the thigh posterior to the adductor longus and observe that it courses between the adductor longus and adductor brevis.
6. Use blunt dissection to gently elevate the adductor longus.
7. On one side of the cadaver, transect the adductor longus 5 cm inferior to its superior attachment (**Cut 2**) and reflect the muscular portions superiorly and inferiorly to expose the **adductor brevis**.
8. On the same side of the cadaver where the adductor longus was transected, use blunt dissection to carefully elevate the pectineus and transect it near the path of the cut through the adductor longus (**Cut 3**).
9. Clean the deep artery of the thigh and identify one or two **perforating arteries**. *Note that the perforating arteries penetrate the adductor brevis and adductor magnus, encircle the femur, and supply the muscles of the posterior compartment of the thigh.*
10. Follow the medial circumflex femoral artery between the pectineus and iliopsoas and identify the underlying **obturator externus**. *Note that to clearly visualize the obturator externus, the pectineus and iliopsoas need to be transected and reflected, a step performed later with dissection of the hip joint.*
11. Review the attachments, actions, and innervation of the obturator externus.
12. Refer to FIGURE 6.13.
13. Identify the **obturator nerve** deep to the cut adductor longus and pectineus.
14. Observe that the obturator nerve splits into anterior and posterior branches around the adductor brevis in the medial compartment of the thigh.
15. On the anterior surface of the adductor brevis, identify the **anterior branch of the obturator nerve**.
16. Follow the anterior branch of the obturator nerve superiorly deep to the pectineus and use the nerve as a landmark to separate the pectineus from the adductor brevis. *Note that the superior border of the adductor brevis is deep to the pectineus.*
17. Use blunt dissection to clean the adductor brevis, paying attention not to damage the anterior branches of the obturator nerve.
18. Identify the **posterior branch of the obturator nerve** where it lies between the adductor brevis and adductor magnus.

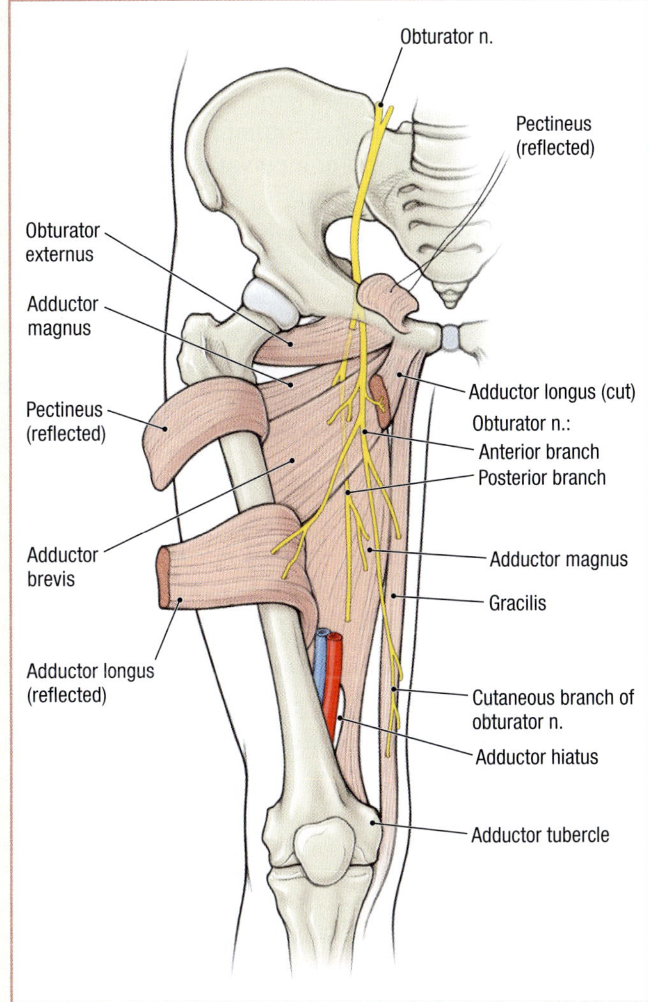

FIGURE 6.13 ● Branches of right obturator nerve. Anterior view.

19. Use blunt dissection to follow the posterior branch of the obturator nerve superiorly and use the nerve as a landmark to separate the adductor brevis from the adductor magnus.
20. Trace the tendon of the hamstring (ischiocondylar) part of the adductor magnus inferiorly to its attachment on the **adductor tubercle**.
21. On the lateral side of the tendon, identify the **adductor hiatus**, an opening in the adductor magnus between its two inferior attachments.
22. Observe that the femoral artery and vein course between the anterior compartment of the thigh and popliteal fossa by passing through the adductor hiatus. *Note that the adductor hiatus is the landmark where the femoral artery and vein change names to popliteal artery and vein.*

Dissection Follow-up

1. Review the attachments and actions of the muscles of the medial compartment of the thigh as shown in **TABLE 6.2**.
2. Trace the deep artery of the thigh from its origin to its termination as the fourth perforating artery.
3. Trace the medial circumflex femoral artery from its origin to where it passes between the iliopsoas and pectineus.
4. Review the branches of the obturator nerve and their respective relationships to the adductor brevis.
5. Recall the pattern of motor innervation to the muscles of the medial compartment of the thigh, noting the muscles that receive dual innervation.
6. Replace the medial thigh muscles in their correct anatomical positions.

TABLE 6.2 Muscles of Medial Thigh (Adductors)

Muscle	*Proximal Attachments*	*Distal Attachments*	*Actions*	*Innervation*
Gracilis	Body of pubis and inferior pubic ramus	Superior part of medial surface of tibia	Adducts the thigh; flexes and internally rotates the leg	Obturator n.
Pectineus	Superior pubic ramus	Pectineal line	Adducts the thigh	Obturator n. and femoral n.
Adductor longus	Body of pubis inferior to pubic crest	Middle third of linea aspera		Obturator n.
Adductor brevis	Body of pubis and inferior pubic ramus	Pectineal line and proximal part of linea aspera		
Adductor magnus	Ischiopubic ramus and ischial tuberosity	Gluteal tuberosity, linea aspera, medial supracondylar line (adductor part); adductor tubercle of the femur (hamstring part)	Adducts and extends the thigh	Obturator n. (adductor part); tibial division of the sciatic n. (hamstring part)
Obturator externus	External margins of obturator foramen and obturator membrane (medial attachment)	Trochanteric fossa of femur (lateral attachment)	Laterally rotates the thigh	Obturator n.

Abbreviation: n., nerve.

GLUTEAL REGION

Dissection Overview

The gluteal region is an area of transition between the trunk and the lower limb. The gluteal region lies on the posterior aspect of the pelvis and thus is part of the trunk anatomically; however, it contains muscles that extend, abduct, and laterally rotate the thigh. The two sides are separated by the intergluteal cleft, and each contains the area of the buttock and the hip.

The order of dissection will be as follows: The subcutaneous tissue will be removed from the gluteal region. The borders of the gluteus maximus will be defined, and it will be reflected laterally. Muscles that lie deep to the gluteus maximus will be studied. Arteries and nerves in the region will be studied.

Skeletal Anatomy

Refer to an articulated skeleton or disarticulated lower limb skeleton to identify the following skeletal features.

Posterior Hip

ATLAS 6.2B, 6.30C

1. Refer to FIGURE 6.14.
2. Identify the **iliac crest** on the superior aspect of the **ilium**.

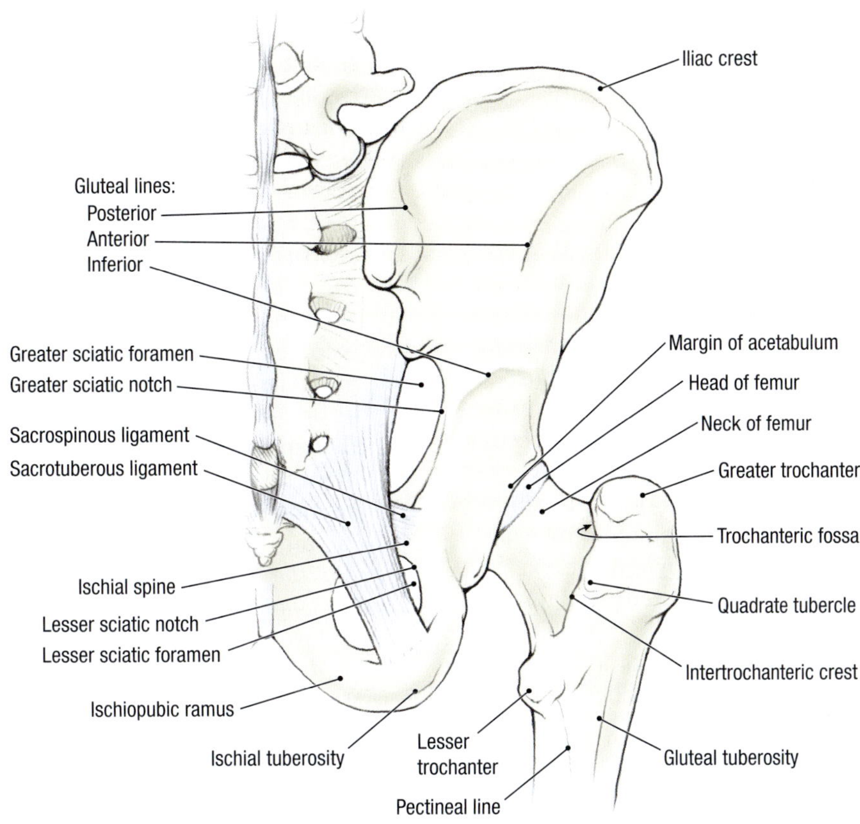

FIGURE 6.14 ● Skeleton of right gluteal region. Posterior view.

3. On the lateral (external) surface of the ilium, identify the **gluteal lines (posterior, anterior, inferior)**.
4. Observe the comparative proximity of the inferior gluteal line to the **margin of the acetabulum**, the rim of the cup-shaped depression of the **acetabulum** forming the socket of the hip joint with the **head of the femur**.
5. On the posterior aspect of the ilium, identify the **greater sciatic notch**.
6. Observe that the greater sciatic notch is located superior to the **ischial spine** and is part of the ilium, whereas the **lesser sciatic notch** is located inferior to the ischial spine and is part of the **ischium**.
7. On an articulated pelvis, identify the **sacrospinous ligament** connecting from the sacrum to the ischial spine. Observe that the greater sciatic notch forms part of the margin of the **greater sciatic foramen** along with the sacrospinous ligament.
8. On an articulated pelvis, identify the **sacrotuberous ligament** connecting from the sacrum to the **ischial tuberosity**. Observe that the lesser sciatic notch forms part of the margin of the **lesser sciatic foramen** with the sacrotuberous and sacrospinous ligaments.

Proximal Posterior Femur

ATLAS 6.2B, 6.30C

1. Refer to FIGURE 6.14.
2. Inferior to the head of the femur, identify the **neck of the femur**. Observe that the neck of the femur is not in line with the shaft of the femur but rather is directed medially at an angle known as the angle of inclination.
3. On the proximal femur, identify the **greater trochanter** posteriorly and laterally.
4. Identify the depression of the **trochanteric fossa** on the medial aspect of the greater trochanter posteriorly.
5. On the posterior aspect of the proximal femur, identify the **intertrochanteric crest** between the greater trochanter and **lesser trochanter**.
6. Approximately midway down the length of the intertrochanteric crest, identify the **quadrate tubercle**.
7. Identify the roughened area of the **gluteal tuberosity** on the posterior aspect of the proximal femur inferior to the intertrochanteric crest.

Dissection Instructions

Gluteus Maximus

ATLAS 6.31B, 6.32C; VIDEO 6.4.1

1. Refer to FIGURE 6.15.
2. Place the cadaver in the prone position.
3. Identify the **gluteus maximus** and observe that it attaches to the IT tract inferiorly, and through it, the lateral condyle of the tibia. *Note that because the gluteus maximus attaches to both the gluteal tuberosity of the femur directly and the fascia lata, which connects to the lateral intermuscular septum, it effectively attaches to the entire length of the femur and therefore acts as a powerful extensor of the thigh.*
4. Identify and clean the entire length of the inferior border of the gluteus maximus beginning medially near its attachments on the sacrum and coccyx.
5. Along the inferior border of the gluteus maximus, identify the inferior cluneal nerves if not done previously but do not spend considerable time doing so.
6. Use blunt dissection to define the superior border of the gluteus maximus.
7. Remove the fascia lata from the posterior surface of the gluteus maximus and clean the entire expanse of the muscle.

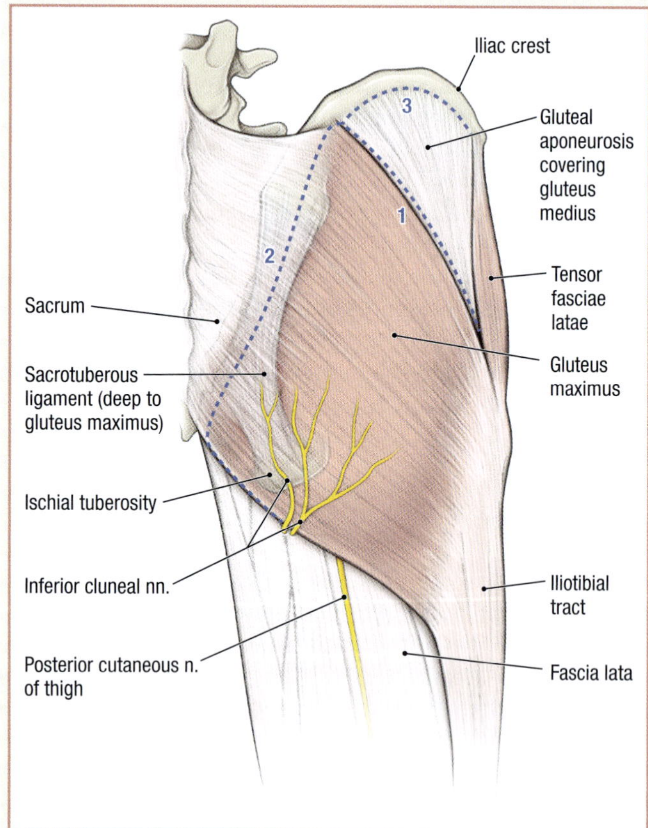

FIGURE 6.15 ■ Superficial dissection of right gluteal region. Posterior view.

8. Observe that the fascia lata is relatively thin over the surface of the gluteus maximus, but superior to the muscle, it becomes thicker to form the **gluteal aponeurosis** overlying the gluteus medius.
9. Separate the gluteus maximus from the gluteal aponeurosis along the superior border of the muscle (**Cut 1**). *Note that the aponeurosis may be strongly connected to the fascia lata and it may be necessary to use sharp dissection to cut the connection.*
10. Near the inferior border of the gluteus maximus, palpate the sacrotuberous ligament through the muscular belly of the gluteus maximus and observe its orientation.
11. Detach the gluteus maximus from its medial attachment beginning superiorly at its superior border and continuing through its attachments to the ilium, sacrum, and sacrotuberous ligament (**Cut 2**). *Note that the gluteus maximus is often tightly adhered along the length of the sacrotuberous ligament and care must be taken not to cut through the ligament while reflecting the muscle laterally.*
12. While reflecting the gluteus maximus, palpate the **inferior gluteal artery**, **vein**, and **nerve** on its deep surface near the center of the muscle. *Note that the inferior gluteal nerve is the only nerve supply to the gluteus maximus, but the muscle receives blood from both the superior and inferior gluteal arteries.*
13. Cut the inferior gluteal vessels and nerve near the muscle belly of the gluteus maximus.
14. Use blunt dissection to loosen the gluteus maximus from the remaining deeper structures and reflect it laterally along its lateral attachments to the IT tract and gluteal tuberosity.
15. Review the attachments and actions of the gluteus maximus (see **TABLE 6.3**).

Gluteus Medius and Minimus

ATLAS 6.31C, 6.31D, 6.32C, 6.32D, 6.32E; VIDEO 6.4.2

1. Refer to FIGURE 6.15.
2. Use a scalpel to cut the gluteal aponeurosis along the iliac crest and use skinning motions to remove it from the underlying gluteus medius (**Cut 3**). *Note that the gluteus medius is firmly attached to the gluteal aponeurosis as it serves as an attachment site for the muscle.*
3. Identify the **gluteus medius** and use blunt dissection to define its borders.
4. Observe that the gluteus medius attaches more superiorly than the gluteus maximus and is visible with the gluteus maximus in anatomical location.
5. Review the attachments, actions, and innervation of the gluteus medius (see **TABLE 6.3**).
6. Refer to FIGURE 6.16.

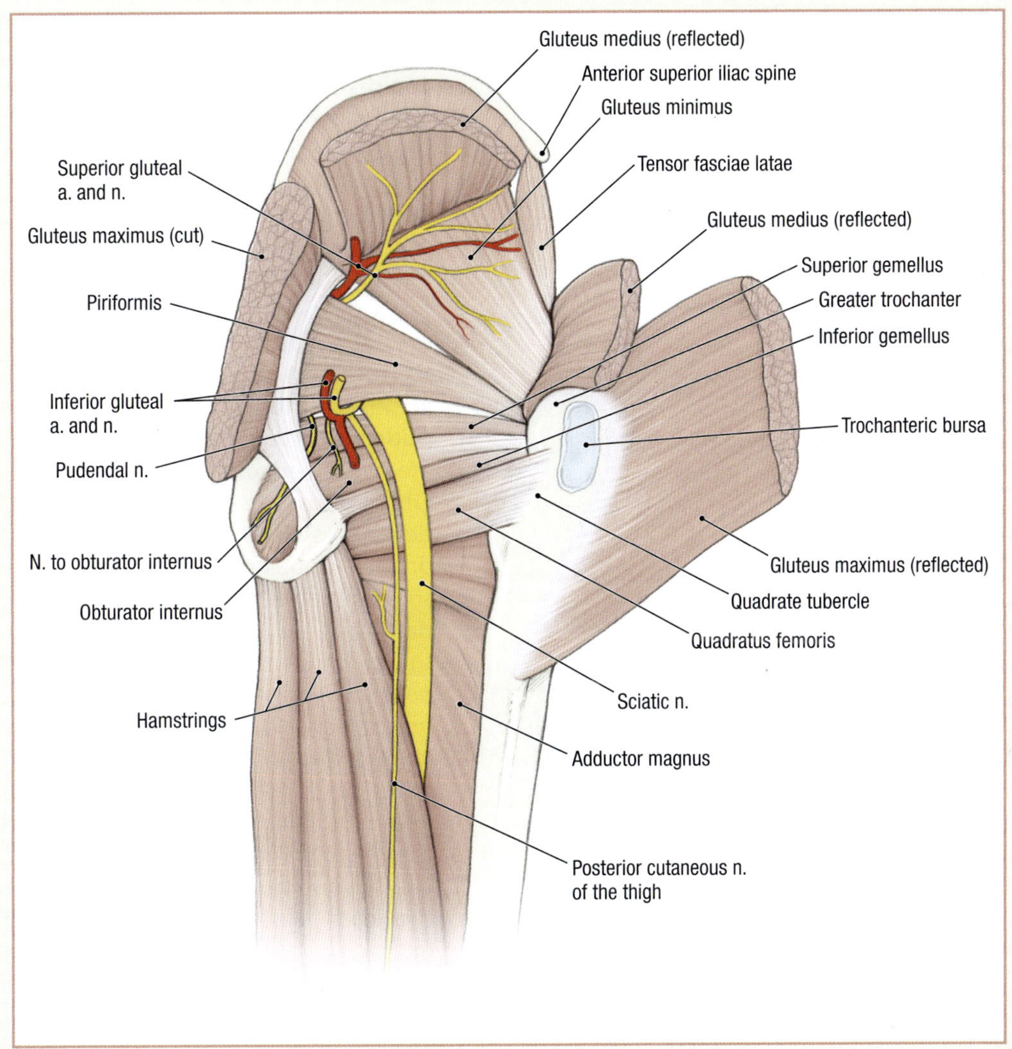

FIGURE 6.16 ● Deep dissection of right gluteal region. Posterior view.

7. Along the inferomedial border of the gluteus medius, identify the **piriformis** and observe its location approximately in the center of the gluteal region.
8. Use blunt dissection to gently expand the interval between the gluteus medius and piriformis to identify the branches of the **superior gluteal vessels**.
9. Follow the course of the superior gluteal vessels for a short distance within the fascial plane between the overlying gluteus medius and the more deeply located gluteus minimus.

Dissection Note: To expose the gluteus minimus, you must reflect the superior part of the gluteus medius.

10. Transect the gluteus medius near its midpoint paralleling the course of the superior gluteal vessels, taking care to not cut the vessels.
11. Gently reflect the cut portions of the gluteus medius and identify the **gluteus minimus**.
12. Identify the branches of the **superior gluteal nerve** and follow them to both the gluteus medius and minimus. *Note that branches of the superior gluteal nerve course laterally to innervate the TFL within the fascia lata on the anterior aspect of the hip inferior to the ASIS.*
13. Review the attachments, actions, and innervation of the gluteus minimus and TFL (see **TABLE 6.3**).

External Rotators of Hip

ATLAS 6.31D, 6.34A; VIDEO 6.4.3

1. Refer to FIGURE 6.16.
2. Use blunt dissection to clean the superior border of the piriformis and observe that the **superior gluteal artery**, **vein**, and **nerve** exit the pelvic cavity and enter the gluteal region by passing superior to the superior border of the piriformis.
3. Use blunt dissection to clean the inferior border of the piriformis and observe that it lies superior to the cut edge of the **inferior gluteal artery** and **vein**.

4. Inferior to the piriformis, identify the **sciatic nerve**, the largest nerve in the body, consisting of a tibial division and a common fibular division which may or may not be distinguishable at this point in the dissection (see **Clinical Correlation 6.4**).

CLINICAL CORRELATION 6.4

Intragluteal Injections

ATLAS 6.34

The gluteal region is commonly subdivided into quadrants for delineation of safe regions to use for intramuscular injections. To create the quadrants, a vertical line is drawn down from the highest point of the iliac crest, and a horizontal line is drawn halfway between the high point of the iliac crest and the level of the ischial tuberosity.

Intragluteal injections into the superior lateral quadrant are relatively safe as the superior gluteal nerve and vessels are well branched in this region and rarely is the sciatic nerve in danger of penetration in this location. Injections into the two inferior quadrants of the gluteal region would endanger the sciatic nerve or the nerves and vessels that pass inferior to the piriformis. Injections into the superior medial quadrant could similarly risk the superior gluteal nerve and vessels.

Dissection Note: Occasionally, the sciatic divisions may emerge from the pelvis separately with the common fibular division passing over the superior border or through the center of the piriformis and the tibial division passing inferior to the piriformis.

5. Make a vertical cut through the fascia lata overlying the sciatic nerve in the posterior thigh.
6. Follow the sciatic nerve inferiorly into the posterior compartment of the thigh until the point where it courses deep to the hamstrings.
7. On the medial side of the sciatic nerve, identify the **posterior cutaneous nerve of the thigh**.
8. Follow the posterior cutaneous nerve of the thigh superiorly and observe that it lies lateral to the **inferior gluteal vessels** and **nerve**.
9. Identify the **superior gemellus** inferior to the piriformis. Observe that the piriformis passes through the greater sciatic foramen nearly filling it, whereas the superior gemellus originates from the ischial spine.
10. Identify the **nerve to obturator internus**, **internal pudendal artery** and **vein**, and **pudendal nerve** near the medial end of the inferior border of the piriformis.
11. Observe that the pudendal nerve and internal pudendal vessels exit the pelvis by passing through the greater sciatic foramen, between the piriformis and superior gemellus, and then enter the perineum by passing through the lesser sciatic foramen deep to the sacrotuberous ligament. *Note that the pudendal nerve and internal pudendal vessels supply the anal and urogenital triangles.*
12. Identify the tendon of the **obturator internus** inferior to the superior gemellus and superior to the **inferior gemellus**. *Note that the two gemellus muscles attach to the obturator internus tendon and might obscure it.*
13. Use a probe to verify that the obturator internus exits the lesser pelvis by passing through the lesser sciatic foramen.
14. Inferior to the inferior gemellus, identify and clean the **quadratus femoris**.
15. Review the attachments, actions, and innervation of the obturator internus, the superior gemellus, the inferior gemellus, and the quadratus femoris (see **TABLE 6.3**).

Dissection Follow-up

1. Review the attachments and innervation of the gluteal muscles as shown in **TABLE 6.3**.
2. Study the functions of the muscles in the gluteal region including extension, abduction, and lateral rotation of the thigh.
3. Review the site where a safe intragluteal injection may be performed.
4. Identify the piriformis and use it as a guide to review the neurovascular relationships of the gluteal region.
5. Review the sacral plexus and its contributions to the sciatic nerve and note that branches of the sacral plexus innervate the muscles of the gluteal region.
6. Replace the muscles of the gluteal region in their correct anatomical positions.

TABLE 6.3 Muscles of Gluteal Region

<table>
<tr><th>Muscle</th><th>Proximal Attachments</th><th>Distal Attachments</th><th>Actions</th><th>Innervation</th></tr>
<tr><td>Gluteus maximus</td><td>Ilium posterior to posterior gluteal line, dorsal surface of the sacrum and coccyx, and sacrotuberous ligament</td><td>Iliotibial tract and gluteal tuberosity</td><td>Extends and laterally rotates the thigh</td><td>Inferior gluteal n.</td></tr>
<tr><td>Gluteus medius</td><td>External surface of ilium between anterior and posterior gluteal lines and gluteal fascia</td><td>Lateral surface of greater trochanter of the femur</td><td rowspan="2">Abducts and medially rotates the thigh</td><td rowspan="3">Superior gluteal n.</td></tr>
<tr><td>Gluteus minimus</td><td>Lateral surface of the ilium between the anterior gluteal and inferior gluteal lines</td><td>Anterior surface of greater trochanter of the femur</td></tr>
<tr><td>Tensor of fascia lata</td><td>Anterior superior iliac spine</td><td>Iliotibial tract</td><td>Abducts, medially rotates, and flexes the thigh</td></tr>
<tr><td>Piriformis</td><td>Anterior surface of the sacrum</td><td rowspan="2">Greater trochanter of the femur (lateral)</td><td rowspan="5">Laterally rotates the thigh</td><td>Anterior rami of S1 and S2</td></tr>
<tr><td>Obturator internus</td><td>Internal margin of the obturator foramen and inner surface of the obturator membrane</td><td rowspan="3">Nerve to obturator internus</td></tr>
<tr><td>Superior gemellus</td><td>Ischial spine (medial)</td><td rowspan="2">Greater trochanter of the femur (lateral) and obturator internus tendon</td></tr>
<tr><td>Inferior gemellus</td><td>Ischial tuberosity (medial)</td></tr>
<tr><td>Quadratus femoris</td><td>Ischial tuberosity (medial)</td><td>Quadrate tubercle (lateral)</td><td>Nerve to quadratus femoris</td></tr>
</table>

Abbreviation: n., nerve; S, sacral vertebrae.

POSTERIOR COMPARTMENT OF THIGH AND POPLITEAL FOSSA

Dissection Overview

The posterior compartment of the thigh contains the posterior thigh muscles: biceps femoris, semimembranosus, and semitendinosus. The muscles of the posterior group extend the thigh and flex the leg. The posterior thigh muscles are commonly referred to as the "hamstrings," although this excludes the short head of the biceps femoris, which only crosses the knee.

The order of dissection will be as follows: The muscles of the posterior compartment of the thigh will be studied. The course and branches of the sciatic nerve will be studied. The dissection will be extended inferiorly to include the popliteal fossa. The muscular boundaries of the popliteal fossa will be identified, and the contents of the popliteal fossa will be studied.

Skeletal Anatomy

Refer to an articulated or disarticulated skeleton of the lower limb to identify the following skeletal features.

Posterior Hip and Femur

ATLAS 6.30C

1. Refer to FIGURE 6.17.
2. Identify the roughened area of the **ischial tuberosity** on the inferior aspect of the ischium.
3. On the posterior aspect of the femur, identify the **medial lip** and **lateral lip of the linea aspera**.
4. Follow the medial lip of the linea aspera superiorly to the **pectineal line**, which angles medially toward the **lesser trochanter** of the femur.
5. Follow the linea aspera inferiorly to the point where it widens into the **medial** and **lateral supracondylar lines** to either side of the **popliteal surface**, which in turn transition to the **medial** and **lateral epicondyles**.

6. On the medial epicondyle, identify the **adductor tubercle**.
7. Observe that the medial and lateral epicondyles are located just proximal to the large terminal projections of bone distally on the femur, the **medial** and **lateral condyles**.

Proximal Posterior Tibia and Fibula

ATLAS 6.30C, 6.68A

1. Refer to FIGURE 6.17.
2. On the proximal end of the fibula, identify the **head of the fibula** and observe that it narrows toward the **apex**.
3. Just inferior to the head of the fibula, identify the narrowed region of the **neck of the fibula**.
4. On the proximal tibia, identify the **medial condyle** and the **lateral condyle**.
5. On the proximal tibia posteriorly, identify the obliquely oriented **soleal line**.
6. Observe on an articulated skeleton that the condyles of the femur and tibia align and form the articular surfaces for the weight-bearing portion of the knee joint.
7. Confirm on an articulated skeleton that the fibula does not articulate at the knee.

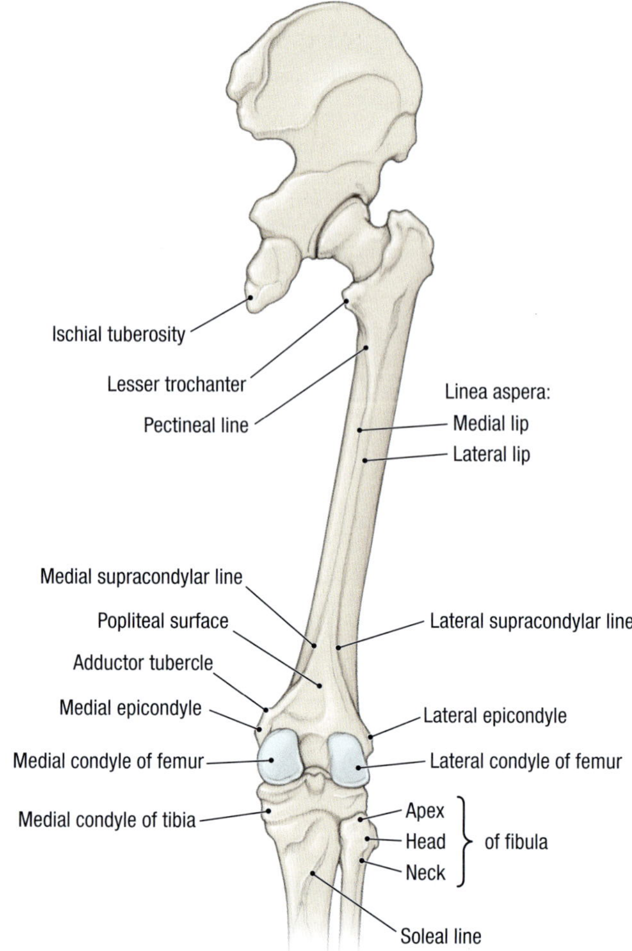

FIGURE 6.17 ■ Skeleton of right hip, thigh, and knee. Posterior view.

Dissection Instructions

Posterior Compartment of Thigh

ATLAS 6.31, 6.33; VIDEO 6.5.1

1. Refer to FIGURE 6.18.
2. Place the cadaver in the prone position.
3. Use scissors to continue the vertical incision made through the fascia lata on the posterior thigh to expose the sciatic nerve and extend the incision from the level of the gluteus maximus to the knee.
4. Spread open the fascia lata medially and laterally and follow the **sciatic nerve** until it branches into the **tibial** and **common fibular nerves**. *Note that prior to the physical point of separation, the portions of the sciatic nerve are typically referred to as the tibial and common fibular divisions as the fibers remain organized along the length of the nerve.*
5. Clean the fascia off the sciatic nerve and observe that it passes deep (anterior) to the **long head of the biceps femoris** and courses inferiorly to the area posterior to the knee, the **popliteal fossa**. *Note that the sciatic nerve may split into the tibial and common fibular divisions in the gluteal region, at any level in the posterior thigh, or in the popliteal fossa.*
6. Locate the **posterior cutaneous nerve of the thigh** in the gluteal region and follow it inferiorly to observe that it sends cutaneous branches through the fascia lata to the posterior surface of the thigh.
7. On the lateral aspect of the posterior thigh, identify and clean the **long head of the biceps femoris.**
8. Retract the long head of the biceps femoris and identify and clean the **short head of the biceps femoris.**
9. Review the attachments and actions of the biceps femoris (see **TABLE 6.4**).
10. On the medial side of the thigh, identify and clean the **semimembranosus**. *Note that the semimembranosus ("half membrane") is named for the broad, flat, membrane-like tendon at its superior end.*

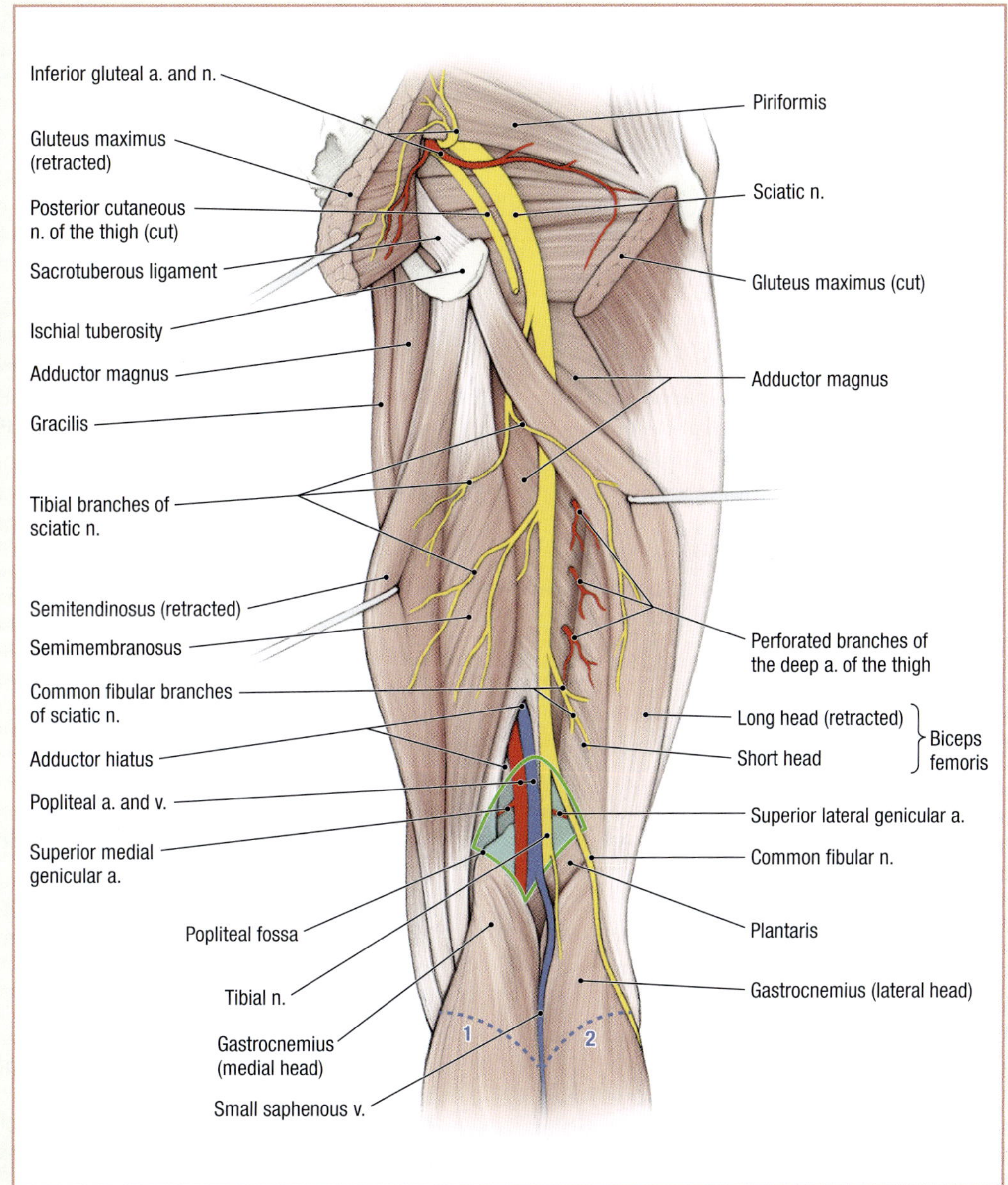

FIGURE 6.18 ■ Contents of posterior compartment of right thigh and popliteal fossa. Posterior view.

11. Lateral to the semimembranosus, identify and clean the **semitendinosus**. *Note that the semitendinosus ("half tendon") is named for the long, cord-like tendon at its inferior end.*
12. Observe that inferiorly, the semitendinosus tendon passes posterior to the semimembranosus.
13. Review the attachments and actions of the semimembranosus and semitendinosus (see **TABLE 6.4**).
14. Follow the branches of the sciatic nerve and observe that it supplies the hamstrings through its **tibial division** and the short head of the biceps femoris through its **common fibular division** (see **Clinical Correlation 6.5**).

CLINICAL CORRELATION 6.5

Sciatic Nerve Injury

ATLAS 6.31C, 6.36A, 6.36B

Sciatic nerve injury may result in significant peripheral neurologic deficits including paralysis of the flexors of the knee and all muscles below the knee, along with possible widespread numbness of the skin on the posterior aspect of the lower limb, the anterior side of the leg, and the dorsal and plantar surfaces of the foot. Sciatica refers to radiating pain along the path of the sciatic nerve and is often caused by a herniated disc, spinal stenosis, or bone spurs.

15. Verify that the **hamstring part of the adductor magnus** arises from the ischial tuberosity inferior to the superior attachments of the hamstrings.
16. Observe that the adductor magnus is in the medial compartment of the thigh and forms the anterior boundary of the posterior compartment of the thigh.

Popliteal Fossa

ATLAS 6.44B, 6.45, 6.46; VIDEO 6.5.2

1. Refer to FIGURE 6.18.
2. Identify the borders of the diamond-shaped **popliteal fossa** beginning with the superolateral border formed by the biceps femoris and the superomedial border formed by the semitendinosus and semimembranosus.
3. At the medial side of the knee, observe that the tendons of the **sartorius, gracilis,** and **semitendinosus** converge on the proximal end of the tibia in an arrangement named the pes anserinus for its goose-foot-like appearance. *Note that one muscle from each of the three compartments of the thigh is involved in the pes anserinus, making knee flection an action of each.*
4. Identify the inferolateral border of the popliteal fossa formed by the **lateral head of the gastrocnemius** and **plantaris,** and the inferomedial border formed by the **medial head of the gastrocnemius.**
5. Observe that the popliteal fossa is bounded posteriorly by the skin and deep (popliteal) fascia and that anteriorly it is limited by the popliteal surface of the femur, posterior surface of the knee joint capsule, and popliteus.
6. Observe that near the superior apex of the popliteal fossa, the sciatic nerve typically divides into the **tibial** and **common fibular nerves,** although this subdivision may occur higher in the posterior compartment or even in the gluteal region.
7. Use blunt dissection to follow the common fibular nerve laterally along the superolateral border of the popliteal fossa.
8. Observe that the common fibular nerve parallels the biceps femoris tendon and passes superficial to the lateral head of the gastrocnemius and plantaris.
9. Use blunt dissection to separate the **tibial nerve** from the loose connective tissue that surrounds it and follow the nerve inferiorly.
10. Observe that the tibial nerve passes deep to the plantaris and gastrocnemius at the inferior apex of the popliteal fossa.
11. Remove the remnants of the deep (popliteal) fascia and overlying fat to expose the medial and lateral heads of the gastrocnemius while sparing the branches of the tibial nerve.
12. At the inferior apex of the popliteal fossa, separate the two bellies of the gastrocnemius and gently pull the muscle bellies apart for a distance of 5 to 10 cm.

Dissection Note: Perform dissection steps 13 to 15 on only one lower limb.

13. On one lower limb, place a probe deep to the two heads of the gastrocnemius just superior to the point where they join.
14. Transect both the medial and lateral heads of the muscle while sparing the branches of the **tibial nerve** and **popliteal artery (Cuts 1** and **2).**
15. Use blunt dissection to reflect the two cut muscular heads superiorly and the bulk of the muscle belly inferiorly.
16. Refer to FIGURE 6.19.
17. Identify the **popliteal artery** and **vein** deep to the tibial nerve and observe that the popliteal artery and vein are enclosed by a connective tissue sheath.
18. Use scissors to cut the sheath of connective tissue enclosing the popliteal artery and vein and spread it open.
19. Use blunt dissection to separate the popliteal artery from the more superficially located popliteal vein.
20. Identify the **small (lesser) saphenous vein** draining into the posterior aspect of the popliteal vein. Remove the other venous tributaries in the region to clear the dissection field.
21. Identify and clean the **superior lateral genicular artery** and **superior medial genicular artery** deep in the popliteal fossa proximal to the attachments of the gastrocnemius.
22. Follow the popliteal artery distally and observe that it passes deep to the plantaris and gastrocnemius to enter the posterior compartment of the leg.
23. Retract the popliteal artery posteriorly and identify the **inferior lateral genicular artery** and **inferior medial genicular artery** deep to the medial and lateral heads of the gastrocnemius.

Dissection Note: The genicular anastomosis formed by branches of the popliteal artery receives contributions from the femoral artery, lateral circumflex femoral artery, and anterior tibial artery.

24. Retract the inferior end of the popliteal artery and vein and identify the **popliteus.**
25. Observe that the floor of the popliteal fossa is partially formed by the popliteus, which will be seen better when the posterior muscles of the leg are dissected.

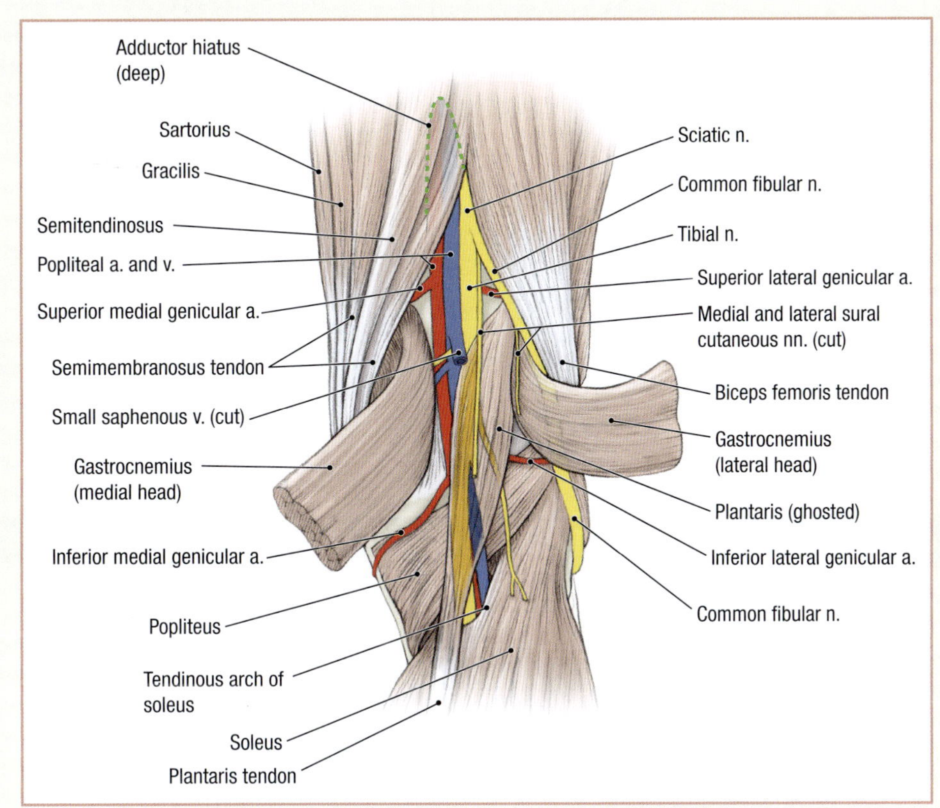

FIGURE 6.19 ■ Contents of right popliteal fossa. Posterior view.

Dissection Follow-up

1. Review the attachments and actions of the posterior thigh muscles as shown in **TABLE 6.4**.
2. Trace the course of the sciatic nerve from the pelvis to the knee and review its terminal branches.
3. Trace the femoral artery from the level of the inguinal ligament to the popliteal fossa through the adductor canal and hiatus, naming its branches.
4. Review the course of the deep artery of the thigh through the medial compartment of the thigh and review the course of its perforating vessels, which pass through the adductor magnus and brevis to reach the posterior compartment of the thigh.
5. Review the genicular anastomosis around the knee.
6. Review the principal functions and innervations of the muscular compartments of the thigh.
7. Replace the muscles of the posterior compartment of the thigh into their correct anatomical positions.

TABLE 6.4 Muscles of Posterior Thigh and Popliteal Fossa

Muscle	*Proximal Attachments*	*Distal Attachments*	*Actions*	*Innervation*
Biceps femoris	Ischial tuberosity (long head) Lateral lip of the linea aspera of femur (short head)	Head of the fibula	Extends the thigh (only long head) and flexes the leg	Tibial division of the sciatic n. (long head) and common fibular division of the sciatic n. (short head)
Semitendinosus	Ischial tuberosity	Medial surface of the superior part of the tibia	Extends the thigh and flexes and medially rotates the leg	Tibial division of the sciatic n.
Semimembranosus		Posterior part of the medial condyle of the tibia		
Popliteus	Lateral surface of lateral condyle of femur and lateral meniscus	Posterior surface of tibia superior to soleal line	Unlocks fully extended leg, weak flexor of leg	Tibial n.

Abbreviation: n., nerve.

POSTERIOR COMPARTMENT OF LEG

Dissection Overview

The two bones of the leg are unequal in size, although similar in length. The larger medially located tibia is the weight-bearing bone of the leg. The thinner laterally located fibula is surrounded by muscles except at its proximal and distal ends. The tibia and fibula are joined by an interosseous membrane as shown in FIGURE 6.20. The crural fascia is attached to the fibula by two intermuscular septa: anterior and posterior. The tibia, fibula, interosseous membrane, and intermuscular septa divide the leg into three compartments: posterior, lateral (fibular), and anterior.

The posterior compartment of the leg lies posterior to the tibia, interosseous membrane, and fibula. A transverse intermuscular septum divides the muscles of the posterior compartment into superficial and deep groups. The superficial posterior group contains three muscles: gastrocnemius, soleus, and plantaris. The combined action of the superficial posterior group is flexion of the knee and plantar flexion of the ankle. The deep posterior group contains four muscles: popliteus, tibialis posterior, flexor digitorum longus, and flexor hallucis longus. The shared actions of the deep posterior muscle group are inversion of the foot, plantar flexion of the foot, and flexion of the toes. The tibial nerve innervates both the superficial and deep posterior muscle groups.

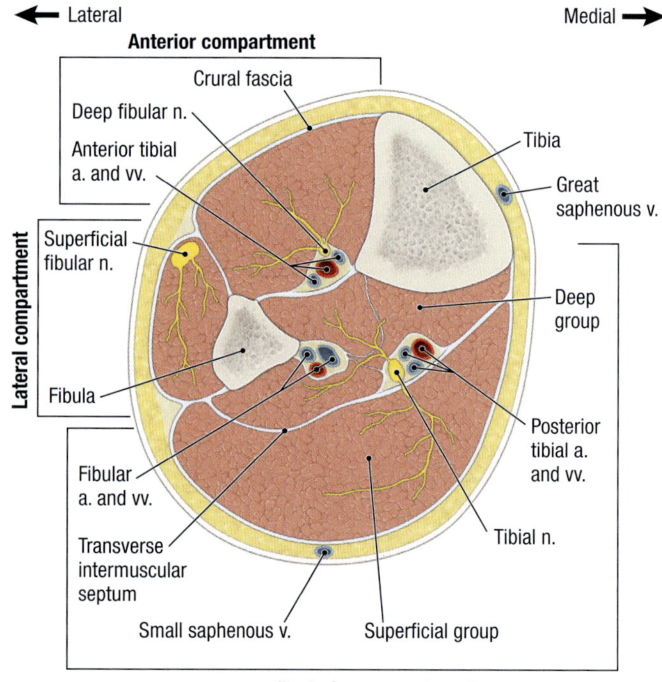

FIGURE 6.20 ● Axial section through right leg. Inferior view.

The order of dissection will be as follows: The superficial veins and cutaneous nerves of the posterior side of the leg will be reviewed. The crural fascia of the posterior side of the leg will be opened, and the superficial posterior group of leg muscles will be examined. The muscles in the superficial posterior group will be reflected to expose the muscles of the deep posterior group. The vessels and nerves of the posterior compartment will be dissected. The muscles of the deep posterior group will be identified.

Skeletal Anatomy

Refer to an articulated skeleton or disarticulated tibia and fibula to identify the following skeletal features.

Posterior Tibia and Fibula

ATLAS 6.68A

1. Refer to FIGURE 6.21.
2. On the proximal aspect of the **tibia**, identify the flattened articular surfaces of the **medial condyle** medially and **lateral condyle** laterally.
3. Between the medial and lateral condyles, identify the **intercondylar eminence**, the roughened process for attachment of the cruciate ligaments of the knee.
4. On the posterior aspect of the proximal tibia, identify the obliquely oriented **soleal line**.
5. On the inferior aspect of the tibia medially, identify the large protrusion of the **medial malleolus**.
6. On the proximal aspect of the **fibula**, identify the boxlike **head** of the fibula superior to the narrowed region of the **neck**.
7. Follow the length of the fibula inferiorly along the **shaft (body)** to the triangular-shaped **lateral malleolus**.
8. Place the tibia and fibula side by side in anatomical position and observe that the fibula does not align with the superior surface of the tibia, extends further inferiorly, does not articulate at the knee, and functions as a non–weight-bearing bone at both the ankle and knee.

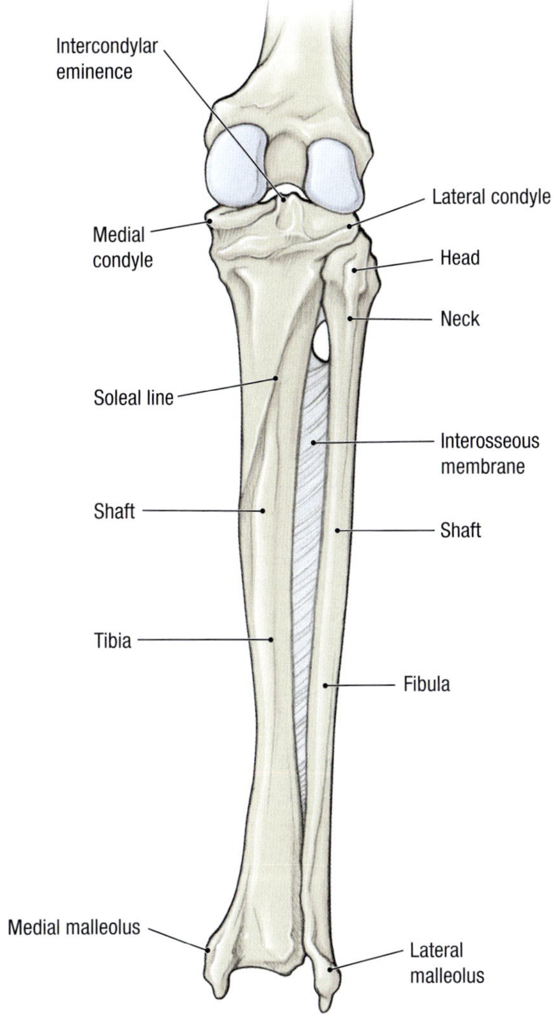

FIGURE 6.21 ■ Skeleton of right leg. Posterior view.

Dissection Instructions

Superficial Compartment of Posterior Leg

ATLAS 6.69B, 6.69C; VIDEO 6.6.1

1. Refer to FIGURE 6.22.
2. With the cadaver in the prone position, use scissors to make a vertical cut through the crural fascia from the popliteal fossa to the calcaneal tuberosity.
3. Use blunt dissection to spread the crural fascia and expose the posterior compartment of the leg.
4. Reflect the cut portions of the **gastrocnemius** superiorly and inferiorly on the side where the incisions were made and identify the **soleus**.
5. Identify the tendon of the **plantaris** between the lateral head of the gastrocnemius and soleus.
6. Follow the tendon of the plantaris superiorly and observe that the muscle belly lies in the popliteal fossa. *Note that the plantaris may be absent in a small percentage of individuals.*
7. Follow the plantaris tendon inferiorly and observe that it either joins the **calcaneal (Achilles) tendon**, the common tendon of the gastrocnemius and soleus, or attaches to the calcaneal tuberosity independently.
8. Review the attachments and actions of the superficial posterior group of leg muscles (see **TABLE 6.5**).

Deep Compartment of Posterior Leg

ATLAS 6.70A, 6.70C, 6.71A; VIDEO 6.6.2

1. Refer to FIGURE 6.22.
2. Follow the **tibial nerve** and **posterior tibial vessels** from where they exit the popliteal fossa inferiorly and observe that they pass deep (anterior) to the tendinous arch of the soleus.
3. Observe that the **tibial nerve** and **posterior tibial vessels** course distally within the **transverse intermuscular septum**, separating the superficial and deep posterior groups.

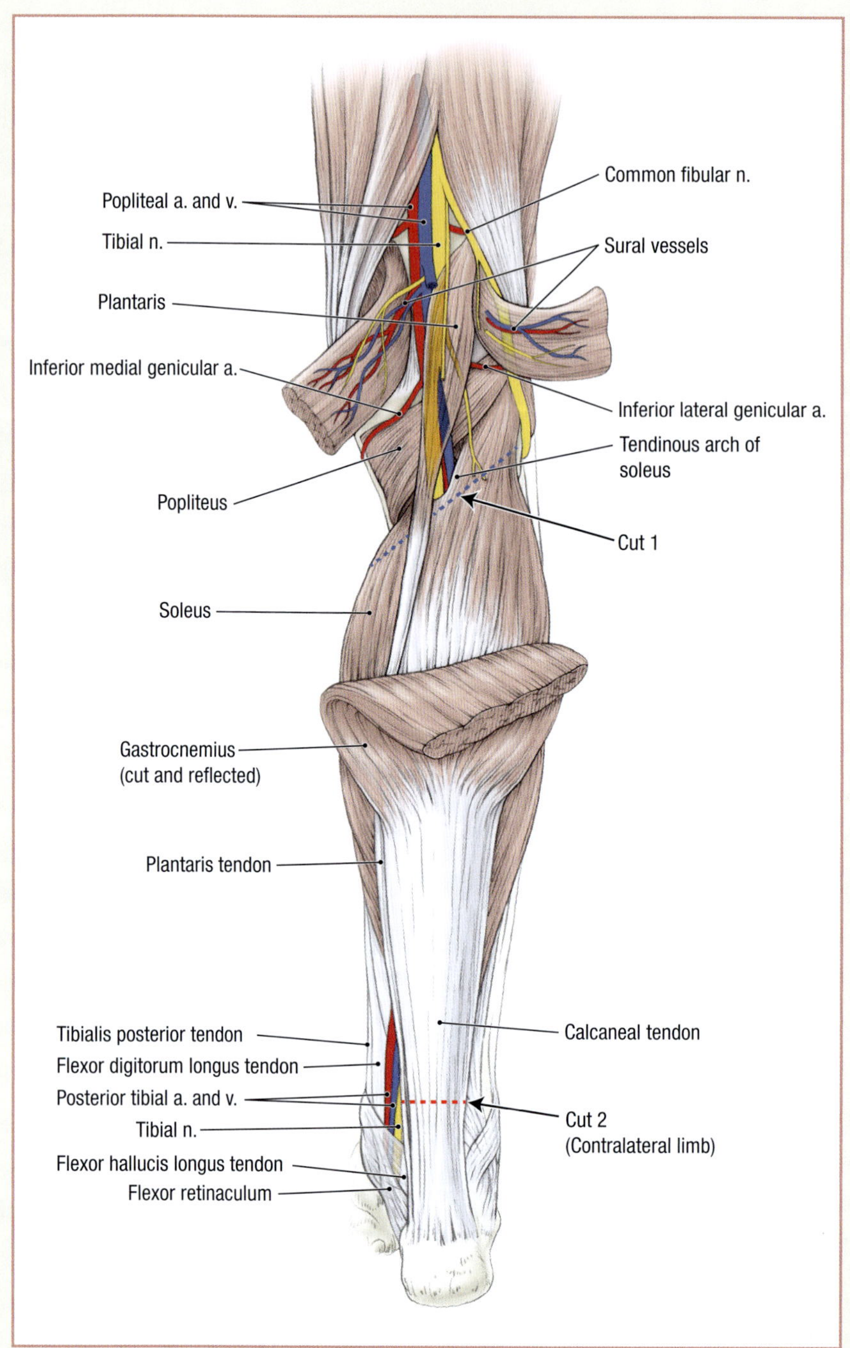

FIGURE 6.22 ● Superficial posterior compartment of right leg. Posterior view.

Dissection Note: To better see the deep muscle layer, the soleus will be reflected in two methods. Steps 4 and 5 should be performed on same limb where the gastrocnemius was transected, while steps 6 and 7 should be performed on the contralateral limb.

4. On the ipsilateral side of the body where the gastrocnemius was transected, cut the soleus beginning at its tibial (medial) attachment extending across the leg to its fibular attachment (**Cut 1**). This cut should pass 2 cm inferior to the tendinous arch of the soleus.
5. Leave the soleus attached to both the calcaneal tendon and the fibula and reflect the soleus and the distal part of the gastrocnemius laterally to expose the transverse intermuscular septum.
6. On the contralateral side of the body where the gastrocnemius was transected, cut the calcaneal tendon about 5 cm superior to the tuberosity of the calcaneus (**Cut 2**).
7. Elevate the calcaneal tendon superiorly and use your fingers to separate the calcaneal tendon from the muscles in the deep posterior group of leg muscles.
8. Refer to FIGURE 6.23.

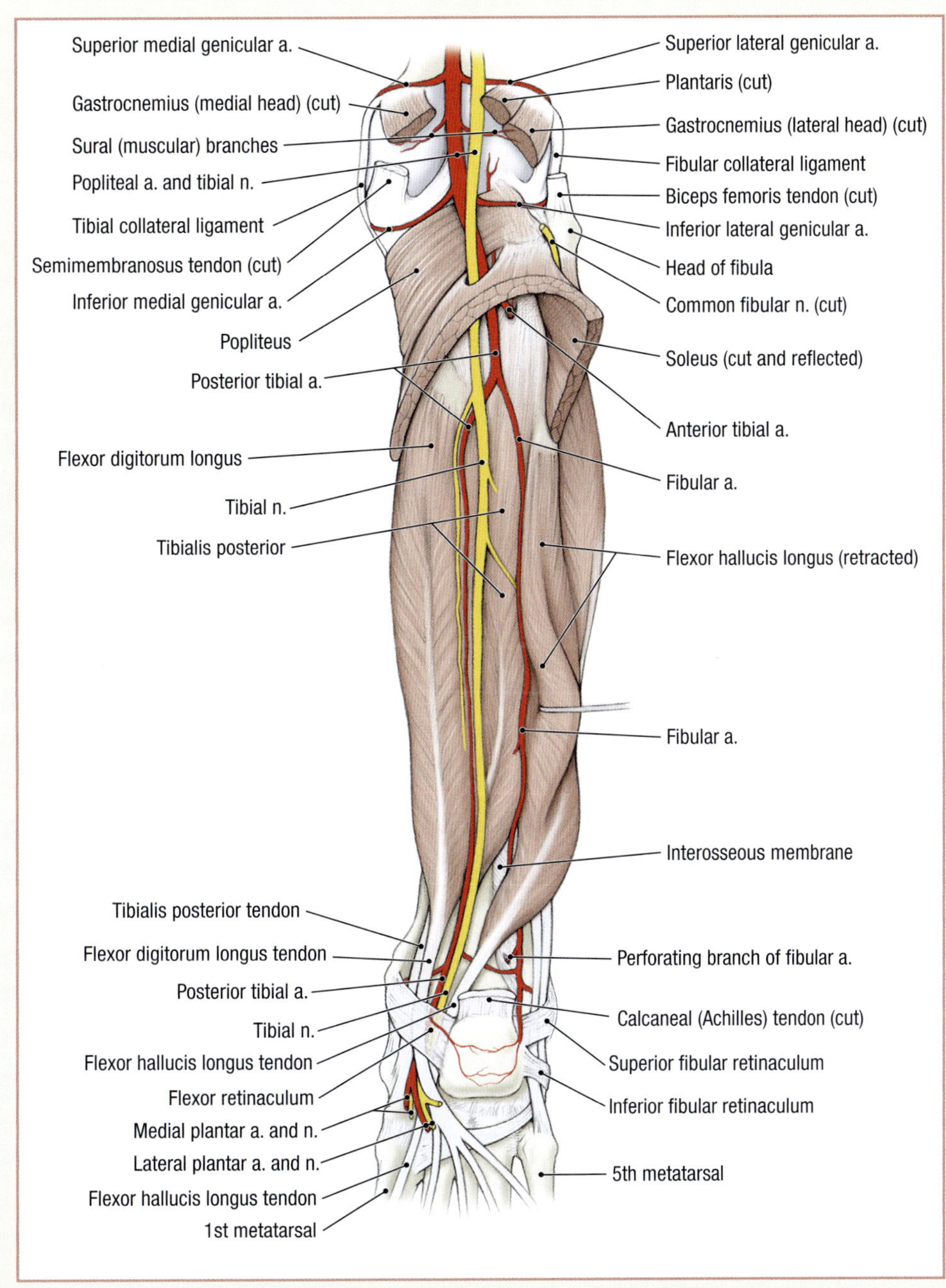

FIGURE 6.23 ■ Deep posterior compartment of right leg. Posterior view.

9. Identify the **posterior tibial artery** and **vein** and **tibial nerve** within the transverse intermuscular septum.
10. Observe that the posterior tibial artery is usually accompanied by two veins, venae comitantes, and thus can be distinguished from the tibial nerve. Remove the veins to clear the dissection field.
11. Use blunt dissection to follow the posterior tibial artery proximally and observe that it bifurcates at the inferior border of the popliteus to the **anterior** and **posterior tibial arteries.**
12. Superior to the superior extent of the soleus, identify the **popliteus**.
13. To better visualize the popliteus, gently retract the contents of the popliteal fossa laterally.
14. Observe that the popliteus fibers course through the popliteal fossa at an oblique angle from inferomedial to superolateral.
15. Deep to the soleus, identify and clean the **tibialis posterior** directly posterior to the tibia.
16. Medial to the tibialis posterior, identify and clean the **flexor digitorum longus.**
17. Observe that the tibialis posterior tendon crosses deep to the flexor digitorum longus tendon as they course posterior to the medial malleolus.

18. Lateral to the tibialis posterior, identify and clean the **flexor hallucis longus**. Observe that the bulk of the muscle belly of the flexor hallucis longus lies deep to the soleus on the lateral side of the leg but its tendon crosses the ankle to the medial side with the tendons of the other deep posterior group muscles.
19. Review the attachments and actions of the deep posterior group of leg muscles (see **TABLE 6.5**).
20. Posterior to the medial malleolus and deep to the flexor retinaculum, observe that the **posterior tibial artery** and **tibial nerve** lie between the tendons of the flexor digitorum longus and flexor hallucis longus.

Dissection Note: The following mnemonic device may be used to identify the tendons and vessels posterior to the medial malleolus in anterior to posterior order: **T**om, **D**ick, and **A** **V**ery **N**ervous **H**arry (**T**ibialis posterior, flexor **D**igitorum longus, posterior tibial **A**rtery, posterior tibial **V**ein, tibial **N**erve, flexor **H**allucis longus).

21. In the upper part of the posterior leg, between the tibialis posterior and the flexor hallucis longus, identify the **fibular artery** arising from the posterior tibial artery about 2 or 3 cm distal to the inferior border of the popliteus. *Note that the fibular artery supplies blood to the muscles of the lateral compartment of the leg and lateral side of the posterior compartment of the leg by means of several small branches.*
22. Identify the **perforating branch of the fibular artery** just superior to the ankle joint where it passes through the interosseous membrane. *Note that the perforating branch of the fibular artery anastomoses with a branch of the anterior tibial artery and will occasionally give rise to the dorsalis pedis artery.*

Dissection Follow-up

1. Review the attachments and actions of each muscle in the posterior compartment of the leg as shown in **TABLE 6.5**.
2. Review the distribution of the arteries of the posterior compartment of the leg beginning at the popliteal fossa with the popliteal artery.
3. Follow the tibial nerve through the popliteal fossa and posterior compartment of the leg, observing that it gives numerous muscular branches to the posterior compartment of the leg.
4. Review the relationships of the nerve, tendons, and vessels posterior to the medial malleolus using this pattern to organize the contents of the deep posterior compartment of the leg.
5. Replace the muscles of the posterior compartment of the leg into their correct anatomical positions.

TABLE 6.5 Muscles of Posterior Leg

SUPERFICIAL GROUP				
Muscle	*Proximal Attachments*	*Distal Attachments*	*Actions*	*Innervation*
Gastrocnemius	Superior to the lateral and medial femoral condyles	Posterior surface of calcaneus via calcaneal tendon	Plantarflexes the foot and flexes the knee	Tibial n.
Plantaris	Lateral supracondylar line of the femur			
Soleus	Soleal line of the tibia and head of the fibula		Plantarflexes the foot	
DEEP GROUP				
Muscle	*Proximal Attachments*	*Distal Attachments*	*Actions*	*Innervation*
Popliteus	Lateral surface of lateral condyle of femur and lateral meniscus	Posterior surface of tibia superior to soleal line	Unlocks fully extended leg; weakly flexes the knee	Tibial n.
Tibialis posterior	Tibia, fibula, and interosseous membrane	Navicular, cuneiform, cuboid, and bases of metatarsals 2–4	Inverts and plantarflexes the foot	
Flexor digitorum longus	Medial part of posterior surface of tibia inferior to the soleal line	Bases of the distal phalanges of the lateral four toes	Flexes toes 2–5 and plantarflexes the foot	
Flexor hallucis longus	Inferior two-thirds of the fibula and interosseous membrane	Base of the distal phalanx of the great toe	Flexes the great toe and plantarflexes the foot	

Abbreviation: n., nerve.

LATERAL COMPARTMENT OF LEG

Dissection Overview

The lateral compartment of the leg contains two muscles: fibularis longus and fibularis brevis. The two muscles of the lateral compartment of the leg are innervated by the superficial fibular nerve and combine to produce eversion and plantarflexion of the foot.

The order of dissection will be as follows: The lateral aspect of the crural fascia will be examined and opened. The fibular retinaculum will be studied. The superficial fibular nerve will be examined on the lateral surface of the leg. The tendons of each muscle of the lateral compartment will be followed posterior to the lateral malleolus.

Dissection Instructions

Lateral Compartment of Leg

ATLAS 6.62B, 6.62C; VIDEO 6.7.1

Dissection Note: Depending on the orientation of the foot, the lateral compartment of the leg may be easier to access with the body either prone or supine. Turn the cadaver to whichever orientation facilitates the dissection.

1. Refer to FIGURE 6.24.
2. Examine the crural fascia on the lateral side of the leg and identify the **fibular retinaculum**, a thickening of the fascia on the lateral side of the ankle between the lateral malleolus and calcaneus which assists in holding down the fibularis longus and brevis tendons.
3. Observe that the fibular retinaculum may be subdivided into a **superior** portion attaching to the lateral malleolus of the fibula, and an **inferior** portion attaching to the extensor retinaculum of the foot.
4. About two-thirds of the way down the leg, identify the **superficial fibular nerve** where it penetrates the crural fascia. Recall that the superficial fibular nerve is a branch of the common fibular nerve.
5. Follow the superficial fibular nerve distally to the dorsum of the foot and observe that it gives rise to several **dorsal digital branches**. *Note that the superficial fibular nerve is the primary cutaneous nerve of the dorsum of the foot.*
6. Use scissors to cut the crural fascia overlying the lateral compartment of the leg as far inferiorly as the superior fibular retinaculum sparing the superficial fibular nerve.
7. In the superior leg, observe that the **fibularis longus** is attached to the inner surface of the crural fascia.
8. Use a scalpel to carefully detach the fibularis longus from the crural fascia using a similar technique to skinning.

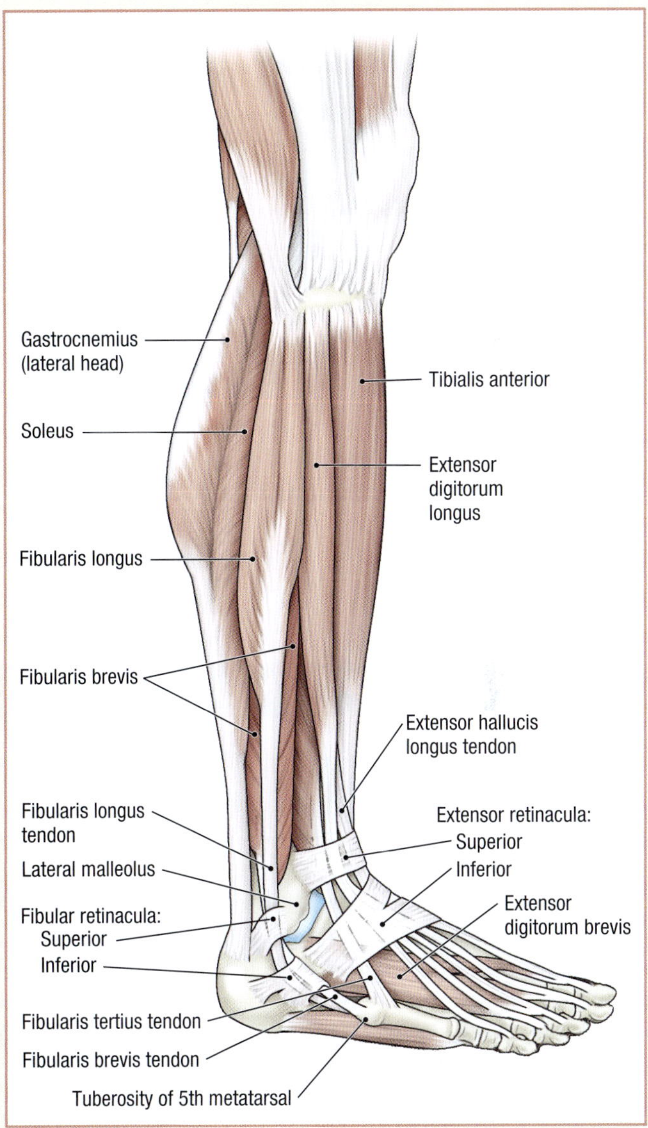

FIGURE 6.24 ■ Lateral compartment of right leg. Lateral view.

9. Deep to the fibularis longus, identify the **fibularis brevis**.
10. Use blunt dissection to follow and separate the tendons distally and observe that the fibularis longus and brevis tendons pass posterior to the lateral malleolus, deep to the superior and inferior fibular retinacula. *Note that the tendon of the fibularis brevis is anterior to the tendon of the fibularis longus where they pass posterior to the lateral malleolus.*
11. Follow the tendon of the fibularis brevis inferiorly to its distal attachment on the **tuberosity of the 5th metatarsal bone** on the lateral aspect of the foot.
12. Follow the tendon of the fibularis longus inferiorly to the point where it courses around the lateral side of the cuboid bone to enter the sole of the foot. *Note that the tendon of the fibularis longus attaches to the plantar surface of the medial cuneiform and 1st metatarsal.*
13. Review the attachments and actions of the lateral group of leg muscles (see **TABLE 6.6**).

Dissection Follow-up

1. Review the attachments and actions of the muscles in the lateral compartment of the leg as shown in **TABLE 6.6**.
2. Review the blood supply to the muscles of the lateral compartment of the leg.
3. Review the pattern of innervation for the lateral compartment of the leg.
4. Replace the muscles of the lateral compartment of the leg into their correct anatomical positions.

TABLE 6.6 Muscles of Lateral Leg

Muscle	*Proximal Attachments*	*Distal Attachments*	*Actions*	*Innervation*
Fibularis longus	Head and superior two-thirds of lateral surface of fibula	Base of 1st metatarsal and medial cuneiform	Everts and plantarflexes the foot	Superficial fibular n.
Fibularis brevis	Inferior two-thirds of lateral surface of fibula	Tuberosity of the 5th metatarsal		

Abbreviation: n., nerve.

ANTERIOR COMPARTMENT OF LEG AND DORSUM OF FOOT

Dissection Overview

The anterior compartment of the leg contains four muscles: tibialis anterior, extensor hallucis longus, extensor digitorum longus, and fibularis tertius. The muscles of the anterior compartment of the leg are innervated by the deep fibular nerve and produce dorsiflexion and inversion of the foot and extension of the toes.

The order of dissection will be as follows: The distribution of cutaneous nerves over the lower anterior surface of the leg and dorsal surface of the foot will be reviewed. The anterior aspect of the deep fascia of the leg and foot will be examined and the extensor retinacula identified. The anterior compartment of the leg will be opened and the relationships of tendons, vessels, and nerves will be examined on the anterior surface of the ankle. The tendon of each muscle of the anterior compartment will be followed into the foot. The intrinsic muscles of the dorsum of the foot will be identified. The deep vessels and nerve of the leg and dorsum of the foot will be dissected.

Skeletal Anatomy

Refer to an articulated skeleton of the bones of the foot to identify the following skeletal features.

Anterior Tibia and Fibula

ATLAS 6.61B

1. Refer to FIGURE 6.25.
2. On the proximal aspect of the **tibia**, identify the flattened articular surfaces of the **medial condyle** medially and **lateral condyle** laterally.

3. On the anterior aspect of the proximal tibia, identify the **tibial tuberosity**, the roughened portion of bone serving as the distal attachment of the patellar tendon.
4. On the anterior aspect of the **shaft of the tibia**, identify the sharp ridge of the **anterior border**.
5. On the proximal aspect of the **fibula**, identify the box-like **head of the fibula** superior to the narrowed region of the **neck**.
6. Observe that the head of the fibula has a pointed **apex**, which articulates with the lateral condyle of the tibia.
7. Follow the length of the fibula inferiorly along the **shaft (body)** to the triangular-shaped **lateral malleolus**.
8. Place the tibia and fibula side by side in anatomical position and observe that the fibula does not align with the superior surface of the tibia, extends further inferiorly, does not articulate at the knee, and functions as a non–weight-bearing bone at both the ankle and the knee.
9. On an articulated skeleton, observe that the **patella** articulates with the femur.

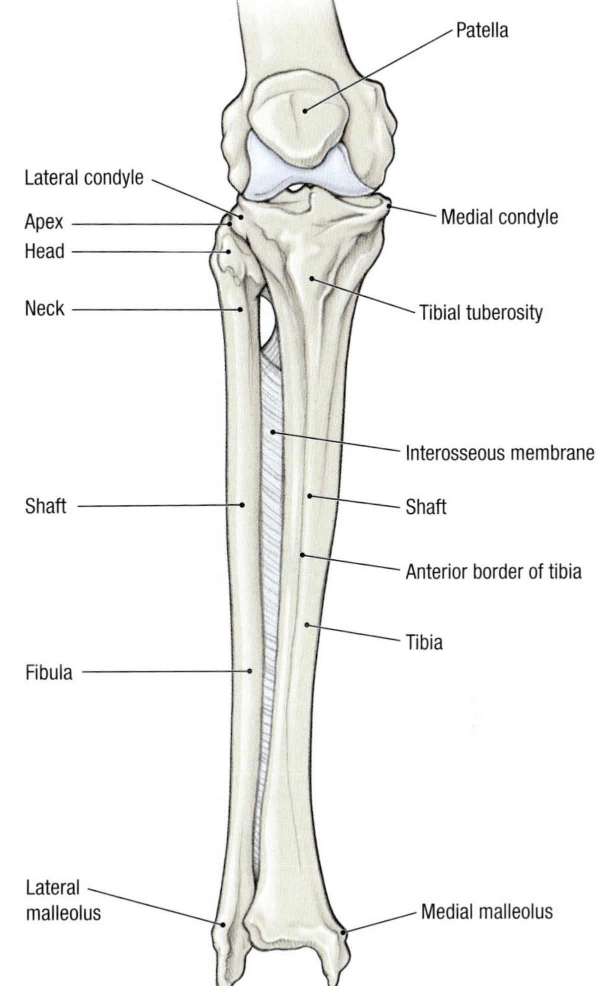

FIGURE 6.25 ■ Skeleton of right leg. Anterior view.

Skeleton of Dorsum of Foot

ATLAS 6.64A, 6.66D

1. Refer to FIGURE 6.26.
2. In an articulated skeleton of the foot, identify the seven tarsal bones beginning with the "heel bone," the **calcaneus**.
3. Superior to the calcaneus, identify the **talus** and observe that the superior aspect of the talus articulates with the inferior aspect of the tibia.
4. Anterior to the talus medially, identify the "boat-shaped" **navicular** bone.
5. Observe that on the medial aspect of the foot, the navicular articulates on its anterior surface with the three **cuneiform bones**: 1st (medial), 2nd (intermediate, middle), and 3rd (lateral).
6. On the lateral aspect of the foot, lateral to the lateral cuneiform and navicular bones, identify the last of the tarsal bones, the **cuboid**.
7. Observe that the cuboid articulates with the anterior aspect of the calcaneus on the lateral aspect of the foot.
8. Distal to the tarsal bones, identify the five **metatarsal bones** beginning with the 1st metatarsal on the medial aspect of the foot and ending with the 5th metatarsal on the lateral aspect of the foot.

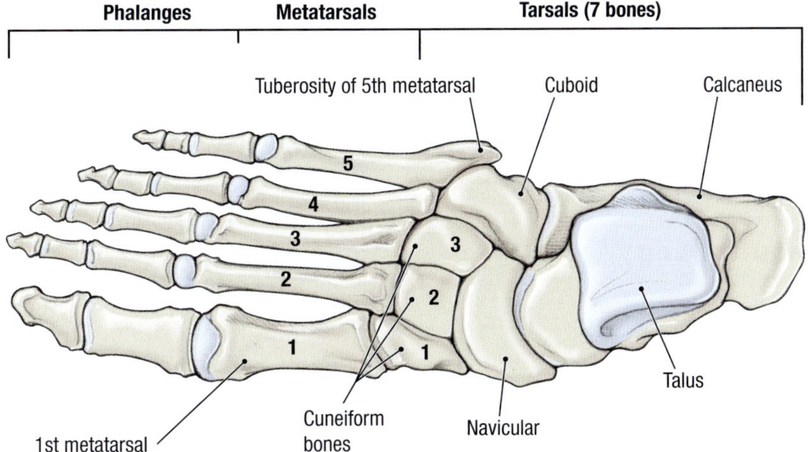

FIGURE 6.26 ■ Skeleton of right foot. Superior (dorsal) view.

9. Identify the **tuberosity of the 5th metatarsal bone** and observe that it extends laterally past the cuboid and serves as a site of muscle attachment.
10. Distal to the metatarsals, identify the 14 **phalanges** and observe that the 1st toe has only two phalanges, whereas the other toes each have three phalanges.
11. On an articulated skeleton, identify the bones of the three subdivisions of the foot: the hindfoot (calcaneus and talus), midfoot (cuboid, navicular, and cuneiforms), and forefoot (metatarsals and phalanges).

Dissection Instructions

Crural Fascia

ATLAS 6.18A, 6.65B; VIDEO 6.8.1

1. Refer back to FIGURE 6.4.
2. Place the cadaver in the supine position.
3. Remove the remnants of subcutaneous tissue on the anterior surface of the leg and dorsum of the foot to clearly expose the **crural fascia** and deep fascia of the foot while preserving the branches of the **superficial fibular nerve**. *Note that the superficial fibular nerve provides most of the cutaneous innervation to the anterior surface of the ankle and dorsum of the foot.*
4. Observe that the crural fascia is firmly attached to the anterior border of the tibia.
5. Refer to FIGURE 6.27.
6. Identify the **superior** and **inferior extensor retinacula** on the anterior surface of the ankle, the transverse thickenings of crural fascia near the ankle.
7. Observe that the **superior extensor retinaculum** extends across the tendons of the anterior compartment muscles superior to the ankle.
8. Observe that the **inferior extensor retinaculum** is at the level of the ankle and is Y-shaped with the stem of the "Y" directed laterally to the calcaneus.
9. Make a vertical cut through the crural fascia just below the lateral condyle of the tibia paralleling the anterior tibial border.
10. Use forceps to lift the edges of the crural fascia and observe that the muscles of the anterior compartment attach to its deep surface.
11. Extend the vertical cut distally through the crural fascia while sparing the extensor retinacula.
12. Reflect and remove the crural fascia by peeling it away from the muscles of the anterior compartment. *Note that the superior attachments of the anterior muscles of the leg are on the proximal tibia, fibula, and interosseous membrane. Do not attempt to dissect the superior attachments.*

Anterior Compartment of Leg

ATLAS 6.60, 6.62B; VIDEO 6.8.2

1. Refer to FIGURE 6.27.
2. Use blunt dissection to separate the vessels, nerves, and tendons of the anterior muscles of the leg where they pass deep to the extensor retinacula.
3. Identify the **tibialis anterior tendon** anterior to the medial malleolus.
4. Observe that the tibialis anterior and tibialis posterior tendons are the two tendons closest to the medial malleolus and are named according to their location relative to the bone.
5. Follow the tendon of the tibialis anterior into the foot toward its attachments to the 1st cuneiform and base of the 1st metatarsal.
6. Lateral to the tibialis anterior, identify the **extensor hallucis longus tendon** and follow it into the foot toward its attachment to the base of the distal phalanx of the great toe.
7. At the level of the superior extensor retinaculum deep to the extensor hallucis longus tendon, identify the **anterior tibial artery** and follow it proximally.
8. Use blunt dissection to separate the extensor digitorum longus from the tibialis anterior.
9. Use blunt dissection to clean the anterior tibial artery where it passes posteriorly over the superior border of the interosseous membrane.
10. Observe that the **deep fibular nerve** travels with the anterior tibial artery in the anterior compartment of the leg. *Note that the deep fibular nerve is the motor nerve of the anterior compartment of the leg and muscles in the dorsum of the foot.*
11. Trace the deep fibular nerve proximally and confirm that it is a branch of the **common fibular nerve** (see **Clinical Correlation 6.6**).

CLINICAL CORRELATION 6.6

Common Fibular Nerve Injury

ATLAS 6.62C, 6.65B

The common fibular nerve is one of the most frequently injured nerves in the body due to its superficial position and relationship to the head and neck of the fibula. When the common fibular nerve is injured, it may impair eversion and dorsiflexion of the foot and extension of the toes in a condition called "foot drop." In foot drop, or steppage gait, the advancing foot hangs with the toes pointed toward the ground necessitating the knee to be lifted high enough so the toes may clear the ground. Foot drop is also commonly accompanied by sensory loss on the dorsum of the foot and toes.

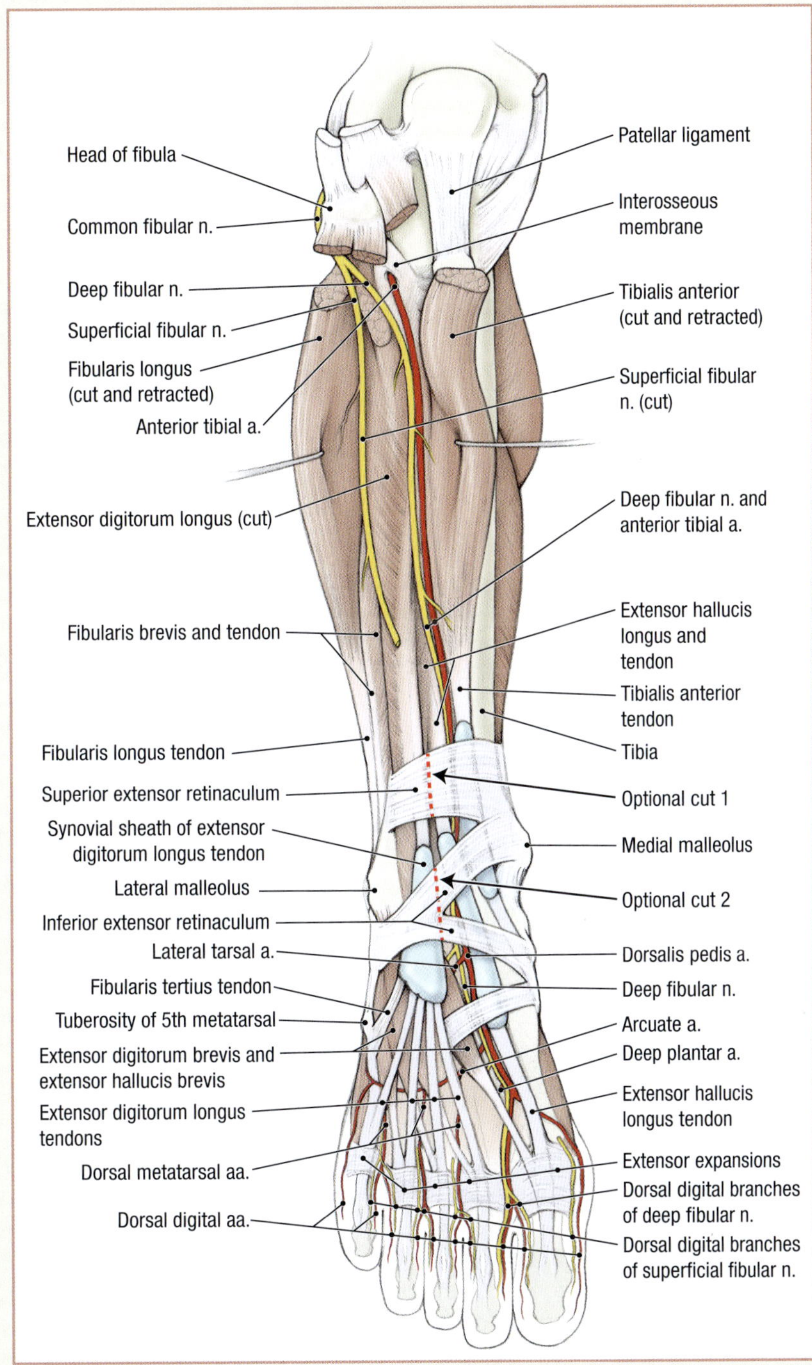

FIGURE 6.27 ● Anterior compartment of right leg and dorsum of foot. Anterior view.

12. Lateral to the extensor hallucis longus tendon, identify the tendons of the **extensor digitorum longus** and follow them distally to confirm they attach to the **extensor expansions** of the lateral four toes.
13. On the lateral aspect of the extensor digitorum longus, identify the tendon of the **fibularis tertius** and follow it distally to confirm its attachment on the dorsal surface of the shaft of the 5th metatarsal. *Note that the fibularis tertius is absent in some individuals.*
14. If the neurovascular structures and tendons of the anterior compartment are not clearly visible, use scissors to cut the superior (**Optional Cut 1**) and inferior extensor retinacula (**Optional Cut 2**) between the extensor digitorum longus and extensor hallucis

longus tendons. Retract the tendons of the extensor digitorum longus in the lateral direction.

15. Review the attachments and actions of the anterior group of leg muscles (see **TABLE 6.7**).

Dorsum of Foot

ATLAS 6.63B, 6.65B; VIDEO 6.8.3

1. Refer to FIGURE 6.27.
2. On the dorsum of the foot deep to the tendons of the extensor digitorum longus, identify the **extensor digitorum brevis** and **extensor hallucis brevis,** which share a common muscle belly attaching to the calcaneus.
3. Identify the four tendons arising from the common muscle belly to attach to the extensor expansions of toes 2 to 5. *Note that the portion of this muscle that attaches on the great toe is called the extensor hallucis brevis.*
4. Review the attachments and actions of the muscles on the dorsum of the foot (see **TABLE 6.7**).
5. Return to the anterior leg and trace the anterior tibial artery deep to the inferior extensor retinaculum where it crosses the ankle joint and its name changes to **dorsalis pedis artery**.
6. Follow the dorsalis pedis artery onto the dorsum of the foot and observe that it lies on the lateral side of the extensor hallucis longus tendon at the ankle. *Note that in the living person, the pulse of the dorsalis pedis artery can be palpated between the tendons of the extensor hallucis longus and extensor digitorum longus.*
7. Deep to the tendons on the dorsum of the foot, identify the **arcuate artery**, a branch of the dorsalis pedis artery that crosses the proximal ends of the metatarsal bones.
8. Identify the **dorsal metatarsal arteries** branching from the arcuate artery.
9. Identify the **lateral tarsal artery** arising from the dorsalis pedis artery near the ankle passing deep to the extensor digitorum brevis and extensor hallucis brevis. *Note that the lateral tarsal artery joins the lateral end of the arcuate artery to complete an arterial arch.*
10. Identify the **deep plantar artery** arising from the dorsalis pedis artery near the origin of the arcuate artery passing between the 1st and 2nd metatarsals to enter the sole of the foot. *Note that the deep plantar artery anastomoses with the plantar arch.*
11. At the level of the ankle, identify the **deep fibular nerve** between the tendons of the extensor hallucis longus and extensor digitorum longus.
12. Use blunt dissection to follow the deep fibular nerve onto the dorsum of the foot. *Note that the deep fibular nerve innervates the extensor digitorum brevis and extensor hallucis brevis.*
13. Trace the cutaneous branch of the deep fibular nerve to the region of skin between the great toe and 2nd toe and identify its two **dorsal digital branches.** *Note that the skin between the great toe and the 2nd toe is the only skin on the dorsum of the foot innervated by the deep fibular nerve.*

Dissection Follow-up

1. Review the attachments and actions of the muscles in the anterior compartment of the leg as shown in **TABLE 6.7**.
2. Trace the anterior tibial artery through the anterior compartment of the leg to the foot and identify where its name changes to the dorsalis pedis artery.
3. Review the pattern of innervation for the anterior compartment of the leg and dorsum of the foot.
4. Review the principal functions and innervations of the muscle groups of the leg.
5. Replace the muscles of the anterior compartment of the leg and dorsum of the foot into their correct anatomical positions.

TABLE 6.7 Muscles of Anterior Leg and Dorsum of Foot

ANTERIOR LEG				
Muscle	*Proximal Attachments*	*Distal Attachments*	*Actions*	*Innervation*
Tibialis anterior	Lateral condyle and superior half of lateral surface of tibia	Base of 1st metatarsal and medial and inferior surfaces of medial cuneiform	Dorsiflexes and inverts the foot	Deep fibular n.
Extensor hallucis longus	Middle part of anterior surface of fibula and interosseous membrane	Dorsal aspect of base of distal phalanx of great toe	Extends great toe and dorsiflexes foot	
Extensor digitorum longus	Lateral condyle of tibia and superior three-fourths of anterior surface of interosseous membrane	Extensor expansion to distal phalanges of lateral four digits	Extends lateral four digits and dorsiflexes foot	
Fibularis tertius	Inferior third of anterior surface of fibula and interosseous membrane	Dorsum of base of 5th metatarsal	Dorsiflexes and everts foot	
DORSUM OF FOOT				
Muscle	*Proximal Attachments*	*Distal Attachments*	*Actions*	*Innervation*
Extensor digitorum brevis	Calcaneus, floor of the tarsal sinus	Extensor expansions of digits 2–5	Extends digits	Deep fibular n.
Extensor hallucis brevis	Calcaneus, floor of the tarsal sinus	Extensor expansion of digit 1	Extends great toe	

Abbreviation: n., nerve.

SOLE OF FOOT

Dissection Overview

The foot is arched both longitudinally and transversely, with the weight-bearing points at the calcaneus posteriorly and heads of the five metatarsal bones anteriorly. The plantar aponeurosis supports the longitudinal arch along with the deeper located long and short plantar ligaments and spring ligament. Deep to the plantar aponeurosis are four layers of intrinsic foot muscles with their associated tendons, vessels, and nerves. The axis of reference for the toe movements of abduction and adduction is through the 2nd digit (2nd toe), which differs from the hand where movements of the fingers are described around an axis passing through the 3rd digit.

The order of dissection will be as follows: The skin and fat pad on the sole of the foot will be removed. The plantar aponeurosis will be cleaned of subcutaneous tissue, studied, and reflected to expose the first muscle layer of the sole. The dissection will proceed from superficial to deep, and each of the four layers of the sole will be dissected.

Skeletal Anatomy

Skeleton of Sole of Foot

ATLAS 6.66D, 6.70E, 6.77A

1. Refer to FIGURE 6.28.
2. In the articulated foot, identify the seven tarsal bones beginning with the "heel bone," the **calcaneus**.
3. On the posterior superior surface of the calcaneus, identify the roughened region of the **calcaneal tuberosity**.
4. From the calcaneal tuberosity, palpate medially and anteriorly to the shelf-like projection of the **sustentaculum tali**.
5. Identify the **talus** superior to the calcaneus and observe that in an articulated skeleton, the superior aspect of the talus articulates with the inferior aspect of the tibia. *Note that the talus is the only tarsal bone without sites of muscle attachment.*
6. Anterior to the talus medially, identify the "boat-shaped" **navicular** bone.
7. Observe that on the medial aspect of the foot, the navicular articulates on its anterior surface with the three **cuneiform bones**: 1st (medial), 2nd (intermediate, middle), and 3rd (lateral).
8. On the lateral aspect of the foot, lateral to the lateral cuneiform and navicular, identify the last of the tarsal bones, the **cuboid**.
9. Observe that the cuboid articulates with the anterior aspect of the calcaneus on the lateral aspect of the foot.

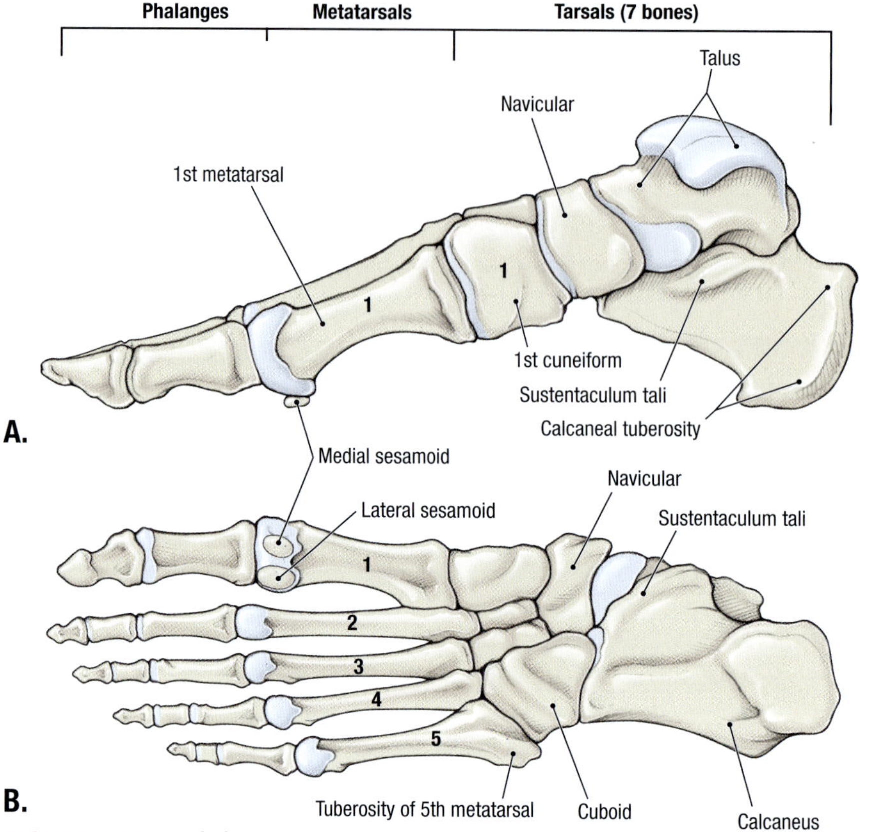

FIGURE 6.28 ■ Skeleton of right foot. **A.** Medial view. **B.** Inferior (plantar) view.

10. Distal to the tarsal bones, identify the five **metatarsal bones** beginning with the 1st metatarsal on the medial aspect of the foot and ending with the 5th metatarsal on the lateral aspect of the foot.
11. Identify the **tuberosity of the 5th metatarsal bone** and observe that it extends laterally past the cuboid and serves as a site of muscle attachment.
12. Distal to the metatarsals, identify the 14 **phalanges**. Observe that the 1st toe has only two phalanges, whereas the other toes each have three phalanges.

Dissection Instructions

Skin Incisions of Sole of Foot

ATLAS 6.71A, 6.76A, 6.76B; VIDEO 6.9.1

Dissection Note: Perform the following dissection sequence bilaterally.

1. Refer to FIGURE 6.29.
2. Place the cadaver in the prone position.
3. Make a midline incision extending from the heel (I) to the base of the 2nd digit (M).
4. Make a horizontal incision arching from the base of the 1st digit to the base of the 5th digit (H to H).
5. Remove the skin beginning at the midline incision and working toward the edges of the foot. Observe that the skin is thick over the heel and heads of the metatarsal bones but is thinner on the toes and instep.
6. Remove the skin on the plantar surface of the toes on at least two digits by making a midline incision down the digit to its distal extent (P).

Plantar Aponeurosis and Cutaneous Nerves

ATLAS 6.71A, 6.76B; VIDEO 6.9.2

1. Refer to FIGURE 6.30.
2. Observe that the plantar fascia over the medial and lateral sides of the sole of the foot is thin, whereas in the center, it is thickened to form the **plantar aponeurosis**.
3. Use the side of a scalpel blade to scrape the subcutaneous tissue off the plantar aponeurosis.
4. Observe that the plantar aponeurosis is attached to the calcaneus posteriorly and that it divides distally into five bands as **digital slips** to each toe. *Note that the five bands are joined by the superficial transverse metatarsal ligaments.*
5. Use a probe to elevate the plantar aponeurosis longitudinally. *Note that to fully elevate the plantar aponeurosis, it may be necessary to carefully cut along its lateral edges with a scalpel. Do not cut too deeply.*

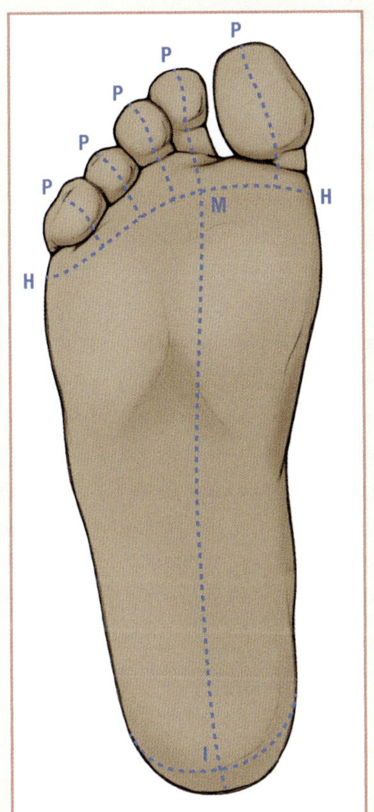

FIGURE 6.29 ■ Skin incisions of sole of right foot. Inferior view.

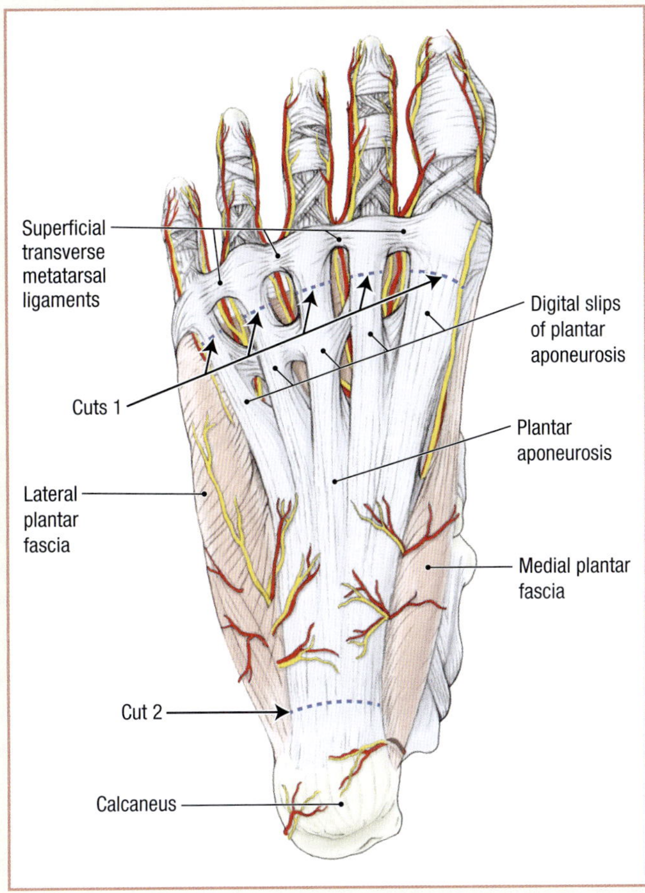

FIGURE 6.30 ■ Sole of right foot. Inferior view.

6. Make transverse cuts through the plantar aponeurosis distally in the anterior one-third of the foot through each digital slip (**Cuts 1**).
7. Reflect the plantar aponeurosis proximally toward the calcaneus.
8. Observe that tough bands of connective tissue attach the plantar aponeurosis to the metatarsal bones. Use a scalpel to cut these bands and release the plantar aponeurosis from the underlying structures.
9. Remove the plantar aponeurosis from the sole of one foot by making a horizontal incision near its attachment to the calcaneus (**Cut 2**).

First Layer of Sole of Foot

ATLAS 6.77; VIDEO 6.9.3

Dissection Note: Perform the following dissection sequence bilaterally.

1. Refer to FIGURE 6.31.
2. Identify the **flexor digitorum brevis**, which lies in the center of the foot immediately deep to the plantar aponeurosis.
3. Trace the flexor digitorum brevis tendons toward their distal attachments, removing remnants of the plantar aponeurosis as necessary.
4. On the plantar surface of at least two digits, carefully make a vertical incision along the length of the toe through the synovial sheaths overlying the flexor digitorum brevis tendons, making an effort to not cut too deeply (**Cut 3**).
5. Spread open the synovial sheath to expose the "Y" shaped tendinous attachment of the flexor digitorum brevis to the middle phalanx.
6. Identify the **abductor hallucis** on the medial side of the flexor digitorum brevis and use blunt dissection to follow its tendon toward its distal attachment on the great toe.
7. Identify the **abductor digiti minimi** on the lateral side of the flexor digitorum brevis and use blunt dissection to follow its tendon toward its distal attachment on the 5th (small) toe.
8. Review the attachments, actions, and innervation of the muscles of the first layer of the foot (see **TABLE 6.8**).
9. Cut the flexor digitorum brevis close to the calcaneus (**Cut 4**) and reflect it distally.
10. Identify the **posterior tibial artery** and **tibial nerve** near the medial malleolus and follow them a short distance into the sole of the foot.

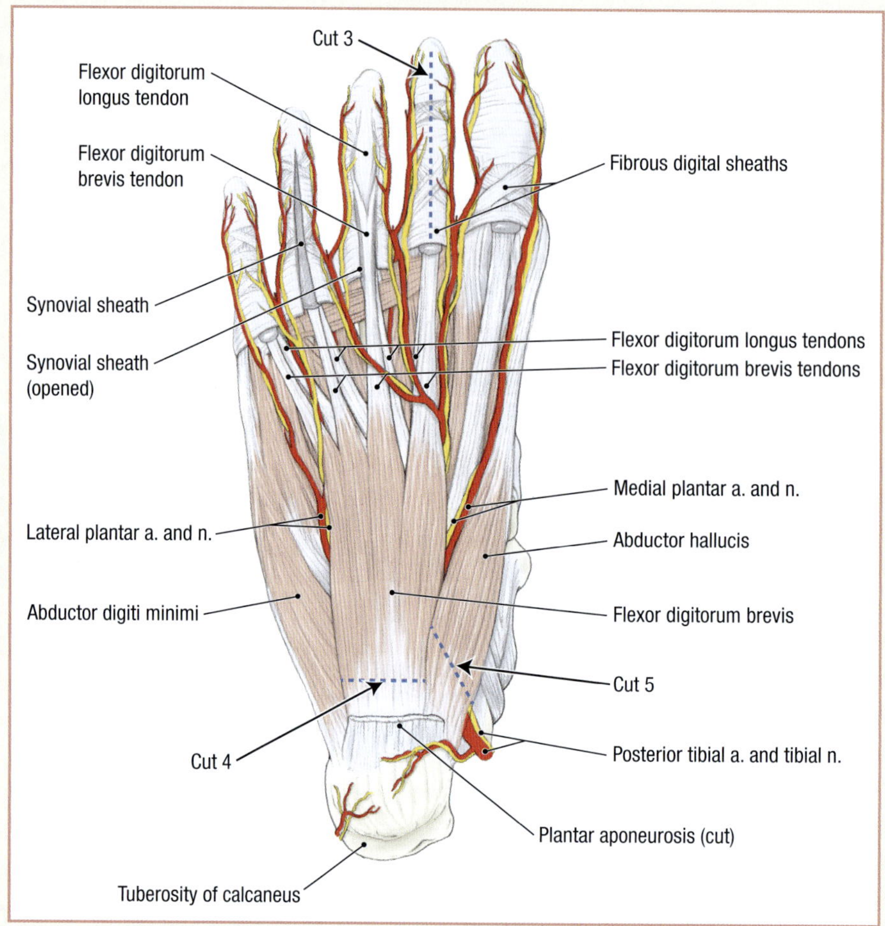

FIGURE 6.31 ■ First muscle layer of sole of right foot. Inferior view.

11. Push a probe deep to the abductor hallucis along the course of the posterior tibial artery and tibial nerve.
12. Cut the abductor hallucis over the probe (**Cut 5**) sparing the neurovasculature and reflect the muscle distally.

Second Layer of Sole of Foot

ATLAS 6.78; VIDEO 6.9.4

Dissection Note: Perform the following deep dissection steps for the second through fourth layers of the sole on only one foot.

1. Refer to FIGURE 6.32.
2. Use blunt dissection to follow the posterior tibial artery and tibial nerve into the sole of the foot and identify the **medial** and **lateral plantar arteries** and **nerves.**
3. Follow the **medial plantar artery** and **nerve** until they branch into **common plantar digital arteries** and **nerves.**
4. Clean the common plantar digital arteries and identify the **proper plantar digital arteries** branching from them in the web of the toes. Observe that branches from the medial plantar artery supply the first three toes and medial aspect of the 4th.
5. Observe that the **common** and **proper plantar digital nerves** parallel the vessels to supply the peripheral aspects of each toe and that they lie between the tendons of the muscles of the first and second layers of the foot.
6. Identify the **quadratus plantae** deep to the flexor digitorum brevis.
7. Use blunt dissection to isolate the **flexor digitorum longus tendons** in the sole of the foot.
8. Observe that the four tendons of the flexor digitorum longus pass through the tendons of the flexor digitorum brevis near the proximal interphalangeal joints to reach the distal phalanges.
9. Observe that four **lumbricals** arise from the tendons of the flexor digitorum longus.
10. Observe that the first lumbrical arises from the medial surface of the first tendon of flexor digitorum longus, whereas the remaining three arise between two adjacent tendons.

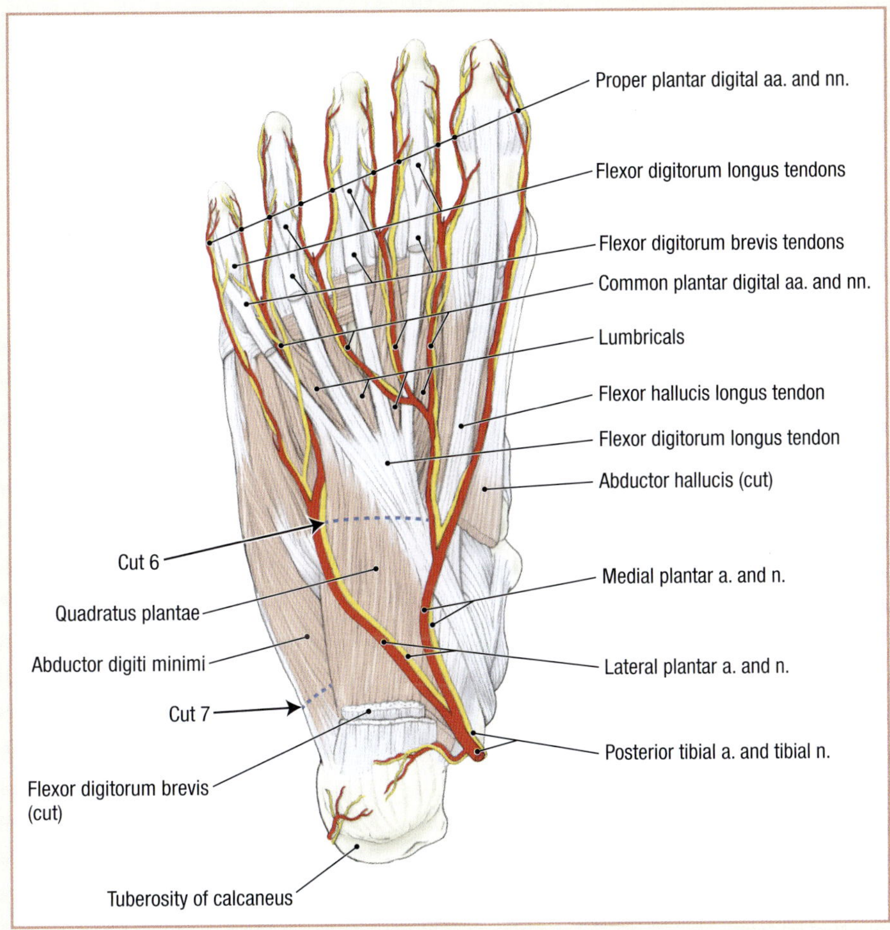

FIGURE 6.32 ● Second muscle layer of sole of right foot. Inferior view.

11. Review the attachments, actions, and innervation of the muscles of the second layer of the foot (see **TABLE 6.8**).
12. Cut the flexor digitorum longus tendon where it is joined by the quadratus plantae (**Cut 6**) and reflect the tendons distally along with the attached lumbricals.

Dissection Note: To reflect the tendons of the muscles in the second layer of the foot, it may be necessary to also cut the medial plantar artery and nerve and reflect them distally.

13. Transect the abductor digiti minimi near its attachment to the calcaneus (**Cut 7**) and reflect it distally.

Third Layer of Sole of Foot

ATLAS 6.79; VIDEO 6.9.5

1. Refer to FIGURE 6.33.
2. Identify and clean the **flexor hallucis brevis** coursing along the deep surface of the **flexor hallucis longus tendon** near the distal attachment site of the **tibialis posterior tendon**.
3. Observe that the flexor hallucis brevis is composed of a **medial head** and a **lateral head** and that each head has its own tendon. *Note that a sesamoid bone is found in each of the tendons.*
4. Observe that the tendon of the flexor hallucis longus lies superficial to the flexor hallucis brevis, is positioned between the two flexor hallucis brevis tendons and associated sesamoid bones, and attaches to the base of the distal phalanx of the great toe.
5. In the central compartment of the foot, identify and clean the **adductor hallucis**.
6. Observe that the adductor hallucis has a **transverse head** and an **oblique head** attaching to the lateral side of the base of the proximal phalanx of the great toe.
7. On the lateral aspect of the foot, identify and clean the **flexor digiti minimi brevis**.
8. Observe the proximity of the flexor digiti minimi to the distal attachment of the **fibularis brevis tendon** and path of the **fibularis longus tendon**.

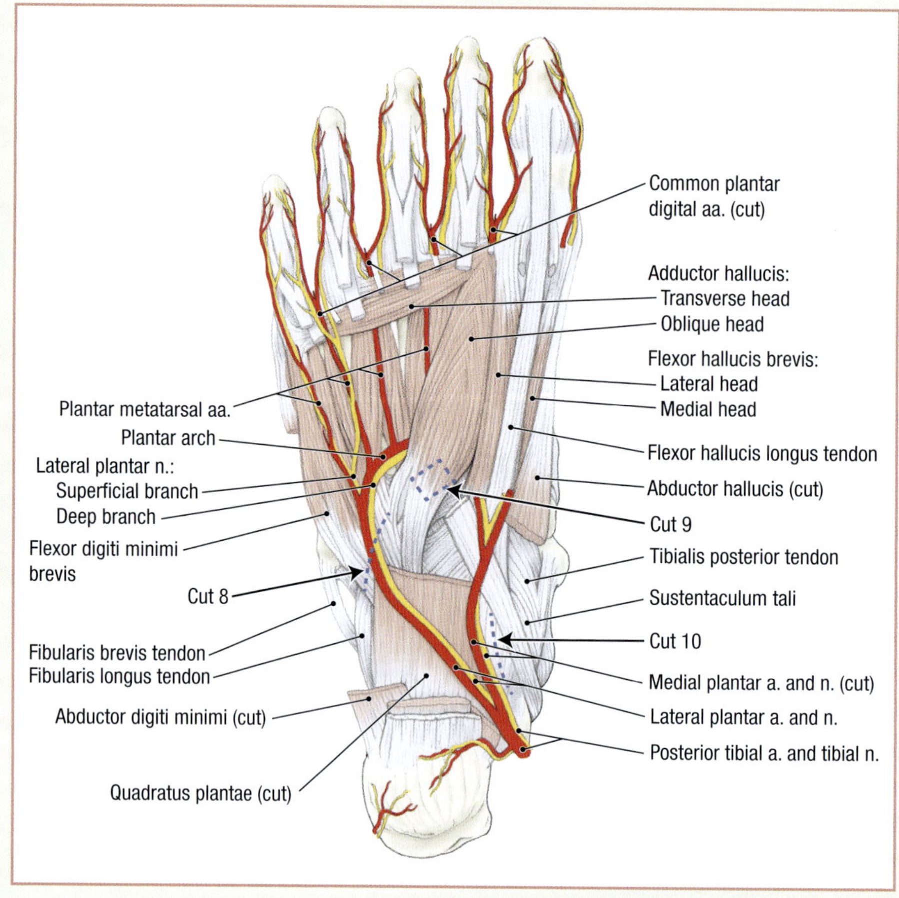

FIGURE 6.33 ■ Third muscle layer of sole of right foot. Inferior view.

9. Review the attachments, actions, and innervation of the muscles of the third layer of the foot (see **TABLE 6.8**).
10. Use blunt dissection to trace the **lateral plantar artery** distally and observe that at the level of the base of the metatarsal bones, it splits into **superficial** and **deep branches.**
11. Trace the deep branch and observe that it turns sharply medially to form the **plantar arch.**
12. Continue to follow the plantar arch medially until it passes deep to the oblique head of the adductor hallucis. *Note that the medial end of the plantar arch is formed by the deep plantar artery arising from the dorsalis pedis artery.*
13. Identify the **plantar metatarsal arteries** arising from the plantar arch coursing between the muscles in the third and fourth muscular layers.
14. Follow the plantar metatarsal arteries distally and observe that they anastomose with the more superficially located common plantar digital arteries.
15. Follow the **lateral plantar nerve** to where it splits into **superficial** and **deep branches** and observe that its branches supply the 5th toe and lateral aspect of the 4th digit.

Fourth Layer of Sole of Foot

ATLAS 6.80; VIDEO 6.9.6

1. Refer to FIGURE 6.33.
2. Locate the **fibularis longus tendon** posterior to the lateral malleolus and insert a probe along its superficial surface deep to the flexor digiti minimi brevis near the cut edge of the abductor digiti minimi.
3. Transect the flexor digiti minimi brevis over the probe (**Cut 8**) and reflect it distally, sparing the overlying lateral plantar artery and nerve.
4. Follow the fibularis longus tendon into the sole of the foot and observe that it turns deeply around the lateral surface of the cuboid bone.
5. Insert a probe along the superficial surface of the fibularis longus tendon (into its tendon sheath) and

gently push the probe medially across the sole of the foot. Wiggle the probe so you can see where the tip is located and observe that the fibularis longus tendon crosses the sole of the foot at its deepest plane.

6. To better visualize the path of the fibularis longus tendon, cut a small window into the tendon sheath (**Cut 9**) and then gently pull on the tendon near the ankle to view it moving through the cut window.
7. On the medial aspect of the foot, follow the **tibialis posterior tendon** distally and verify that it has a broad distal attachment on the navicular, all three cuneiforms, and the bases of the 2nd, 3rd, and 4th metatarsals.
8. Locate the **flexor hallucis longus** in the posterior compartment of the leg and follow its tendon distally until it disappears into an osseofibrous tunnel at the medial side of the ankle.
9. Push a probe into the osseofibrous tunnel superficial to the flexor hallucis longus tendon and open the tunnel by cutting down to the probe with a scalpel (**Cut 10**).
10. Lift the tendon of the flexor hallucis longus with a probe and verify that it crosses the inferior surface of the **sustentaculum tali**. *Note that the sustentaculum tali acts as a pulley to change the direction of force of the flexor hallucis longus.*
11. Refer to FIGURE 6.34.
12. Observe that the **interossei** are located superior (deep) to the plantar arch.

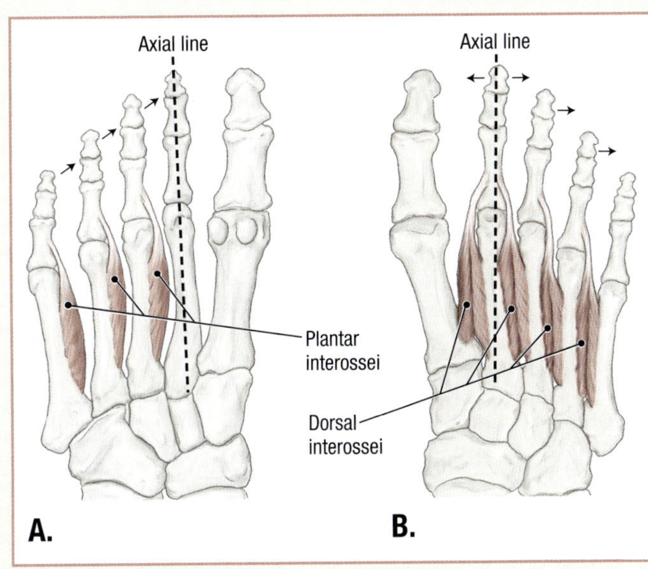

FIGURE 6.34 ● Fourth muscle layer of sole of right foot isolated. **A.** Plantar view. **B.** Dorsal view.

13. Identify but do not isolate the four bipennate **Dorsal interossei**, which are **AB**ductors **(DAB)**, and the three unipennate **Plantar interossei**, which are **AD**ductors **(PAD)**, of the toes.

Dissection Note: Recall that the reference axis for abduction and adduction of the foot passes through the 2nd metatarsal and toe.

14. Review the attachments, actions, and innervation of the muscles of the fourth layer of the foot (see **TABLE 6.8**).

Dissection Follow-up

1. Review the attachments and action of each muscle in the four layers of the foot as shown in **TABLE 6.8**.
2. Follow the posterior tibial artery from its origin in the leg to its bifurcation in the sole of the foot and review the distribution of the medial and lateral plantar arteries.
3. Review the connection between the deep plantar arch and deep plantar branch of the dorsalis pedis artery.
4. Follow the tibial nerve from the popliteal fossa to its bifurcation in the sole of the foot and review the distribution of the medial and lateral plantar nerves.
5. Replace the structures of the four layers of the sole of the foot into their correct anatomical positions.

TABLE 6.8 Muscles of Sole of Foot

Muscle	Proximal Attachments	Distal Attachments	Actions	Innervation
FIRST LAYER				
Muscle	*Proximal Attachments*	*Distal Attachments*	*Actions*	*Innervation*
Flexor digitorum brevis	Calcaneal tuberosity and plantar aponeurosis	Middle phalanges of the lateral four toes	Flexes toes 2–5	Medial plantar n.
Abductor hallucis	Medial process of tuberosity of calcaneus, flexor retinaculum, and plantar aponeurosis	Medial side of base of proximal phalanx of 1st digit	Abducts and flexes 1st digit	
Abductor digiti minimi	Medial and lateral processes of tuberosity of calcaneus, plantar aponeurosis, and intermuscular septa	Lateral side of base of proximal phalanx of 5th digit	Abducts and flexes 5th digit	Lateral plantar n.
SECOND LAYER				
Muscle	*Proximal Attachments*	*Distal Attachments*	*Actions*	*Innervation*
Quadratus plantae	Medial surface and lateral margin of plantar surface of calcaneus	Posterolateral margin of tendon of flexor digitorum longus	Flexes lateral four digits	Lateral plantar n.
Lumbricals	Tendons of flexor digitorum longus	Medial aspect of extensor expansion of lateral four digits	Flexes proximal phalanges and extends middle and distal phalanges of digits 2–4	Medial plantar n. (first) Lateral plantar n. (second to fourth)
THIRD LAYER				
Muscle	*Proximal Attachments*	*Distal Attachments*	*Actions*	*Innervation*
Flexor hallucis brevis	Plantar surfaces of cuboid and lateral cuneiforms	Both sides of base of proximal phalanx of 1st digit	Flexes proximal phalanx of 1st digit	Medial plantar n.
Adductor hallucis	Bases of metatarsals 2–4 (oblique head), plantar ligaments of MTP (transverse head)	Lateral side of base of proximal phalanx of 1st digit	Adducts 1st digit	Deep branch of lateral plantar n.
Flexor digiti minimi	Base of 5th metatarsal	Base of proximal phalanx of 5th digit	Flexes proximal phalanx of 5th digit	Superficial branch of lateral plantar n.
FOURTH LAYER				
Muscle	*Proximal Attachments*	*Distal Attachments*	*Actions*	*Innervation*
Plantar interossei	Plantar surface of metatarsals 3–5	Medial sides of bases of phalanges of digits 3–5	Adducts digits 3–5 and flexes MTP joints	Lateral plantar n.
Dorsal interossei	Adjacent sides of metatarsals 1–5	Medial side of proximal phalanx of 2nd digit (first), lateral sides of proximal phalanx of digits 2–4 (second to fourth)	Abducts digits 2–4 and flexes MTP joints	

Abbreviations: MTP, metatarsophalangeal joint; n., nerve.

JOINTS OF LOWER LIMB

Dissection Overview

In order to dissect the joints in the lower limb, it will be necessary to reflect or remove a majority of the surrounding muscles. Because the joint dissections will make it difficult to review key muscular relationships later, it is recommended to limit the joint dissections to one lower limb and to keep the soft tissue structures of the other limb intact for review purposes. Alternatively, if enough cadaveric specimens are available in the lab, perform only select dissections on each limb and alternate the dissections performed on each cadaver. While removing the muscles of the selected lower limb, take advantage of this opportunity to review the attachments, actions, and innervation of each muscle as it is removed.

The order of dissection will be as follows: The hip joint will be dissected. The knee joint will be dissected. The ankle joint will be dissected. The intermetatarsal joints, which are responsible for inversion and eversion, will be studied.

Dissection Instructions

Hip Joint

ATLAS 6.39, 6.40, 6.43D; VIDEO 6.10.1

Dissection Note: Perform the following dissection sequence on only one lower limb.

1. Refer back to FIGURE 6.12 and FIGURE 6.13 and refer to FIGURE 6.35.
2. On the cadaver, identify the three bones that form the acetabulum: **ilium**, **ischium**, and **pubis**.
3. Detach the sartorius from its superior attachment to the ASIS and reflect the muscle inferiorly.
4. Detach the rectus femoris from its superior attachment to the AIIS and reflect the muscle inferiorly.
5. Cut the tendon of the **iliopsoas** close to the lesser trochanter and reflect the muscle superiorly.
6. Remove the **pectineus** completely from the dissection field to expose the anterior aspect of the joint capsule of the hip.
7. Identify the ligaments that contribute to the formation of the **fibrous joint capsule**: **iliofemoral ligament, ischiofemoral ligament**, and **pubofemoral ligament**.
8. Examine the **iliofemoral ligament** and verify that its distal end attaches to the intertrochanteric line of the femur and its proximal end attaches to the AIIS and margin of the acetabulum.
9. Flex and extend the femur and observe that the iliofemoral ligament becomes lax in flexion and taut in extension. *Note that the iliofemoral ligament prevents overextension of the hip joint.*
10. Open the anterior aspect of the **joint capsule** by cutting through the iliofemoral ligament anteriorly and pubofemoral ligament inferiorly (**Cut 1**).
11. Within the joint capsule, identify the **cartilage on the articular surface of the head of the femur.** Rotate the femur and observe that you can see more of the articular surface of the head in lateral rotation, while the articular surface disappears into the **acetabulum** during medial rotation.
12. Abduct and laterally rotate the femur and identify the **ligament of the head of the femur**.
13. Identify the obturator externus and observe that it passes inferior to the neck of the femur.
14. Remove the obturator externus to expose the **pubofemoral ligament** and **obturator membrane**.
15. Observe that the **obturator artery and nerve** pass through the obturator canal, a gap within the obturator membrane, to supply the medial compartment of the thigh.
16. Insert a probe under the ligament of the head of the femur and cut the ligament with a scalpel over the path of the probe (**Cut 2**).
17. Refer to FIGURE 6.36.
18. Turn the cadaver to the prone position.
19. Reflect the gluteus maximus laterally.
20. Reflect the gluteus medius and gluteus minimus laterally.

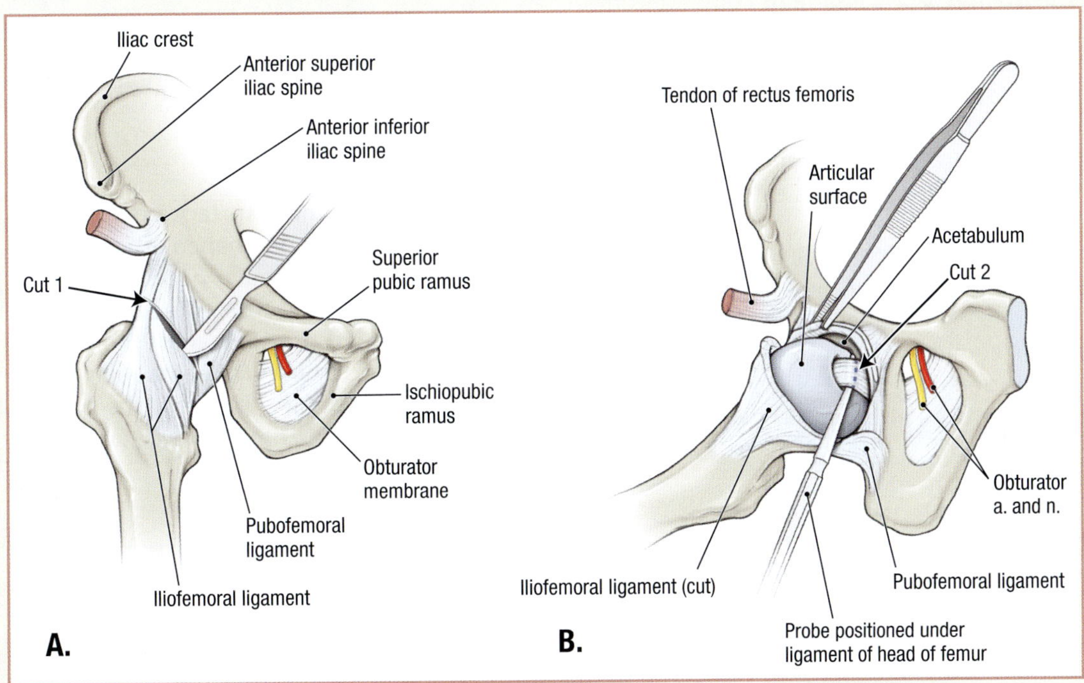

FIGURE 6.35 Opening anterior surface of right hip joint capsule. **A.** Initial incision. **B.** Exposed head of femur. Anterior views.

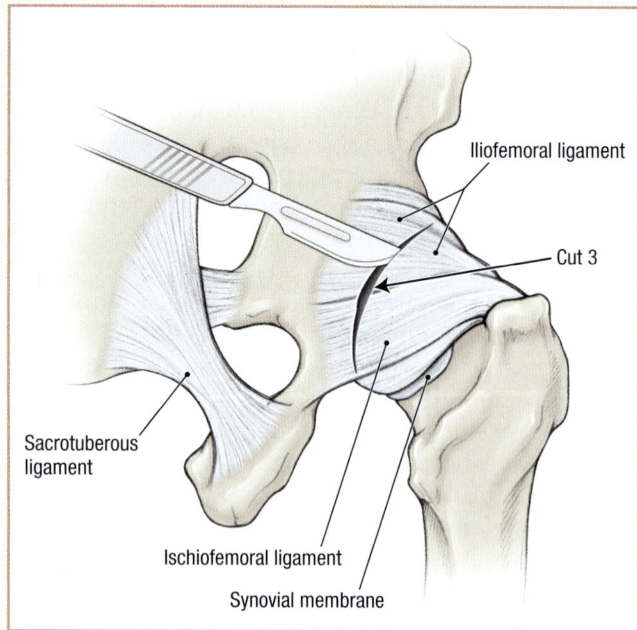

FIGURE 6.36 ● Opening posterior surface of right hip joint capsule. Posterior view.

21. Detach the piriformis, superior gemellus, obturator internus, inferior gemellus, and quadratus femoris from their lateral attachments to the femur and reflect them medially.

Dissection Note: To increase visibility of the hip joint posteriorly, completely remove the lateral rotators of the hip from the dissection field.

22. Clean the posterior surface of the **joint capsule**.
23. Identify the **ischiofemoral ligament** coursing from the acetabular margin to the neck of the femur. *Note that the ischiofemoral ligament does not attach to the intertrochanteric crest, leaving an area where the synovial membrane of the hip joint is exposed.*
24. Extend the femur and observe that the ischiofemoral ligament becomes taut and limits extension of the hip joint.
25. Open the posterior wall of the joint cavity by cutting the joint capsule through the iliofemoral ligament superiorly and ischiofemoral ligament posteriorly, thus making a complete circumferential cut with the incisions made anteriorly (**Cut 3**).
26. Spread apart the two halves of the now bisected joint capsule and observe its thickness.
27. Refer to FIGURE 6.37.
28. Return the specimen to the supine position.
29. Rotate the femur laterally until the head of the femur comes out of the acetabulum.
30. Observe that the joint capsule encloses both the **neck** and **head of the femur**.
31. Examine the articular surface of the head of the femur and identify the depression of the **fovea capitis**, the attachment site of the **ligament of the head of the femur**.

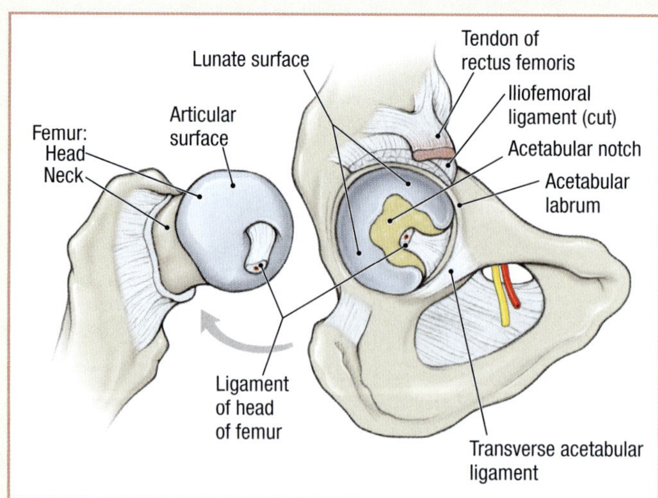

FIGURE 6.37 ● Disarticulated right hip joint. Anterior view.

32. Observe the cut end of the ligament of the head of the femur and identify the **artery of the ligament of the head of the femur** in its center (see **Clinical Correlation 6.7**).

CLINICAL CORRELATION 6.7

Neck of Femur Fracture

ATLAS 6.43

A fracture of the neck of the femur disrupts the blood supply to the head of the femur. If the blood supply (via the artery of the ligament of the head) is insufficient, the head of the femur will become necrotic and need replacing. Necrosis of the femoral head is a common complication in femoral neck fractures particularly in the elderly.

33. Identify the **lunate surface** in the acetabulum, the smooth half-moon–shaped articular surface.
34. Identify the **acetabular notch**, a gap in the lunate surface anteriorly around the medial attachment of the **ligament of the head of the femur**.
35. Identify the **transverse acetabular ligament** bridging the acetabular notch and the **acetabular labrum** surrounding the rim of the acetabulum deepening the socket.

Knee Joint Posterior Approach

ATLAS 6.51A, 6.55C; VIDEO 6.10.2

Dissection Note: Perform the following dissection sequence on the lower limb with the transected medial and lateral heads of the gastrocnemius.

1. Refer to FIGURE 6.38.
2. Turn the cadaver to a prone position.

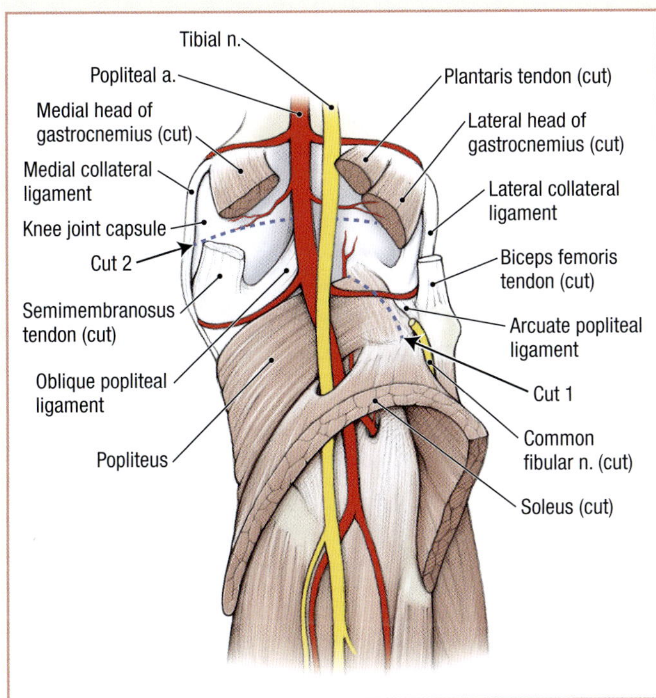

FIGURE 6.38 ● Right knee. Posterior view.

3. In the cadaver, identify the **medial condyle**, **lateral condyle**, and **intercondylar fossa** on the distal end of the femur.
4. Identify the **medial** and **lateral condyles** on the proximal end of the tibia.
5. Identify the tendons of the sartorius, gracilis, and semitendinosus attaching at their distal attachments (pes anserinus) on the medial side of the knee. Recall that these three muscles arise from different compartments of the thigh and have different motor innervations, yet all work together to flex the knee and medially rotate the tibia.
6. Elevate the muscles attaching to the pes anserinus and identify the **medial (tibial) collateral ligament (MCL)** of the knee. *Note that the MCL is attached to the medial meniscus through the joint capsule.*
7. On the lateral side of the knee, identify the **tendon of the biceps femoris** close to its distal attachment on the head of the fibula.
8. Identify the **lateral (fibular) collateral ligament (LCL)** of the knee and observe that it is not attached to the external surface of the joint capsule.
9. On the posterior aspect of the knee, observe that the popliteus tendon passes between the LCL and the joint capsule.
10. On the posterior aspect of the knee, identify the **oblique popliteal ligament** that sweeps superiorly and laterally from the tendon of the semimembranosus. *Note that the oblique popliteal ligament reinforces the posterior surface of the knee joint capsule.*
11. If the oblique popliteal tendon is not clearly visible, remove the popliteal vessels, tibial nerve, and common fibular nerve from the popliteal fossa.
12. Identify the popliteus and observe the presence of the **arcuate popliteal ligament** spanning the superficial surface of the popliteus tendon. *Note that the popliteus reinforces the posterior wall of the joint capsule.*
13. Cut the popliteus tendon (**Cut 1**) and reflect the muscle inferiorly to expose the posterior surface of the capsule enclosing the knee.
14. Make a horizontal incision through the joint capsule (**Cut 2**) and remove the posterior aspect of the joint capsule from the dissection field.
15. Refer to FIGURE 6.39A.
16. From a posterior perspective, identify the cruciate ligaments, which cross each other within the joint capsule.
17. Observe that the **posterior cruciate ligament (PCL)** attaches to the tibia posteriorly and that the **anterior cruciate ligament (ACL)** attaches to the tibia anteriorly.
18. Identify the **medial** and **lateral menisci**. Observe that the **medial meniscus** is firmly attached to the MCL, while in contrast, the **lateral meniscus** is not attached to the LCL (see **Clinical Correlation 6.8**).

CLINICAL CORRELATION 6.8

Knee Injuries

ATLAS 6.50, 6.51

Forced abduction and lateral rotation of the leg may result in the simultaneous injury of the MCL, medial meniscus, and ACL, otherwise known as the "unhappy triad." Typically, an unhappy triad injury is caused by a blow to the lateral side of the knee forcing the inner aspect of the knee to rapidly expand, a common injury in contact sports. As the medial meniscus is firmly attached to the MCL, while the lateral meniscus is separated from the LCL by the popliteal tendon, the medial meniscus is injured six to seven times more often than the lateral meniscus.

Knee Joint Anterior Approach

ATLAS 6.49, 6.50, 6.52; VIDEO 6.10.3

Dissection Note: Perform the following dissection sequence on the contralateral lower limb to where the posterior knee joint approach was performed.

1. Refer to FIGURE 6.39B and FIGURE 6.39C.
2. On the anterior surface of the knee, identify the tendon of the quadriceps femoris superior to the patella and the **patellar ligament** inferior to the patella.

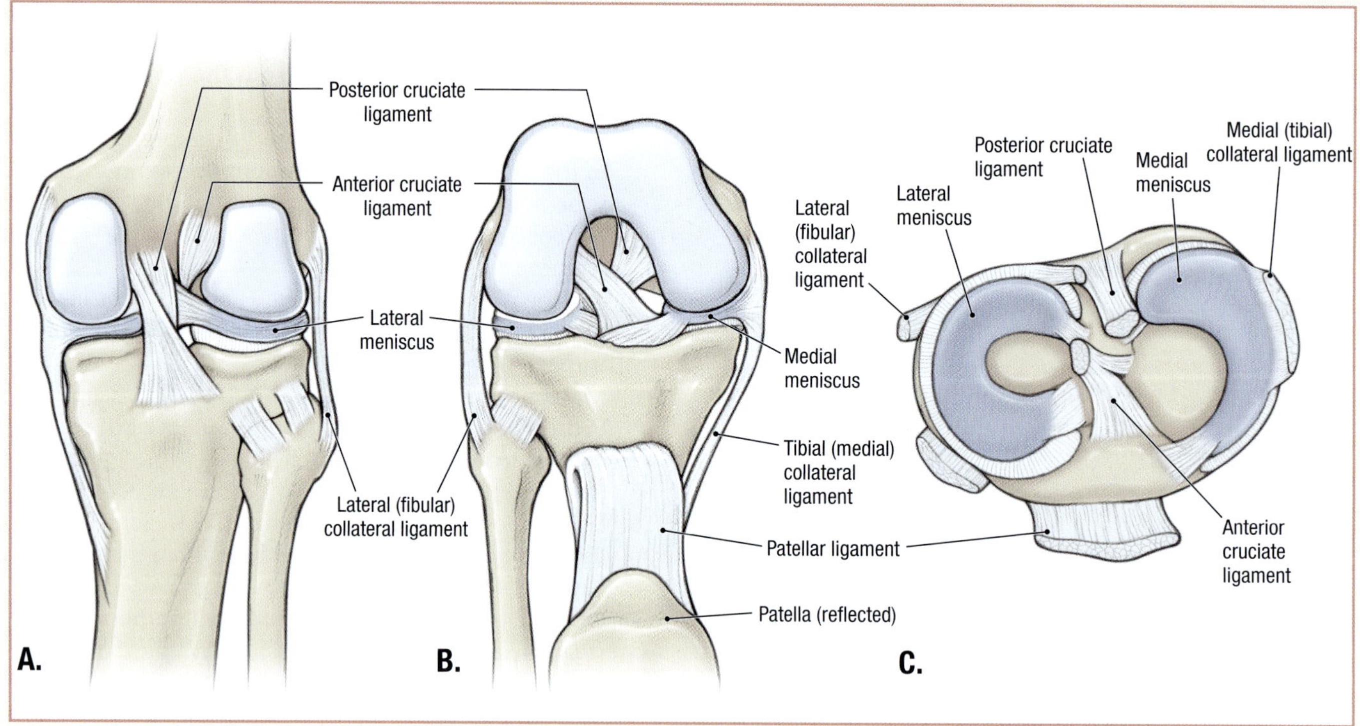

FIGURE 6.39 ■ Right knee joint. **A.** Posterior view. **B.** Anterior view. **C.** Superior view.

3. Observe that the quadriceps tendon has **patellar retinacula** that help keep the patella centered in the knee.
4. Make a transverse incision superior to the patella through the quadriceps femoris tendon.
5. Continue the transverse incision around the sides of the knee, stopping short of the MCL and LCL.
6. Reflect the patella and patellar ligament inferiorly to expose the joint cavity anteriorly.
7. Confirm that the femur and tibia remain attached to each other by **two collateral ligaments** on the periphery of the knee, **two cruciate ligaments** crossing within the joint capsule, and by the oblique and arcuate popliteal ligaments posteriorly.
8. Verify that the cruciate ligaments are located *outside* of the synovial cavity but *inside* the joint capsule.
9. Verify from an anterior perspective that the cruciate ligaments cross each other to reach the intercondylar eminence of the tibia.
10. Flex the knee and observe that the **ACL** attaches to the tibia anteriorly and that the **PCL** attaches to the tibia posteriorly.
11. Extend the leg and observe that the articular surfaces of the femur and tibia are in maximum contact in an extended position. *Note that when the knee is fully extended, the joint is "locked" in its most stable position and that the ACL is taut and prohibits further extension.*
12. Flex the leg and observe that there is less contact between the articular surfaces of the femur and tibia in a flexed position. Observe that when the knee is flexing, some rotation occurs in the knee joint.
13. With the knee flexed, pull the tibia forward (anterior drawer test) and observe that the ACL prevents the tibia from being pulled anteriorly. *Note that if the tibia has a large degree of forward movement, it may indicate a ruptured ACL, an important clinical sign.*
14. In the same position, push on the tibia (posterior drawer test) and observe that the PCL prevents the tibia from being pushed posteriorly.
15. Observe from an anterosuperior view that the **medial meniscus** is more "C" shaped, whereas the **lateral meniscus** is more rounded.
16. Confirm from an anterosuperior view that the **MCL** attaches to the medial meniscus, whereas the **LCL** does not attach to the lateral meniscus.

Ankle Joint

ATLAS 6.82, 6.83A, 6.85A, 6.85C; VIDEO 6.10.4

Dissection Note: Perform the following dissection sequence on the lower limb where the calcaneal tendon was cut.

1. Refer back to FIGURE 6.23 and FIGURE 6.27.
2. On the distal end of the fibula, identify the **lateral malleolus**.

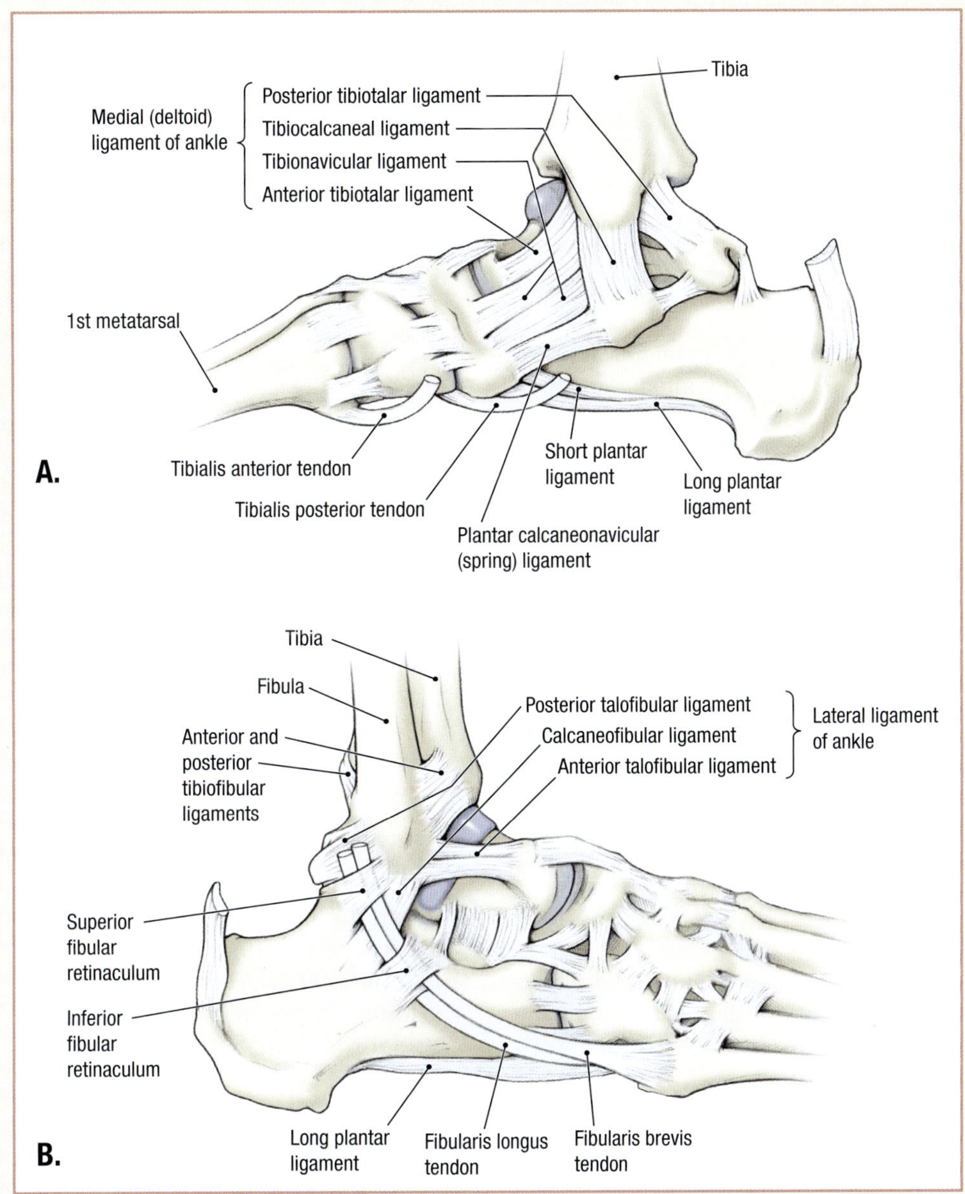

FIGURE 6.40 ● Right ankle joint. **A.** Medial view. **B.** Lateral view.

3. On the distal end of the tibia, identify the **medial malleolus**.
4. On the medial aspect of the ankle joint, cut and reflect the flexor digitorum longus.

Dissection Note: When cutting the tendons around the ankle, leave approximately 2 cm of each tendon attached to their respective distal attachments on the skeleton of the foot and reflect the remaining portion of the tendon and muscle away from the ankle to increase exposure of the underlying ligaments.

5. Retract the tendon of the tibialis posterior anteriorly but do not cut it.
6. Cut and reflect the tendons, vessels, and nerves that cross the anterior aspect of one ankle joint.
7. Refer to FIGURE 6.40.
8. On the medial side of the ankle, clean and define the **medial (deltoid) ligament of the ankle**.
9. Observe that the deltoid ligament has four parts named according to their skeletal attachments: **anterior tibiotalar, tibionavicular, tibiocalcaneal,** and **posterior tibiotalar**.
10. On the lateral side of the ankle, make a vertical incision through the superior and inferior fibular retinacula and retract the tendons of the fibularis longus and brevis anteriorly.

11. Clean and define the **lateral ligament of the ankle** (see **Clinical Correlation 6.9**).

CLINICAL CORRELATION 6.9

Ankle Injuries

ATLAS 6.85

The ankle is the most frequently injured major joint in the body. The lateral ligament of the ankle is injured when the foot is forcefully inverted, resulting in an ankle sprain with swelling around the lateral malleolus. In severe cases, the calcaneofibular and anterior talofibular ligaments are torn, and the inferior tip of the lateral malleolus may be avulsed (pulled off).

12. Observe that the lateral ligament of the ankle has three parts named according to their skeletal attachments: **anterior talofibular**, **calcaneofibular**, and **posterior talofibular**.
13. Dorsiflex and plantarflex the ankle and observe that these are the primary actions of the joint.

Joints of Inversion and Eversion

ATLAS 6.81, 6.94A, 6.94B; VIDEO 6.10.5

Dissection Note: Perform the following dissection sequence on the lower limb where the deep dissection of the foot was performed.

1. Refer to FIGURE 6.41.
2. With one hand, immobilize the ankle joint by holding the talus stationary between the tibia and fibula and use the other hand to invert and evert the foot. Observe that during inversion and eversion, the talus remains fixed in the ankle joint and the foot rotates about the inferior surface of the talus (subtalar joint) and anterior surface of the talus (talonavicular and talocuboid joints).
3. Stabilize the ankle and make an effort to produce **eversion** by pulling on the tendons of the fibularis longus and fibularis brevis.
4. Stabilize the ankle and make an effort to produce **inversion** by simultaneously pulling on the tendons of the tibialis anterior and tibialis posterior.
5. Observe that the movements of inversion and eversion occur at the **transverse tarsal joint** (calcaneocuboid and talonavicular joints) and **subtalar joint**.
6. In the sole of the foot where the deep dissection was performed, remove the flexor digitorum brevis and quadratus plantae.
7. Observe that the longitudinal arch of the foot is supported by ligaments spanning the tarsal bones.
8. Identify and clean the more superficially located **long plantar (calcaneocuboid) ligament** extending from the calcaneal tuberosity to the cuboid bone. *Note that the long plantar ligament is the longest of the tarsal ligaments.*
9. Observe that superficial fibers of the long plantar ligament extend from the cuboid to the base of the 2nd through 5th metatarsals.
10. Deep to the long plantar ligament, identify the **short plantar (calcaneocuboid) ligament** extending from the calcaneus to the cuboid. Observe that the short plantar ligament terminates on the

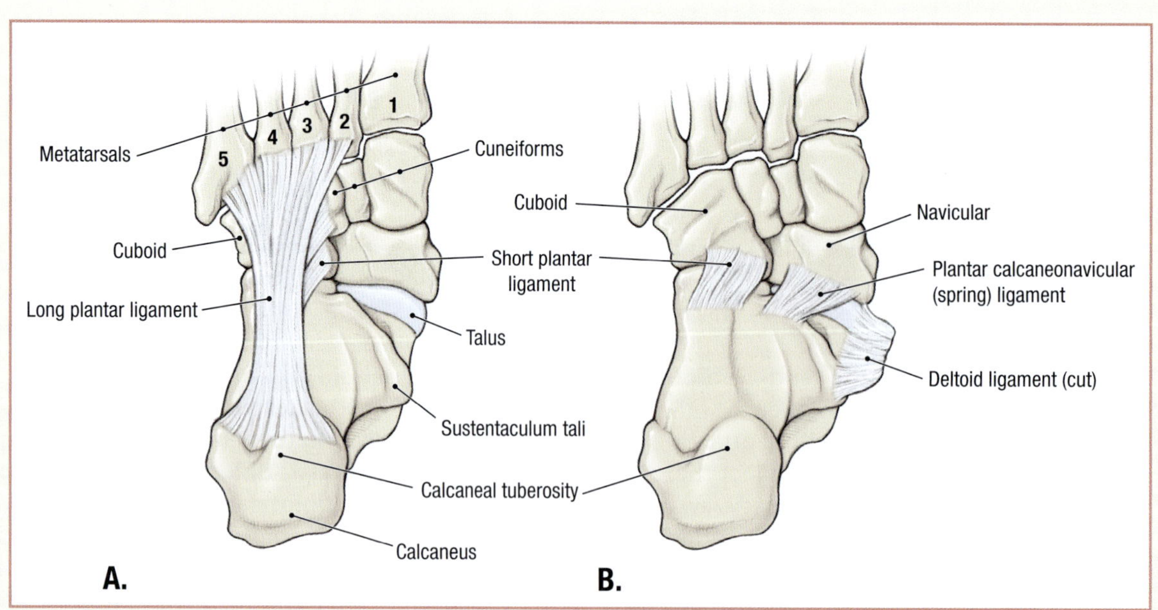

FIGURE 6.41 ■ **A.** Long plantar ligament. **B.** Short plantar and spring ligaments. Inferior views.

cuboid prior to the groove for the fibularis longus tendon.

11. Cut the tendon of the tibialis posterior near its distal attachment and remove the portion of the tendon crossing inferior to the talus.
12. Identify the **plantar calcaneonavicular (spring) ligament** attaching from the sustentaculum tali of the calcaneus to the plantar surface of the navicular.
13. Observe that the spring ligament has three parts named according to their skeletal attachments: **superomedial, intermedial (medioplantar),** and **lateral (inferoplantar).** *Note that the spring ligament and tibialis posterior tendon support the head of the talus and longitudinal arch of the foot and that the spring ligament bears the bulk of the body weight in a normally functioning foot.*

Dissection Follow-up

1. Review the names of the bones articulating at each joint of the lower limb.
2. Review the movements permitted at each joint of the lower limb.
3. Use the dissected specimen to identify the key ligaments associated with each joint and review their respective points of attachment.
4. Return the reflected muscles of the lower limb back to their anatomical positions.

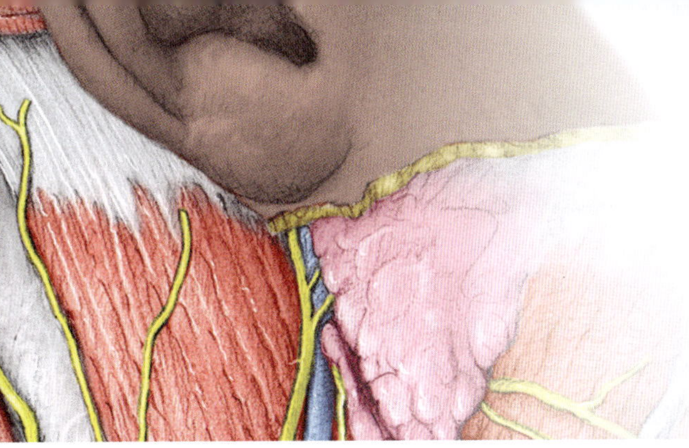

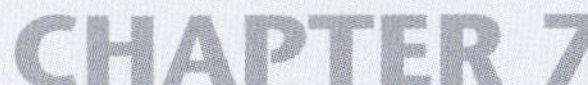

CHAPTER 7

Neck and Head

REFERENCES

ATLAS = *Grant's Atlas of Anatomy*, 16th ed., figure number

VIDEO = *Grant's Dissection Videos*, video sequence number

The study of neck and head anatomy provides a considerable intellectual challenge because the region is packed with small, clinically relevant structures. Dissection of the neck and head requires that peripheral structures are dissected long before their parent structure can be identified. Thus, a full understanding of the region cannot be gained until the final dissection is completed.

The neck is a region of transition between the head and thorax. The major vessels supplying the head and the nerves innervating the organs within the thorax and abdomen pass through the neck. Portions of several systems are located in the neck including gastrointestinal (pharynx and esophagus), respiratory (larynx and trachea), cardiovascular (major vessels to the head and upper limbs), central nervous (spinal cord), and endocrine (thyroid and parathyroid glands). Finally, nerves and vessels to the upper limbs also pass through the inferior part of the neck.

The dissection of the head is foremost a dissection of the course and distribution of the cranial nerves (CN) and branches of the external carotid artery. As the cranial nerves and many blood vessels pass through openings in the skull, it is an important tool with which to organize the study of the soft tissues of the head and neck. Parts of the skull will be studied as needed, and details will be added as the dissection of the head proceeds.

The superficial aspects of the neck (superficial fascia, fat, superficial veins, and cutaneous nerves) will be dissected first. The triangles of the neck will be described, and the anatomy will be discussed within these boundaries. The vascular structures that go to the head as well as the endocrine glands in the neck will then be dissected. The head will begin with superficial and then deep dissections of the face. The calvaria will be detached, and the brain removed from the cranial cavity. The orbit will then be examined from both a superior and an anterior perspective. The head will either be bisected or reflected to study the anatomy of the nasal and oral cavities. Aspects of the pharynx and larynx will be dissected after the head because they cannot be mobilized until after the head is dissected.

CLINICAL CORRELATIONS

During your dissection protocol, you may encounter anatomical variations, clinical conditions, disease processes, or medical devices in your cadaveric donor. The following select clinical correlations will be described in more detail throughout this chapter.

Neck and Head

7.1. Diaphragmatic Referred Pain, see the **Lateral Cervical Region** sequence. ATLAS 4.85, 7.8B, 7.8D, 7.8E
7.2. Tracheostomy, see the **Muscular Triangle** sequence. ATLAS 7.4, 7.7A
7.3. Recurrent Laryngeal Nerve Injury, see the **Thyroid and Parathyroid Glands** sequence. ATLAS 7.21, 7.22
7.4. Thyroidectomy, see the **Thyroid and Parathyroid Glands** sequence. ATLAS 7.19, 7.21
7.5. Thoracic Outlet Syndrome, see the **Subclavian Artery** sequence. ATLAS 7.8G, 7.22
7.6. Bell Palsy, see the **Subcutaneous Tissue of Face and Facial Nerve** sequence. ATLAS 8.13, 8.15B, 9.22E
7.7. Parotidectomy, see the **Parotid Region** sequence. ATLAS 8.13
7.8. Scalp Injuries and Infections, see the **Scalp** sequence. ATLAS 8.20
7.9. Dental Anesthesia, see the **Infratemporal Fossa** sequence. ATLAS 8.50, 8.52
7.10. Epidural Hemorrhage, see the **Cranial Meninges** sequence. ATLAS 8.21, 8.22B
7.11. Subdural and Subarachnoid Hemorrhages, see the **Cranial Meninges** sequence. ATLAS 8.22C, 8.22D

7.12. Cranial Base Fracture, see the **Middle Cranial Fossa** sequence. ATLAS 8.30, 8.31, 8.34
7.13. Cavernous Sinus Thrombosis, see the **Contents of Orbit** sequence. ATLAS 8.30B, 8.44B
7.14. Tarsal Gland Cysts, see the **Eyelid and Lacrimal Apparatus** sequence. ATLAS 8.37, 8.39C
7.15. Tonsillectomy and Adenoids, see the **Internal Aspect of Pharynx** sequence. ATLAS 8.65, 8.66, 8.67
7.16. Pituitary Tumor Removal, see the **Lateral Wall of Nasal Cavity** sequence. ATLAS 8.30C, 8.77
7.17. Maxillary Sinus Infection, see the **Lateral Wall of Nasal Cavity** sequence. ATLAS 8.79A, 8.80, 8.83
7.18. Carotid Endarterectomy and Hypoglossal Nerve Injury, see the **Sublingual Region** sequence. ATLAS 7.14, 7.16, 9.22F
7.19. Laryngospasm, see the **Interior of Larynx** sequence. ATLAS 7.32, 7.35
7.20. Otitis Media, see the **Walls of Tympanic Cavity** sequence. ATLAS 8.87, 8.88, 8.90

SUPERFICIAL NECK

Dissection Overview

The structures of the neck are surrounded by multiple fascial layers, with superficial fascia connecting to structures in the face, and deep fascia dividing to enclose muscles, visceral compartments, and neurovasculature as shown in FIGURE 7.1. Deep to the investing fascia, the neck may be subdivided into anterior and posterior parts. The larger posterior part contains the cervical vertebral column and associated muscles and is surrounded by prevertebral fascia. The smaller anterior part of the neck contains the cervical viscera and is surrounded by pretracheal fascia. Posteriorly, the pretracheal fascia becomes the buccopharyngeal fascia anterior to the point of separation between the prevertebral and pretracheal fasciae. The point of separation between the pretracheal and prevertebral fasciae is the retropharyngeal space, a potential space subdivided by the alar fascia, a sheet of connective tissue connecting bilaterally to the carotid sheaths. The posterior aspect of the subdivided retropharyngeal space is often referred to as the "danger space" because infections from the neck and head can spread into this space posterior to the alar fascia and pass inferiorly into the posterior mediastinum.

The order of dissection will be as follows: The skin will be removed from the anterior and lateral surfaces of the neck. The platysma will be studied and reflected. The external jugular vein will be identified. Several cutaneous branches of the cervical plexus (great auricular nerve, lesser occipital nerve, transverse cervical nerve, and supraclavicular nerves) will be dissected. The accessory nerve (CN XI) will be identified and followed from the sternocleidomastoid (SCM) to the trapezius.

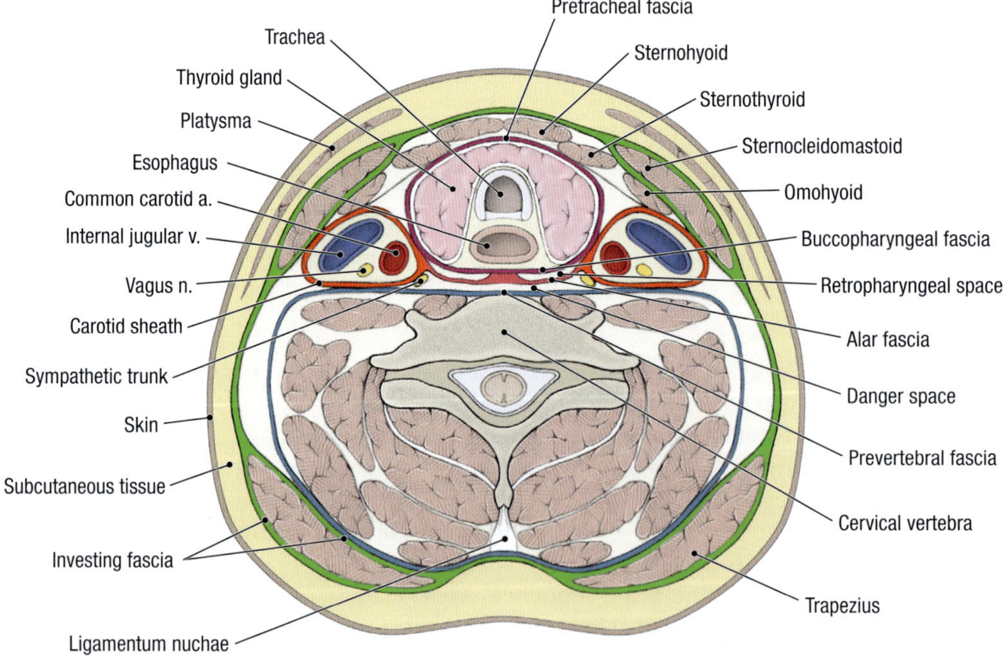

FIGURE 7.1 ● Transverse section through neck at level of thyroid gland. Inferior view.

Skeletal Anatomy

Refer to a skeleton or disarticulated cervical vertebrae to identify the following skeletal features.

Cervical Vertebrae

ATLAS 7.5E, 7.5F

1. Refer back to FIGURE 1.11 and to FIGURE 7.2.
2. Observe that cervical vertebrae have small vertebral bodies, relatively large vertebral foramina, **bifid spinous processes**, and transverse processes that contain a **transverse foramen (foramen transversarium)**.
3. On the isolated **atlas (C1)**, identify the **posterior tubercle** at the midpoint of the **posterior arch**. Recall that unlike the other cervical vertebrae, the atlas does not have a body but rather an **anterior arch and tubercle**.
4. On the superior aspect of the transverse process of C1, identify the groove for the vertebral artery, a smooth depression directed posteromedially along the posterior arch.
5. On the isolated **axis (C2)**, identify the **dens (odontoid process)**, a "toothlike" process extending superiorly from its vertebral body. *Note that the dens is the embryological remnant of the vertebral body of C1, which has fused with the vertebral body of C2.*
6. On the posterior aspect of C2, identify the **bifid spinous process** between the two **laminae**.
7. On **vertebrae C3–C7**, identify the **body**, **transverse processes** with associated **transverse foramina**, laminae, and **spinous process** of each vertebra.
8. On the articulated skeleton, observe that C7 has the longest cervical spinous process **(vertebra prominens)**.

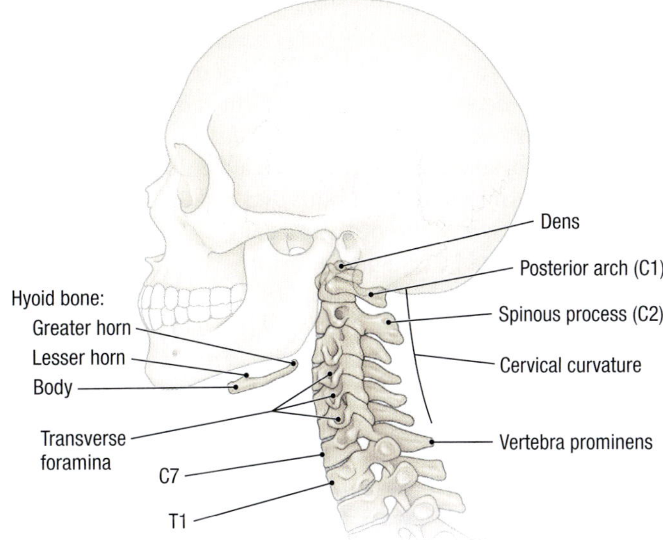

FIGURE 7.2 ● Cervical vertebrae. Left lateral view.

Hyoid Bone

ATLAS 7.5A, 7.5C, 7.5D

1. Refer to FIGURE 7.2.
2. On an articulated skeleton, observe that the **hyoid bone** is the only bone in the body that does not directly articulate with another bone.
3. On an isolated hyoid bone, identify the large bilateral prominences of the **greater horns** projecting posteriorly from the centrally located **body**.
4. Identify the shorter **lesser horns** of the hyoid projecting superiorly near the junction of the greater horns and the body.

Surface Anatomy

The surface anatomy of the neck may be studied on a living subject or on a cadaver. On the cadaver, note that fixation of tissue during embalming may make it difficult to distinguish bone from well-preserved soft tissues in some specimens.

Cervical Triangles

ATLAS 7.3, 7.6

1. Refer to FIGURE 7.3.
2. Place the cadaver in the supine position.
3. Palpate the large diagonally oriented **SCM** on the anterolateral aspect of the neck.
4. Follow the SCM superiorly and palpate its superior attachment to the **mastoid process** on the base of the skull posterior to the ear.
5. Follow the SCM inferiorly and palpate its two inferior attachments to the **sternal end of the clavicle** and **manubrium of the sternum**.

6. Palpate along the lateral aspect of the neck for the anterior border of the **trapezius**.
7. Observe that the **lateral cervical region (posterior triangle of the neck)** is bounded **anteriorly** by the posterior border of the SCM, **posteriorly** by the superior border of the trapezius, and **inferiorly** by the middle one-third of the clavicle. *Note that the lateral cervical region of the neck has a superficial boundary (roof) formed by the investing layer of deep cervical fascia and a deep boundary (floor) formed by the muscles of the neck covered by prevertebral fascia.*
8. Observe that the **anterior cervical region (anterior triangle of the neck)** is bounded **medially** by the median plane of the neck, **laterally** by the anterior border of the SCM, and **superiorly** by the inferior border of the mandible. *Note that the anterior cervical region has a superficial boundary (roof) formed by the investing layer of deep cervical fascia and a deep boundary (floor) formed by the larynx and pharynx.*

Dissection Note: For descriptive purposes, the anterior cervical region is divided by the digastric and omohyoid into smaller triangles: muscular, carotid, submandibular, and submental, which will be studied later in more detail.

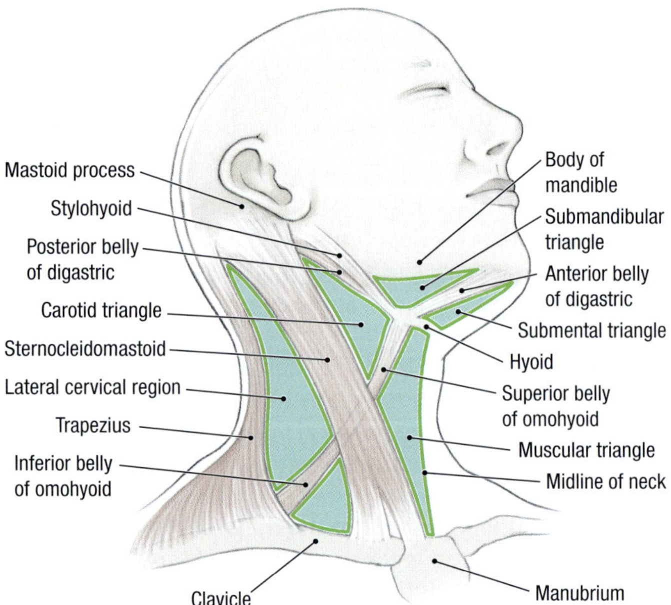

FIGURE 7.3 ● Boundaries of cervical triangles. Right anterolateral view.

Dissection Instructions

Skin Incisions of Neck

VIDEO 7.1.1

Dissection Note: Prior to commencing with skin incisions, note that the superficial veins and cutaneous nerves are easily damaged in the neck if skin incisions are made too deeply. It is thus recommended that a partial-thickness skinning technique be implemented in the neck.

1. Refer to FIGURE 7.4.
2. Make an anterior midline skin incision from the chin (C) to the jugular notch of the sternum (E).
3. Make a horizontal skin incision beginning from the midline incision at the chin (C) along body of the mandible that arches superiorly along the jaw line to a point just anterior to the ear lobe (D).
4. Make a skin incision in the transverse plane from the point anterior to the ear lobe (D) to the external occipital protuberance (X). *Note that if the back has been dissected previously, part of this incision has been made.*
5. If the back has not been dissected, make a skin incision along the superior border of the trapezius from the external occipital protuberance (X) to the acromion process of the scapula (I).
6. If the thorax has not been dissected, make an incision from the jugular notch (E) along the anterior surface of the clavicle laterally to the acromion process (I).
7. Beginning at the anterior midline, reflect the skin in the lateral direction as far as the anterior border of the trapezius, paying particular attention to not disrupt the superficially located veins or platysma descending from the face.
8. Detach the skin of the neck and place it in the tissue container.

Dissection Note: Reflecting the skin with portions still attached will block views of the underlying anatomy; thus, it is recommended to completely remove the skin. If the skin is removed in large portions, it may, however, be used later to wrap the neck post dissection to prevent desiccation.

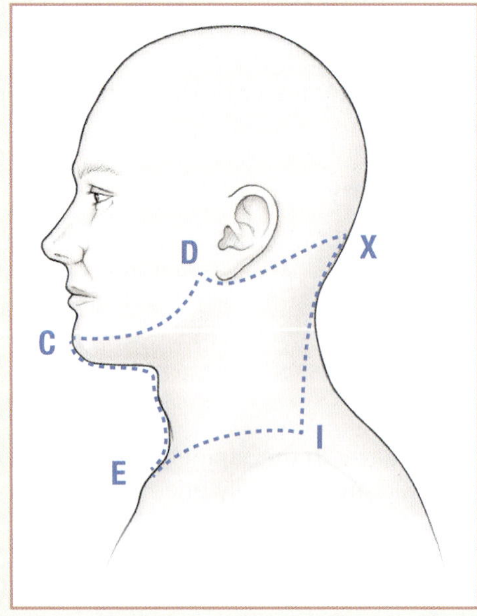

FIGURE 7.4 ● Skin incisions of neck. Left lateral view.

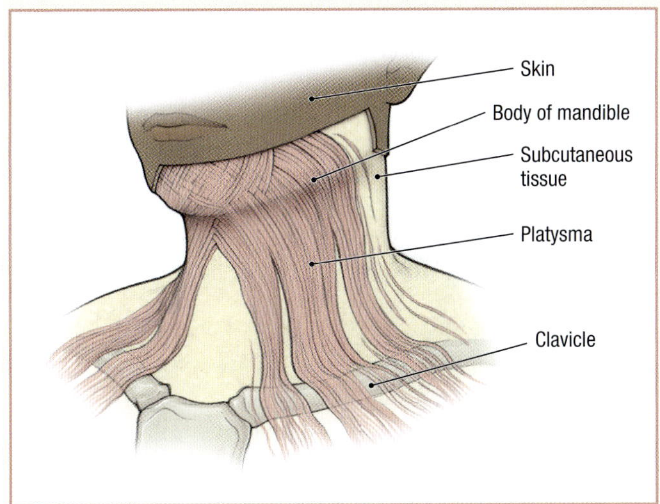

FIGURE 7.5 ● Platysma and subcutaneous tissue of neck. Left anterolateral view.

Lateral Cervical Region

ATLAS 7.1, 7.3, 7.8A, 7.8B; VIDEO 7.1.2

1. Refer to FIGURE 7.5.
2. Identify the **platysma** in the **subcutaneous tissue** of the neck.
3. Observe that the platysma is very thin and covers the bulk of the anterior and lateral cervical regions.
4. Observe that the platysma passes superficial to the **clavicle** as it descends toward its inferior attachment in the subcutaneous tissue of the thorax. *Note that some of the structures to be dissected in steps 5 and 6 are in contact with the deep surface of the platysma and care must be taken to preserve them (i.e., supraclavicular nerves, transverse cervical nerve, and external jugular vein).*
5. Near the clavicle, raise the inferior border of the platysma near the midline of the neck.
6. Carefully use sharp dissection to free the platysma from the vessels and nerves on its deep surface and reflect the muscle superiorly as far as the mandible, leaving it attached along the body of the mandible.
7. Refer to FIGURE 7.6.
8. Identify and clean the **external jugular vein** in the subcutaneous tissue deep to the platysma.
9. Observe that the external jugular vein begins posterior to the angle of the mandible and crosses the superficial surface of the SCM as it descends toward the thorax.
10. Follow the external jugular vein inferiorly and observe that about 3 cm superior to the clavicle, it pierces the **investing layer of deep cervical fascia** (roof of the lateral cervical region) to drain into the subclavian vein. *Note that the external jugular vein will be followed superiorly during the anterior cervical region dissection.*
11. Along the posterior border of the SCM, identify the **nerve point of the neck**, which contains cutaneous nerve branches of the **cervical plexus**. The cutaneous nerves arising from the nerve point of the neck pass through the lateral cervical region to enter the subcutaneous tissue near the midpoint of the SCM to innervate the skin of the neck and part of the posterior head (see **Clinical Correlation 7.1**).

CLINICAL CORRELATION 7.1

Diaphragmatic Referred Pain

ATLAS 4.85, 7.8B, 7.8D, 7.8E

Pain and sensory information due to irritation of the mediastinal or diaphragmatic parietal pleura, or the parietal peritoneum lining the inferior aspect of the diaphragm, is carried by the phrenic nerves (C3–C5). The internal information of pain is referred to the somatic region of the shoulder via the supraclavicular cutaneous nerves arising from the same vertebral levels.

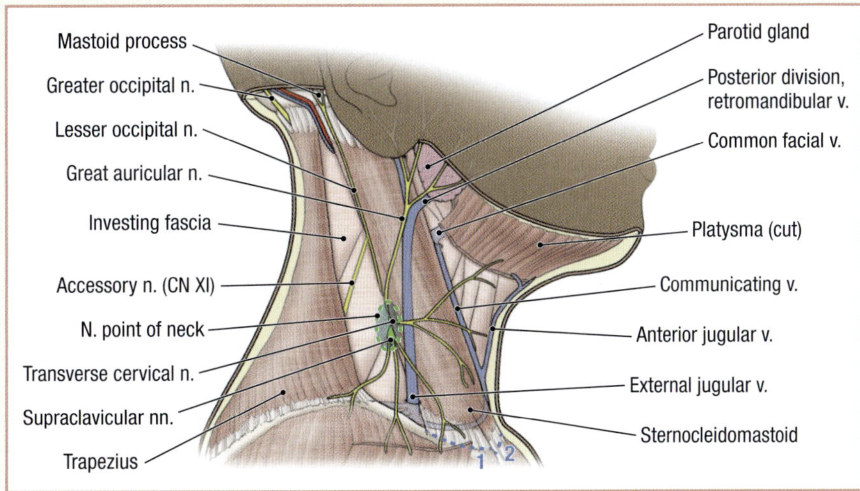

FIGURE 7.6 ● Boundaries and contents of lateral cervical region. Right lateral view.

12. Identify and clean the **lesser occipital nerve (C2)**, which parallels the posterior border of the SCM as it passes superiorly. *Note that the lesser occipital nerve supplies the part of the scalp that is immediately posterior to the ear.*
13. Identify and clean the **great auricular nerve (C2, C3)**, which crosses the superficial surface of the SCM parallel to the external jugular vein. *Note that the great auricular nerve supplies the skin of the lower part of the ear, skin over the parotid gland, and an area of skin extending from the angle of the mandible to the mastoid process.*
14. Identify and clean the **transverse cervical nerve (C2, C3)**, which passes transversely across the SCM and neck. *Note that the transverse cervical nerve supplies the skin of the anterior cervical region and may have been removed during reflection of the platysma if not seen.*
15. Last, identify and clean the **supraclavicular nerves (C3, C4)**, which pass inferiorly to innervate the skin over the shoulder. Observe medial, intermediate, and lateral branches of the supraclavicular nerves.
16. Identify the **accessory nerve (CN XI)**, which crosses the lateral cervical region deep to the investing layer of deep cervical fascia. Observe that the accessory (spinal accessory) nerve courses from slightly superior to the midpoint of the posterior border of the SCM to the superior border of the trapezius.
17. Use blunt dissection to free the accessory nerve from the surrounding connective tissue to verify that it innervates both the SCM and trapezius. *Note that the accessory nerve is a cranial nerve and thus does not originate from the cervical plexus.*
18. Observe that branches of spinal nerves C3 and C4 join the accessory nerve in the posterior cervical triangle to provide proprioceptive sensory innervation to the trapezius. If the back has been dissected, confirm that the accessory nerve may be found on the deep surface of the trapezius.

Dissection Follow-up

1. Review the boundaries and contents of the lateral cervical region.
2. Review the attachments, actions, and innervations of the muscles in the lateral cervical region in **TABLE 7.1**.
3. Review the fascial distribution of the neck and structures surrounded by each layer.
4. Review the path and distribution of the accessory nerve and its relationship to the fasciae of the neck.
5. Review the area of distribution of the cutaneous branches of the cervical plexus noting their relationship to the SCM and platysma.
6. Replace the reflected tissues of the lateral cervical region of the neck in their correct anatomical positions.

TABLE 7.1 Muscles of Lateral Cervical Region

Muscle	*Superior Attachments*	*Inferior Attachments*	*Actions*	*Innervation*
Trapezius	Superior nuchal line, external occipital protuberance, ligamentum nuchae, SP C7–T12	Lateral one-third of clavicle and acromion and spine of scapula	Rotates scapula to tilt glenoid cavity superiorly, elevates (superior part), retracts (middle part), and depresses (inferior part) scapula	Motor: spinal accessory n. (CN XI) Proprioception: C3–C4
Sternocleidomastoid	Mastoid process, lateral half of superior nuchal line	Anterior surface of manubrium of sternum (sternal head), superior surface of medial one-third of clavicle (clavicular head)	Laterally flexes head and rotates face to opposite side (unilateral); extends head (bilateral)	Spinal accessory n. (CN XI)
Platysma	Mandible, skin of cheek, angle of mouth, and orbicularis oris	Superficial fascia of deltoid and pectoral regions	Tenses skin of neck; depresses mandible	Cervical branch of facial n. (CN VII)

Abbreviations: C, cervical vertebrae; CN, cranial nerve; n., nerve; SP, spinous process; T, thoracic vertebrae.

ANTERIOR CERVICAL REGION

Dissection Overview

The cervical viscera are located within the anterior cervical region and include the thyroid and parathyroid glands, larynx and trachea (the superior parts of the respiratory tract), and pharynx and esophagus (the superior parts of the digestive tract). Refer back to FIGURE 7.1 to confirm that the visceral part of the neck is bound posteriorly by the cervical vertebrae, anteriorly by the thin infrahyoids, and bilaterally by the SCM and scalenes. To either side of the cervical viscera and pretracheal fascia are the spaces of the right and left carotid sheaths. The carotid sheath contains the carotid artery (internal carotid artery at more superior levels), internal jugular vein, and vagus nerve.

The order of dissection will be as follows: The superficial veins of the anterior cervical region will be studied. The contents of each subdivision of the anterior cervical region will be dissected in the following order: muscular triangle, submandibular triangle, submental triangle, and carotid triangle.

Dissection Instructions

Superficial Anterior Cervical Region

ATLAS 7.8A, 7.9; VIDEO 7.2.1

1. Refer back to FIGURE 7.6.
2. Identify the **external jugular vein** lateral to the SCM. *Note that superiorly, the external jugular vein is formed by the joining of the posterior division of the retromandibular vein and the posterior auricular vein but do not attempt to identify these vessels at this time.*
3. Identify and clean the superior portion of the **anterior jugular vein** in the subcutaneous tissue near the anterior midline. *Note that inferiorly, the anterior jugular vein passes laterally, deep to the SCM, to join the external jugular vein in the root of the neck.*
4. Observe that the anterior jugular vein begins near the hyoid bone and courses inferiorly near the midline of the neck to the suprasternal region where it penetrates the **investing layer of deep cervical fascia.**
5. Look for a **communicating vein** connecting the common facial vein with the anterior jugular vein along the anterior border of the SCM. *Note that the communicating vein, if present, can be very large.*

Muscular Triangle

ATLAS 7.9, 7.10, 7.12; VIDEO 7.2.2

1. Refer to FIGURE 7.7.
2. Palpate the **hyoid bone** at the angle between the floor of the mouth and superior extent of the neck. *Note that the hyoid bone is unique in that it does not articulate with another bone.*

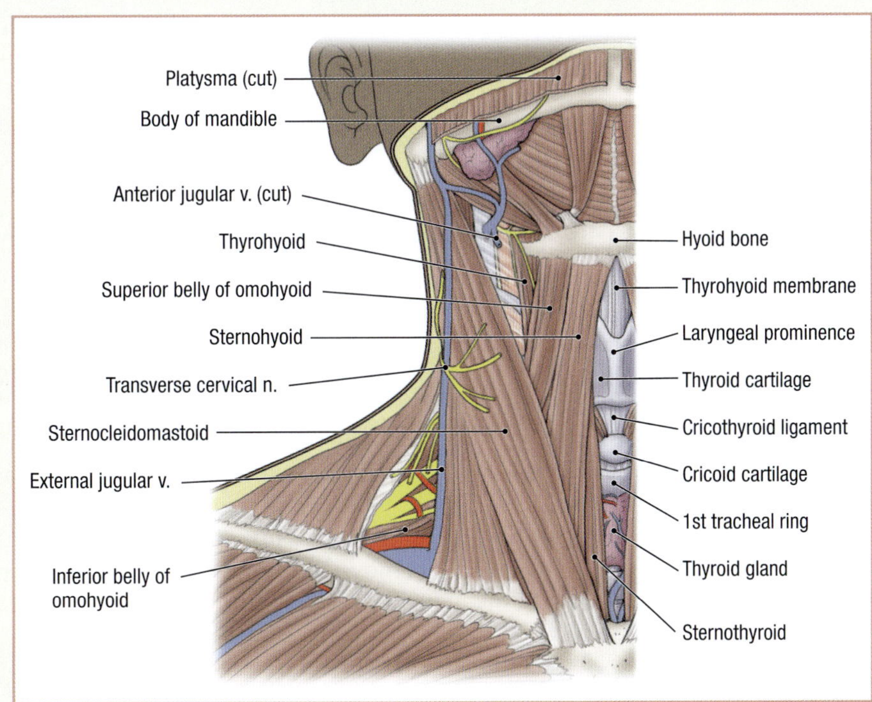

FIGURE 7.7 ● Boundaries and contents of muscular triangle. Anterior view.

3. Near the midline of the neck, use blunt dissection to separate the investing layer of the deep cervical fascia and identify the **sternohyoid**.
4. Loosen the medial border of the sternohyoid from the structures that lie deep to it. Make an effort not to disrupt the lateral border of the sternohyoid as the nerves providing motor innervation enter the muscle along the lateral edge.
5. Detach the sternohyoid from its inferior attachment to the sternum and reflect the muscle superiorly. *Note that if the thorax has been dissected previously, the sternohyoid has already been detached from the sternum.*
6. Lateral to the sternohyoid, identify the **superior belly of the omohyoid**.
7. Use blunt dissection to raise the medial border of the superior belly of the omohyoid and loosen it from deeper structures. Make an effort not to disrupt the lateral border of the omohyoid as the nerves providing motor innervation enter the muscle along the lateral edge.
8. Observe that the **muscular triangle** is bounded medially by the **median plane of the neck**, superolaterally by the **superior belly of the omohyoid**, and inferolaterally by the anterior border of the **SCM**.
9. Deep to the reflected sternohyoid, identify the **sternothyroid** inferiorly and **thyrohyoid** superiorly.

Dissection Note: The ansa cervicalis innervates three of the four infrahyoid muscles (omohyoid, sternohyoid, and sternothyroid) and will be identified later with the dissection of the carotid sheath. The nerve to the thyrohyoid innervates the thyrohyoid and will similarly be identified at a later stage in the dissection of the neck.

10. Review the attachments and actions of the infrahyoid (see **TABLE 7.2**).
11. Gently retract the right and left sternothyroids to widen the gap in the midline of the neck.
12. Inferior to the hyoid, identify the **thyroid cartilage** in the anterior midline of the neck.
13. On the thyroid cartilage, identify the **laryngeal prominence**, an extension of cartilage demarking the location of the vocal cords.
14. Identify the **thyrohyoid membrane** stretching between the thyroid cartilage and hyoid bone.
15. Continue inferiorly from the laryngeal prominence and identify the **cricothyroid ligament (membrane)**. Observe that the cricothyroid ligament attaches along the inferior border of the thyroid cartilage and superior border of the **cricoid cartilage** (see **Clinical Correlation 7.2**).

CLINICAL CORRELATION 7.2

Tracheostomy

ATLAS 7.4, 7.7A

Tracheostomy is the placement of a tube through an incisional opening into the airway to ensure airflow in the upper respiratory tract during obstruction or respiratory failure. Surgically, the opening is made in the midline of the neck between the infrahyoids through the tracheal cartilage after careful separation of the isthmus of the thyroid gland.

In life-threatening situations of airway obstruction (e.g., aspiration of a foreign body, edema of the larynx, or paralysis of the vocal folds), an emergency cricothyrotomy (cricothyroidotomy) must be performed. In this procedure, an incision is made superior to the cricoid cartilage (i.e., through the median cricothyroid membrane/ligament). Using this location prevents damage to the vocal cords superiorly and thyroid gland inferiorly.

16. Inferior to the cricoid cartilage, identify the **1st tracheal ring** and observe its proximity to the **isthmus of the thyroid gland**.
17. Observe that the **thyroid gland** is positioned bilaterally on either side of the trachea, deep to the sternothyroid.

Submandibular Triangle

ATLAS 7.13, 7.14; VIDEO 7.2.3

1. Refer to FIGURE 7.8.
2. On the cadaver, identify the **submandibular gland** and use a probe to gently define its borders. *Note that a portion of the gland extends deep to the posterior border of mylohyoid and will not be visible at this time.*
3. Elevate the platysma and identify the **facial artery** and **facial vein** crossing over the margin of the body of the mandible. Observe that the facial artery courses more anteriorly and is more tortuous than the facial vein.
4. Use blunt dissection to separate the facial artery and vein from the submandibular gland. Observe that the facial vein passes superficial to the submandibular gland and follows a relatively straight path, whereas the facial artery courses deep to the gland and will thus only be visible for a short distance at this time.

Dissection Note: If visibility of the vessels is limited, remove the platysma and superficial part of the submandibular gland on one side of the face. Do not disturb the deep part of the gland.

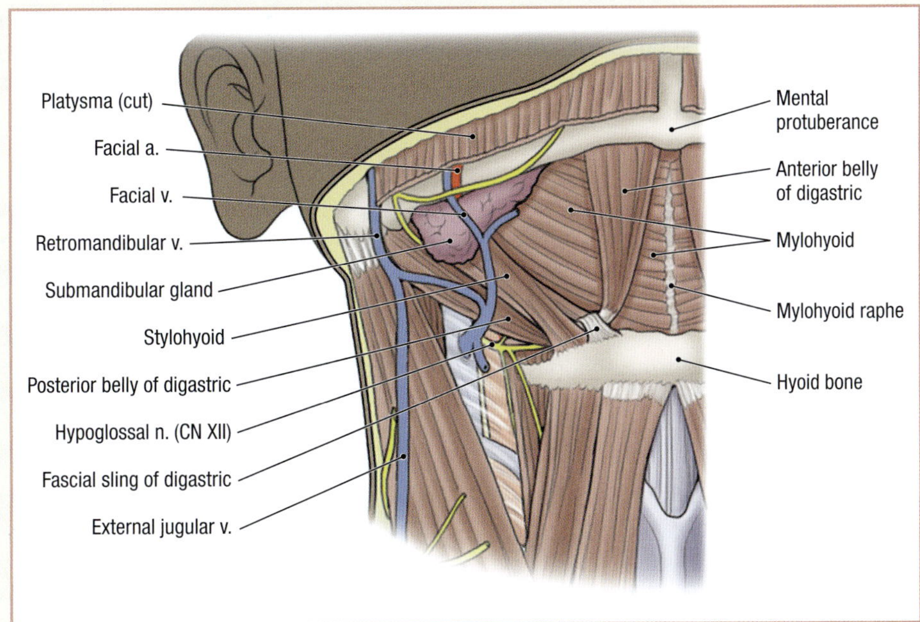

FIGURE 7.8 ● Boundaries and contents of submandibular and submental triangles. Anterior view.

5. Identify and clean the superficial surfaces of the **anterior** and **posterior bellies of digastric.**
6. Observe that the digastric bellies attach to each other by an intermediate tendon that is held to the body and the greater horn of the hyoid bone by a **fascial sling**.
7. Identify and clean the **stylohyoid** located anterior to the posterior belly of digastric. Observe that the **tendon of the stylohyoid** attaches to the body of the hyoid bone by straddling the intermediate tendon of the digastric.
8. Lateral to the carotid arteries, identify the **hypoglossal nerve (CN XII)**.
9. Observe that the hypoglossal nerve enters the submandibular triangle by passing deep to the posterior belly of digastric and the **mylohyoid** to enter the floor of the mouth.
10. Use blunt dissection to follow the hypoglossal nerve through the submandibular triangle for a short distance toward the tongue.
11. Observe that the **submandibular triangle** is bounded superiorly by the **inferior border (body) of the mandible**, anteroinferiorly by the **anterior belly of digastric**, and posteroinferiorly by the **posterior belly of digastric**. *Note that the submandibular triangle has a superficial boundary (roof) formed by the investing layer of the deep cervical fascia and a deep boundary (floor) formed by the mylohyoid and hyoglossus.*

Submental Triangle

ATLAS 7.9, 7.11, 7.12A; VIDEO 7.2.4

1. Refer to FIGURE 7.8.
2. Identify the **mylohyoid** in the midline of the neck deep to the anterior bellies of right and left digastrics. Observe that the right and left mylohyoids fuse in the midline at the **mylohyoid raphe**.
3. Clean the surface of the right and left mylohyoids, removing any remnants of superficial fascia, fat, or lymphatics in the region.
4. Observe that the **submental triangle** is bounded **inferiorly** by the hyoid bone and on the **right and left** by the anterior bellies of the right and left digastrics. *Note that the submandibular triangle has a superficial boundary (roof) formed by the investing layer of deep cervical fascia and a deep boundary (floor) formed by the mylohyoid.*

Carotid Triangle

ATLAS 7.13, 7.14, 7.15C; VIDEO 7.2.5

1. Refer back to FIGURE 7.6.
2. Clean the anterior border of the SCM from its superior attachment on the **mastoid process** to its inferior attachments to the **clavicle** and **sternum** if not previously detached.
3. Observe that at its superior end, the SCM is in contact with the parotid gland. Separate the SCM superiorly

from the **parotid gland** using sharp dissection leaving the superior attachment of the SCM intact.

4. If the thorax has not been dissected, detach the SCM from the medial third of the clavicle (**Cut 1**) and manubrium of the sternum (**Cut 2**), cutting as close to the bone as possible.
5. Use blunt dissection to separate the SCM from the investing fascia that lies posterior to it and reflect the muscle superiorly while preserving the cutaneous branches of the cervical plexus radiating along its posterior border.
6. Use blunt dissection to free the SCM from the investing fascia as far superiorly as the mastoid process to facilitate future dissection of the parotid region.
7. Refer to FIGURE 7.9.
8. Find the **accessory nerve (CN XI)** where it crosses the deep surface of the SCM near the base of the skull and trace it superiorly as far as possible. *Note that the accessory nerve passes through the jugular foramen to exit the skull, but this relationship is too far superior to be seen at this time.*
9. Place the SCM back in anatomical position and observe that the **carotid triangle** is bounded superiorly by the **posterior belly of digastric**, inferomedially by the **superior belly of omohyoid**, and inferolaterally by the anterior border of the **SCM**.
10. Use blunt dissection to clean the **inferior belly of omohyoid**.
11. Observe that the omohyoid bellies attach to each other by an **intermediate tendon** that is held to the clavicle by a **fascial sling**.
12. Review the attachments and actions of the omohyoid (see **TABLE 7.2**).
13. Palpate the **tip of the greater horn of the hyoid** and observe its proximity to the **hypoglossal nerve (CN XII)**.
14. Identify the **nerve to thyrohyoid**, which appears to branch from the hypoglossal nerve. *Note that the nerve to thyrohyoid originates from spinal nerve C1, although it travels with the hypoglossal nerve to reach the thyrohyoid.*
15. Clean a portion of the carotid sheath and identify the **superior root of ansa cervicalis**, which travels with the hypoglossal nerve. *Note that the superior root of ansa cervicalis is mainly composed of fibers from the anterior ramus of the C1 spinal nerve.*
16. Identify the **inferior root of ansa cervicalis** (anterior rami of C2, C3), which passes around the lateral side of the carotid sheath to join the superior root forming a "loop" for which it is named.
17. Clean the ansa cervicalis and trace its delicate branches to the lateral borders of the infrahyoids.
18. Use blunt dissection to raise the posterior border of the thyrohyoid and identify the **thyrohyoid membrane** extending between the thyroid cartilage and hyoid bone.
19. Identify the **internal branch of the superior laryngeal nerve** where it passes through the thyrohyoid membrane. *Note that the internal branch of the superior laryngeal nerve supplies sensory fibers to the mucosa of the larynx superior to the level of the vocal cords.*
20. Follow the internal branch of the superior laryngeal nerve superiorly to the point where the superior laryngeal nerve divided into **internal** and **external branches**. *Note that the superior laryngeal nerve may be too far superior to be seen at this stage of the dissection; if this is the case, continue to look for it as you work superiorly in later dissections.*
21. Refer to FIGURE 7.10.
22. Trace the external branch of the superior laryngeal nerve inferiorly to the **cricothyroid**. *Note that the*

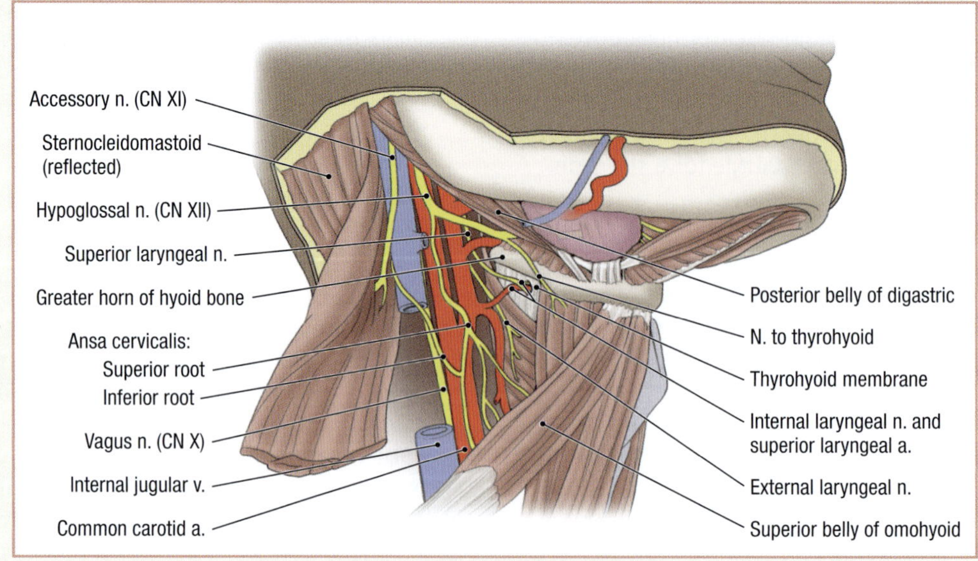

FIGURE 7.9 ● Boundaries and contents of carotid triangle. Right lateral view.

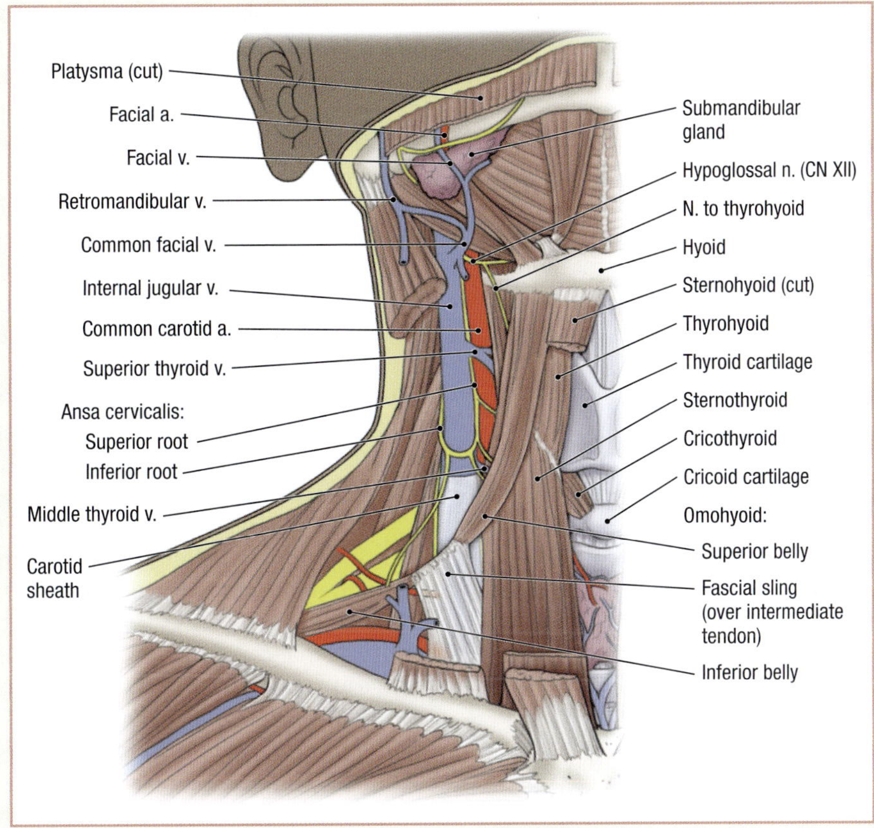

FIGURE 7.10 ● Contents of carotid sheath. Anterior view.

external branch of the superior laryngeal nerve innervates the cricothyroid and part of the inferior pharyngeal constrictor.

23. While preserving the ansa cervicalis, use scissors to open the **carotid sheath** by making a vertical incision through the fascia of the sheath paralleling the underlying large vessels.
24. Within the carotid sheath, identify the **internal jugular vein, common carotid artery**, and **vagus nerve (CN X)**. Observe that the internal jugular vein is located lateral to the common carotid artery and vagus nerve within the carotid sheath.
25. Follow the common carotid artery superiorly and identify its point of bifurcation into the **internal** and **external carotid arteries**, observing that the external carotid artery is located anterior to the internal carotid artery.
26. Use blunt dissection to separate the internal jugular vein from the common and internal carotid arteries.
27. Identify the largest tributaries of the internal jugular vein, the **common facial vein, superior thyroid vein**, and **middle thyroid vein**. To clear the dissection field, you may remove the tributaries of the internal jugular vein.
28. Refer to FIGURE 7.11.
29. Identify and clean the **vagus nerve (CN X)** within the carotid sheath where it lies between and deep to the common carotid artery and internal jugular vein. To see the vagus nerve, retract the internal jugular vein laterally and the common carotid artery medially.
30. Follow the vagus nerve superiorly to identify the point of origin of the superior laryngeal nerve near the **inferior vagal (nodose) ganglion**, a dilation of the vagus nerve near the height of the 1st cervical vertebra. *Note that the nodose ganglion is often difficult to find but is near the point of origin for the laryngeal, pharyngeal, and palatal branches of the vagus nerve and contains the sensory cell bodies for the heart, lungs, and gastrointestinal tract.*

External Carotid Artery

ATLAS 7.15, 7.16, 7.18A; VIDEO 7.2.6

1. Refer to FIGURE 7.11.
2. Identify the origin of the external carotid artery near the level of the superior border of the thyroid cartilage and use blunt dissection to follow it superiorly until it passes deep to the posterior belly of digastric.
3. The external carotid artery has six branches in the carotid triangle. *Note that each branch of the external carotid artery has a companion vein, which may be removed to clear the dissection field.*
4. Beginning inferiorly, identify and clean the **superior thyroid artery** arising from the anterior surface of the external carotid artery near the level of the

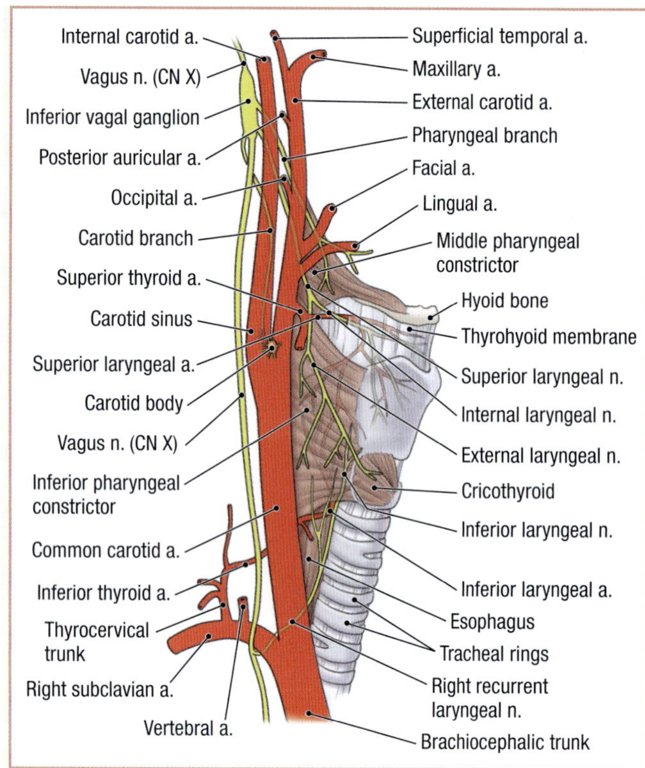

FIGURE 7.11 ● Branches of external carotid artery and right vagus nerve (CN X) in neck. Right lateral view.

superior horn of the thyroid cartilage. Follow the superior thyroid artery inferiorly toward the superior pole of the lobe of the thyroid gland.

5. Identify the **superior laryngeal artery**, a branch of the superior thyroid artery which pierces the thyrohyoid membrane with the internal branch of the superior laryngeal nerve.
6. Superior to the origin of the superior thyroid artery, identify the **lingual artery** arising off the anterior surface of the external carotid artery.
7. Clean the lingual artery for a short distance and observe it arises near the level of the greater horn of the hyoid bone and courses in parallel to the **hypoglossal nerve (CN XII)**. *Note that the lingual artery passes deeply into the muscles of the tongue and will be isolated during a future dissection.*
8. Identify the **facial artery** arising from the anterior surface of the external carotid artery immediately superior to the lingual artery.
9. Follow the facial artery along its path and observe that it passes medial to the posterior belly of digastric and deep to the superficial part of the submandibular gland. Recall that the facial artery crosses the inferior border of the mandible to enter the face anterior to the corresponding facial vein. Do not follow it into the face at this time. *Note that in some individuals, the lingual and facial arteries arise from a common trunk.*
10. On the posterior surface of the external carotid artery, identify the **occipital artery**, which supplies blood to part of the posterior scalp. If the suboccipital region was previously dissected, the distal portion of this vessel was previously identified.
11. Superior to the origin of the occipital artery, identify the **posterior auricular artery**. The posterior auricular artery arises from the posterior surface of the external carotid artery and passes posterior to the ear to supply part of the scalp. *Note that this branch may not be visible if the SCM was not reflected completely in the earlier part of the dissection.*
12. Use blunt dissection to clean the bifurcation of the common carotid artery and identify the **carotid sinus**, a dilation of the internal carotid artery near its origin. *Note that the wall of the carotid sinus contains baroreceptor that monitors blood pressure and that it is innervated by the glossopharyngeal nerve (CN IX) and vagus nerve (CN X).*
13. On the medial aspect of the carotid bifurcation, make an effort to identify the **carotid body**, a small mass of nerve tissue containing chemoreceptors to monitor changes in oxygen and carbon dioxide concentration of the blood. *Note that the carotid body is innervated by the glossopharyngeal nerve (CN IX) and vagus nerve (CN X).*
14. Identify the **ascending pharyngeal artery**, arising from the medial surface of the external carotid artery close to the bifurcation of the common carotid artery. *Note that the ascending pharyngeal artery is quite small and is often difficult to see from this orientation.*

Dissection Follow-up

1. Review the boundaries and contents of the anterior cervical region as well as the subdivisions of the carotid, muscular, submental, and submandibular triangles.
2. Review the attachments, actions, and innervations of the muscles of the anterior cervical region in **TABLE 7.2**.
3. Review the contents and respective locations of the contents of the carotid sheath.
4. Review the branches of the external carotid artery, noting their relationships to muscles, nerves, and glands in the region.
5. Review the branches of the superior laryngeal nerve and note their distribution.
6. Review the course of the hypoglossal nerve and its relation to the vessels in the neck.
7. Review the structures forming the ansa cervicalis and its relationship to the hypoglossal nerve and carotid sheath.
8. Replace the reflected tissues of the anterior cervical region in their correct anatomical positions.

TABLE 7.2 Muscles of Anterior Cervical Region

INFRAHYOID MUSCLES				
Muscle	***Superior Attachments***	***Inferior Attachments***	***Actions***	***Innervation***
Sternohyoid	Body of hyoid bone	Posterior surface of manubrium of sternum	Depresses hyoid bone	Ansa cervicalis (C1–C3)
Omohyoid	Inferior border of hyoid bone	Superior border of scapula near suprascapular notch	Depresses and retracts hyoid bone	
Sternothyroid	Oblique line of thyroid cartilage	Posterior surface of manubrium of sternum	Depresses thyroid cartilage and larynx	
Thyrohyoid	Inferior border of body and greater horn of hyoid bone	Oblique line of thyroid cartilage	Depresses hyoid bone and elevates thyroid cartilage and larynx	C1 via hypoglossal n. (CN XII)
SUPRAHYOID MUSCLES				
Muscle	***Superior Attachments***	***Inferior Attachments***	***Actions***	***Innervation***
Digastric	Mastoid process and digastric groove of temporal bone (posterior belly)	Digastric fossa of mandible (anterior belly)	Elevates hyoid bone and depresses mandible	Nerve to mylohyoid (CN V_3) (anterior belly), facial n. (CN VII) (posterior belly)
Stylohyoid	Styloid process	Body of hyoid bone	Elevates hyoid bone	Facial n. (CN VII)
Mylohyoid	Mylohyoid line of mandible (lateral attachment)	Hyoid bone and mylohyoid raphe (medial attachment)	Elevates hyoid bone and tongue during swallowing and speaking	Nerve to mylohyoid (CN V_3)

Abbreviations: C, cervical vertebrae; CN, cranial nerve; n., nerve.

THYROID AND PARATHYROID GLANDS

Dissection Overview

The thyroid and parathyroid glands are located in the visceral compartment of the neck deep to the infrahyoids and superficial to the larynx and trachea. As endocrine organs, the thyroid and parathyroid glands secrete their hormones without ducts directly into the cardiovascular system and thus have a rich arterial supply and venous drainage. The thyroid gland is regulated by the pituitary gland and produces triiodothyronine (T_3) and thyroxine (T_4) to control the rate of metabolic function, and calcitonin to regulate calcium metabolism. The parathyroid glands produce parathyroid hormone (PTH), which assists in the metabolism of calcium and phosphorous.

The order of dissection will be as follows: The thyroid gland and associated vasculature will be identified. The recurrent laryngeal nerve will be identified and studied. The parathyroid glands will be identified.

Dissection Instructions

Thyroid and Parathyroid Glands

ATLAS 7.18, 7.19, 7.21; VIDEO 7.3.1

1. Refer to FIGURE 7.12.
2. Reflect the SCM, sternohyoid, and sternothyroid superiorly.
3. Identify the **right** and **left lobes** of the **thyroid gland** anterior to the trachea at vertebral levels C5–T1.
4. Observe that the two lobes are connected by the **isthmus**, which crosses the anterior surface of tracheal rings 2 and 3.
5. Identify the **pyramidal lobe**, if present, extending superiorly from the isthmus. *Note that the pyramidal lobe is a remnant of glandular tissue along the route of descent of the thyroid gland during embryonic development from the oral region.*
6. Observe that laterally, the thyroid gland is in contact with the carotid sheath and thus in proximity to the common carotid artery and internal jugular vein.
7. Follow the **superior thyroid artery** from the external carotid artery to the superior extent of the thyroid gland. *Note that the inferior thyroid artery will be dissected later.*
8. Identify and clean the **superior and middle thyroid veins,** tributaries of the internal jugular vein.

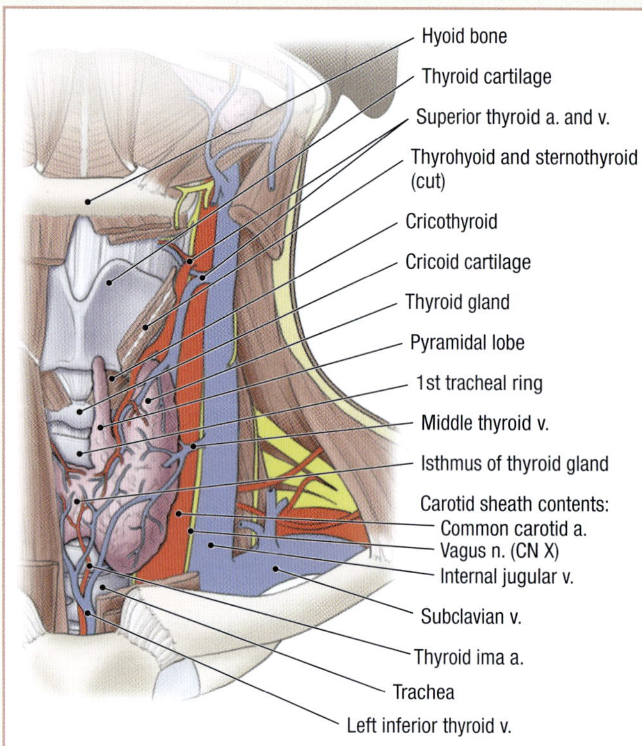

FIGURE 7.12 ● Arterial supply and venous drainage of thyroid gland. Anterior view.

9. Identify the **inferior thyroid veins**, which descend into the thorax on the anterior surface of the trachea to drain into the right and left brachiocephalic veins.
10. Look for the **thyroid ima artery**, if present, entering the thyroid gland inferiorly near the midline. Follow the thyroid ima artery inferiorly toward its point of origin from either the arch of the aorta, right common carotid artery, or right subclavian artery. *Note that the thyroid ima artery is a relatively rare but clinically significant variant as punctures through the trachea may pierce this vessel.*
11. Use sharp dissection to cut the isthmus of the thyroid gland.
12. Use blunt dissection to detach the separated isthmus from the tracheal rings and spread the lobes of the thyroid gland apart.
13. On both sides of the cadaver, use blunt dissection to display the **recurrent laryngeal nerves** that pass immediately posterior to the lobes of the thyroid gland in the groove between the trachea and esophagus (see **Clinical Correlation 7.3**).

CLINICAL CORRELATION 7.3

Recurrent Laryngeal Nerve Injury

ATLAS 7.21, 7.22

The recurrent laryngeal nerve may be injured during thyroidectomy (removal of the thyroid gland) or compressed by a thyroid tumor, causing full or partial paralysis of the laryngeal muscles on the affected side resulting in hoarseness of the voice.

14. Cut all blood vessels leading to or from the left lobe of the thyroid gland and, using blunt dissection, free the left lobe from the surrounding connective tissue to remove it from the dissection field.
15. Examine the posterior aspect of the left lobe of the thyroid gland and attempt to identify the **parathyroid glands**. The parathyroid glands are about 5 mm in diameter and may be darker in color and harder in texture than the thyroid gland. Usually, there are two parathyroid glands on each side of the thyroid gland, but the number can vary from one to three (see **Clinical Correlation 7.4**).

CLINICAL CORRELATION 7.4

Thyroidectomy

ATLAS 7.19, 7.21

The thyroid gland plays a key role in metabolic function for the body. A thyroidectomy is the surgical removal of the thyroid gland, commonly performed for malignancy (cancer). During a thyroidectomy, the small parathyroid glands located on the thyroid's posterior surface are in danger of being damaged or removed. As the parathyroid glands play an important role in the regulation of calcium metabolism, to maintain proper serum calcium levels without medication, at least one parathyroid gland must be retained during surgical removal of the thyroid.

Dissection Follow-up

1. Review the relationship of the thyroid gland to the infrahyoids, carotid sheath, larynx, and trachea.
2. Review the blood supply and venous drainage of the thyroid gland noting the variation between the arteries and veins.
3. Review the relationship of the parathyroid glands to the thyroid gland.
4. Use an embryology textbook to review the origin and migration of the thyroid and parathyroid glands during development.
5. Place the removed left thyroid lobe in a tissue container and replace any reflected tissues of the neck in their correct anatomical positions.

ROOT OF NECK

Dissection Overview

The root (base) of the neck is located inferiorly at the junction with the thorax. The root of the neck is an important area because it lies superior to the superior thoracic aperture, and all structures that pass between the head and thorax, or the upper limb and thorax, must pass through the root of the neck.

The order of dissection will be as follows: The veins of the root of the neck will be identified and studied. The lymphatic drainage into the venous angles will be studied. The vagus and phrenic nerves and the sympathetic trunk will be studied. The muscles that form the floor of the posterior cervical triangle will be studied. The subdivisions and branches of the subclavian artery will be dissected.

Dissection Instructions

Root of Neck

ATLAS 7.22, 7.23, 7.24A; VIDEO 7.4.1

Dissection Note: If the clavicle was cut at its mid length and the thoracic wall removed during dissection of the thorax, remove the anterior thoracic wall and set it aside.

1. Refer to FIGURE 7.13.
2. Reflect the SCM, sternohyoid, and sternothyroid superiorly.
3. Use scissors to cut the fascial sling binding the intermediate tendon of the omohyoid to the clavicle.
4. Follow the **external jugular vein** inferiorly from the upper part of the neck until it passes through the investing layer of deep cervical fascia near the clavicle. *Note that the external jugular vein is the only tributary of the subclavian vein.*
5. To expose the blood vessels in the root of the neck, remove the investing layer of deep cervical fascia forming the roof of the lower part of the lateral cervical region while preserving the external jugular vein.
6. Identify the **subclavian vein** and use blunt dissection to loosen it from the surrounding deep structures.
7. Follow the subclavian vein medially to the point where it is joined by the **internal jugular vein** to form the **brachiocephalic vein**. *Note that the vertebral vein joins the posterior surface of the brachiocephalic vein in the root of the neck but it cannot be seen at this time.*

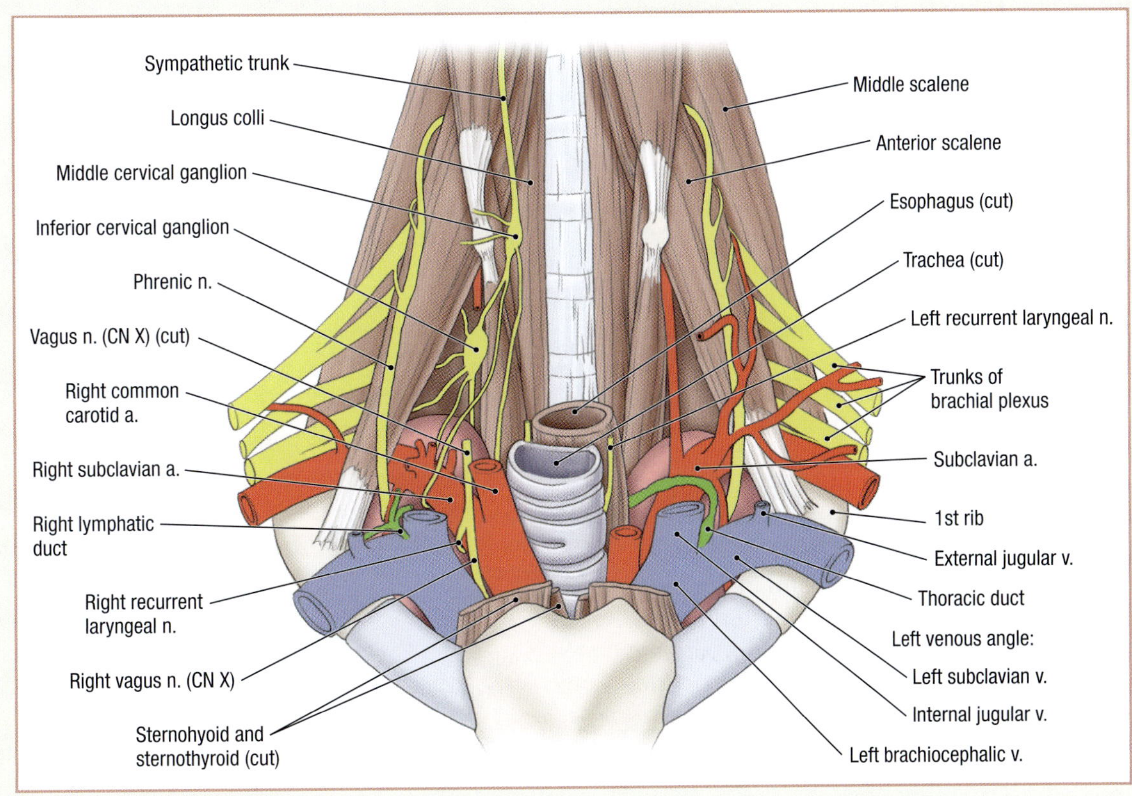

FIGURE 7.13 ● Root of neck with clavicles removed. Anterior view.

8. Identify the **subclavian artery** and observe that the right subclavian artery is a branch of the brachiocephalic trunk and that the left subclavian artery is a branch of the aortic arch.
9. Identify the **thoracic duct** near the **left venous angle** at the junction of the **left subclavian vein** and **left internal jugular vein**. *Note that the thoracic duct is usually a single structure, which has the diameter of a small vein, but it may be represented by several smaller ducts.*
10. Observe that the thoracic duct is posterior to the esophagus at the level of the superior thoracic aperture and then arches anteriorly and to the left to join the venous system.
11. On the right side of the neck, observe that several small lymphatic vessels join with lymph vessels from the right upper limb and right side of the thorax to form the **right lymphatic duct**.
12. Observe that the right lymphatic duct drains into the **right venous angle**, the junction of the right subclavian vein and right internal jugular vein.
13. On both sides of the neck, find the **vagus nerve (CN X)** in the carotid sheath and follow it inferiorly into the thorax. Recall that the vagus nerve passes posterior to the root of the lung while it descends through the thorax toward the esophagus.
14. As the right vagus nerve passes anterior to the subclavian artery, it gives off the **right recurrent laryngeal nerve**. Similarly, as the left vagus nerve descends on the left side of the thorax anterior to the aortic arch, it gives off the **left recurrent laryngeal nerve**.
15. Follow the right and left recurrent laryngeal nerves superiorly along the lateral surface of the trachea and esophagus as far as the 1st tracheal ring. Do not follow them into the larynx at this time.
16. Verify that the **phrenic nerve** crosses the anterior surface of the anterior scalene. Recall that the phrenic nerve arises from vertebral levels C3–C5 and provides motor innervation to the diaphragm and sensory innervation to the mediastinal and diaphragmatic parietal pleura.
17. Follow the phrenic nerve into the thorax and confirm that it passes anterior to the root of the lung along its path to the diaphragm.
18. Identify the cervical portion of the **sympathetic trunk** and verify that it is continuous with the thoracic sympathetic trunk.
19. Identify the **inferior cervical ganglion** in the root of the neck near the superior thoracic aperture. *Note that the inferior cervical ganglion often fuses with the 1st thoracic ganglion to form the cervicothoracic (stellate) ganglion.*
20. Identify the **middle cervical ganglion** midway up the cervical sympathetic chain and the **superior cervical ganglion** high in the neck near the level of the mastoid process.
21. Examine the muscles forming the floor of the posterior cervical triangle and identify the splenius capitis; levator scapulae; and **anterior, middle**, and **posterior scalenes.**
22. Use blunt dissection to define the borders of the anterior and middle scalenes and follow them inferiorly to observe that they attach to the 1st rib.
23. Identify the location of the **interscalene triangle** bounded by the 1st rib and adjacent borders of the anterior and middle scalenes.
24. Review the attachments, actions, and innervations of the scalenes (see **TABLE 7.3**).
25. Observe that the **subclavian artery** and **roots of the brachial plexus** pass between the anterior and middle scalenes through the interscalene triangle.
26. Crossing over the anterior surface of the anterior scalene, identify the **subclavian vein, transverse cervical artery**, and **suprascapular artery**.
27. Use blunt dissection to clean the **roots of the brachial plexus** at the level of the interscalene triangle. Identify the parts of the **supraclavicular portion of the brachial plexus: five roots, three trunks**, and **six divisions.**
28. If the upper limb has been dissected previously, follow the suprascapular nerve as far laterally as the suprascapular notch where it is joined by the suprascapular artery.

Subclavian Artery

ATLAS 7.15, 7.22, 7.23B; VIDEO 7.4.2

1. Refer to FIGURE 7.14.
2. The subclavian artery has three parts that are defined by its relationship to the anterior scalene. Identify the **first part** of the subclavian artery, from its origin to the medial border of the anterior scalene. The first

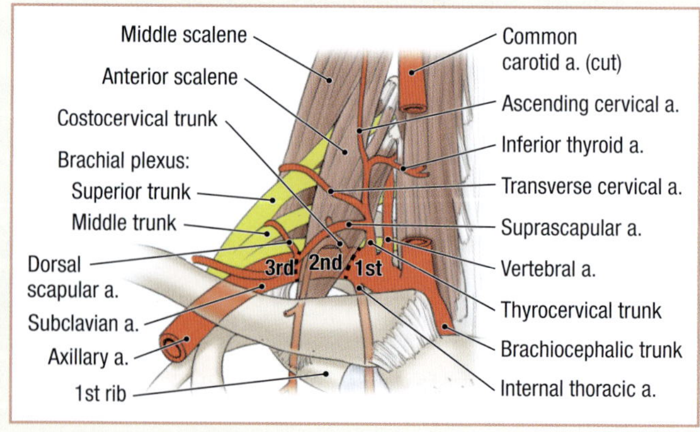

FIGURE 7.14 ● Branches of subclavian artery. Anterior view.

part of the subclavian artery has three branches: the vertebral artery, internal thoracic artery, and thyrocervical trunk.

3. Identify the **vertebral artery**, which courses superiorly between the anterior scalene and longus colli. Trace the vertebral artery superiorly to where it typically passes into the transverse foramen of vertebra C6 to then ascend toward the base of the skull.
4. Identify the **internal thoracic artery**, which arises from the anteroinferior surface of the subclavian artery and passes inferiorly to supply the anterior thoracic wall. *Note that the internal thoracic artery was cut with the removal of the anterior thoracic wall.*
5. Identify the **thyrocervical trunk**, which arises from the anterosuperior surface of the subclavian artery. The thyrocervical trunk typically has three branches named according to their respective paths or targets.
6. Branching off the thyrocervical trunk, identify the **transverse cervical artery**. The transverse cervical artery crosses the root of the neck 2 to 3 cm superior to the clavicle deep to the omohyoid and supplies the trapezius.
7. Branching off the thyrocervical trunk, identify the **suprascapular artery**, which passes laterally and posteriorly to the region of the suprascapular notch. In the shoulder, the suprascapular artery passes superior to the transverse scapular ligament and supplies the supraspinatus and infraspinatus.
8. Identify the last branch off the thyrocervical trunk, the **inferior thyroid artery**, which courses medially toward the thyroid gland often posterior to the cervical sympathetic trunk.
9. Branching off the inferior thyroid artery, identify the **ascending cervical artery**.
10. Return to the subclavian artery and identify the **second part**, which lies posterior to the anterior scalene within the interscalene triangle (see **Clinical Correlation 7.5**).

CLINICAL CORRELATION 7.5

Thoracic Outlet Syndrome

ATLAS 7.8G, 7.22

Thoracic outlet syndrome is a collective term for compression of the neurovascular structures passing to the upper limb via the thoracic outlet (superior thoracic aperture) at the root of the neck. Symptoms of thoracic outlet syndrome include pain, numbness, discoloration, tingling, or weakness of the upper limb associated with the ischemia or nerve dysfunction. Because the interscalene triangle is the point of emergence for the brachial plexus and the pathway of the subclavian artery, it is a common site of compression and of particular clinical concern. Additional muscular slips, shortening and widening of the scalenes, or an accessory cervical rib may all narrow the interval within the interscalene triangle.

11. The second part of the subclavian artery has one branch, the **costocervical trunk**, which arises from its posterior surface. Use blunt dissection to elevate the subclavian artery from the surface of the 1st rib and use blunt dissection to look for the costocervical trunk passing posteriorly near the cervical pleura.
12. The costocervical trunk divides into the **deep cervical artery** and **supreme intercostal artery**. The supreme intercostal artery gives rise to posterior intercostal arteries 1 and 2.
13. Return to the subclavian artery and identify the **third part** between the lateral border of the anterior scalene and the lateral border of the 1st rib.
14. The third part of the subclavian artery has one branch, the **dorsal scapular artery**, which passes between the superior and middle trunks of the brachial plexus to supply the muscles of the scapular region. *Note that in some individuals, the dorsal scapular artery arises from the transverse cervical artery instead of from the subclavian artery.*

Dissection Follow-up

1. Review the boundaries and contents of the interscalene triangle.
2. Review the attachments, actions, and innervation of the scalenes in **TABLE 7.3**.
3. Review the paths of the vagus, recurrent laryngeal, and phrenic nerves.
4. Review the pattern of lymphatic drainage into the venous system at the root of the neck.
5. Review the course of sympathetic fibers to the head and neck.
6. Review the branches arising from the arch of the aorta within the thorax to supply the upper limbs and head and neck.
7. Review the three parts and respective branches of the subclavian artery.
8. Replace the anterior thoracic wall and any reflected tissue back in its correct anatomical position.

TABLE 7.3 Scalene Muscles

Muscle	Superior Attachments	Inferior Attachments	Actions	Innervation
Anterior scalene	TP of C4–C6	1st rib	Flexes neck, elevates 1st rib during inspiration	Anterior rami C4–C6
Middle scalene	Posterior tubercles of TP of C2–C7			Anterior rami C2–C6
Posterior scalene	Posterior tubercles of TP of C4–C6	2nd rib	Flexes neck laterally, elevates 2nd rib during inspiration	Anterior rami C7–C8

Abbreviations: C, cervical vertebrae; TP, transverse process.

FACE

Dissection Overview

Sensory innervation for the skin of the face is provided by three divisions (branches) of the trigeminal nerve (CN V) as shown in FIGURE 7.15. The ophthalmic division (CN V_1) innervates the skin of the forehead, upper eyelids, and nose. The maxillary division (CN V_2) innervates the skin of the lower eyelid, cheek, and upper lip. The mandibular division (CN V_3) innervates the skin of the lower face and part of the side of the head. Branches of the second and third cervical spinal nerves (C2–C3) innervate the skin of the neck and posterior part of the head.

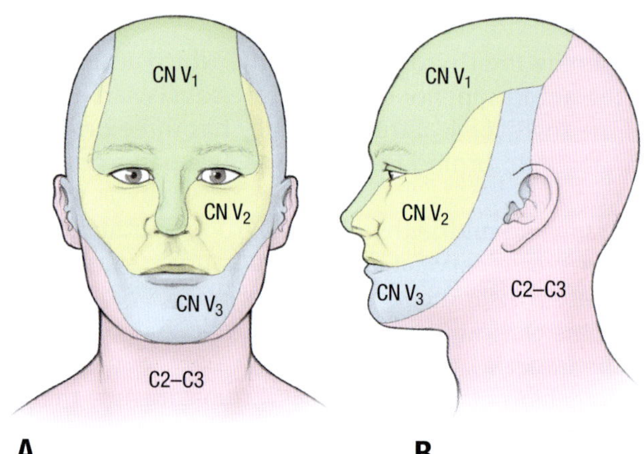

FIGURE 7.15 ● Dermatome map of face and neck. **A.** Anterior view. **B.** Left lateral view.

The subcutaneous tissue of the face contains the parotid gland, fat, muscles of facial expression and associated fascia, branches of the facial nerve (CN VII), branches of the trigeminal nerve (CN V), and branches of the facial artery and vein. The motor innervation to the muscles of facial expression is provided by the facial nerve (CN VII).

The order of dissection will be as follows: The skin of the face will be removed to expose the subcutaneous tissue. The parotid duct and gland will be identified. Branches of the facial nerve will be identified as they emerge from the anterior border of the parotid gland. The muscles of facial expression will be studied. The terminal branches of the three divisions of the trigeminal nerve will be exposed where they emerge from openings in the skull.

Skeletal Anatomy

Refer to an articulated skeleton or disarticulated lower limb skeleton to identify the following skeletal features.

Anterior Skull

ATLAS 8.2

Dissection Note: All parts of the skull are fragile, but the bones of the orbit and nasal cavity are exceptionally delicate. Because the medial wall of the orbit is very easily broken, **never hold a skull by placing your fingers into the orbits.** Similarly, the small bony projections (processes) extending from the inferior surface of the skull can easily be broken by resting the skull on its base without the support of the mandible.

1. Refer to FIGURE 7.16.
2. Identify the **orbit**, the bony cavity protecting the eye, and observe that the **orbital margin** and walls are thickest laterally.
3. Observe that the **orbital margin** is formed by three bones (**frontal**, **maxilla**, and **zygomatic**).
4. Superior to the orbit, identify the **frontal bone** and observe that it extends superiorly to protect the anterior aspect of the brain and posteroinferiorly to form the roof of the orbit.
5. Identify the **superciliary arch**, a thickened ridge along the superior margin of the orbit.
6. Observe that right and left superciliary arches contain the **supraorbital notch (foramen)** and are separated by a small depression, the **glabella**.
7. Inferior to the glabella, identify the **nasion**, the junction between the frontal and **nasal bones**.

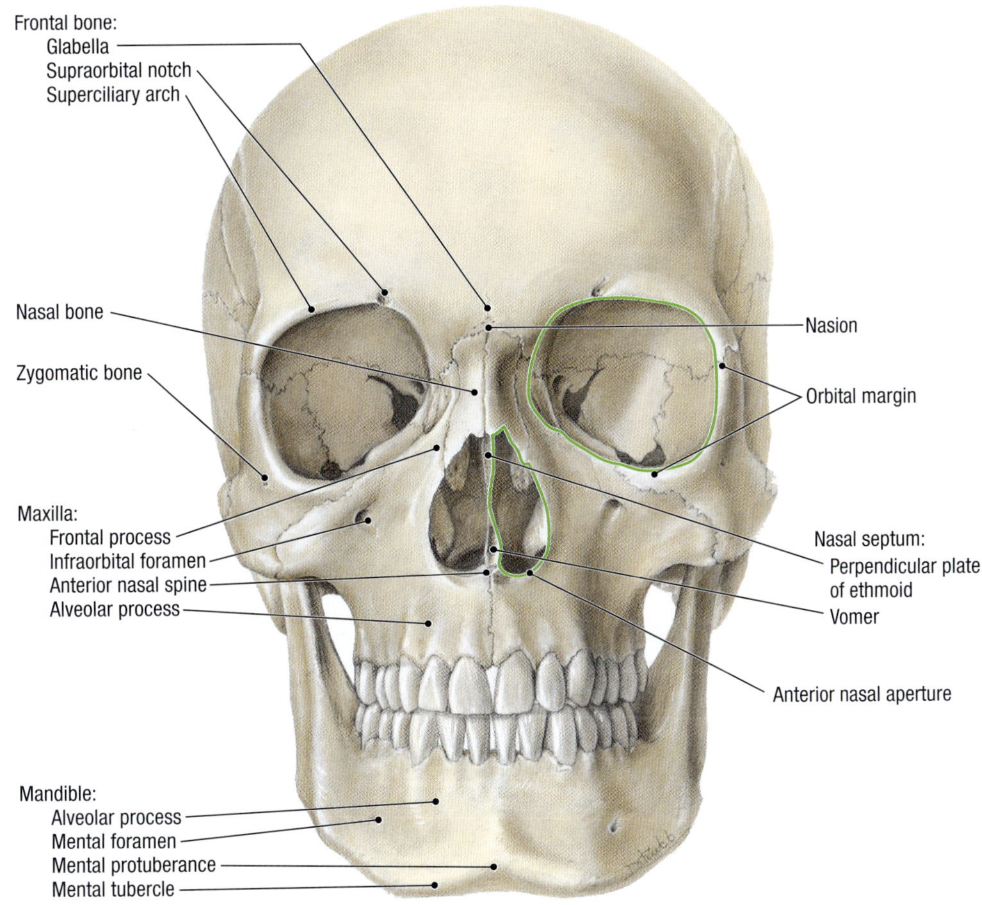

FIGURE 7.16 ■ Skull. Anterior view.

8. Observe that the right and left **nasal bones** form the superior extent of the bridge of the nose.
9. Posterior to the nasal bones, identify the thin **frontal process of the maxilla** extending superiorly to the frontal bone.
10. On the anterior surface of the maxilla, identify the **infraorbital foramen** and the **alveolar processes**, the thickened ridges corresponding to the attachment sites for the upper dentition (upper teeth).
11. In the midline where the maxillae meet, identify the small bony projection of the **anterior nasal spine**, oriented anterior and inferior to the **nasal septum**.
12. Observe that the **anterior nasal aperture** is bounded by the nasal bones and maxillae.
13. Lateral to the maxillae, near the region of the cheek, identify the right and left **zygomatic bones**.
14. Identify the **mandible**, the jaw, and observe that it has **alveolar processes** for the lower dentition (lower teeth).
15. In the midline of the mandible, identify the **mental protuberance**, the thickened ridge marking the fusion point of the right and left portions of the mandible during development.
16. Observe that the shape of a person's chin is related to the shape of the mental protuberance and the bilaterally located ridge-like **mental tubercles** located to either side of the protuberance.
17. On the anterior surface of the mandible, identify the bilateral openings of the **mental foramen**.
18. Observe that the mental foramen is almost in a direct line with the infraorbital foramen and the supraorbital foramen, the exit points of the cutaneous branches of the trigeminal nerve, which, in addition to other functions, provide sensory innervation to the face.

Lateral Skull

ATLAS 8.3

1. Refer to FIGURE 7.17.
2. Posterior to the **frontal bone**, identify the paired **parietal bones**. Observe that a parietal bone is relatively smooth apart from the **superior temporal line** and **inferior temporal line**, which demarcate the superior attachment of the temporalis, a large muscle of mastication.

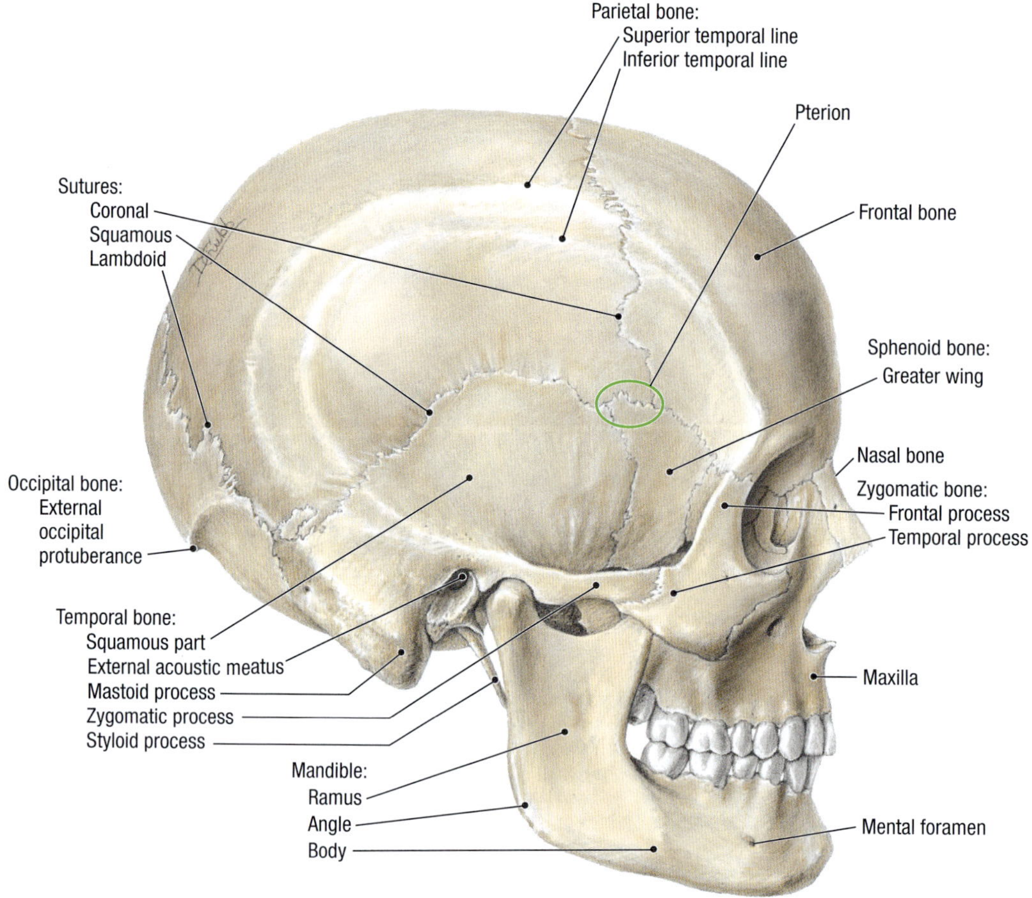

FIGURE 7.17 ● Skull. Lateral view.

3. Identify the **sutures** of the skull, the immobile fibrous joints located along the edges of the bones of the skull where they meet.
4. Observe that the parietal bones articulate anteriorly with the frontal bone along the **coronal suture** and posteriorly with the occipital bone along the **lambdoid (lambdoidal) suture**.
5. On the posterior aspect of the skull, identify the **external occipital protuberance** along the midline of the **occipital bone**. The portion of the occipital bone that extends anteriorly along the base of the skull will be studied at a later time.
6. On the lateral aspect of the skull, identify the **temporal bone**. Observe that the temporal bone meets the parietal bone nearly along the entire length of the flat part of the bone, the **squamous part**, along the **squamous (squamosal) suture**. The other portion of the temporal bone, the "rocklike" petrous part, extends into the cranial cavity and will be seen later.
7. On the lateral aspect of the temporal bone, identify the opening of the **external acoustic meatus** anterior to the large bony extension of the **mastoid process** and posterior to the **zygomatic process** extending toward the zygomatic bone.
8. Observe that the zygomatic process of the temporal bone meets the **temporal process** of the **zygomatic bone** to form the **zygomatic arch**. *Note that the processes forming the arch are named for the bone they are directed at and not the bone from which they originate.*
9. Observe that the zygomatic bone has a vertically oriented **frontal process**, named for its extension toward, and articulation with, the frontal bone.
10. In the depression of the "temple," identify the **greater wing of the sphenoid bone**.
11. Superior to the greater wing of the sphenoid, identify the **pterion**, the junction of the frontal, parietal, greater wing of sphenoid, and squamous part of the temporal bones. *Note that the pterion is of clinical importance because it is a common site of fracture, putting the patient at risk of hemorrhage as it overlies a key artery inside the skull: the middle meningeal artery.*

12. From a lateral perspective, observe that the **mandible** has a **ramus** (vertical portion) and a **body** (horizontal portion), which are differentiated by the **angle**.
13. Follow the **base (inferior border)** of the body of the mandible anteriorly and confirm that the **mental foramen** is visible from the lateral perspective.

Superior Skull

ATLAS 8.4B

1. Refer to FIGURE 7.18.
2. Identify the **calvaria**, the "skull cap," formed by parts of the frontal, parietal, and occipital bones connected through sutures.
3. Observe that the **coronal suture**, the suture between the frontal and paired parietal bones, is perpendicular to the **sagittal suture**, the suture between the two parietal bones, which connect at the **bregma**.
4. On the posterior aspect of the calvaria, identify the **lambdoid suture**, between the occipital and paired parietal bones, and the **lambda**, the point where the sagittal and lambdoid sutures meet.
5. Observe that most of the sutures of the calvaria are readily identifiable; however, the **frontal (metopic) suture**, which forms between the ossification centers of the paired frontal bones, is usually not seen in the adult.

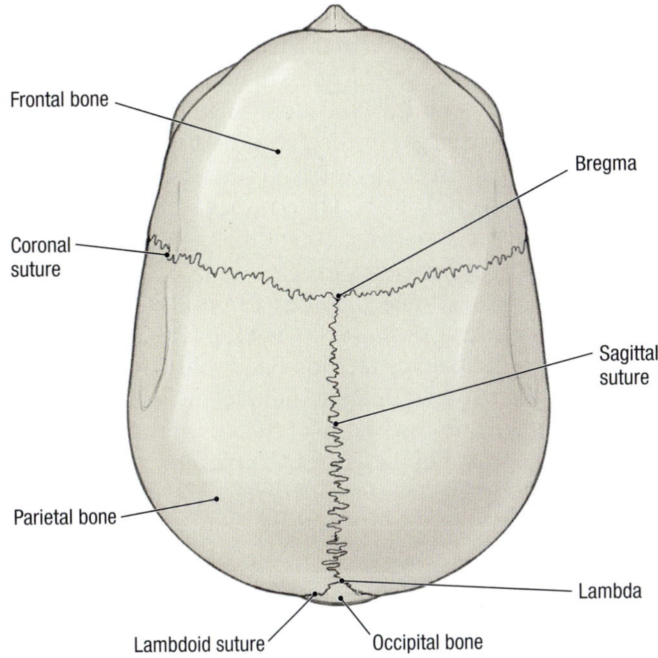

FIGURE 7.18 ■ Calvaria of skull. Superior view.

Surface Anatomy

Face

ATLAS 8.14, 8.73A, 8.73B

The surface anatomy of the face may be studied on a living subject or on a cadaver. On the cadaver, fixation may make it difficult to distinguish bone from well-preserved soft tissues.

1. Refer to FIGURE 7.19.
2. Place the cadaver in the supine position.
3. Palpate the **vertex** of the head, the most superior aspect.
4. Superior to the orbit, palpate the **supraorbital margin** and the location of the **supraorbital notch**.
5. Observe that the eyes are protected by thin extensions of skin over their anterior surfaces, the **upper (superior)** and **lower (inferior) eyelids**.
6. Along the superior aspect of the nose, palpate the transitions between the **nasal bones** and the **nasal cartilage**.
7. Work your fingers inferiorly from the midline of the nose toward the lips and identify the **philtrum**, the small depression superior to the **upper (superior) lip**.
8. Inferior to the **lower (inferior) lip** at the chin, palpate from the **mental protuberance of the mandible** along the **body of the mandible** to the **angle of the mandible**.
9. Palpate the **zygomatic bone** at the cheeks and palpate posterolaterally along the **zygomatic arch** toward the external ear.

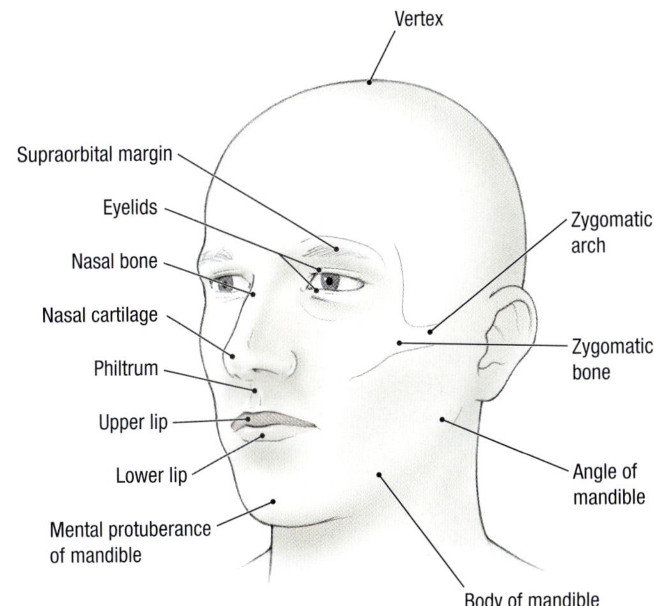

FIGURE 7.19 ■ Surface anatomy of face. Left anterolateral view.

Dissection Instructions

Skin Incisions of Face

VIDEO 7.5.1

Dissection Note: The skin of the face is very thin and firmly attached to the cartilage of the nose and ears but is mobile over other parts of the face. The muscles of facial expression are attached to the skin superficially and the bones of the skull deeply. While making the skin incisions of the face, care must be taken to not cut too deeply and thus damage the underlying structures.

1. Refer to FIGURE 7.20.
2. In the midline, make a shallow (2 mm) skin incision beginning near the vertex (A) that passes inferiorly through the hairline and forehead to the nasion (B).
3. From the nasion, continue the midline incision inferiorly along the bridge of the nose to a point just superior to the upper lip at the philtrum.
4. Encircle the mouth at the margin of the upper and lower lips.
5. Make a midline incision from the inferior border of the lower lip to the mental protuberance (C).
6. Make an incision from the mental protuberance (C) along the inferior border of the mandible to a point just superior to the angle of the mandible. *Note that if the neck was previously dissected, this incision has already been made.*
7. On the lateral surface of the head, make a skin incision from the vertex (A) toward the upper part of the ear on the lateral aspect of the head (D).

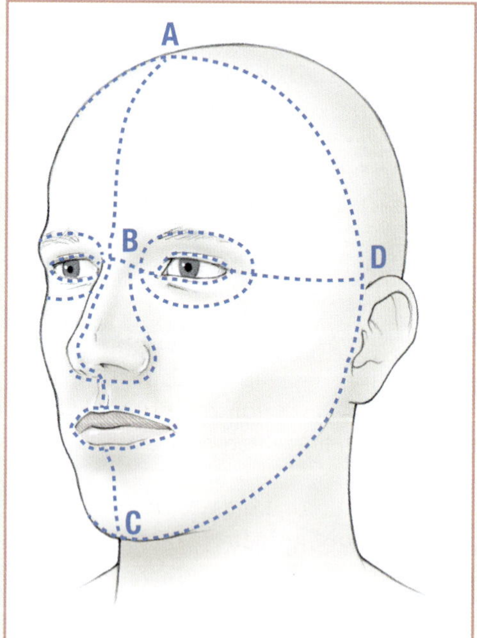

FIGURE 7.20 ■ Skin incisions of face. Left anterolateral view.

8. Continue the incision inferiorly from the lateral aspect of the head (D) by passing anterior to the ear toward the angle of the mandible to connect with the horizontal incision along the margin of the mandible.
9. Starting at the nasion (B), carefully make a shallow incision that encircles the orbital margin. *Do not yet remove the skin overlying the eyelids because this will be removed later.*
10. Extend the incision from the lateral angle of the eye to the incision on the lateral aspect of the head (D).
11. Beginning at the midline, remove the skin of the forehead, making an effort to leave the connective tissue intact and to not remove the thin frontalis with the skin. *Note that the skin of the region adheres tightly to the tough subcutaneous connective tissue and sharp dissection may be required.*
12. Remove the skin of the lower face, beginning at the midline and proceeding laterally, observing that the subcutaneous tissue of the face contains the muscles of facial expression.
13. Detach the skin laterally and place it in the tissue container.

Subcutaneous Tissue of Face and Facial Nerve

ATLAS 8.13, 8.15; VIDEO 7.5.2

Dissection Note: Because the deeper dissection of the face will take place on the right side of the cadaver, make special effort to clearly identify the following superficial structures on the left side of the face.

1. Refer to FIGURE 7.21.
2. Observe that the superior part of the **platysma** extends into the face along the inferior border of the mandible. Recall that the inferior attachment of the platysma is the superficial fascia of the upper thorax and that it forms a sheet of muscle covering the anterior and lateral cervical regions.
3. Use blunt dissection to define the superior attachment of the platysma on the inferior border of the mandible, skin of the cheek, and angle of the mouth.
4. Identify the **masseter**, a large muscle of mastication on the lateral aspect of the face near the angle of the mandible. The masseter will be cleaned at a later stage in the dissection.
5. Identify the **parotid duct** where it crosses the lateral surface of the masseter about 2 cm inferior to the zygomatic arch. *Note that the parotid duct is larger than the nearby nerves, approximately the diameter of a probe handle, and often looks like a pale vein.*
6. Use blunt dissection to follow the parotid duct anteriorly just past the anterior border of the masseter where the duct turns medially into the cheek to pierce the **buccinator**. Clean the portion of the parotid duct lateral to the masseter, the remaining

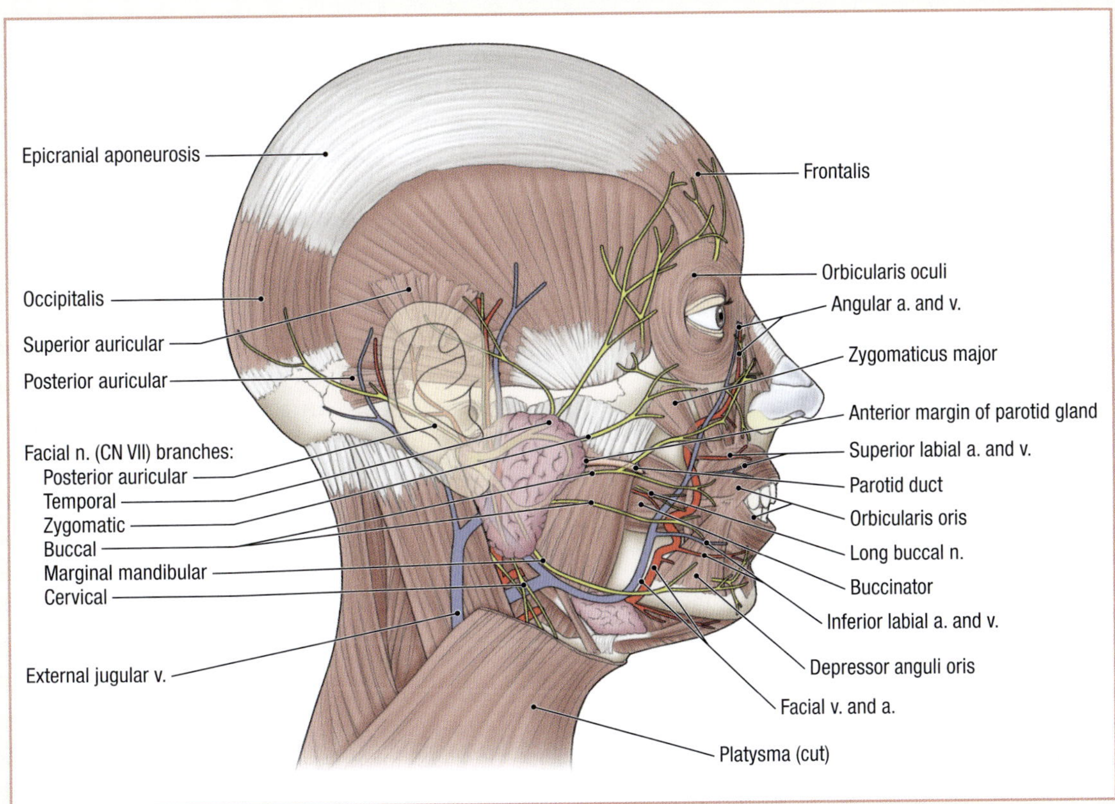

FIGURE 7.21 ■ Superficial dissection of face. Right lateral view.

anterior portion of the duct will be cleaned at a later stage in the dissection. *Note that the parotid duct drains into the oral vestibule lateral to the 2nd maxillary molar tooth.*

7. Use blunt dissection to follow the parotid duct posteriorly and identify the anterior margin of the **parotid gland**. *Note that in some individuals, an accessory parotid gland is present, which courses anteriorly along the parotid duct.*
8. Observe that the parotid gland is enclosed within the **parotid sheath**. *Note that the parotid sheath and the stroma of the parotid gland (connective tissue, blood vessels, nerves, and ducts) are continuous with the investing layer of the deep cervical fascia.*

Dissection Note: The tough connective tissue surrounding the parotid gland will not yield to blunt dissection; thus, scissors or the tip of the scalpel are recommended to remove this layer.

9. Identify a **buccal branch of the facial nerve** coursing parallel to the parotid duct. *Note that the buccal branch is typically not isolated but rather contains multiple branches coursing toward the cheek.*
10. Use blunt dissection to follow a buccal branch into the parotid gland, removing the parotid tissue superficial to the nerve piece by piece. Within the parotid gland, the nerve will join other facial nerve branches to form the **parotid plexus** (see **Clinical Correlation 7.6**).

CLINICAL CORRELATION 7.6

Bell Palsy

ATLAS 8.13, 8.15B, 9.22E

Bell palsy, idiopathic facial paralysis, is the sudden loss of control of the muscles of facial expression, usually on one side of the face. The exact cause of Bell palsy is unknown but is believed to be associated with a virus, including inflammation and swelling around the facial nerve which controls the muscles of facial expression. The patient presents with drooping of the mouth and an inability to close the eyelid on the affected side.

11. From the parotid plexus, follow the other facial nerve branches peripherally toward the muscles of facial expression beginning superiorly with the **temporal branch**, which crosses the zygomatic arch.
12. Between the temporal branch and buccal branch, identify the **zygomatic branch** crossing the zygomatic bone.
13. Inferior to the buccal branch, identify the **mandibular branch** coursing parallel to the inferior margin of the mandible, and the **cervical branch** crossing the angle of the mandible to enter the neck.

14. Make a brief effort to identify the **posterior auricular branch** of the facial nerve, which passes posterior to the ear. *Note that the posterior auricular branch is often difficult to find because it is the first branch to emerge from the stylomastoid foramen and courses deep to the external ear.*
15. Follow the parotid plexus branches posteriorly and deeply (below the ear lobe) until they combine to form a single nerve, the **facial nerve (CN VII)**. *Note that the facial nerve emerges from the base of the skull through the stylomastoid foramen in the temporal bone. Do not attempt to follow the facial nerve to the foramen at this time.*
16. Define the anterior border of the masseter while preserving the parotid duct and branches of the facial nerve.
17. Anterior to the masseter, identify the **buccal fat pad** within the hollow depression of the cheek.
18. Use blunt dissection to remove the buccal fat pad and expose the **buccinator** and verify that it is pierced by the parotid duct.
19. Coursing on the lateral surface of the buccinator, identify the **buccal (long buccal) nerve**, a branch of the mandibular division of the trigeminal nerve (CN V_3) emerging from deep to the masseter. *Note that the buccal nerve is a sensory nerve that pierces the buccinator to provide sensory innervation to the mucosa and skin of the cheek. Recall that motor innervation to the buccinator was provided by the buccal branch of the facial nerve.*

Facial Artery and Vein

ATLAS 8.12, 8.18B, 8.19; VIDEO 7.5.3

Dissection Note: The facial artery and vein follow a winding course across the face and may pass either superficial or deep to the muscles of facial expression.

1. Refer to FIGURE 7.21.
2. Find the **facial artery** where it crosses the inferior border of the mandible at the anterior border of the masseter.
3. Observe that the facial artery is more tortuous and usually located anterior to the facial vein. *Note that at this location, the facial artery and vein are covered only by the platysma and skin.*
4. On the right side of the face, if not already done, cut the platysma along the inferior border of the mandible while preserving the facial vessels. Detach the platysma from the angle of the mouth and place it in the tissue container.
5. Follow the facial vein inferiorly, observing that it passes superficial to the submandibular gland in the neck. The facial vein may have been cut when a portion of the gland was removed earlier.
6. Follow the facial artery inferiorly to the point where it passes deep to the submandibular gland in the neck where it crosses the inferior border of the mandible.
7. Use blunt dissection to trace the facial artery superiorly toward the angle of the mouth and identify the **inferior labial** and **superior labial arteries** arising from it.
8. Continue to trace the facial artery superiorly as far as the lateral side of the nose, where its name changes to **angular artery**, and observe that the facial artery has several loops or bends in this part of its course.
9. Observe that the facial vein receives tributaries corresponding to the branches of the facial artery including the **superior** and **inferior labial veins** and the **angular vein**. *Note that the angular vein has a clinically important anastomotic connection with the ophthalmic veins in the orbit, which will be described when the orbit is dissected.*

Muscles around Orbital Opening

ATLAS 8.12, 8.14A, 8.15; VIDEO 7.5.4

1. Refer to FIGURE 7.22.
2. Carefully remove the skin of the upper and lower eyelids, taking particular care as the skin of the eyelids is the thinnest skin in the body at only 1 to 2 mm in thickness.
3. Identify the **orbicularis oculi** encircling the **palpebral fissure**, the opening between the eyelids.
4. Identify the **orbital part** of the orbicularis oculi surrounding the orbital margin, the more peripherally located portion responsible for the tight closure of the eyelids.
5. Identify the **palpebral part** of the orbicularis oculi, the thinner, more centrally located portion contained in the eyelids responsible for blinking.
6. Review the attachments and actions of the orbicularis oculi (see **TABLE 7.4**).

Muscles around Oral Opening

ATLAS 8.12, 8.15A, 8.16; VIDEO 7.5.5

Dissection Note: Several muscles alter the shape of the mouth and lips. Delineating the boundaries of the muscles of facial expression in this region is often difficult, and care must be taken to avoid damaging these thin muscles.

1. Refer to FIGURE 7.22.
2. Identify the **orbicularis oris** (both superior and inferior portions), which surrounds the opening of the oral cavity.
3. Use blunt dissection to define the borders of the **zygomaticus major** and **minor** angling from the corner of the mouth toward the zygomatic bone of the cheek. *Note that the zygomaticus major is typically larger and more laterally and inferiorly located.*

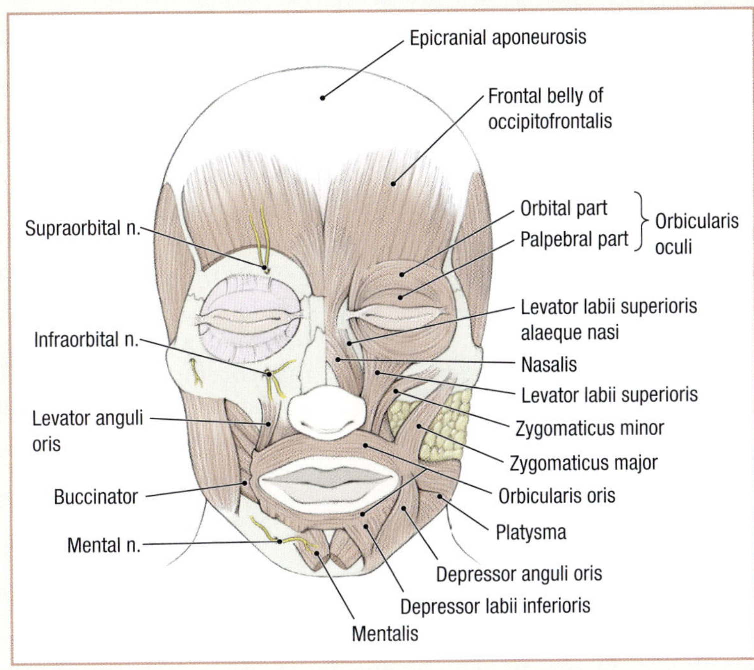

FIGURE 7.22 ■ Muscles of facial expression. Anterior view.

4. Superior to the upper lip, use blunt dissection to define the borders of the **levator labii superioris**, and the extension of muscle tissue coursing along the lateral aspect of the nose, the **levator labii superioris alaeque nasi**.
5. Identify the **levator anguli oris** attaching near the angle of the mouth medial and somewhat deep to the medial aspect of the zygomaticus major.
6. Inferior to the lower lip, use blunt dissection to define the borders of the **depressor anguli oris** and **depressor labii inferioris**.
7. Open the oral cavity and palpate the thickness of the **buccinator** lining the cheek. Recall that the buccinator is a muscle of facial expression and not only contributes to the actions of whistling, sucking, and blowing but also assists mastication by providing tension to hold food between the teeth.
8. Review the attachments, actions, and innervations of the muscles of facial expression (see **TABLE 7.4**).

Sensory Nerves of Face

ATLAS 8.16, 8.17; VIDEO 7.5.6

1. Refer to FIGURE 7.22 and to FIGURE 7.23.
2. Observe that three branches of the trigeminal nerve supply sensory innervation to the face, the supraorbital, infraorbital, and mental nerves which supply the forehead, cheek, and chin, respectively.
3. Identify the location of the **supraorbital nerve**, a branch of the ophthalmic division of the trigeminal nerve (CN V_1), which passes through the supraorbital notch (foramen) of the frontal bone to reach the skin above the eye. *Note that the supraorbital nerve lies deep to the frontal belly of the occipitofrontalis and will be seen in the cadaver when the scalp is studied.*

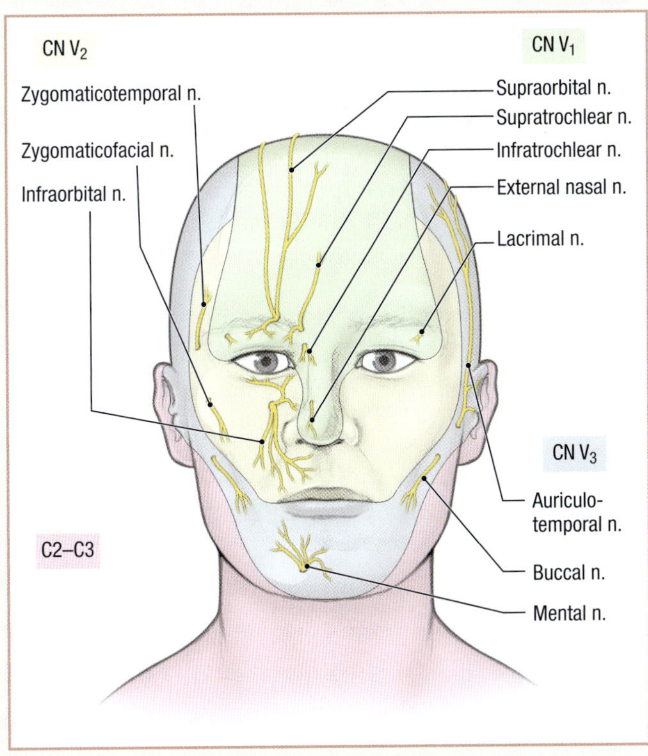

FIGURE 7.23 ■ Cutaneous nerves of face. Anterior view.

4. On the right side of the face, transect the levator labii superioris close to the infraorbital margin and reflect it inferiorly.
5. Deep to the reflected levator labii superioris, identify the **infraorbital nerve**, a branch of the maxillary division of the trigeminal nerve (CN V_2), which passes through the infraorbital foramen of the maxilla. *Note that the infraorbital nerve supplies sensory innervation to the inferior eyelid, side of the nose, and upper lip.*
6. Observe that the **infraorbital artery** and **vein** also emerge from the infraorbital foramen.
7. On the right side of the face, transect the depressor anguli oris near the angle of the mouth and reflect it inferiorly.
8. Deep to the reflected depressor anguli oris, identify the **mental nerve,** a branch of the mandibular division of the trigeminal nerve (CN V_3), which emerges from the mental foramen of the mandible. *Note that the mental nerve supplies sensory innervation to the skin of the lower lip and chin as well as the gingiva covering the outer mandible in the oral cavity.*
9. Observe that the **mental artery** and **vein** also emerge from the mental foramen.
10. Several smaller branches of the trigeminal nerve (**lacrimal, infratrochlear, zygomaticofacial, zygomaticotemporal,** and **external nasal**) also innervate the facial region. Do not attempt to dissect these small branches at this time.

Dissection Follow-up

1. Review the path of the branches of the facial nerve from the parotid plexus to the muscles of facial expression.
2. Review the attachments, action, and innervation of the muscles of facial expression in **TABLE 7.4**.
3. Use a skull and the dissected specimen to review the branches of the trigeminal nerve supplying the face and their associated foramina of the skull which they pass through.
4. Review the origin and course of the facial artery and vein as well as their branches and tributaries.
5. Replace the reflected muscles and tissues of the face back in their correct anatomical position.

TABLE 7.4 Muscles of Facial Expression

Muscle	*Medial Attachments*	*Lateral Attachments*	*Actions*	*Innervation*
Orbicularis oculi	Medial orbital margin, medial palpebral ligament, and lacrimal bone	Skin around orbital margin	Tightly closes eyelids and winking (orbital part) Loosely closes eyelids and blinking (palpebral part)	Facial n. (CN VII)
Levator labii superioris	Upper lip (inferior attachment)	Maxilla just below orbital margin (superior attachment)	Elevates upper lip	
Zygomaticus major	Angle of mouth	Zygomatic bone	Draws angle of mouth superiorly and posteriorly	
Orbicularis oris	Maxilla, mandible, and skin in median plane	Angle of mouth	Sphincter of mouth	
Buccinator	Angle of mouth	Pterygomandibular raphe and lateral surfaces of alveolar processes of maxilla and mandible	Compresses cheek against molar teeth, keeping food on occlusal surfaces during chewing	
Depressor anguli oris	Angle of mouth	Mandible	Depresses angle of mouth	
Depressor labii inferioris	Lower lip (superior attachment)		Depresses lower lip	

Abbreviations: CN, cranial nerve; n., nerve.

PAROTID REGION

Dissection Overview

The parotid gland is the largest of three paired salivary glands and is located in the parotid region, the area on the side of the face inferior to the zygomatic arch anterior to the ear. Secretions from the parotid gland reach the oral cavity via the parotid duct. The parotid gland is surrounded by the thick investing layer of deep cervical fascia known as the parotid sheath and occupies an irregular space known as the parotid bed. The parotid gland surrounds the posterior edge of the ramus of the mandible and therefore is in close contact with nerves, vessels, muscles, bones, and ligaments in the region. The superficial portion of the parotid gland was removed to expose branches of the facial nerve. The goal of this dissection is to remove the remainder of the parotid gland piece by piece, preserving the nerves and vessels that pass through it.

The order of dissection will be as follows: The branches of the facial nerve will be reviewed and followed posteriorly toward the stylomastoid foramen. The motor root of the facial nerve will be transected near the lobe of the ear and parotid plexus, and its branches will be reflected anteriorly. The retromandibular vein will be followed superiorly through the parotid gland. The external carotid artery will then be followed superiorly as additional parotid tissue is removed.

Skeletal Anatomy

Refer to a skeleton or disarticulated skull to identify the following skeletal features.

Temporal Bone and Mandible

ATLAS 8.48

Dissection Note: Recall that the small bony projections (processes) extending from the inferior surface of the skull can easily be broken by resting the skull on its base without the support of the mandible.

1. Refer to FIGURE 7.24.
2. Identify the opening of the **external acoustic meatus** on the lateral aspect of the temporal bone, the depression aligned with the outer (external) ear.
3. Anterior to the external acoustic meatus, identify the depression of the **mandibular fossa** on the inferior aspect of the temporal bone. If a mandible is present, articulate it with the base of the skull and observe that the mandibular fossa serves as the socket for the **temporomandibular joint (TMJ)**.
4. Medial to the mandibular fossa, identify the **styloid process**, a thin bony extension named for its pen-like "stylus" appearance descending from the base of the skull.
5. Posterior to the external acoustic meatus and posterolateral to the styloid process, identify the large round mass of the **mastoid process**.
6. Between the styloid and mastoid processes, identify the **stylomastoid foramen**, the exit point of the facial nerve (CN VII) at the base of the skull.
7. On the mandible, review the location of the **head**, **neck**, **ramus**, **angle**, and **body**.

Boundaries of Parotid Bed

ATLAS 8.47

Refer to a skull with an articulated mandible and an illustration to identify the boundaries of the parotid bed.

1. Refer to FIGURE 7.24.
2. Identify the superior boundary of the parotid bed formed by the **zygomatic arch**.
3. Identify the anterior boundary of the parotid bed formed by the **ramus of the mandible**, medial pterygoid, and masseter.
4. Identify the medial boundary of the parotid bed formed by the **styloid process** and associated muscles (stylopharyngeus, styloglossus, and stylohyoid).
5. Identify the posterior boundary of the parotid bed formed by the **external acoustic meatus**, **mastoid process**, and posterior belly of the digastric.

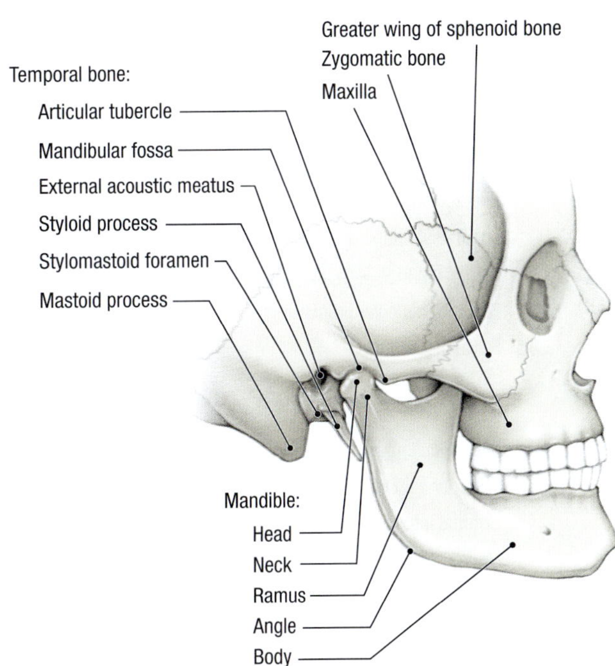

FIGURE 7.24 ■ Skeleton of parotid region. Right lateral view.

Dissection Instructions

Parotid Region

ATLAS 8.47; VIDEO 7.6.1

Dissection Note: Perform the following dissection steps on only the right side of the head. Preserve the superficial structures on the left side of the head for review.

1. Refer to FIGURE 7.25.
2. Identify the **great auricular nerve** where it crosses the SCM and angle of the mandible. Detach the great auricular nerve superiorly and reflect it inferiorly off the surface of the SCM while leaving it attached to the cervical plexus.
3. Review the branches of the **facial nerve (CN VII)** previously dissected: **temporal**, **zygomatic**, **buccal**, **mandibular**, and **cervical**.
4. Trace the facial nerve branches posteriorly toward the parotid plexus and identify the two larger subdivisions of the plexus, the **temporofacial** and **cervicofacial divisions**.
5. Trace the divisions of the plexus toward the lobe of the ear and identify the main stem of the **motor root of the facial nerve**.
6. Cut the facial nerve as far posteriorly as possible (**Cut 1**), leaving a stump emerging from the stylomastoid foramen, and reflect the parotid plexus of facial nerve branches anteriorly (see **Clinical Correlation 7.7**).

CLINICAL CORRELATION 7.7

Parotidectomy

ATLAS 8.13

Swelling of the parotid gland (as occurs in mumps) may be quite painful due to the increased pressure on the parotid sheath irritating branches of the facial nerve including the great auricular nerve. The enlarged parotid gland pushes the ear lobe superiorly and laterally and may cause compression of the facial nerve along its course through the gland. During parotidectomy (surgical excision of the parotid gland), the facial nerve is in danger of being injured and the branches must carefully be avoided. If the facial nerve is damaged, the muscles of facial expression will become paralyzed as seen in Bell palsy.

7. Review the course of the **parotid duct**.
8. Make a vertical cut through the parotid gland to leave a portion of the gland attached to the parotid duct near where it exits the gland and reflect the duct and attached glandular tissue anteriorly, leaving its passage through the buccinator undisturbed (**Cut 2**).
9. Near the superior extent of the parotid gland, identify the **auriculotemporal nerve**, a branch of the mandibular division of the trigeminal nerve (CN V_3), which passed between the head of the mandible and external acoustic meatus. *Note that as the auriculotemporal nerve passes through the parotid gland, it delivers postsynaptic parasympathetic nerve fibers from the otic ganglion.*
10. Follow the auriculotemporal nerve superiorly where it crosses the zygomatic process of the temporal bone alongside the **superficial temporal artery** and **vein** to reach the skin of the anterior side of the ear and temporal region.
11. Use blunt dissection to follow the **external jugular vein** superiorly to the point where it is formed by the joining of the **posterior auricular vein** and **retromandibular vein**.
12. Use blunt dissection to follow the retromandibular vein superiorly into the parotid gland.

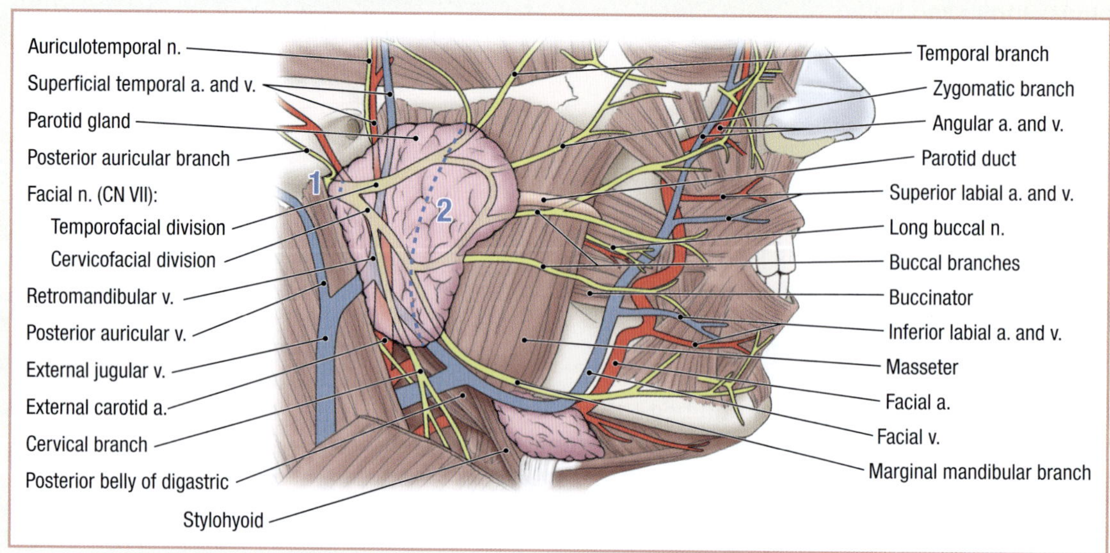

FIGURE 7.25 ■ Parotid region. Right lateral view.

13. Trace the retromandibular vein to the point where it is formed by the joining of the **maxillary vein** and **superficial temporal vein**, removing parotid tissue as you progress superiorly.
14. Follow the **superficial temporal vein** superiorly until it crosses the superficial surface of the zygomatic arch, continuing to remove the parotid gland as you proceed. Do not follow the maxillary vein at this time because it will be dissected later.
15. Use blunt dissection to follow the **external carotid artery** superiorly as far as the angle of the mandible, removing the lower part of the parotid gland.
16. Verify that the external carotid artery passes superiorly along the posterior edge of the ramus of the mandible. *Note that near the neck of the mandible, the external carotid artery divides into its two terminal branches, the maxillary artery and superficial temporal artery, although the terminal branches may not yet be visible as the retromandibular vein lies superficially.*
17. On the lateral aspect of the head, identify and clean the **superficial temporal artery** where it crosses the zygomatic process of the temporal bone just anterior to the external acoustic meatus. Observe that at this location, the superficial temporal artery is anterior to the auriculotemporal nerve.
18. Make an effort to clean and follow one or two of the branches of the superficial temporal artery, which distribute blood supply to the lateral part of the scalp. *Note that the branches of the superficial temporal artery are named according to their target region of distribution and include transverse facial, auricular, zygomatico-orbital, middle temporal, frontal, and parietal arterial branches.*
19. Remove any remaining parotid tissue from the zygomatic arch and lateral surface of the masseter.
20. Follow the **posterior belly of the digastric** and **stylohyoid** superiorly toward the base of the skull and clean any parotid tissue that remains on their anterior borders or lateral surfaces. Expose the digastric all the way to its attachment on the mastoid process.
21. Remove all remaining parotid tissue and the investing layer of deep cervical fascia that binds the SCM to deeper structures while preserving the posterior division of the retromandibular vein.

Dissection Follow-up

1. Review the boundaries of the parotid bed.
2. Review the branches of the facial nerve supplying the muscles of facial expression.
3. Review the superficial venous drainage of the lateral side of the head and neck, beginning with the superficial temporal veins and ending with the subclavian vein in the root of the neck.
4. Review the origin, course, and branches of the external carotid artery.
5. Replace the facial nerve in its correct anatomical position and approximate the cut ends.
6. Replace the parotid duct and any other reflected tissue in its correct anatomical position.

SCALP

Dissection Overview

The scalp consists of five layers, which can be remembered from superficial to deep by the mnemonic ***SCALP***. The first layer, or most superficial layer, of the scalp is the ***S****kin*. Deep to the skin, dense subcutaneous **C***onnective* tissue containing the vessels and nerves of the scalp forms the second layer. The third layer of the scalp is the ***A****poneurosis* (epicranial aponeurosis, L. galea aponeurotica) connecting the frontal belly to the occipital belly of the occipitofrontalis. The first three layers of the scalp are tightly bound to each other and are difficult to separate. Deep to the epicranial aponeurosis is the fourth layer formed by ***L****oose* connective tissue which permits the scalp to move over the skull. The fifth and last layer is the ***P****ericranium* or periosteum of the cranial bones.

The order of dissection will be as follows: The layers of the scalp will be reflected. The muscles of the scalp will be examined. The underlying neurovasculature of the scalp will be studied.

Dissection Instructions

Scalp

ATLAS 8.15B, 8.20; VIDEO 7.7.1

Dissection Note: The following cuts may be made through the entire thickness of the scalp with the scalpel contacting the bone of the calvaria or through the initial three layers of the scalp only to approach the layers of the scalp sequentially.

1. Refer to FIGURE 7.26.
2. Make a midline cut from the nasion (B) through the vertex (A) to the external occipital protuberance (X). *Note that if the face was previously dissected, a portion of this cut was already made.*
3. Make a cut in the coronal plane bilaterally from the vertex (A) to a point anterior to the ear (D). *Note that if the face was previously dissected, a portion of this cut was made previously.*
4. Beginning at the vertex, use forceps to grasp one corner of the cut scalp.
5. If reflecting all layers at once, slide the edge of a chisel between the scalp and calvaria to loosen and raise the flaps of skin.
6. Once the flap of scalp is raised, grasp the flap with both hands or a pair of locking hemostats and pull it inferiorly.
7. If reflecting the first three layers only, grasp the cut edge of skin and dense connective tissue and separate them from the underlying aponeurosis remaining over the skull. *Note that the separation of these layers is difficult as they are quite thin and firmly attached.*
8. Refer to FIGURE 7.27.
9. In either technique, reflect all four flaps of scalp down to the level that a hatband would occupy but do not yet detach the flaps.
10. If all layers were cut and reflected together, examine the cut edge of the scalp and identify the **occipitofrontalis**. *Note that the occipitofrontalis is a muscle of facial expression and innervated by branches of the facial nerve (CN VII).*
11. If the skin and connective tissue was reflected in isolation, identify the occipitofrontalis on the superior aspect of the skull.
12. Observe that the occipitofrontalis is composed of two muscular bellies, **frontalis** and **occipitalis**, connected over the vertex of the skull by the **epicranial aponeurosis**.
13. Observe that the inferior attachment of the occipital belly is the occipital bone and its superior attachment is the epicranial aponeurosis. Similarly, observe that the superior attachment of the frontal belly is the epicranial aponeurosis and its inferior attachment is the skin of the forehead and eyebrows.
14. If the skin and connective tissue was reflected in isolation, make cuts through the epicranial aponeurosis (**Cut 1**) paralleling the skin incision lines.
15. Reflect the four sections of muscular and aponeurotic tissue inferiorly to the same level as the reflected skin.
16. Refer to FIGURE 7.28.

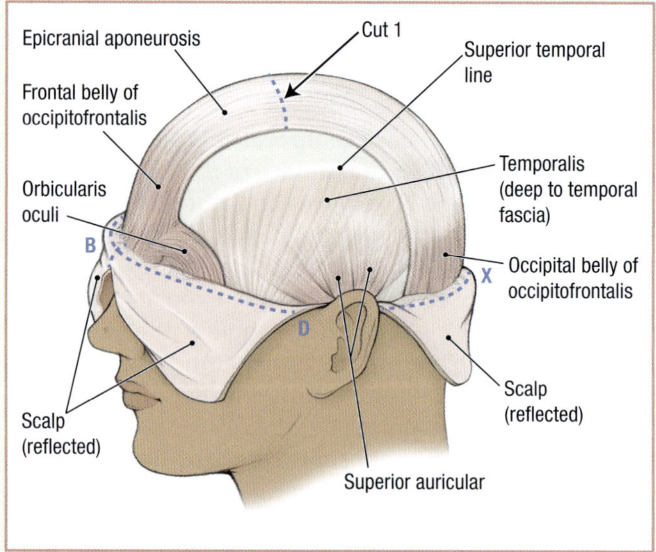

FIGURE 7.27 ● Reflection of scalp. Left lateral view.

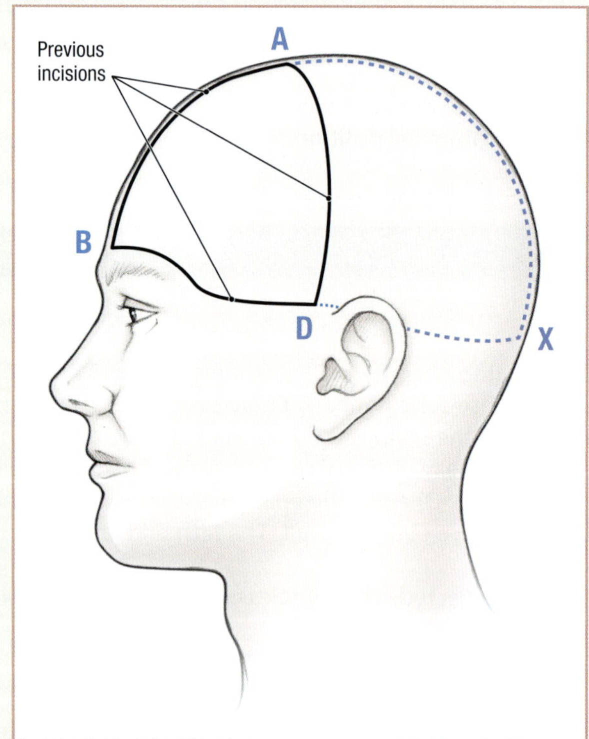

FIGURE 7.26 ● Skin incisions of scalp. Left lateral view.

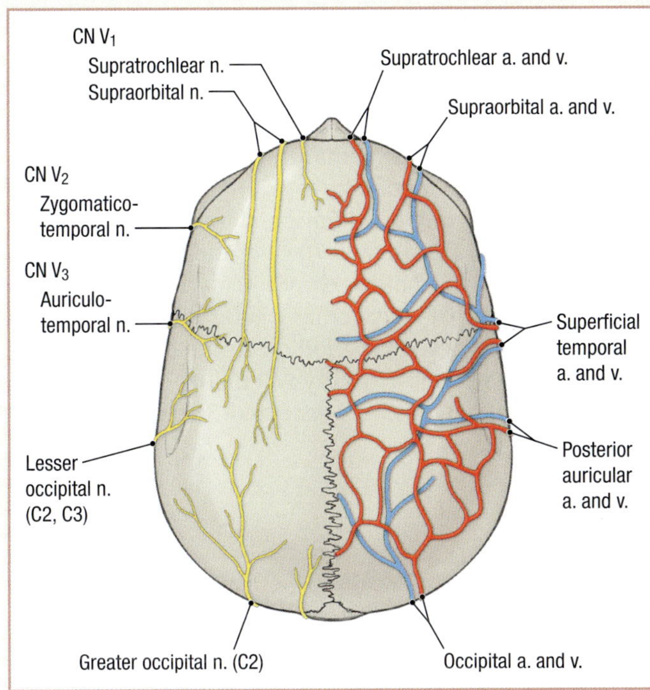

FIGURE 7.28 ■ Cutaneous nerves (*left side*) and blood vessels (*right side*) of scalp. Superior view.

17. Observe that nerves and vessels contained within the layers of the scalp enter it from more inferior regions around the circumference of the head (see **Clinical Correlation 7.8**).

CLINICAL CORRELATION 7.8

Scalp Injuries and Infections

ATLAS 8.20

A proper understanding of the layers of the scalp is critical when diagnosing an epicranial hemorrhage or hematoma due to head trauma, delivery, or infection and the associated level of risk. A caput succedaneum occurs superficial to the aponeurotic layer and thus may spread within the subcutaneous tissue to the forehead, face, side of the head, or neck. Although worrisome in appearance, a caput succedaneum is typically caused by the rupture of small vessels in the scalp during birth, resulting in benign edema. A subgaleal (subaponeurotic) hemorrhage occurs deep to aponeurosis and is thus limited by the attachments of the occipitofrontalis. Subgaleal bleeds are of far more concern as they are often caused by severing of emissary veins resulting in significant blood loss or communication with the intracranial cavity leading to life-threatening pressure on the brain. A cephalohematoma occurs deep to the periosteum, is localized by adherence of this layer to the sutures of the skull, and often spontaneously resolves.

18. Pull an anterior scalp flap and muscular tissue inferiorly to expose the supraorbital margin.
19. Identify the **supraorbital** and **supratrochlear nerves and vessels** where they exit the orbit to enter the deep surface of the reflected scalp.
20. On the lateral aspect of the head, identify the **superficial temporal vessels** accompanying the branches of the **auriculotemporal nerve** and observe that the scalp has separated from the fascia covering the **temporalis.**
21. Make a brief effort to identify the thin muscle bellies of the **anterior**, **superior**, and **posterior auricular** overlying the fascia of the temporalis.
22. Posterior to the ear, identify the **posterior auricular vessels** accompanying the branches of the **lesser occipital nerve.**
23. Pull the posterior scalp flap and muscular tissue inferiorly to expose the region of the external occipital protuberance and identify the **occipital vessels** accompanying the branches of the **greater occipital nerve.**
24. Refer back to FIGURE 7.27.
25. If the scalp and underlying muscles were reflected together, carefully separate the layers of the scalp superficial to the occipitofrontalis and epicranial aponeurosis while preserving the branches of the superficial temporal artery and auriculotemporal nerve.
26. Remove the skin and dense connective tissue from the dissection field by making horizontal incisions around the periphery of the head from the nasion (B) to the lateral aspect of the head (D) just above the ear until you reach the external occipital protuberance (X) and place them in the tissue container. Take care to leave the muscular tissue layer intact.

Dissection Follow-up

1. Review the layers of the scalp.
2. Review the course of nerves and vessels supplying the scalp.
3. Use a skull and the dissected specimen to review the course of the supraorbital nerve through the supraorbital notch.
4. Review the attachments and innervations of the occipitofrontalis.
5. Replace the flaps of remaining scalp in their correct anatomical positions.

TEMPORAL AND INFRATEMPORAL REGIONS

Dissection Overview

The temporal region consists of two fossae: temporal and infratemporal. The temporal fossa is located superior to the zygomatic arch and contains the temporalis. The infratemporal fossa is inferior to the zygomatic arch, deep to the ramus of the mandible, and contains the medial and lateral pterygoids, branches of the mandibular division of the trigeminal nerve (CN V_3), and maxillary vessels with their associated branches. The infratemporal and temporal fossae are in open communication with each other through the area between the zygomatic arch and lateral surface of the skull.

The order of dissection will be as follows: The masseter will be studied. The zygomatic arch will be cut. The masseter will be reflected inferiorly while remaining attached to a portion of the cut arch. The temporalis will be studied. The coronoid process will be detached from the mandible, and the temporalis will be reflected superiorly with the attached coronoid. The superior part of the ramus of the mandible will be removed, and the maxillary artery will be traced across the infratemporal fossa. The branches of the mandibular division of the trigeminal nerve will be dissected. The medial and lateral pterygoids will be studied, and the TMJ will be dissected.

Skeletal Anatomy

Refer to a disarticulated mandible to identify the following skeletal features.

Mandible

ATLAS 8.48

1. Refer to FIGURE 7.29.
2. From a lateral view, review the location of the **ramus**, **angle**, and **body of the mandible**.
3. Follow the ramus of the mandible superiorly and identify the **head (mandibular condyle, condyloid process)**, the projection of bone located on the posterior and superior extent of the bone superior to the thinner **neck**.
4. Identify the **coronoid process**, the thinner "bladelike" projection of bone extending superiorly from the anterior portion of the ramus.
5. Observe that the two superior projections of bone, the coronoid and condyloid processes, are separated from one another by the **mandibular notch**.
6. Inferiorly along the body of the mandible, review the location of the **mental foramen** and **mental tubercle**.
7. On the internal surface of the ramus of the mandible, identify the small projection of the **lingula**, the inferior attachment site of the sphenomandibular ligament.
8. Posterior to the lingula, identify the opening of the **mandibular foramen**, a passage for the inferior alveolar nerves and vessels to the lower dentition.

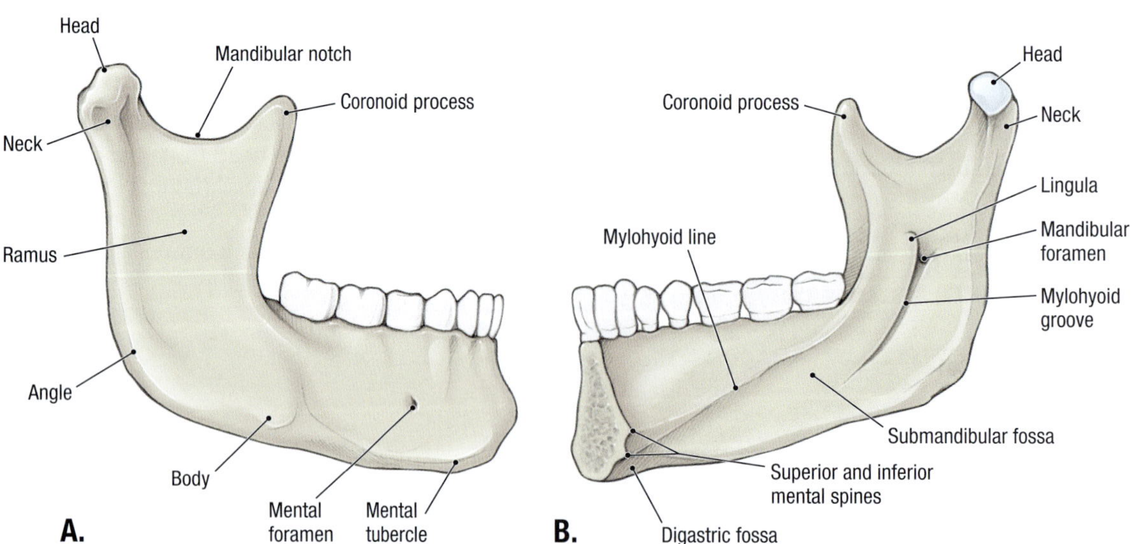

FIGURE 7.29 ● External and internal features of right side of mandible. **A.** Right lateral view. **B.** Right medial view.

9. On the inner surface of the body of the mandible beginning at the mandibular foramen, identify the **mylohyoid groove**, a thin depression for the nerve to mylohyoid and mylohyoid vessels.
10. Identify the **mylohyoid line** slightly superior to the mylohyoid groove, coursing anteriorly toward the small projections of bone near the midline of the mandible on its inner surface, the **superior** and **inferior mental spines (glenoid tubercles)**.
11. Inferior to the mylohyoid line, identify the depression of the **submandibular fossa** laterally and the **digastric fossa** more anteriorly.

Temporal and Infratemporal Fossae

ATLAS 8.48A, 8.50B

Dissection Note: Review the following skeletal features on a skull with the mandible removed.

1. Refer back to FIGURE 7.17.
2. From a lateral perspective, identify the **superior and inferior temporal lines** on the parietal bone.
3. Observe that the **temporal fossa** is formed by parts of four cranial bones: parietal, frontal, squamous part of temporal, and greater wing of sphenoid. Recall that the junction point of these bones forms the **pterion**.
4. Observe that the **zygomatic arch** is formed by the **zygomatic process of the temporal bone** and **temporal process of the zygomatic bone**.
5. Refer to FIGURE 7.30.
6. Review the location of the **mandibular fossa** and **articular tubercle** on the temporal bone.
7. Deep to the zygomatic arch, identify the **pterygomaxillary fissure** between the **lateral pterygoid plate** of the sphenoid bone and **maxilla**.
8. Carefully insert a thin wooden stick, or wire, through the superior end of the pterygomaxillary fissure into the space of the **pterygopalatine fossa**.
9. On the medial wall of the pterygopalatine fossa, identify the opening of the **sphenopalatine foramen**. Carefully pass the wire through the sphenopalatine foramen and observe from an anterior view that this opening connects the nasal cavity to the pterygopalatine fossa.

Dissection Note: **To reach the nasal cavity, structures from the infratemporal fossa will pass through a fissure (pterygomaxillary), a fossa (pterygopalatine), and a foramen (sphenopalatine).**

10. Anterior to the pterygomaxillary fissure, observe that the maxilla has an **infratemporal surface** inferior to the **inferior orbital fissure**, a gap between the greater wing of the sphenoid bone and maxilla. Pass the wire through the inferior orbital fissure and observe that this opening connects the infratemporal fossa to the orbit.
11. From an inferior perspective, identify the **foramen ovale** and **foramen spinosum** on the **greater wing of the sphenoid bone**.
12. Reposition the mandible on the skull and identify the **bony boundaries of the infratemporal fossa** beginning with the lateral boundary formed by the **ramus** of the mandible.
13. Observe that the infratemporal fossa has an anterior boundary formed by the **infratemporal surface of the maxilla** and a medial boundary formed by the **lateral pterygoid plate**.
14. Observe that the roof of the infratemporal fossa is formed by the **greater wing of the sphenoid bone** curving out laterally superior to the space.

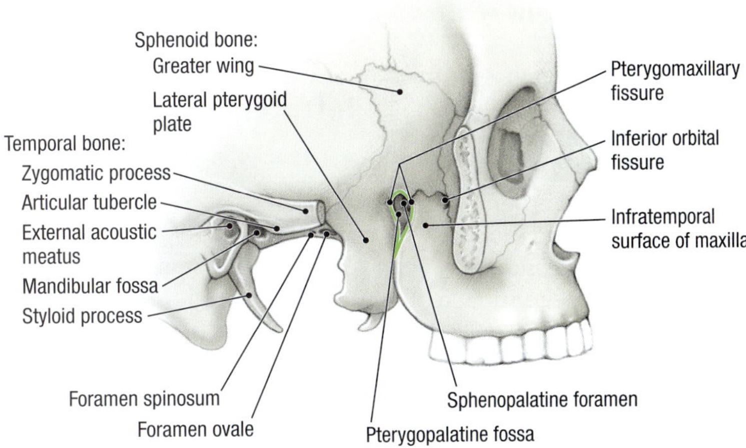

FIGURE 7.30 ■ Skeleton of infratemporal region. Right lateral view.

Dissection Instructions

Masseter and Removal of Zygomatic Arch

ATLAS 8.49, 8.50, 8.53A; VIDEO 7.8.1

Dissection Note: Perform the following dissection steps on only the right side of the head. Preserve the superficial structures on the left side of the head for review.

1. Refer back to FIGURE 7.25.
2. Reflect the cut **facial nerve** with its associated branches and the cut **parotid gland** and **parotid duct** anteriorly.
3. Clean the lateral surface of the **masseter** and define its borders inferiorly along the ramus of the mandible and superiorly along the inferior border of the zygomatic arch.
4. Review the attachments and actions of the masseter (see **TABLE 7.5**).
5. Review the course of the **superficial temporal vessels** and **auriculotemporal nerve** across the zygomatic arch.
6. Make a vertical incision through the temporal fascia overlying the temporalis and use blunt dissection to elevate a portion of the fascia from the surface of the muscle.
7. Cut through the temporal fascia along the superior temporal line and reflect it inferiorly. Observe that the temporalis is firmly attached to the deep surface of the temporal fascia, and it may be necessary to use a scalpel to cut the fascia from the surface of the muscle.
8. Cut the temporal fascia along the superior border of the zygomatic arch to remove it from the dissection field.
9. Refer to FIGURE 7.31.
10. Near the anterior end of the zygomatic arch, insert a probe deep to the zygomatic arch as close to the orbit as possible. The probe should follow a slightly oblique path if inserted properly.
11. Use a saw to cut through the zygomatic bone along the oblique line paralleling the probe (**Cut 1**). *Wear eye protection for all steps that require the use of a bone saw.*
12. Insert the probe deep to the zygomatic arch near the anterior border of the head of the mandible.
13. Use a saw to cut through the zygomatic arch posteriorly in a line parallel to the probe (**Cut 2**).
14. Gently pull the masseter and attached portion of the zygomatic arch laterally and inferiorly and look for the masseteric vessels and nerve crossing superior to the mandibular notch to enter the deep surface of the muscle.
15. Reflect the masseter and zygomatic arch in the inferior direction and cut through the masseteric nerve and vessels.

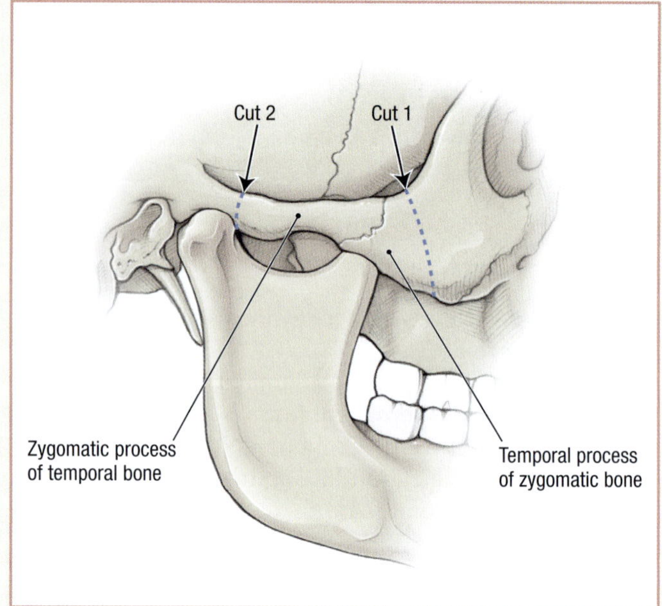

FIGURE 7.31 ● Removal of zygomatic arch. Right lateral view.

16. Use a scalpel to detach the masseter from the superior part of the ramus of the mandible but leave the masseter attached to the mandible near the angle.

Temporal Region

ATLAS 8.49, 8.50, 8.53B; VIDEO 7.8.2

1. Refer back to FIGURE 7.21 and FIGURE 7.30.
2. On the right side of the cadaver, identify the **temporalis**.
3. Remove the overlying fascia and connective tissue to clean the inferior attachment of the temporalis to the coronoid process of the mandible.
4. On the left side of the cadaver, observe that the **superficial boundary** of the temporal region is the **temporal fascia**.
5. Review the attachments and actions of the temporalis (see **TABLE 7.5**).

Infratemporal Fossa

ATLAS 8.49, 8.50; VIDEO 7.8.3

Dissection Note: Wear eye protection for all steps that require the use of the bone saw, chisel, or bone cutters.

1. Refer to FIGURE 7.32.
2. Gently insert a probe through the mandibular notch posterior to the temporalis tendon and push the probe anteroinferiorly toward the 3rd mandibular molar tooth. While advancing the probe, keep it in close contact with the deep surface of the mandible

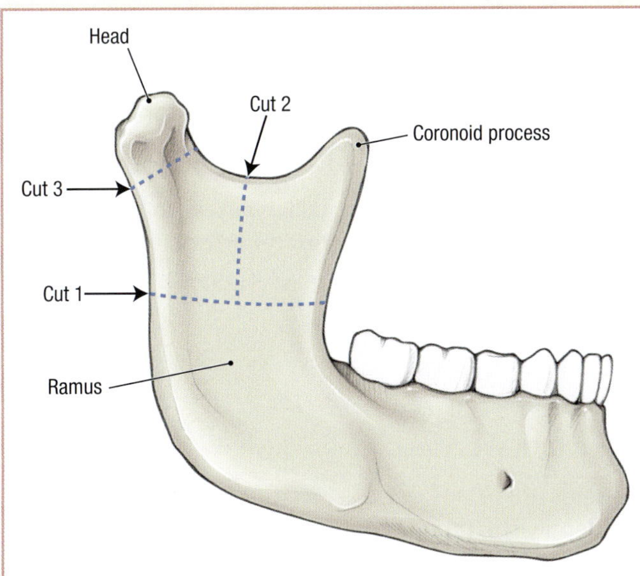

FIGURE 7.32 ■ Removal of superior aspect of ramus of mandible. Right lateral view.

to create separation from the underlying structures deep to the mandible.

3. Use a saw to score a line (cut halfway) horizontally through the ramus of the mandible just above the level of the lower dentition near the midpoint of the ramus (**Cut 1**).
4. Use a saw to score a line (cut halfway) vertically through the ramus of the mandible at the midpoint of the horizontal cut, which bisects the lowest point of the mandibular notch (**Cut 2**).

Dissection Note: The two cuts through the ramus of the mandible should create an inverted "T"-shaped cut. Pay attention to not cut through the full depth of the bone while making the score lines.

5. Use bone cutters, or a chisel, to carefully break the bone along the score lines.
6. Insert a probe medial to the neck of the mandible and create separation between the underlying structures and the bone.
7. Use a saw to cut halfway through the neck of the mandible (**Cut 3**).
8. Use bone cutters to break the bone along the score line.
9. Refer to FIGURE 7.33.
10. Gently reflect the coronoid process, portions of the anterior superior corner of the ramus, and the attached temporalis superiorly.
11. Use blunt dissection to release the temporalis from the skull and observe that the **anterior** and **posterior deep temporal nerves** (branches of the mandibular division of the trigeminal nerve) and **arteries** enter the muscle on its deep surface. *Note that the deep temporal nerves, branches from CN V_3, provide motor innervation to the temporalis.*
12. Deep to the mandible, identify the **inferior alveolar nerve** and **vessels** (see **Clinical Correlation 7.9**).

CLINICAL CORRELATION 7.9

Dental Anesthesia

ATLAS 8.50, 8.52

An inferior alveolar block is a commonly used method of providing dental anesthesia to the mandibular teeth. The needle is inserted through the oral mucosa near the opening of the mandibular foramen to anesthetize the lower dentition, oral mucosa, and lower lip innervated by the inferior alveolar nerve.

Similarly, a mandibular nerve block may be performed by injecting an anesthetic agent into the infratemporal fossa. A mandibular nerve block will anesthetize not only the inferior alveolar nerve but also the lingual, buccal, and possibly auriculotemporal nerves, resulting in anesthesia of the mandibular teeth, lower lip, chin, cheek, tongue, and TMJ.

13. Use bone cutters to carefully remove the superior posterior part of the mandible, beginning at the mandibular notch and proceeding inferiorly, stopping at the level of the lingula.

Dissection Note: While removing the bone, make small cuts and stop periodically to verify that you are staying on the lateral side of the muscles, nerves, and vessels.

14. Remove the portions of bone superior to the horizontal score line and place it in the tissue container.
15. Clean the inferior alveolar nerve and artery and follow them inferiorly to the **mandibular foramen** where they enter the bone to reach the teeth via the **mandibular canal**. *Note that the inferior alveolar nerve provides sensory innervation to the mandibular teeth.*
16. Identify the **nerve to mylohyoid** arising from the posterior aspect of the inferior alveolar nerve prior to entering the mandibular foramen. *Note that the nerve to mylohyoid is a useful way to differentiate the inferior alveolar nerve from the nearby neurovascular structures.*
17. Near the chin, identify the **mental nerve** and recall that it is a branch of the inferior alveolar nerve, which passes through the mental foramen to innervate the chin and lower lip.
18. Medial to the cut ramus of the mandible, identify the **lingual nerve** anterior to the inferior alveolar nerve. Observe that the lingual nerve does not enter the mandibular foramen but remains medial to the mandible near the 3rd mandibular molar. *Note that the lingual nerve provides sensory innervation to the mucosa of the anterior two-thirds of the tongue, mucosa of the floor of the mouth, and lingual alveolar mucosa.*

Maxillary Artery

ATLAS 8.50, 8.51; VIDEO 7.8.4

1. Refer to FIGURE 7.33.
2. Identify the **maxillary artery** where it arises from the termination of the external carotid artery.
3. Observe that the maxillary artery courses horizontally through the infratemporal fossa and crosses either the superficial surface (two-thirds of cases) or the deep surface (one-third of cases) of the lateral pterygoid. *If the maxillary artery in your specimen passes deep to the lateral pterygoid, it may be necessary to remove portions of the muscle while you identify the following branches of the maxillary artery.*
4. Use blunt dissection to trace the maxillary artery through the infratemporal fossa.
5. Near the point of origin of the maxillary artery from the external carotid artery, if visible, identify the **middle meningeal artery**. *Note that as the middle meningeal artery lies quite deep in the temporal fossa, it will be isolated at a later stage in the dissection.*
6. Identify and clean the **deep temporal arteries (anterior and posterior)**. Observe that deep temporal arteries arise from the superior aspect of the maxillary artery and pass superiorly and laterally across the roof of the infratemporal fossa near the bone to enter the deep surface of the temporalis.
7. Identify and clean the remaining portion of the **masseteric artery** (cut in a previous dissection step). The masseteric artery courses laterally from the maxillary artery and passes through the mandibular notch to enter the deep surface of the masseter.
8. Identify the **inferior alveolar artery** and follow it from where it entered the mandibular foramen with the inferior alveolar nerve, back to its origin from the maxillary artery.
9. The last branch of the maxillary artery to be dissected at this time is the **buccal artery**, which passes anteriorly onto the buccinator to supply the cheek. *Note that the buccal artery may be quite small and is often difficult to dissect.*

Pterygoids

ATLAS 8.50, 8.53C; VIDEO 7.8.5

1. Refer to FIGURE 7.33.
2. Identify the **lateral pterygoid** coursing horizontally through the infratemporal fossa.
3. Use blunt dissection to clean the surface of the lateral pterygoid and identify the plane of separation between its superior and inferior heads. *Note that the lateral pterygoid is innervated by branches of CN V_3 along with the other muscles of mastication; however, it is unique in that it acts to open the jaw.*
4. Review the attachments and actions of the lateral pterygoid (see **TABLE 7.5**).
5. Inferior and deep to the lateral pterygoid, identify the **medial pterygoid**. Reflect the masseter back and forth to observe that the medial pterygoid has a similar fiber orientation and thus acts in a similar fashion to close the jaw.

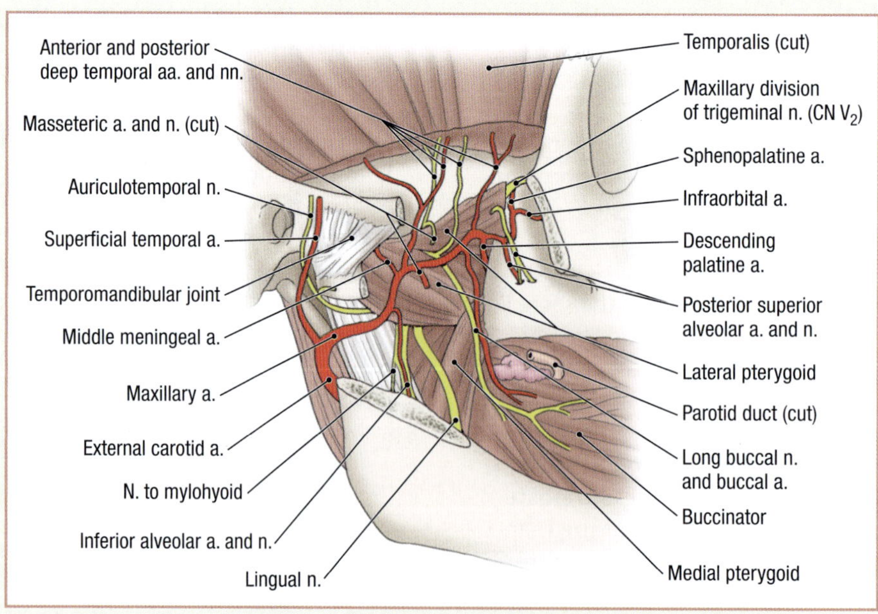

FIGURE 7.33 ● Superficial dissection of infratemporal fossa. Lateral view.

6. Observe that the lingual and inferior alveolar nerves pass between the medial and lateral pterygoids.
7. Clean the surface of the medial pterygoid using the lingual and inferior alveolar nerves as a guide to assist in identification of the plane of separation between the pterygoids.
8. Review the attachments and actions of the medial pterygoid (see **TABLE 7.5**).
9. Define the inferior border of the lateral pterygoid by inserting a probe between it and the medial pterygoid.
10. Use scissors to cut the lateral pterygoid close to its posterior attachments to the neck of the mandible and articular disc.
11. Remove the muscle in a piecemeal fashion to preserve superficially positioned nerves and vessels.

Dissection Note: If the maxillary artery courses deep to the lateral pterygoid, then it may be possible to simply reflect the lateral pterygoid anteriorly and avoid removing it completely from the dissection field.

12. Use blunt dissection to follow the lingual and inferior alveolar nerves superiorly toward the foramen ovale in the roof of the infratemporal fossa.
13. Refer to FIGURE 7.34.
14. Return to the proximal end of the maxillary artery and identify the **middle meningeal artery** arising medial to the neck of the mandible and lateral pterygoid, where it ascends toward the base of the skull.
15. Observe that just below the base of the skull, the middle meningeal artery is encircled by the **auriculotemporal nerve** prior to passing through the foramen spinosum to enter the middle cranial fossa and supply the dura mater.
16. Use blunt dissection to carefully separate the loop of nervous tissue encircling the middle meningeal artery, noting that the auriculotemporal nerve is the only posteriorly oriented branch of the **mandibular division of trigeminal nerve (CN V_3)**.
17. Identify the **chorda tympani**, a thin nerve joining the posterior aspect of the **lingual nerve** high in the infratemporal fossa.
18. Follow the maxillary artery anteromedially toward the **pterygopalatine fossa**.
19. Observe that prior to entering the pterygopalatine fossa, the maxillary artery divides into four arterial branches: posterior superior alveolar, infraorbital, descending palatine, and sphenopalatine. At this time, identify only the **posterior superior alveolar artery**, which enters the infratemporal surface of the maxilla. The other branches will be dissected later.

Temporomandibular Joint

ATLAS 8.47C, 8.50A, 8.55, 8.56; VIDEO 7.8.6

1. Refer to FIGURE 7.34.
2. Identify the capsule of the TMJ and observe while mobilizing the mandible that the joint capsule is loose, allowing for increased mobility.
3. Observe that the lateral surface of the joint capsule is reinforced by the **lateral ligament**.
4. Preserve the superficial temporal vessels and auriculotemporal nerve by gently pulling them away from the TMJ.
5. Use a scalpel to trim away the lateral side of the joint capsule and lateral ligament.

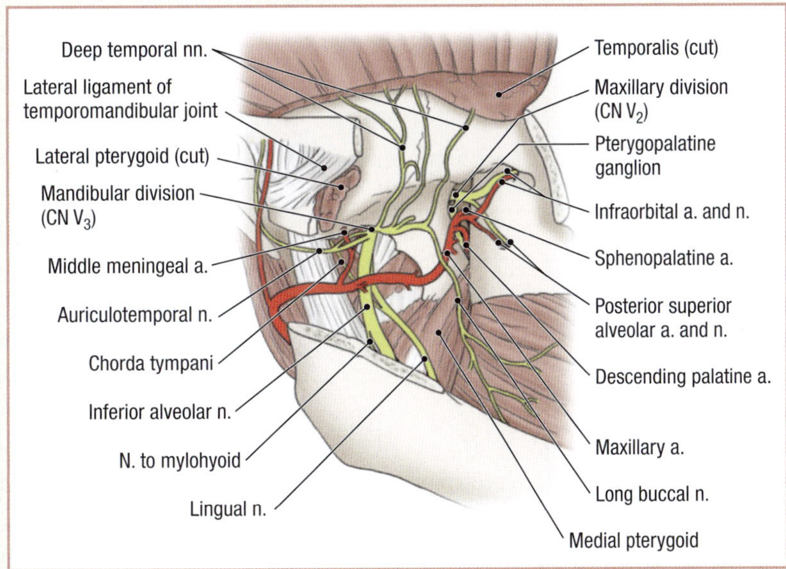

FIGURE 7.34 ● Deep dissection of infratemporal fossa. Lateral view.

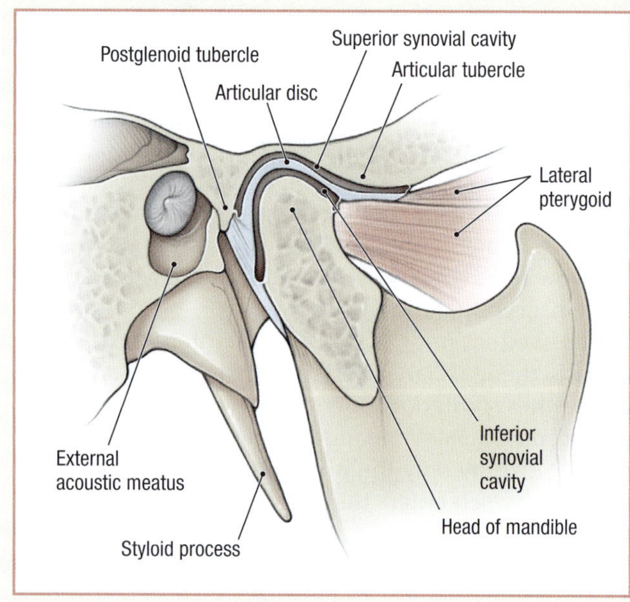

FIGURE 7.35 ● Sagittal section of right temporomandibular joint. Right lateral view.

6. Refer to FIGURE 7.35.
7. Within the joint, identify the **articular disc** and observe its location between the mandibular fossa of the temporal bone and head of the mandible. *Note that the tendon of the lateral pterygoid is attached to both the neck of the mandible and the articular disc, which may assist in its identification by following the muscle fibers posteriorly.*
8. Examine the articular disc and observe that it is thin near its center and thicker near its edges.
9. Insert a probe both superior and inferior to the disc to identify the **superior** and **inferior synovial cavities.**
10. Move the small remaining portion of the head of the mandible and observe the two types of movements occurring in the TMJ. Verify that in the superior synovial cavity, gliding movements occur between the articular disc and mandibular fossa (protrusion and retrusion), and that in the inferior synovial cavity, hinge movements occur between the head of the mandible and articular disc.

Dissection Follow-up

1. Review the attachments and actions of the muscles of mastication in **TABLE 7.5**.
2. Review the path of the mandibular division of the trigeminal nerve through the foramen ovale into the infratemporal fossa.
3. Review the sensory and motor branches of the mandibular division of the trigeminal nerve.
4. Follow the external carotid artery from its origin near the hyoid bone to the infratemporal fossa, reviewing the location of its two terminal branches.
5. Review the course and regions of supply of the branches of the maxillary artery.
6. Review the relationship of the middle meningeal artery and auriculotemporal nerve.
7. Replace the reflected muscles of mastication and tissues of the infratemporal region in their correct anatomical positions.

TABLE 7.5 Muscles of Mastication

Muscle	*Superior Attachments*	*Inferior Attachments*	*Actions*	*Innervation*
Masseter	Inferior border and medial surface of zygomatic arch	Lateral surface of ramus and angle of mandible	Elevates and protrudes mandible	CN V_3 via masseteric n.
Temporalis	Floor of temporal fossa and deep surface of temporal fascia	Tip and medial surface of coronoid process and anterior border of ramus of mandible	Elevates and retrudes mandible	CN V_3 via deep temporal nn.
Medial pterygoid	Medial surface of lateral pterygoid plate (deep head) Tuberosity of maxilla (superficial head)	Medial surface of ramus of mandible	Elevates and protrudes mandible (bilateral) Side to side movement of mandible (unilateral)	CN V_3 via medial pterygoid n.
Lateral pterygoid	Infratemporal surface and infratemporal crest of greater wing of sphenoid (superior head) Lateral surface of lateral pterygoid plate (inferior head)	Neck of mandible, articular disc, and capsule of TMJ	Depresses and protrudes mandible (bilateral) Side-to-side movement of mandible (unilateral)	CN V_3 via lateral pterygoid n.

Abbreviations: CN, cranial nerve; n., nerve; nn., nerves; TMJ, temporomandibular joint.

INTERIOR OF SKULL

Dissection Overview

Some schools remove the brain prior to the cadaveric dissection. If the brain has been removed in your cadaver, skip ahead to the **Cranial Meninges** section. If you must remove the brain yourself, proceed with the following instructions.

The bones of the calvaria provide a protective covering for the cerebral hemispheres. The bones of the calvaria are classified as flat bones and thus consist of an outer lamina and inner lamina composed of compact bone, which encase the diploë, the core of spongy bone as shown in FIGURE 7.36.

Within the cranial cavity, the brain is covered by three protective and supportive membranes called meninges. The meninges serve as the framework for cerebral arteries and veins and form the spaces containing venous blood draining from the brain (dural venous sinuses) and the space containing cerebrospinal fluid (CSF) (subarachnoid space). The dura mater is the tough outermost membrane, the arachnoid mater is the "cobweb"-like intermediate membrane, and the pia mater is the innermost delicate membrane intimately adhered to the surface of the brain.

The order of dissection will be as follows: The calvaria will be exposed by reflecting the scalp and temporalis. The calvaria will be cut with a saw and removed. The dura mater will be examined and opened to reveal the underlying arachnoid and pia mater.

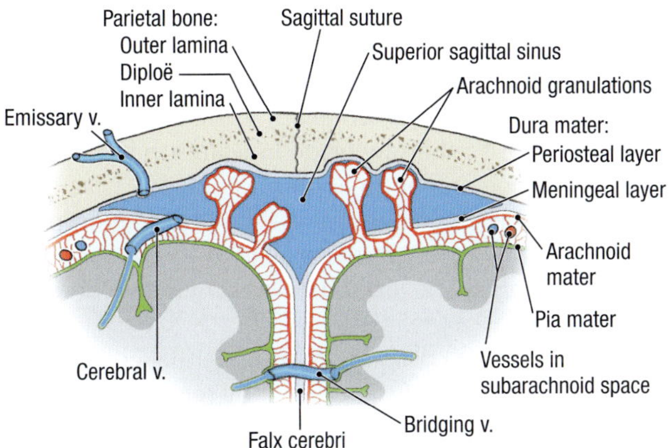

FIGURE 7.36 Coronal section through superior sagittal sinus and cranial meninges. Anterior view.

Dissection Instructions

Removal of Calvaria

VIDEO 7.9.1

1. Refer to FIGURE 7.37.
2. With the cadaver in the supine position, reflect the **frontalis** and **occipitalis** (frontal and occipital bellies of the occipitofrontalis) and any remaining layers of the scalp inferiorly.
3. Use a scalpel to detach the **temporalis** from the calvaria by cutting it from its attachments at the **superior** and **inferior temporal lines** and reflect the muscle inferiorly.
4. Identify the **pericranium (periosteum)**, the deepest layer of the scalp covering the surface of each bone of the calvaria.
5. Use a scalpel or chisel to scrape the bones of the calvaria clean of pericranium and any remaining muscle fibers.
6. Place a rubber band or tie a string around the circumference of the skull about 2 cm superior to the supraorbital margin anteriorly and at the level of the external occipital protuberance posteriorly.
7. Trace the circumference of the calvaria with a pencil or marker, following the circumferential path of the rubber band or string. Once the complete circumference of the skull has been traced, remove the rubber band or string.
8. Draw a vertical line from above the ear on one side of the head up and over the vertex of the skull to a similar location on the opposite side. The vertical line

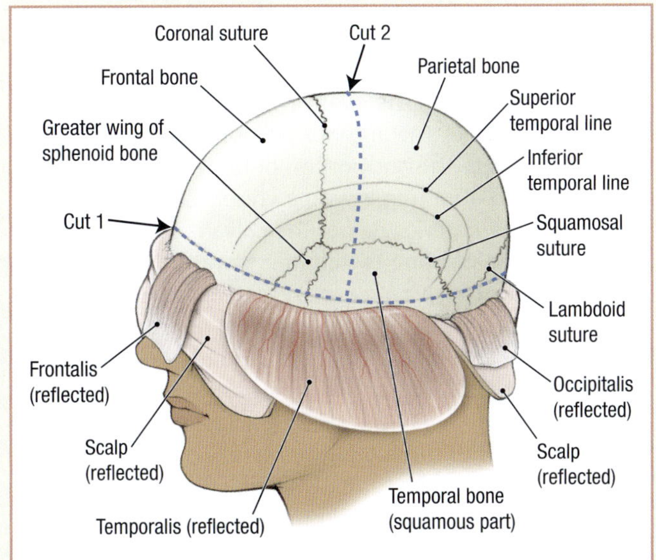

FIGURE 7.37 Reflection of temporalis and occipitofrontalis and cuts for calvaria removal. Left lateral view.

should effectively divide the skull into anterior and posterior halves.

9. Use a saw to cut along the marked lines around the circumference of the skull (**Cut 1**), passing only through the outer lamina of the calvaria but not completely through the bone. If you saw through the inner lamina, you may damage the underlying dura mater or the brain.
10. To facilitate the cuts through the calvaria, turn the body alternately from supine to prone and back as needed.

Dissection Note: Be particularly careful when cutting the squamous part of the temporal bone, which is very thin. Moist red bone on the saw blade indicates that the saw is within the diploë and at an appropriate depth.

11. Use a saw to cut along the vertical line arching over the superior aspect of the skull (**Cut 2**) connecting to the horizontal line around its circumference on each side.
12. After making a complete circumferential cut, break the inner lamina of the calvaria by repeatedly inserting a chisel into the saw cut and striking the chisel gently with a mallet. Once the skull has been completely cut through, you should see a small amount of movement between the portions of cut skull.
13. Use a "T-tool," if available, or the edge of a chisel to create a small amount of movement and increase the space between the cut pieces of bone and the circumference of the skull by inserting and twisting the instrument in the created gap. While doing so, you may hear a distinct tearing sound as the dura mater is separated from the overlying bone.
14. Beginning with the anterior portion of sectioned bone, elevate the cut portion of bone by prying it from the dura mater with a chisel. Continue to elevate the anterior half of the calvaria and remove the portion of bone by tilting it toward the forehead. *Note that excessive force may result in tearing the dura mater and damage to the underlying brain.*
15. Using the cut edge of bone as a guide, insert the handle of a forceps under the posterior portion of bone to push away the periosteal layer of dura mater from the deep surface of the bone.
16. Repeat the process to remove the remaining posterior half of the calvaria using a chisel as leverage against the bones.

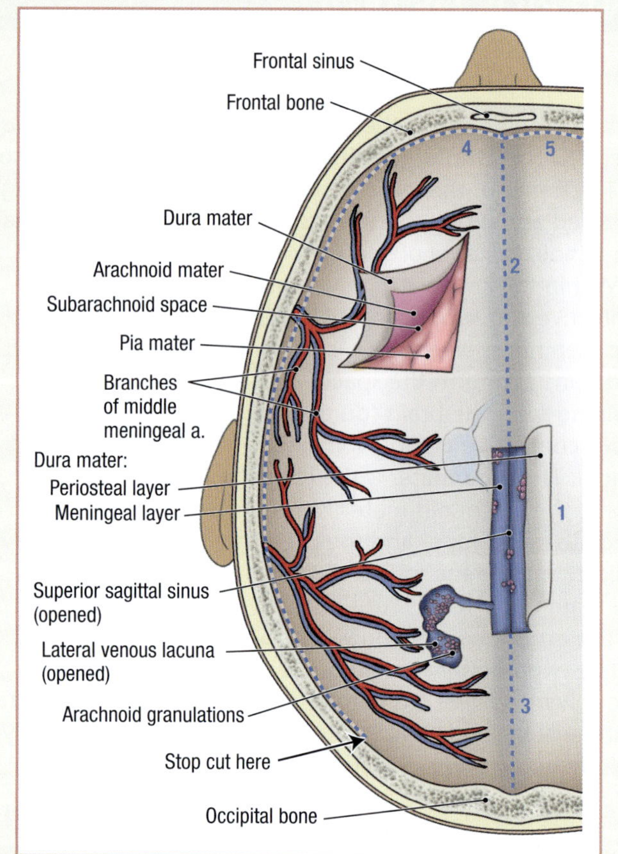

FIGURE 7.38 ● Cranial meninges and opening of superior sagittal sinus. Superior view.

Cranial Meninges

ATLAS 8.22, 8.23, 8.24; VIDEO 7.9.2

1. Refer to FIGURE 7.38.
2. Identify the **dura mater**, which consists of two layers, an external **periosteal layer** and internal **meningeal layer**. *Note that the two dural layers are indistinguishable except where they separate to enclose the dural venous sinuses and form the falx cerebri and falx cerebelli.*
3. Identify the **superior sagittal sinus**, a dural venous sinus coursing along the superior extent of the cranial cavity in the midsagittal plane.
4. Use scissors to make a longitudinal incision through the periosteal layer of dura mater overlying the superior sagittal sinus near the vertex for a short distance (**Cut 1**). Use forceps to gently spread open the sinus and verify that its inner surface is smooth because it is lined by endothelium.
5. Extend the incision through the periosteal layer of dura to the frontal bone anteriorly (**Cut 2**) and to the cut edge of the occipital bone posteriorly (**Cut 3**). Observe that the caliber of the superior sagittal sinus increases from anterior to posterior following the direction of venous blood flow.
6. Gently insert a probe into the lateral expansions along the wall of the sinus and identify the **lateral venous lacunae**. Within a lateral venous lacuna, identify the **arachnoid granulations** responsible for the return of CSF to the venous system.

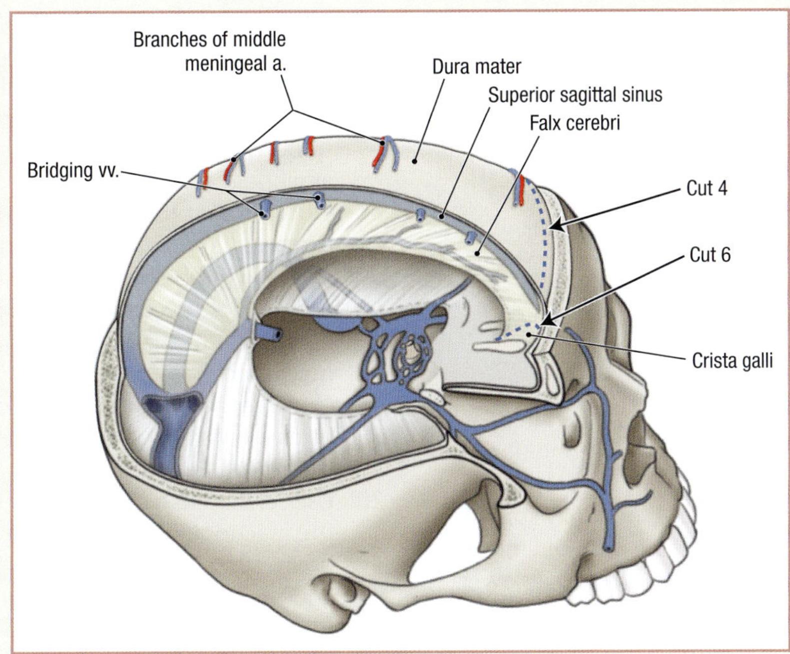

FIGURE 7.39 ■ Reflection of dura mater. Right superolateral view.

7. Examine the surface of the dura mater covering the cerebral hemispheres and observe the branches of the **middle meningeal artery**. The middle meningeal artery supplies the dura mater and adjacent calvaria (see **Clinical Correlation 7.10**). *Note that the anterior branch of the middle meningeal artery crosses the inner surface of the pterion, where it may tunnel through the bone.*

CLINICAL CORRELATION 7.10

Epidural Hemorrhage

ATLAS 8.21, 8.22B

Fractures through the pterion, the weak point of junction of the parietal, frontal, and temporal bones, may result in tearing of the underlying middle meningeal artery. Rupture of the middle meningeal artery results in an epidural hemorrhage (extradural hematoma), the blood accumulation between the skull and periosteal layer of dura mater. Bleeding into the epidural space results in a life-threatening increased pressure on the underlying cerebral cortex within hours if left untreated.

8. On the inner surface of the removed calvaria, identify the grooves formed by the middle meningeal artery, comparing them with the visible vessels on the surface of the dura mater. Recall that the middle meningeal artery arose from the maxillary artery in the infratemporal fossa.
9. On the inner surface of the removed calvaria, identify the **groove for the superior sagittal sinus** and compare it with the path of the sinus within the dura mater.
10. Use scissors to cut through the dura mater along the circumference of the cut edge of the calvaria, stopping at a point posteriorly about 3.5 cm lateral to the midline bilaterally (**Cut 4** and **Cut 5**). The objective is to permit the dura mater to be pulled free from the surface of the brain but to leave it attached posteriorly in the area of the superior sagittal sinus.
11. Refer to FIGURE 7.39.
12. Use blunt dissection to gently retract the anterior aspect of the dura mater and insert scissors between the cerebral hemispheres to cut the **falx cerebri (cerebral falx)** where it attaches to the crista galli (**Cut 6**). The falx cerebri is an extension of the meningeal layer of dura mater, which descends between the cerebral hemispheres along the midline to physically separate the right and left cerebral hemispheres.
13. Grasp the anterior pole of the dura mater and gently pull it posteriorly, gradually working the falx cerebri free from between the cerebral hemispheres as you progress.
14. Identify **cerebral veins** connecting from the surface of the brain to the superior sagittal sinus along its lateral sides (see **Clinical Correlation 7.11**).

CLINICAL CORRELATION 7.11

Subdural and Subarachnoid Hemorrhages

ATLAS 8.22C, 8.22D

Head trauma with rapid acceleration and deceleration, as seen in a car crash, may tear the cerebral veins at the point where they enter the superior sagittal sinus. The venous blood from the tear accumulates in the potential space between the dura mater and the arachnoid mater, creating a "subdural space" in a condition called a subdural hematoma. By comparison, a rupture of a cerebral artery from a burst aneurysm will bleed into the subarachnoid space, a true space occupied by CSF, in a condition called a subarachnoid hemorrhage.

A subdural hematoma of venous blood may spread further than an epidural bleed because it is not limited by the dural adhesions to the sutures. Despite a slower onset, subdural hemorrhage may still lead to loss of consciousness and be life-threatening if left untreated.

15. Cut the cerebral veins as you pull the dura mater posteriorly to permit the falx cerebri to be completely retracted from between the cerebral hemispheres until the dura mater is attached to the skull only near its posterior pole. *Note that the reflected portion of dura mater will be removed along with the brain dissection.*
16. Refer back to FIGURE 7.38.
17. Deep to the location of the now reflected dura mater, identify the **arachnoid mater** covering the surface of the brain, named in reference to the spiderweb-like connective tissue strands in the subarachnoid space.
18. Observe that the arachnoid mater loosely covers the brain and spans across the fissures and sulci. In the living person, the arachnoid mater is closely applied to the internal meningeal layer of the dura mater due to the pressure of CSF in the subarachnoid space.
19. Observe that deep to the arachnoid mater, cerebral veins are visible following the contours of the sulci of the brain.
20. Use scissors to make a small cut (2.5 cm) through the arachnoid mater over the lateral surface of the brain. Use a probe to elevate the arachnoid mater and observe the **subarachnoid space**. In the living person, the subarachnoid space contains CSF. In the cadaver, the arachnoid mater appears "deflated" as the CSF is no longer present.
21. Through the opening in the arachnoid mater, observe the **pia mater** on the surface of the brain. *Note that the pia mater faithfully follows the contours of the brain, covering all gyri, sulci, and fissures, and cannot be separated from the surface of the brain.*

Dissection Follow-up

1. Review the bones comprising the calvaria.
2. Review the features and locations of the two layers of cranial dura mater.
3. Review the features of the spinal dura mater and compare it to the cranial dura mater.
4. Review the location and likely source of blood for an epidural, subdural, and subarachnoid hematoma.
5. Return the reflected portion of dura mater back to its anatomical position.
6. Wrap the head with a moist towel or wrapping soaked with embalming fluid or wetting solution to prevent desiccation of the exposed meninges and brain.

BRAIN REMOVAL, DURAL INFOLDINGS, AND DURAL VENOUS SINUSES

Dissection Overview

The internal meningeal layer of dura mater forms inwardly projecting folds (dural infoldings) that serve as incomplete partitions of the cranial cavity. Three of these folds (falx cerebri, tentorium cerebelli, and falx cerebelli) extend inward between parts of the brain. Recall that the periosteal and meningeal layers of the dura mater separate from each other in several locations to form dural venous sinuses. The dural venous sinuses collect venous drainage from the brain and conduct it out of the cranial cavity.

The order of dissection will be as follows: Bony features of the cranial cavity will be studied on a skull. The dural infoldings will be cut to facilitate brain removal. The brain will be removed with the associated leptomeninges (arachnoid mater and pia mater). The dura mater will be repositioned to recreate its three-dimensional morphology during life. The infoldings of the dura mater and associated dural venous sinuses will be identified.

Skeletal Anatomy

Cranial Fossae

ATLAS 8.6

On a skull with the calvaria removed, review the following skeletal features.

1. Refer to FIGURE 7.40.
2. Within the cranial cavity, identify the three **cranial fossae**.
3. Anteriorly, identify the **anterior cranial fossa** and observe that it is predominantly formed by the right and left **orbital plates of the frontal bone**.
4. Between the orbital plates, identify the **crista galli** of the ethmoid bone, the small ridge-like process serving as the anterior attachment of the falx cerebri. Observe that to either side of the crista galli is the **cribriform plate**, a small depression with multiple apertures superior to the nasal cavity allowing passage of olfactory nerves.

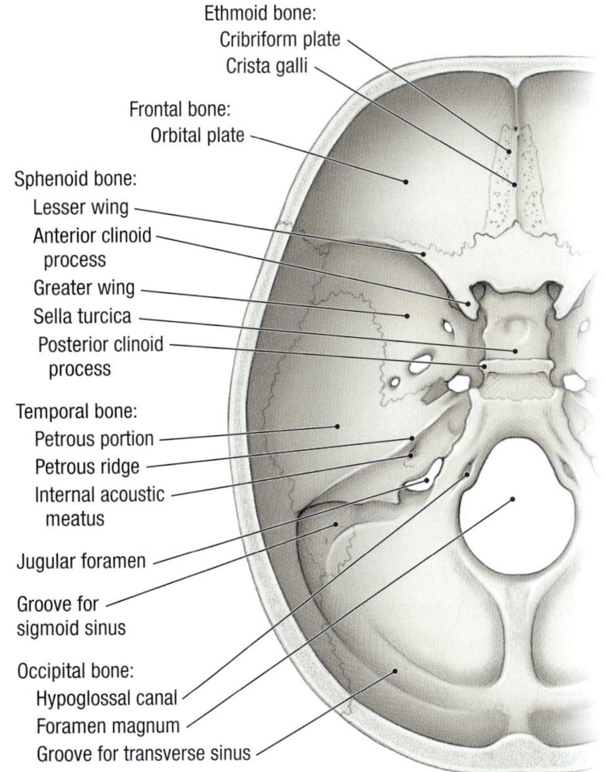

FIGURE 7.40 ● Floor of cranial cavity. Superior view.

5. At the border between the anterior and middle cranial fossae, identify the ridge formed by the **lesser wing of the sphenoid**, which ends medially as the rounded **anterior clinoid process**.
6. Identify the middle cranial fossa and observe that it is formed by the **greater wing of the sphenoid** and **petrous part of the temporal bone**.
7. In the midline of the skull between the right and left middle cranial fossae, identify the saddle-shaped depression of the **hypophyseal fossa (*sella turcica*)**. In the living person, the sella turcica supports the pituitary gland.
8. On the posterior aspect of the **sella turcica**, identify the **posterior clinoid process** demarcating the posterior aspect of the sphenoid bone.
9. Lateral and posterior to the sella turcica, identify the **petrous ridge** of the temporal bone separating the **middle** and **posterior cranial fossae**. *Note that the petrous ridge serves as the anterior attachment of the tentorium cerebelli.*
10. Identify the **internal acoustic meatus** on the vertical part of the petrous part of the temporal bone within the posterior cranial fossa. *Note that the internal acoustic meatus is the medial opening leading to the inner and middle ear.*
11. Identify the **jugular foramen**, a large somewhat bean-shaped hole inferior to the internal acoustic meatus separating the petrous part of the temporal bone from the occipital bone.
12. Observe that the **groove for the sigmoid sinus** as it courses medially follows the inferior border of the petrous part of the temporal bone to terminate at the jugular foramen. *Note that the sigmoid sinus is a dural venous sinus draining cerebral blood to the internal jugular vein.*
13. Trace the groove for the sigmoid sinus laterally and observe that it is continuous with the anterior aspect of the **groove for the transverse sinus**. *Note that the transverse sinus is a dural venous sinus coursing in the peripheral edge of the tentorium cerebelli.*
14. Within the **posterior cranial fossa,** identify the large **foramen magnum** positioned in the midline. *Note that the foramen magnum aligns with the vertebral canal, and is the point of passage of the spinal cord from the inferior extent of the brainstem, and the vertebral arteries, which supply the posterior aspect of the brain.*
15. Within the wall of the foramen magnum, identify the **hypoglossal canal**.

Dissection Instructions

Removal of Brain

ATLAS 8.24, 8.26; VIDEO 7.10.1

Dissection Note: If the brain has been removed from your cadaver, skip ahead to the section entitled **Dural Infoldings**. The structures cut to remove the brain will be reviewed after the brain has been removed.

1. Refer to FIGURE 7.41.
2. Retract the dura mater overlying the surface of the right and left cerebral hemispheres, along with the anterior aspect of the falx cerebri. If the falx proves difficult to elevate, ensure that it was completely detached from the crista galli anteriorly (**previous cut**).
3. Gently elevate the frontal lobes of the brain.
4. Use a probe to lift the olfactory bulb from the cribriform plate on each side of the crista galli.
5. As you elevate the anterior aspect of the cerebral hemispheres, carefully use a scalpel to cut the following structures bilaterally: optic nerve, internal carotid artery, and oculomotor nerve.
6. Cut the stalk of the pituitary gland in the midline.
7. On the right side, gently lift the temporal lobe (lateral part of brain) and identify the horizontally oriented meningeal infolding of the **tentorium cerebelli (cerebellar tentorium)**.
8. Use a scalpel to cut the cerebellar tentorium as close to the superior border of the petrous part of the temporal bone as possible (**Cut 1**). The cut should begin anteriorly near the posterior clinoid process and extend posterolaterally to the end of the superior border of the petrous part of the temporal bone near the groove for the sigmoid sinus.
9. Repeat the cut of the tentorium cerebelli on the left side of the cadaver (**Cut 2**).
10. Inferior to the cut edge of the tentorium, ensure that the trochlear nerve, trigeminal nerve, and abducens nerve were cut bilaterally. With the cerebellar tentorium cut, the brain may be gently moved to gain access to structures that lie inferior to the tentorium.
11. Elevate the cerebrum and brainstem slightly and cut the following structures bilaterally: facial and vestibulocochlear nerves near the internal acoustic meatus; glossopharyngeal, vagus, and accessory nerves near the jugular foramen; and the hypoglossal nerves near the hypoglossal canal within the walls of foramen magnum.
12. Use a scalpel to sever the two vertebral arteries where they enter the skull through the foramen magnum and the cervical spinal cord as low in the foramen magnum (or cervical vertebral canal) as you can reach.
13. Support the cerebral hemispheres from behind with the palm of one hand. Insert the other hand (palm facing superiorly) between the frontal lobes and the skull with your middle finger extending down the ventral surface of the brainstem. Insert the tip of your middle finger into the cut that was made across the cervical spinal cord to support the brainstem and cerebellum.
14. Using upward pressure on the cut end of the cervical spinal cord, roll the brain, brainstem, and cerebellum

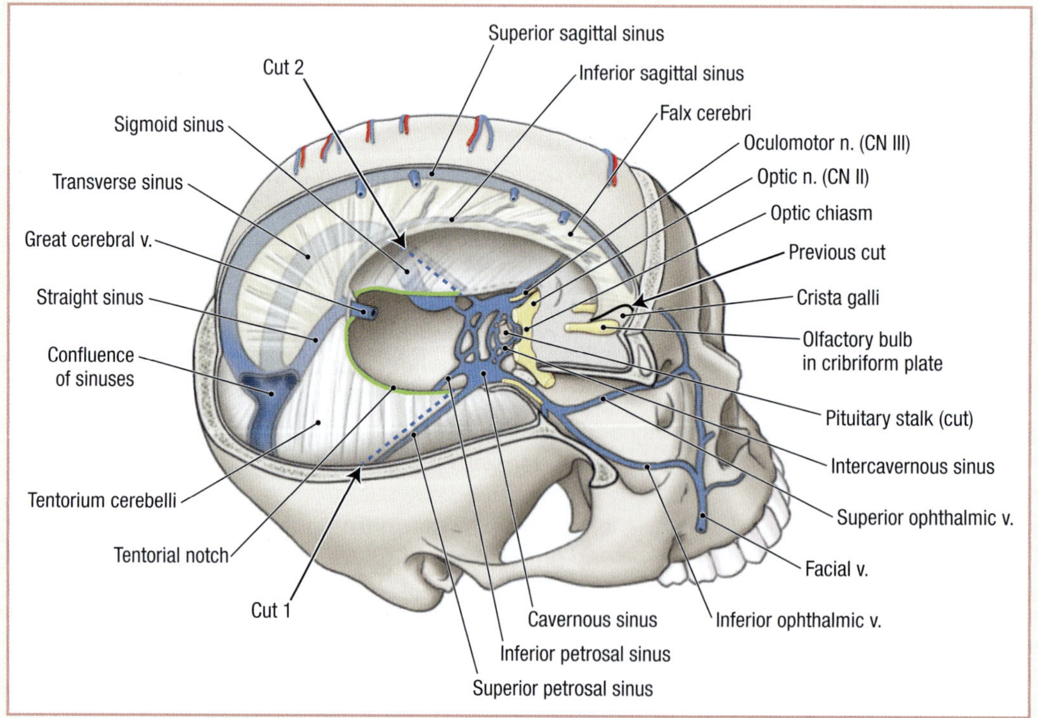

FIGURE 7.41 ● Dural infoldings and dural venous sinuses. Right superolateral view.

posteriorly and out of the cranial cavity in one piece. If done properly, the meningeal infoldings of the dura mater will be left attached to the skull.

15. Return the dura mater to its correct anatomical position.
16. The brain should be stored in a bath of preservative fluid.

Dural Infoldings

ATLAS 8.24A, 8.26; VIDEO 7.10.2

1. Refer to FIGURE 7.41.
2. Identify the **falx cerebri (cerebral falx)** between the cerebral hemispheres.
3. Observe that the falx cerebri is attached to the crista galli at its anterior end, calvaria on both sides of the groove for the superior sagittal sinus, and tentorium cerebelli posteriorly.
4. Identify the **tentorium cerebelli (cerebellar tentorium)**.
5. Observe that the tentorium cerebelli is attached to the clinoid processes of the sphenoid bone, superior border of the petrous part of the temporal bone, and occipital bone on both sides of the groove for the transverse sinus.
6. Identify the **tentorial notch (tentorial incisure)**, the opening in the tentorium cerebelli between the right and left sides allowing passage of the brainstem. *Note that the tentorium cerebelli lies between the cerebral hemispheres and the cerebellum in its anatomical position.*
7. Identify the **falx cerebelli (cerebellar falx)**, a low ridge of dura mater located inferior to the tentorium cerebelli in the midline.
8. Observe that the falx cerebelli is attached to the inner surface of the occipital bone between the cerebellar hemispheres.

Dural Venous Sinuses

ATLAS 8.24A, 8.25, 8.26; VIDEO 7.10.3

1. Refer to FIGURE 7.41.
2. Identify the **superior sagittal sinus** within the superior margin of the falx cerebri and observe that it begins anteriorly near the crista galli and ends posteriorly by draining into the **confluence of sinuses**.
3. Identify the **inferior sagittal sinus** within the inferior margin of the falx cerebri and observe that it ends near the tentorium cerebelli by draining into the anterior end of the **straight sinus**. *Note that the inferior sagittal sinus is smaller in diameter than the superior sagittal sinus.*
4. Identify the location of the straight sinus at the junction of the falx cerebri and tentorium cerebelli. Observe that at its anterior end, the straight sinus receives the inferior sagittal sinus and **great cerebral vein** and that posteriorly, it drains into the confluence of sinuses. *Note that the great cerebral vein was cut when the brain was removed.*
5. Identify the **transverse sinus** (right and left), which transports venous blood from the confluence of sinuses to the sigmoid sinus.
6. On one side, use a scalpel to open the lumen of the transverse sinus and observe that it is lined with smooth endothelium.
7. Identify the **sigmoid sinus** (right and left), which begins at the lateral end of the transverse sinus and ends at the jugular foramen.
8. On one side, use a scalpel to open the lumen of the sigmoid sinus from the transverse sinus to the jugular foramen. *Note that the internal jugular vein forms at the external surface of the jugular foramen.*
9. On the floor of the cranial cavity, identify the dura mater covering all of the bones and observe that it contains openings through which the cranial nerves pass.
10. Observe that additional small dural venous sinuses are located between the layers of the dura mater in the floor of the cranial cavity. Identify the location of the **sphenoparietal sinus**, **cavernous sinus**, **superior petrosal sinus**, **inferior petrosal sinus**, and **basilar plexus**. *Do not make an effort to dissect the cavernous sinus at this point of the dissection as this will be done later.*

Dissection Follow-up

1. Review the bones forming the floor of the cranial cavity.
2. Review the major skeletal features in each of the three cranial fossae.
3. Review the location of the dural infoldings and discuss the portions of the brain separated by each.
4. Naming all venous structures encountered along the way, trace the route of a drop of blood from a superior cerebral vein to the internal jugular vein, from the sphenoparietal sinus to the sigmoid sinus, and from the great cerebral vein to the internal jugular vein.
5. Return the reflected dural infoldings and cut dura mater back to their anatomical position.
6. Wrap the head with a moist towel or wrapping soaked with embalming fluid or wetting solution to prevent desiccation of the exposed meninges and brain.

GROSS ANATOMY OF BRAIN

Dissection Overview

The brain consists of the cerebrum (cerebral hemispheres and diencephalon), brainstem (midbrain, pons, and medulla oblongata), and cerebellum. The study of brain anatomy and its function is highly specialized and usually reserved for a neuroscience course. Because the full extent of brain function is not meant to be covered in most dissection-based courses, the description provided here is intended to relate the major features of the external surface of the brain to parts of the skull that will be studied in subsequent dissections. An additional goal of this study is to establish a mental picture of the continuity of the arteries and nerves of the brain with those same structures left behind in the cranial fossae after brain removal.

The order of dissection will be as follows: The gross anatomy of the brain will be studied including the major lobes, fissures, sulci, and gyri. The blood supply of the brain will be studied including a detailed look at the cerebral arterial circle (circle of Willis). The 12 cranial nerves will be studied from an inferior perspective of the brain.

Dissection Instructions

Brain

ATLAS 8.101, 8.103A; VIDEO 7.11.1

Dissection Note: Review the following neural features on a brain that has been stored in a bath of preservative fluid.

1. Refer to FIGURE 7.42.
2. Observe that the human brain is subdivided according to large points of separation created by two major fissures. Identify the **longitudinal fissure**, which separates the cerebrum into **right** and **left cerebral hemispheres**, and the **transverse fissure**, which separates the cerebrum from the **cerebellum** with the **brainstem** acting as the bridge between the two.
3. Examine the surface of the brain and observe that it is composed of **gyri** (raised regions) and **sulci** (grooves).
4. On the lateral surface of the brain, identify the **central sulcus** between the **precentral gyrus** (primary motor cortex) of the **frontal lobe** and the **postcentral gyrus** (primary sensory cortex) of the **parietal lobe.**
5. Identify the **temporal lobe** of the brain laterally and observe that it is separated from the frontal and parietal lobes by the **lateral sulcus.**
6. On the posterior aspect of the brain, identify the **occipital lobe** superior to the transverse fissure.
7. Refer to a skull and identify the three **cranial fossae: anterior, middle,** and **posterior.**
8. Use the cadaver and brain to verify that the **frontal lobe** is located in the **anterior cranial fossa,** that the **temporal lobe** is located in the **middle cranial fossa,** and that the **cerebellum** is located in the **posterior cranial fossa.**
9. Observe that the **occipital lobe** is located superior to the tentorium cerebelli and therefore superior to the groove of the transverse sinus.
10. Observe that the **brainstem** becomes continuous with the cervical spinal cord at the **foramen magnum.**

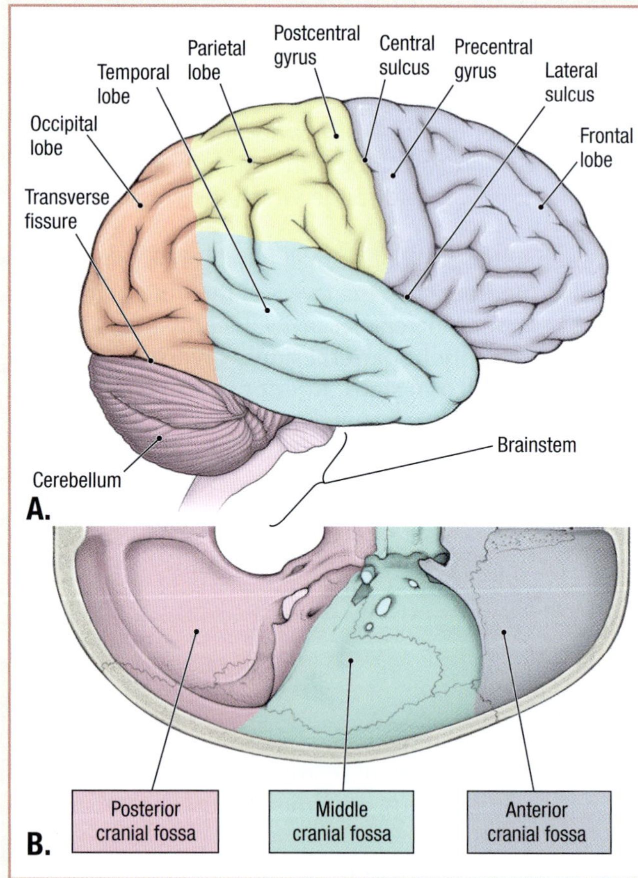

FIGURE 7.42 ● **A.** Surface anatomy of brain. Right lateral view. **B.** Cranial fossae. Superior view.

Blood Supply of Brain

ATLAS 8.26, 8.29, 8.32, 8.33; VIDEO 7.11.2

1. Refer to FIGURE 7.43.
2. Examine the surface of the brain and observe that it is covered by arachnoid mater.
3. Use a probe to peel back the arachnoid mater and expose the arteries on the inferior surface of the brain.
4. Identify the four arteries supplying blood to the brain: the two vertebral arteries posteriorly and the two internal carotid arteries anteriorly.

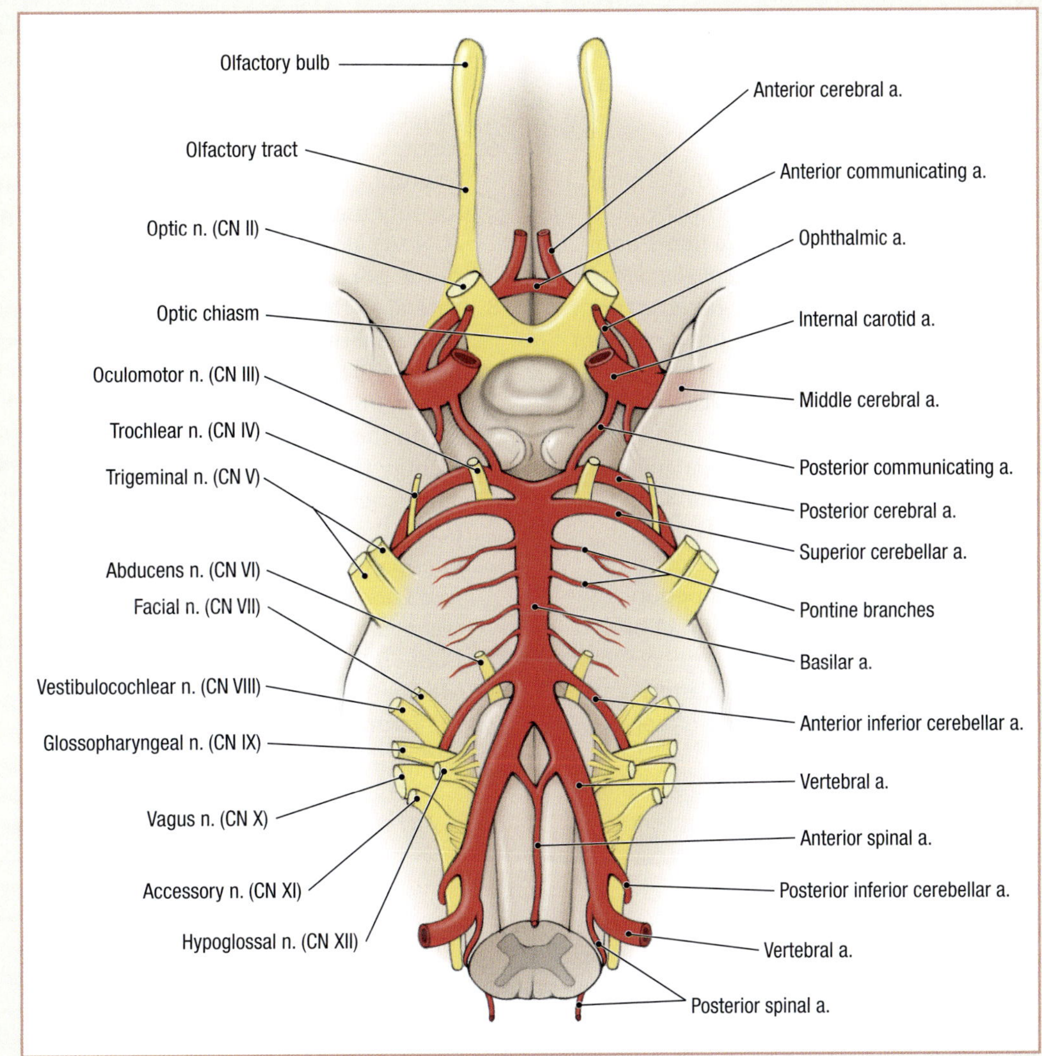

FIGURE 7.43 ● Blood vessels (*left side*) and cranial nerves (*right side*) on inferior surface of brain. Inferior view.

5. Observe that each **vertebral artery** gives rise to one **posterior inferior cerebellar artery (PICA)** prior to combining to form the unpaired **basilar artery** in the approximate midline of the brainstem.
6. Arising from the basilar artery, identify the **anterior inferior cerebellar artery (AICA)**, the **superior cerebellar artery**, and several **pontine branches** arising bilaterally.
7. Follow the basilar artery superiorly and observe that it terminates by branching into the paired **posterior cerebral arteries.**
8. Observe that each posterior cerebral artery has a **posterior communicating artery**, which anastomoses with the **internal carotid artery**.
9. Within the cranial cavity, identify the cut edge of the internal carotid artery.
10. Observe that the first branch of the internal carotid artery, the **ophthalmic artery**, arises medial to the anterior clinoid process and passes through the optic foramen with the **optic nerve**.
11. On the inferior aspect of the brain, observe that each internal carotid artery terminates by dividing into a **middle cerebral artery** and an **anterior cerebral artery**.
12. Gently separate the frontal lobes and observe that the anterior cerebral arteries are joined across the midline by the **anterior communicating artery.**
13. Identify the **cerebral arterial circle (circle of Willis)**, formed by the posterior cerebral, posterior communicating, internal carotid, anterior cerebral, and anterior communicating arteries. *Note that the cerebral arterial circle forms an anastomosis in the brain, ensuring adequate blood supply to all regions.*

Cranial Nerves

ATLAS 8.26, 8.30A, 8.32, 9.1; VIDEO 7.11.3

Dissection Note: It is important to note that the cranial nerves are called such because of their interaction with the skull, or cranium, and not because they originate off the brain. In the following sequence, we will review the **12 cranial nerves** by name and number from an inferior view of the brain. The foramen associated with each cranial nerve will be reviewed with the cranial fossae.

1. Refer to FIGURE 7.43.
2. On the rostral (anterior) inferior surface of the brain, identify the **olfactory bulb and tract** and, if visible, the **olfactory nerve (CN I)**, small nerve fibers originating from the olfactory bulb. *Note that the olfactory nerve fibers are probably not visible because they were likely torn during the separation of the brain from the anterior cranial fossa.*
3. Identify the **optic nerve (CN II)** arising bilaterally from the **optic chiasm**. The optic chiasm is the point where visual information from the medial retina (lateral visual field) of each eye crosses to the contralateral side of the brain prior to reaching the **optic tracts**.
4. Identify the **oculomotor nerve (CN III)** emerging from the midbrain between the cerebral peduncles, which connect the cerebrum to the midbrain of the brainstem. Observe that the oculomotor nerve exits the brain between the posterior cerebral artery and superior cerebellar artery, a potential site of nerve entrapment.
5. Identify the thin **trochlear nerve (CN IV)** and follow it posteriorly around the lateral aspect of the cerebral peduncle to where it originates from the posterior surface of the midbrain.
6. Identify the relatively large **trigeminal nerve (CN V)** arising from the anterolateral aspect of the pons.
7. Identify the thin **abducens (abducent) nerve (CN VI)** along the anterior (ventral) inferior surface of the pons.
8. Lateral to the origin of the abducens nerve, identify the **facial nerve (CN VII)** and **vestibulocochlear nerve (CN VIII)** near the junction of the pons with the medulla.
9. Along the lateral aspect of the medulla posteriorly, identify the **glossopharyngeal nerve (CN IX)**, **vagus nerve (CN X)**, and **spinal accessory nerve (CN XI)** arising in sequential order from superior to inferior. *Note that the spinal accessory nerve contains fibers originating from the spinal cord but is considered a cranial nerve because it exits the base of the skull through the jugular foramen with CN IX and CN X.*
10. Medial (ventral) to CN IX, CN X, and CN XI, identify the **hypoglossal nerve (CN XII)** between the olive and pyramid of the medulla.

Dissection Follow-up

1. Review the lobes of the brain and the cranial fossae in which they are located.
2. Review the infoldings of the dura mater and their relationships to the cerebral hemispheres and cerebellum.
3. Review the formation of the cerebral arterial circle (circle of Willis).
4. Recall the origins of the internal carotid and vertebral arteries and the route that each takes to enter the cranial cavity.
5. Review the location and name of each of the 12 cranial nerves in sequential order.
6. Preserve the brain in a bath of preservative fluid to prevent desiccation.

CRANIAL FOSSAE

Dissection Overview

The skull base provides support for the weight of the brain (assisted largely by CSF encasing the brain in liquid) and passage for the neurovascular structures passing in and out of the skull. The skull base is subdivided into three cranial fossae, or depressions, with the anterior located most superiorly and the posterior most inferiorly.

The order of dissection will be as follows: The bones of the floor of the cranial cavity will be studied, and the boundaries of the cranial fossae identified. The vessels and nerves of each cranial fossa will be studied.

Skeletal Anatomy

Cranial Base

ATLAS 8.6

On a skull with the calvaria removed, review the following skeletal features.

1. Refer to FIGURE 7.44.
2. Review the location of the three cranial fossae.
3. Within the anterior cranial fossa, identify the **crista galli** and **cribriform plate** of the **ethmoid bone** between the **orbital plates of the frontal bones**.

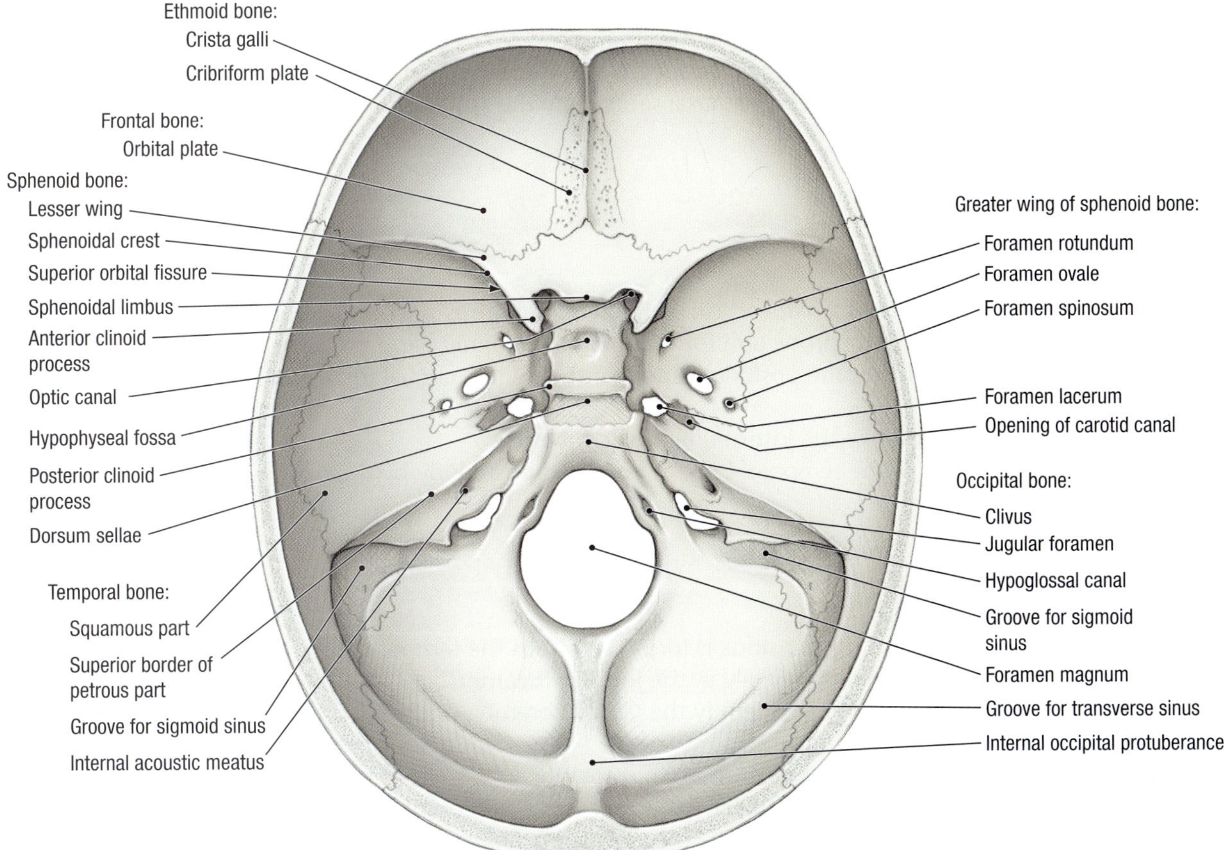

FIGURE 7.44 ● Features of cranial fossae. Superior view.

4. Observe that the **anterior cranial fossa** is separated from the **middle cranial fossa** by the right and left **sphenoidal crests** and **sphenoidal limbus** of the **lesser wing of the sphenoid bone**.
5. Observe that the middle cranial fossa is separated from the **posterior cranial fossa** by the **petrous ridge** of the right and left temporal bones and **dorsum sellae**. *Note that the tentorium cerebelli is attached to the superior border of the petrous part of the temporal bone and forms the roof of the posterior cranial fossa.*

Sphenoid Bone

ATLAS 8.6, 8.11

1. Refer to FIGURE 7.44.
2. Observe that the posterior aspect of the anterior cranial fossa is formed by the **lesser wing of the sphenoid bone**.
3. Identify the **superior orbital fissure** between the lesser wing and **greater wing of the sphenoid**. Pass a wire through the opening and verify that the superior orbital fissure connects the orbit with the cranial cavity.
4. From an anterior perspective through the orbit, identify the smooth round opening of the **optic canal** superior and medial to the superior orbital fissure. Pass a wire through the optic canal and observe that it passes medial to the **anterior clinoid process** within the cranial cavity.
5. In the midline of the sphenoid bone, identify the **hypophyseal fossa (part of the sella turcica)** and recall that this is the location of the pituitary gland.
6. Observe that the hypophyseal fossa is positioned between the two **anterior clinoid processes** anteriorly and the two **posterior clinoid processes** posteriorly.
7. Lateral to the sella turcica, within the floor of the middle cranial fossa, identify the oval-shaped **foramen ovale**.
8. Observe that the foramen ovale is positioned anteromedial to the small round opening of the **foramen spinosum**, the entrance point of the middle meningeal artery. Observe that grooves formed by the middle meningeal artery are visible within the middle cranial fossa emanating from the foramen spinosum.
9. Within the middle cranial fossa anteriorly and medially, identify the **foramen rotundum** inferior to the superior orbital fissure.

10. Identify the **foramen lacerum**, formed by portions of the greater wing of the sphenoid bone and the temporal bone. *Note that in the living individual, the foramen lacerum is covered by cartilage.*
11. Look through the nasal cavity from an anterior perspective and observe that the **body of the sphenoid** is visible. Observe that the sphenoid is connected to the nasal septum by the **sphenoidal crest**, a ridge on the anterior surface of the sphenoid.

Temporal Bone

ATLAS 8.6, 8.10

1. Refer to FIGURE 7.44.
2. Observe that the temporal bone has a flat, vertically oriented **squamous part** and a horizontal, medially oriented **petrous part**, which forms the bony protection for the middle and inner ear.
3. Observe that the petrous part forms the posterior aspect of the middle cranial fossa and the anterior aspect of the posterior cranial fossa.
4. Inferior to the petrous ridge, identify the **internal acoustic meatus**.
5. Observe that the petrous part of the temporal bone is bordered posteriorly by the **groove for the sigmoid sinus**.

Occipital Bone

ATLAS 8.6

1. Refer to FIGURE 7.44.
2. Observe that the **groove for the sigmoid sinus** is formed by both the temporal bone anteriorly and the occipital bone posteriorly and that it terminates medially at the **jugular foramen**.
3. In the center of the posterior cranial fossa, identify the largest foramen of the skull, the **foramen magnum**, which is bound completely by the occipital bone.
4. Within the walls of foramen magnum, identify the **hypoglossal canal** on both the right and left sides.
5. Anterior to the foramen magnum, identify the **clivus**, the smooth portion of the occipital bone posterior to the sella turcica. *Note that the clivus is positioned anterior to the pons of the brainstem.*
6. Follow the groove for the sigmoid sinus laterally and observe that it is continuous with the **groove for the transverse sinus**. Observe that the right and left grooves for the transverse sinuses meet posteriorly at the **internal occipital protuberance**.

Dissection Instructions

Anterior Cranial Fossa

ATLAS 8.6, 8.26; VIDEO 7.12.1

Dissection Note: Because the floor of the cranial cavity is covered by dura mater, the dissection is much easier if a dry skull is held next to the cadaver during dissection to permit direct observation of the foramina.

1. Refer to FIGURE 7.45.
2. On the right side of the cadaver only, use a probe to loosen the dura mater along the cut edge of the frontal bone. Grasp the dura mater and pull it posteriorly as far as the lesser wing of the sphenoid bone.
3. Use scissors to detach the dura mater along the sphenoidal crest and along the midline of the anterior cranial fossa and place it in the tissue container.
4. Observe that the sphenoparietal venous sinus is located along the sphenoidal crest and that its lumen may now be visible where you detached the dura mater.
5. Identify the three bones forming the **anterior cranial fossa**: sphenoid, ethmoid, and frontal.
6. Identify the **crista galli** in the midline of the anterior cranial fossa and recall that before the brain was removed, the falx cerebri was attached here and that the frontal lobe of the brain rested on the orbital part of the frontal bone. *Note that the orbital part of the frontal bone also forms the roof of the orbit.*
7. Identify the openings of the cribriform plate and recall that the **olfactory bulb** arising from the **olfactory tract** rests on the cribriform plate and that the fibers of the **olfactory nerve (CN I)** arising from the bulb pass through these openings to enter the nasal cavity.

Middle Cranial Fossa

ATLAS 8.6, 8.26, 8.30, 8.31; VIDEO 7.12.2

1. Refer to FIGURE 7.45.
2. Identify the **middle cranial fossa** and recall that it contains the temporal lobe of the brain.
3. Observe the dura mater that covers the floor of the middle cranial fossa and hides all of the openings in the skull as well as the nerves and vessels that pass through them.
4. Identify the **middle meningeal artery** visible through the dura mater on the floor of the middle cranial fossa as a dark line extending laterally from the deepest point of the middle cranial fossa.

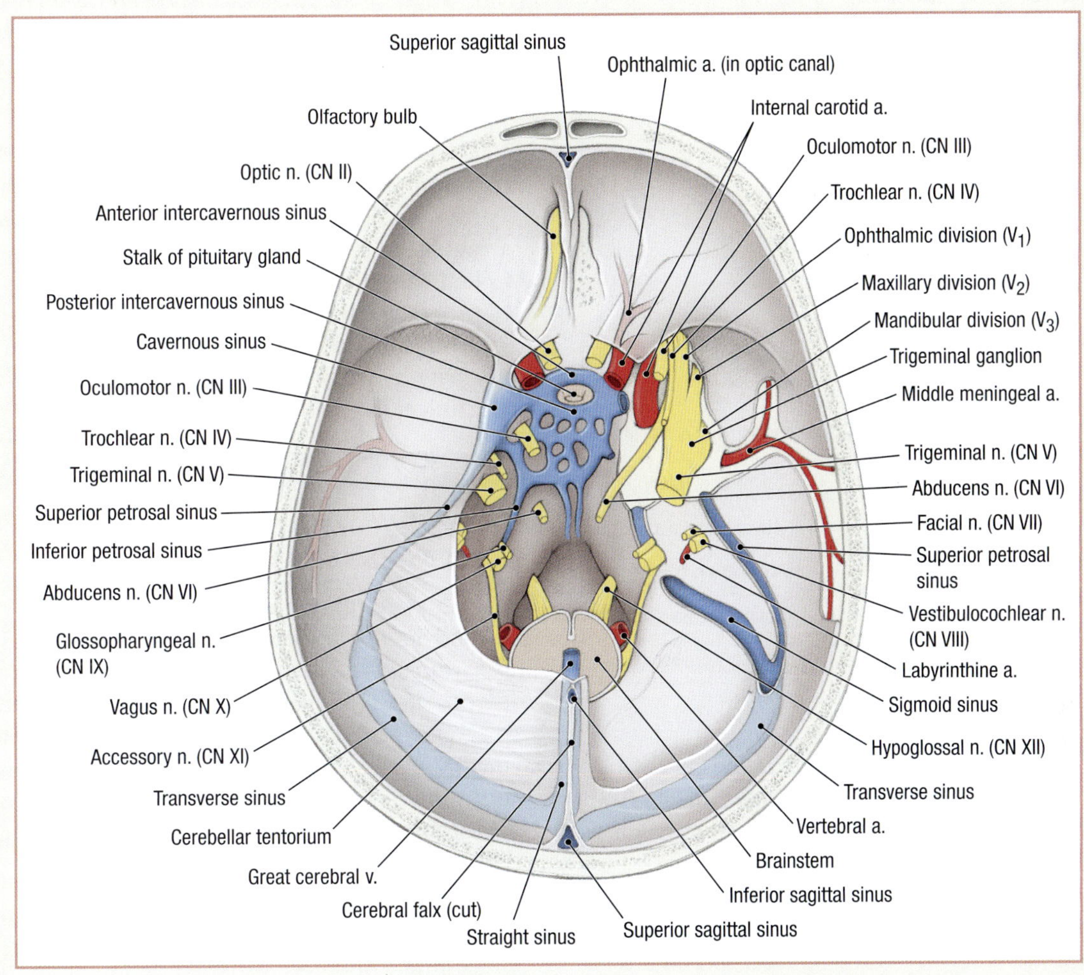

FIGURE 7.45 ■ Cranial nerves and vessels in cranial fossae. Superior view.

5. Grasp the dura mater along the sphenoidal crest and peel it posteriorly as far as the superior border of the petrous part of the temporal bone. Make an effort to not disrupt the nerves lying deep to the dura mater medially or the branches of the middle meningeal artery laterally. Use a probe to tease the proximal part of middle meningeal artery away from the dura mater and leave it in the skull.
6. Clean the middle meningeal artery within the middle cranial fossa and observe that it enters the region by passing through the **foramen spinosum**.
7. Use scissors to detach the dura mater along the superior border of the petrous part of the temporal bone and place it in the tissue container. Pay attention to not cut the cranial nerves that cross the anterior end of the superior border of the petrous part of the temporal bone (oculomotor, trigeminal, trochlear, and abducens).
8. Observe that the lumen of the **superior petrosal sinus** can be seen along the edge of the cut dura mater parallel to the petrous ridge.
9. Identify the two bones forming the floor of the middle cranial fossa: sphenoid and temporal.
10. Identify the **optic nerve (CN II)** passing through the **optic canal** to enter the orbit. *Note that the optic nerve is technically an extension of the brain surrounded by a sleeve of dura mater as it exits the middle cranial fossa and is thus sensitive to intracranial pressure changes.*
11. Use a probe to identify the **superior orbital fissure** inferior to the lesser wing of the sphenoid bone. *Note that three cranial nerves (CN III, CN IV, and CN VI) and part of a fourth cranial nerve (CN V1) exit the middle cranial fossa by passing through the superior orbital fissure.*
12. Refer to FIGURE 7.45 and to FIGURE 7.46.
13. Identify the **oculomotor nerve (CN III)** where it passes over the petrous ridge to pass anteriorly within the lateral wall of the cavernous sinus.
14. Identify the **trochlear nerve (CN IV)** where it courses anteriorly within the lateral wall of the cavernous sinus immediately inferior to the oculomotor nerve. *Note that the trochlear nerve is a very small nerve often found in a sleeve of dura mater at the anterior end of the tentorial notch.*
15. Identify the **abducens nerve (CN VI)** where it enters the dura mater covering the clivus of the occipital bone. Observe that the abducens nerve passes

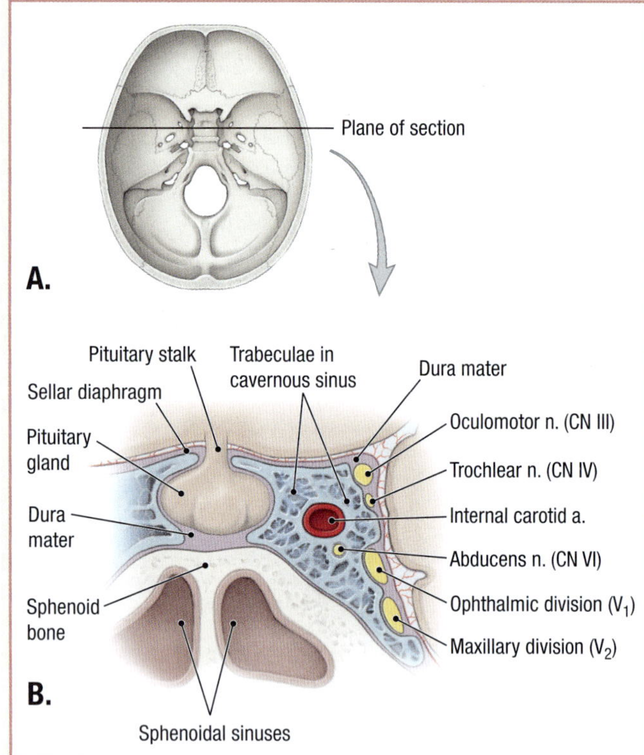

FIGURE 7.46 ● **A.** Plane of section of middle cranial fossa. Superior view. **B.** Coronal section through cavernous sinus. Posterior view.

anteriorly within the cavernous sinus in close relationship to the lateral surface of the internal carotid artery.

16. Identify the **ophthalmic division of the trigeminal nerve (CN V_1)** where it passes through the superior orbital fissure. Observe that the ophthalmic division of the trigeminal nerve arises from the trigeminal ganglion and passes anteriorly along the lateral wall of the cavernous sinus inferior to the trochlear nerve.
17. Use blunt dissection to clean the nerves that pass through the superior orbital fissure.
18. Carefully remove the tightly adhered dura mater overlying the cavernous sinus and identify the three nerves in its lateral wall (CN III, CN IV, and CN V_1) and the one within the space (CN VI).
19. Identify the **trigeminal nerve (CN V)** where it crosses the superior border of the petrous part of the temporal bone.
20. Follow the trigeminal nerve anteriorly and carefully remove the overlying dura mater to identify the **trigeminal (semilunar) ganglion**.
21. Use blunt dissection to define the three divisions (nerves) arising from the anterior border of the trigeminal ganglion (ophthalmic [CN V_1], maxillary [CN V_2], and mandibular [CN V_3]). *Note that the three divisions of the trigeminal nerve are named according to their region of distribution and numbered from superior to inferior.*
22. Identify the **maxillary division of the trigeminal nerve (CN V_2)** and follow it anteriorly to the **foramen rotundum** where it exits the middle cranial fossa. Observe that the maxillary division courses along the lateral wall of the cavernous sinus just inferior to the ophthalmic division of the trigeminal nerve (CN V_1).
23. Identify the **mandibular division of the trigeminal nerve (CN V_3)** and follow it inferiorly to the **foramen ovale** where it exits the middle cranial fossa to enter the infratemporal fossa.
24. Return to the area of the cavernous sinus and use a probe to retract the cranial nerves and identify the **internal carotid artery**, which enters the cranial cavity by passing through the **carotid canal** (see **Clinical Correlation 7.12**).

CLINICAL CORRELATION 7.12

Cranial Base Fracture

ATLAS 8.30, 8.31, 8.34

In fractures of the cranial base of the skull, the internal carotid artery may rupture within the cavernous sinus. As a result of the release of arterial blood into the cavernous sinus, the space dilates and creates an abnormal reflux of blood from the cavernous sinus into the nearby venous structures. Increased ophthalmic venous pressure results in eyeball extrusion (exophthalmos), engorgement of the conjunctiva (chemosis), and possible compression of CN III, CN IV, CN V_1, CN V_2, and CN VI.

25. Observe that the internal carotid artery makes a sagittally oriented S-shaped bend within the cavernous sinus to emerge near the optic nerve. *Note that CN III, CN IV, CN V_1, CN V_2, and CN VI cross the lateral side of the internal carotid artery. Among this group of nerves, the abducens nerve (CN VI) is most closely related to the internal carotid artery.*
26. Identify the region of the **hypophyseal fossa** and observe that it is covered by dural infoldings, the **sellar diaphragm (*diaphragma sellae*)**.
27. Identify the stalk of the pituitary gland passing through an opening in the sellar diaphragm. Recall that the pituitary gland is located in the hypophyseal fossa inferior to the sellar diaphragm.
28. Identify the location of the **anterior** and **posterior intercavernous sinuses**, the two small dural venous sinuses anterior and posterior to the stalk of the pituitary gland. *Note that the intercavernous sinuses connect the right and left cavernous sinuses across the midline.*

Posterior Cranial Fossa

ATLAS 8.6, 8.26, 8.28; VIDEO 7.12.3

Dissection Note: The features of the posterior cranial fossa will be studied with the dura mater intact.

1. Refer back to FIGURE 7.45.
2. Identify the posterior cranial fossa and recall that it contains the cerebellum and brainstem. Observe that

at the foramen magnum, the **brainstem** becomes continuous with the **cervical spinal cord**, which is now visible with the brain removed.

3. Identify the **facial nerve (CN VII)** and **vestibulocochlear nerve (CN VIII)** where they enter the internal acoustic meatus.
4. Identify the **glossopharyngeal nerve (CN IX)**, **vagus nerve (CN X)**, and **accessory nerve (CN XI)** where they enter the jugular foramen.

Dissection Note: Because CN IX and CN X are formed by rootlets, it is difficult to distinguish one nerve from the other as they enter the jugular foramen. However, the cervical root of the accessory nerve can be positively identified because it enters the posterior cranial fossa through the foramen magnum and crosses the inner surface of the occipital bone.

5. Review the course of the transverse and sigmoid sinuses. Observe that the sigmoid sinus ends at the jugular foramen posterior to the exit point of CN IX, CN X, and CN XI.
6. Identify the **hypoglossal nerve (CN XII)** where it enters the **hypoglossal canal.**
7. On the left (undissected) side of the cranial cavity, identify the cranial nerves in order from anterior to posterior.

Dissection Follow-up

1. Review the bones that form the floor of the cranial cavity.
2. In the skull, review the openings through which the cranial nerves pass.
3. In the cadaver, review the course and associated foramina of each cranial nerve.
4. If the brain is still available, review the cranial nerves and severed vessels on its inferior surface.
5. Review the path and pattern of dural venous sinus drainage.
6. Preserve the brain in a bath of preservative fluid to prevent desiccation.
7. Return any reflected tissue back to its anatomical position.
8. Wrap the head with a moist towel or wrapping soaked with embalming fluid or wetting solution to prevent desiccation of the exposed meninges and brain.

ORBIT

Dissection Overview

The orbit is a roughly pyramidal, or cone shaped, bony cavity containing the eyeball and accessory visual structures. The eyeball is about 2.5 cm in diameter and occupies the anterior half of the orbit with the associated mucous membrane, lacrimal apparatus, and eyelids. The posterior half of the orbit contains fat, fascia, muscles, branches of cranial nerves, and blood vessels. Some vessels and nerves pass between the cranial cavity and face through the orbit.

The roof of the orbit is related to the anterior cranial fossa, and the floor of the orbit is related to the maxillary sinus as shown in FIGURE 7.47. The medial wall of the orbit is related to the ethmoid air cells and nasal cavity. The part of the ethmoid bone that forms the medial wall is paper-thin and thus referred to as the lamina papyracea. The lateral wall of the orbit is the thickest and has the largest role in protecting the eye.

The order of dissection will be as follows: The bones of the orbit will be studied. On the right side, the floor of the anterior cranial fossa (roof of the orbit) will be removed, and the orbit dissected from a superior approach. CN III, CN IV, CN V_1, and CN VI will be followed through the superior orbital fissure into the orbit, and the extraocular muscles will be identified. On the left side, the anatomy of the eyelid and lacrimal apparatus will be studied, and the orbit will be dissected from an anterior approach. The eyeball will be removed and the attachments of the extraocular muscles will be studied.

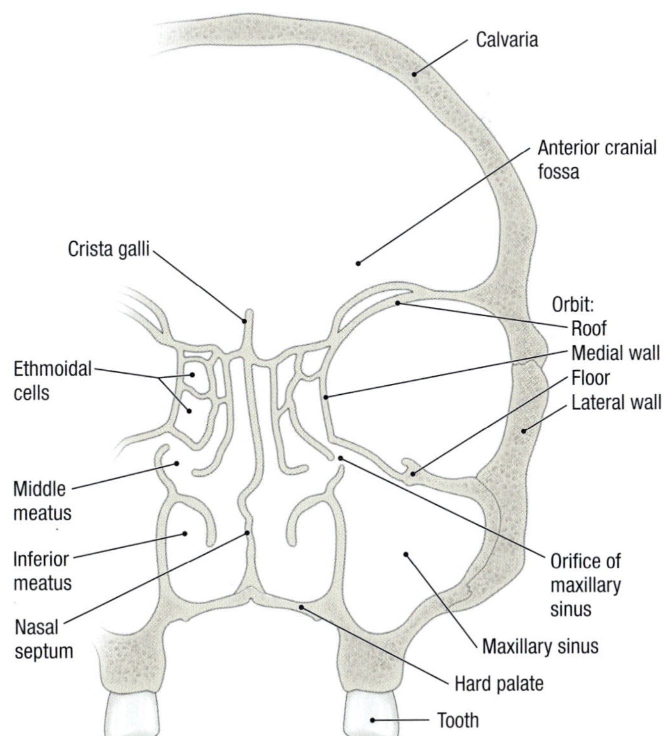

FIGURE 7.47 ● Coronal section of skull. Anterior view.

Skeletal Anatomy

Orbit

ATLAS 8.36A, 8.37A

Refer to a skull and identify the bones that participate in forming the walls of the orbit.

1. Refer to FIGURE 7.48.
2. From an anterior perspective, identify the orbital margin, noting the presence of the **supraorbital notch** along its superior margin.
3. Observe that the bones of the orbit form a four-sided pyramid with the base of the pyramid formed by the **orbital margin** and the apex of the pyramid at the **optic canal** medially.
4. Identify the gap of the **superior orbital fissure** between the **lesser wing** and **greater wing of the sphenoid bone**.
5. Identify the round opening of the **optic canal** superomedial to the superior orbital fissure.
6. Identify the **inferior orbital fissure**, a gap between the maxilla and greater wing of the sphenoid bone.
7. The bones of the orbit are lined with periosteum called **periorbita**, which at the optic canal and superior orbital fissure is continuous with the dura mater of the middle cranial fossa.
8. Observe that when viewed from above, the medial walls of the two orbits are parallel to each other and about 2.5 cm apart and that the lateral walls of the two orbits form an approximate right angle to each other.
9. Identify the **roof of the orbit** formed by the **orbital plate of the frontal bone** and **lesser wing of the sphenoid bone**.
10. Identify the **floor of the orbit** formed by the **maxilla**, **zygomatic bone**, and a small portion of the **palatine bone**.
11. On the floor of the orbit, identify the **infraorbital groove** coursing toward the **infraorbital foramen**.
12. Identify the **medial wall of the orbit** formed by the **orbital plate of the ethmoid bone, lacrimal bone, frontal process of the maxilla**, and a small portion of the **body of the sphenoid**.
13. On the medial wall of the orbit, identify the **anterior** and **posterior ethmoidal foramina**.
14. On the anterior aspect of the medial wall of the orbit, identify the **lacrimal fossa**, a depression between the **anterior** and **posterior lacrimal crests** leading to the **lacrimal canal**, which houses the nasolacrimal duct.
15. Identify the **lateral wall of the orbit** formed by the frontal process of the zygomatic bone and orbital plate of the greater wing of the sphenoid.

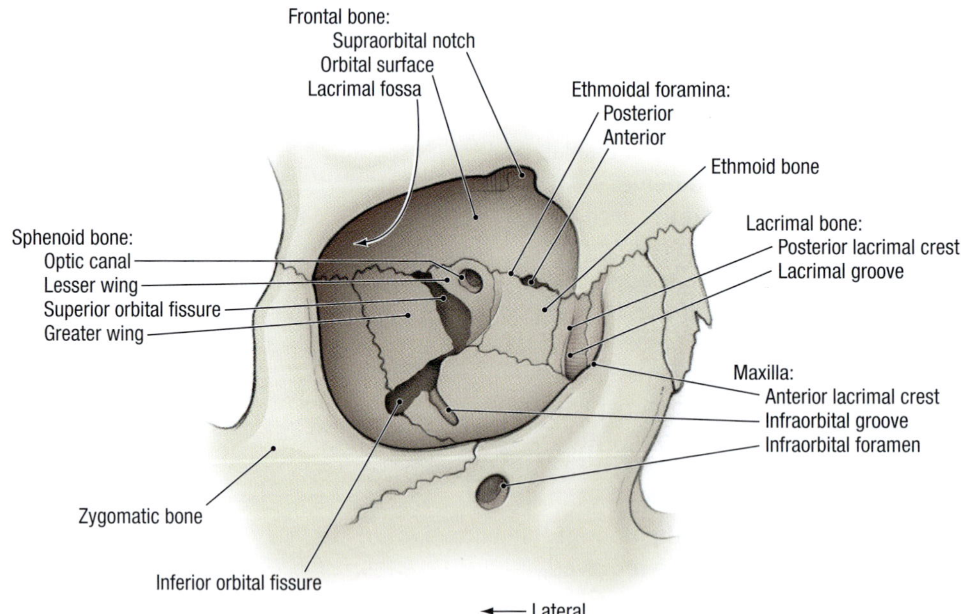

FIGURE 7.48 ● Walls of right orbit. Anterior view.

Surface Anatomy

Eyeball

ATLAS 8.36B, 8.36C, 8.37B

Use a mirror, or recruit the assistance of your lab partner, to inspect the living eye and identify the following features.

1. Refer to FIGURE 7.49.
2. Identify the **palpebral fissure (rima)**, the opening between the eyelids, and observe that it is lined by the **eyelashes (cilia)**.
3. Identify the **medial and lateral palpebral commissures**, the points where the upper and lower eyelids join to form the **medial and lateral angles (canthi)**, or corners of the eye.
4. In the medial angle of the eye, identify the **lacrimal caruncle**, a pink fleshy bump. Observe that fluid accumulates at the **lacrimal lake**, the area surrounding the lacrimal caruncle.
5. On the medial aspect of each eyelid, identify the small bump of the **lacrimal papilla** and observe that each features a small opening at its apex, the **lacrimal puncta**.
6. Identify the **sclera**, the whitish, posterior five-sixths of the fibrous tunic of the eyeball. The sclera is continuous with the **cornea**, the transparent, anterior one-sixth of the fibrous tunic of the eyeball.
7. Identify the **iris**, the colored diaphragm seen through the cornea. Observe that the iris surrounds the **pupil**, the aperture in the center of the eye permitting light to enter the eye.
8. Gently reflect the lower lid slightly and observe that the **margin of the eyelid** is flat and thick and that the **eyelashes (cilia)** are arranged in two or three irregular rows.

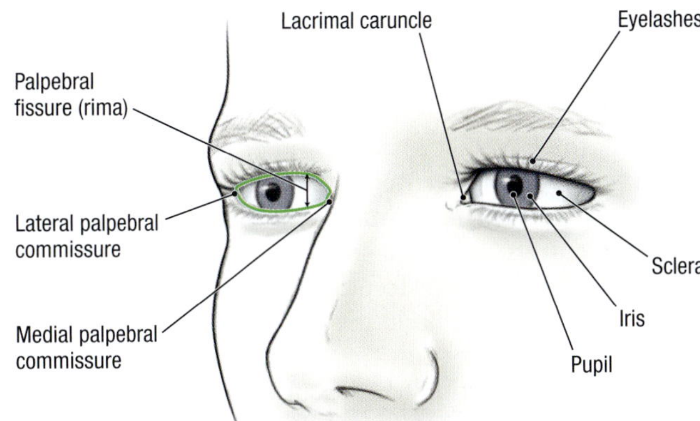

FIGURE 7.49 ● Surface anatomy of eyes and eyelids. Anterolateral view.

Conjunctiva

ATLAS 8.36B, 8.37B, 8.39C

Study the following features on the cadaver and relate them to the living eye.

1. Refer to FIGURE 7.50.
2. Observe that the anterior aspect of the orbit including the eyelids and eyeball are lined by conjunctiva, a specialized, protective mucous membrane.
3. Identify the **bulbar conjunctiva** on the surface of the eyeball and the **palpebral conjunctiva** lining the inner surfaces of the eyelids.
4. Identify the **superior** and **inferior conjunctival fornices**, the recesses where the bulbar conjunctiva reflects as palpebral conjunctiva.
5. Identify the **conjunctival sac**, the space between the eyeball and eyelid surrounded by conjunctiva.

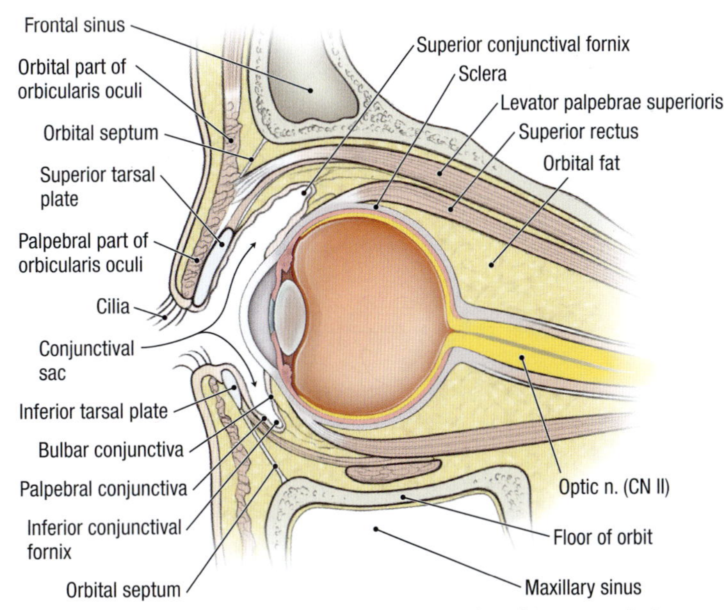

FIGURE 7.50 ● Sagittal section through orbit. Lateral view.

Dissection Instructions

Right Orbit from Superior Approach

ATLAS 8.38A, 8.38C; VIDEO 7.13.2

Dissection Note: Dissect only the right orbit from the superior approach. Wear eye protection for all steps that require the use of bone cutters.

1. Refer to FIGURE 7.51.
2. In the floor of the anterior cranial fossa, tap the **orbital plate of the frontal bone** with the side of the bone cutters, or with a chisel, until the bone cracks (**Cut 1**). Use forceps to pick out the bone fragments.
3. Enlarge the opening in the **roof of the orbit** with the bone cutters (**Cut 2**) and remove the roof of the orbit as far anteriorly as the superior orbital margin.
4. Anteriorly, the **frontal sinus** of the frontal bone may extend into the roof of the orbit. Medially, the **ethmoidal cells** of the ethmoid bone may extend into the roof of the orbit. If either sinus extends into the orbit in your cadaver, use a probe to push the mucous membrane lining the sinuses away from the roof of the orbit and remove the associated layer of thin bone to further expose the orbit (**Cut 3**).
5. Identify the **periorbita,** the periosteal membrane lining the bones of the orbit.
6. Push a probe posteriorly between the roof of the orbit and periorbita. The probe should pass inferior to the **lesser wing of the sphenoid bone** through the **superior orbital fissure** into the middle cranial fossa. Elevate the probe to break the lesser wing of the sphenoid bone.
7. Use bone cutters to remove the fragments of the lesser wing of the sphenoid bone (**Cut 4**).
8. Chip away the roof of the **optic canal** and remove the **anterior clinoid process**.
9. Examine the periorbita and observe that the frontal nerve may be visible through it.
10. Use scissors to incise the periorbita from the apex of the orbit to the midpoint of the superior orbital margin avoiding the frontal nerve.
11. Use forceps to lift the periorbita off deeper structures and make a transverse incision through it close to the superior orbital margin. Use a probe to tease open the flaps of periorbita and use scissors to remove them from the orbit.

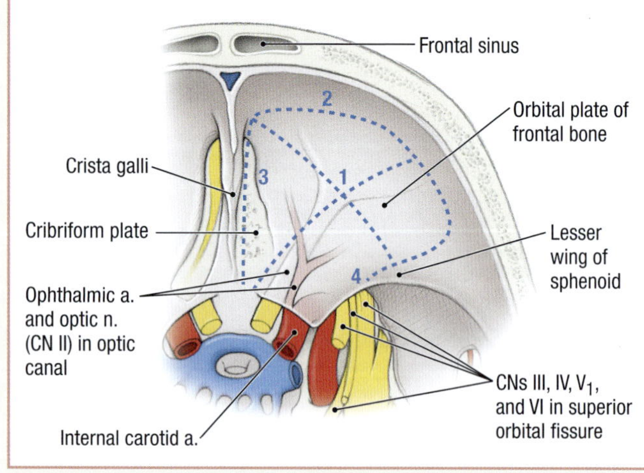

FIGURE 7.51 ■ Superior approach to right orbit. Superior view.

Contents of Orbit

ATLAS 8.38A, 8.38C, 8.44A; VIDEO 7.13.3

Dissection Note: Blunt dissection with a fine probe and forceps is recommended from this point onward in the dissection of the right orbit. Use the forceps to pick out the fat filling the intervals between muscles, nerves, and vessels.

1. Refer to FIGURE 7.52.
2. Observe that branches of three nerves enter the apex of the orbit by passing superior to the extraocular muscles.
3. Identify the **frontal nerve** (a branch of CN V_1) coursing from the apex of the orbit toward the superior orbital margin. Trace the frontal nerve anteriorly and

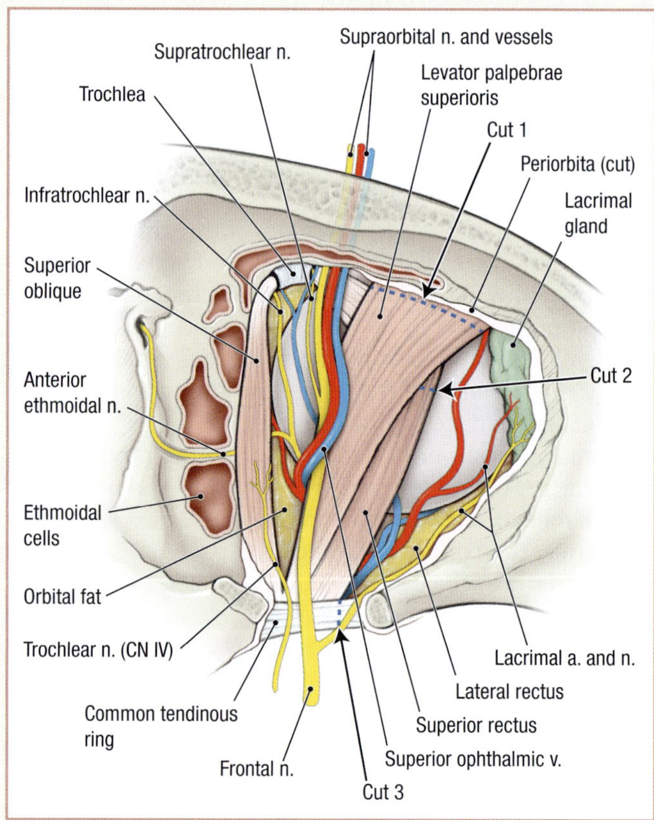

FIGURE 7.52 ■ Superficial dissection of right orbit. Superior view

observe that it divides into the **supratrochlear nerve** and **supraorbital nerve.**

4. On the lateral aspect of the orbit, identify the **lacrimal nerve** (a branch of CN V_1), which passes through the superior orbital fissure lateral to the larger frontal nerve.
5. Follow the lacrimal nerve anterolaterally toward the lacrimal gland.
6. On the medial aspect of the orbit, identify the **trochlear nerve**, which passes through the superior orbital fissure medial to the frontal nerve.
7. Follow the trochlear nerve to the superior border of the **superior oblique**, which it innervates. *Note that the trochlear nerve usually enters the superior border of the superior oblique in its posterior one-third.*
8. While preserving the nerves, use forceps to pick out lobules of fat and expose the superior surface of the **levator palpebrae superioris** attaching to the upper eyelid, which it elevates.
9. Transect the levator palpebrae superioris as far anteriorly as possible (**Cut 1**) and reflect it posteriorly.
10. Identify the **superior rectus** that lies immediately inferior to the levator palpebrae superioris. Clean the superior rectus and observe that it is attached to the eyeball by a thin, broad tendon.
11. Transect the superior rectus close to the eyeball (**Cut 2**) and reflect it posteriorly.
12. Identify the **superior ophthalmic vein** and observe that at the medial angle of the eye, it anastomoses with the angular vein, a tributary of the facial vein (see **Clinical Correlation 7.13**).

CLINICAL CORRELATION 7.13

Cavernous Sinus Thrombosis

ATLAS 8.30B, 8.44B

Anastomoses occur between the facial vein and superior and inferior ophthalmic veins via the angular vein. The venous connections around the orbit are of clinical importance because infections of the upper lip, cheeks, and forehead may spread into the cavernous sinus via the orbit leading to cavernous sinus thrombosis. Thrombosis, a clot in the cavernous sinus, resulting from the facial infection, may lead to involvement of the abducens nerve and dysfunction of the lateral rectus or possible obstruction of the venous drainage of the retina leading to slow painless loss of vision.

13. To increase visibility of the other structures within the orbit, the superior ophthalmic vein may be cut and reflected or removed.
14. On the lateral side of the orbit, identify the **lateral rectus**.

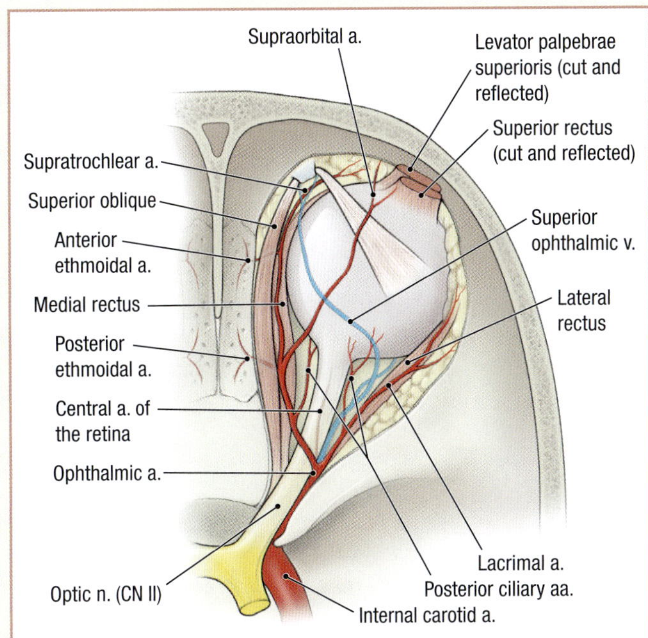

FIGURE 7.53 ● Branches of ophthalmic artery in right orbit. Superior view.

15. Follow the lateral rectus posteriorly and identify the **common tendinous ring**. *Note that the lateral rectus arises by two heads from the common tendinous ring.*
16. Observe that the common tendinous ring surrounds the optic canal and part of the superior orbital fissure and that it is the posterior attachment of the four recti, two of which have now been identified.
17. Cut the common tendinous ring between the attachments of the superior rectus and lateral rectus (**Cut 3**). *Note that the optic nerve (CN II), nasociliary nerve, oculomotor nerve (CN III), and abducens nerve (CN VI) pass through the common tendinous ring.*
18. Refer to FIGURE 7.53.
19. Identify the **ophthalmic artery** where it branches from the internal carotid artery to enter the optic canal.
20. Observe that during its course through the orbit, the ophthalmic artery usually crosses superior to the optic nerve to reach the medial wall of the orbit.
21. Near the medial wall of the orbit, identify the **supraorbital** and **supratrochlear arteries**, the terminal branches of the ophthalmic artery.
22. Use a probe to gently tease out the small **posterior ciliary arteries** supplying the eyeball arising from the ophthalmic artery.
23. On the lateral aspect of the orbit, look for the **lacrimal artery** supplying the **lacrimal gland**.
24. Refer to FIGURE 7.54.
25. Identify the **lacrimal gland** in the anterolateral aspect of the orbit. If necessary, use bone cutters to

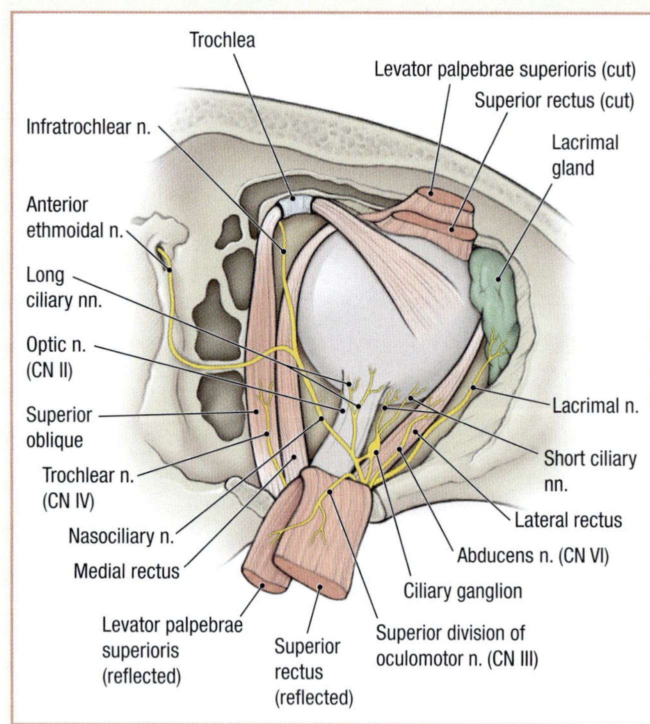

FIGURE 7.54 ● Deep dissection of right orbit. Superior view.

remove additional bone from the orbital plate of the frontal bone to further expose the lacrimal gland.

26. Clean the lateral rectus and identify the **abducens nerve (CN VI)** on its medial surface near the apex of the orbit. Observe that the abducens nerve passes between the two heads of the lateral rectus to enter the muscles medial surface.
27. On the medial side of the orbit, clean the **superior oblique** and trace it anteriorly. Observe that the tendon of the superior oblique passes through the **trochlea**, where it bends at an acute angle to attach to the posterolateral portion of the eyeball.
28. Identify the **medial rectus** inferior to the superior oblique about midway up the height of the eyeball on the medial aspect of the orbit.
29. In the middle cranial fossa, identify the **oculomotor nerve** running along the lateral wall of the cavernous sinus.
30. Follow the oculomotor nerve through the superior orbital fissure into the orbit where it branches into two divisions: the **superior division**, which innervates the levator palpebrae superioris and superior rectus, and the **inferior division**, which innervates the medial rectus, inferior rectus, and inferior oblique. *Note that the inferior rectus and inferior oblique are not easily seen from the superior approach and thus will be identified from the anterior approach.*
31. Review the attachments, actions, and innervations of the extraocular muscles (see **TABLE 7.6**).
32. Identify the **nasociliary nerve,** which is a branch of CN V_1. Observe that the nasociliary nerve courses obliquely through the orbit from lateral to medial and that it is much smaller than the frontal nerve.
33. Identify the large **optic nerve (CN II)** reaching the posterior aspect of the eye at an angle. *Note that the optic "nerve" is actually a brain tract and is thus similarly surrounded by the three meningeal layers: dura mater, arachnoid mater, and pia mater.*
34. Observe that the nasociliary nerve crosses superior to the optic nerve and gives rise to several **long ciliary nerves** supplying the posterior aspect of the eyeball.
35. Follow the nasociliary nerve toward the medial wall of the orbit and identify the **anterior ethmoidal nerve,** which passes through the anterior ethmoidal foramen to supply part of the mucous membrane in the nasal cavity. *Note that the terminal branch of the anterior ethmoidal nerve is the external nasal nerve, which innervates the skin at the apex of the nose.*
36. Identify the **ciliary ganglion,** a small parasympathetic ganglion located between the optic nerve and lateral rectus. Observe that **short ciliary nerves** connect the ciliary ganglion to the posterior surface of the eyeball.

Eyelid and Lacrimal Apparatus

ATLAS 8.37, 8.39A, 8.39E; VIDEO 7.13.1

Perform the following dissection of the eyelid and lacrimal gland only in the left eye.

1. Refer back to FIGURE 7.22 and FIGURE 7.50.
2. Use blunt dissection to raise the lateral part of the **orbital portion of the orbicularis oculi** and reflect the muscle medially.
3. Raise the thin **palpebral portion of the orbicularis oculi** off the underlying **tarsal plates** and reflect it medially.
4. Review the attachments of the **orbicularis oculi** (see **TABLE 7.4**).
5. Refer to FIGURE 7.55.
6. Identify the **orbital septum,** a sheet of connective tissue attached to the tarsal plates and periosteum at the margin of the orbit. *Note that the orbital septum separates the subcutaneous tissue of the face from the contents of the orbit.*
7. Identify the **tarsal plates,** which give shape to the eyelids. Retract the upper eyelid superiorly to see the shape of the **superior tarsal plate** along its posterior surface. Retract the lower eyelid inferiorly to see the shape of the **inferior tarsal plate** along its posterior surface (see **Clinical Correlation 7.14**). *Note that tarsal glands, which secrete an oily substance onto the margin of the eyelid via small orifices posterior to the eyelashes, are embedded in the posterior surface of each tarsal plate.*

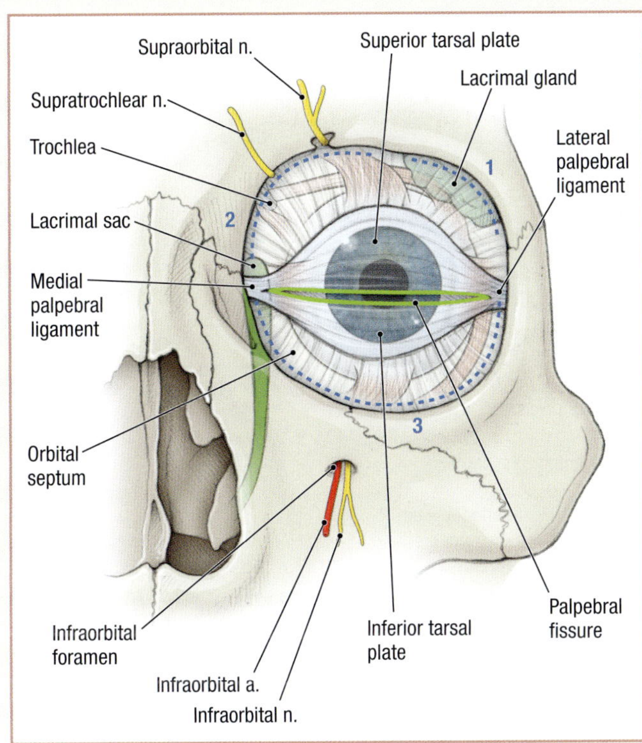

FIGURE 7.55 Orbital septum and tarsal plates of left orbit. Anterior view.

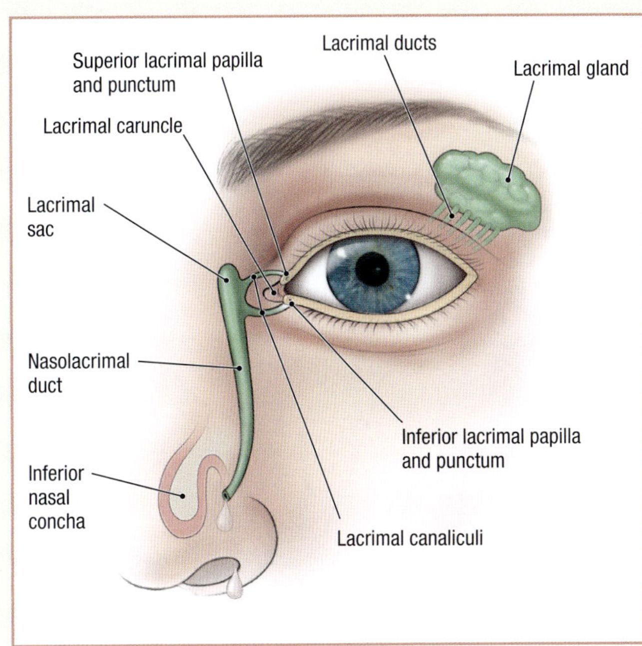

FIGURE 7.56 Components of lacrimal apparatus of left eye. Anterior view.

CLINICAL CORRELATION 7.14

Tarsal Gland Cysts

ATLAS 8.37, 8.39C

If the duct of a tarsal (meibomian) gland becomes obstructed, a chalazion (cyst) may develop deep to the tarsal plate, between the tarsal plate and palpebral conjunctiva. By contrast, if the sebaceous gland associated with a follicle of an eyelash becomes inflamed or obstructed, a hordeolum (stye) may develop superficial to the tarsal plate.

8. Identify the location of the **lacrimal gland** within the lacrimal fossa.
9. To find the lacrimal gland in the cadaver, use a scalpel to carefully cut through the orbital septum adjacent to the orbital margin in the superolateral quadrant of the left orbit (**Cut 1**).
10. Pass a probe through the incision and free the lacrimal gland from the lacrimal fossa. *Note that the lacrimal gland drains into the superior conjunctival fornix by 6 to 10 short ducts.*
11. Use a skull to identify the **lacrimal groove** at the medial side of the orbital margin. Observe that the **anterior lacrimal crest** of the maxilla forms the anterior border of the lacrimal groove. *Note that the medial palpebral ligament is attached to the anterior lacrimal crest and that the lacrimal sac lies posterior to the medial palpebral ligament in the lacrimal groove.*
12. Refer to FIGURE 7.56.
13. Identify the **lacrimal puncta** on the medial aspects of the eyelids, the small openings along the edge of the eyelids. *Note that the lacrimal puncta connect to the two lacrimal canaliculi, which drain lacrimal fluid from the medial angle of the eye into the lacrimal sac. The nasolacrimal duct extends inferiorly from the lacrimal sac to drain into the inferior meatus of the nasal cavity.*
14. Identify the location of the **lacrimal gland** in the superior lateral aspect of the orbit. *Note that lacrimal fluid flows from the lacrimal gland across the eyeball to the medial angle of the eye. During crying, excess lacrimal fluid cannot be emptied through the lacrimal canaliculi and tears overflow the lower eyelids. Increased drainage of tears into the nasal cavity stimulates sniffling, often a characteristic of crying.*

Left Orbit from Anterior Approach

ATLAS 8.37A, 8.39A, 8.41; VIDEO 7.13.4

1. Refer back to FIGURE 7.50 and FIGURE 7.55.
2. Use a probe to explore the **conjunctival sac** via the **palpebral fissure**. Verify that the bulbar conjunctiva is attached to the sclera and is continuous with the palpebral conjunctiva on the inner surface of the eyelids.
3. Use sharp dissection to cut the orbital septum along the periphery of the orbital margin superiorly (**Cut 2**) and inferiorly (**Cut 3**) to remove the orbital septum and attached upper and lower eyelids.
4. Examine the orbit from the anterior view and observe that the **lacrimal gland** is located superolaterally and that the **trochlea** is located superomedially.

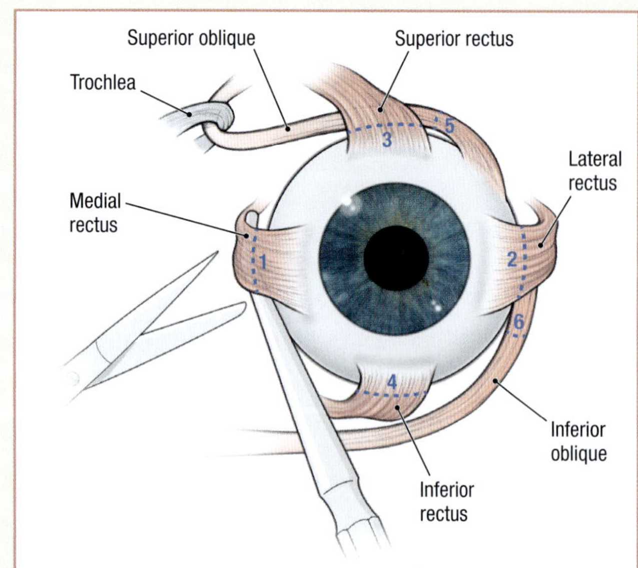

FIGURE 7.57 ● Transection of left extraocular muscles. Anterior view.

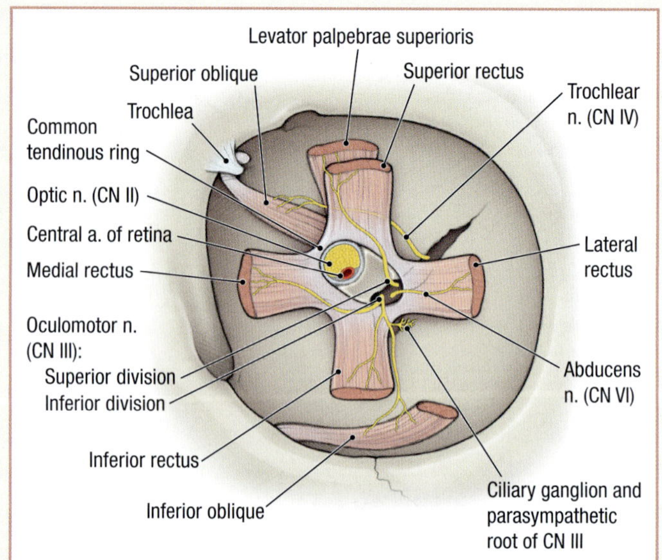

FIGURE 7.58 ● Left orbit with eye removed. Anterior view.

5. Use blunt dissection to remove the visible orbital fat near the orbital margin.
6. Refer to FIGURE 7.57.
7. Use a probe to separate the tendon of the **medial rectus** from the eye and transect it with scissors (**Cut 1**).
8. Use a probe to separate the tendon of the **lateral rectus** from the eye and transect it with scissors (**Cut 2**).
9. Gently depress the eye and use a probe to separate the tendon of the **superior rectus** from the eye and transect it with scissors (**Cut 3**).
10. Gently elevate the eye and use a probe to separate the tendon of the **inferior rectus** from the eye and transect it with scissors (**Cut 4**).
11. Use forceps to grasp the remaining anterior portion of the lateral rectus tendon and pull it anteriorly to adduct the eyeball (turn it medially).
12. Insert scissors into the orbit on the lateral side of the eyeball and transect the optic nerve.
13. Gently elevate the eye and identify the **inferior oblique**, which is attached inferomedially.
14. Pull the eyeball farther anteriorly and transect the superior and inferior oblique tendons near the surface of the eyeball posteriorly (**Cut 5** and **Cut 6**).
15. Remove the eyeball from the orbit.
16. Refer to FIGURE 7.58.
17. Study the enucleated orbit and use forceps to pick out lobules of orbital fat from the posterior portion of the orbit.
18. Trace the four rectus muscles to their attachments on the **common tendinous ring**.
19. From an anterior perspective, identify the structures that pass into the orbit through the common tendinous ring: **optic nerve (CN II)**, **central artery of the retina**, **superior** and **inferior divisions of the oculomotor nerve (CN III)**, **abducens nerve (CN VI)**, and **nasociliary nerve**.
20. From an anterior perspective, identify the structures that pass into the orbit outside the common tendinous ring: **superior** and **inferior ophthalmic veins**, **frontal nerve**, **lacrimal nerve**, and **trochlear nerve (CN IV)**.
21. Trace the motor nerve branches from their point of entrance into the orbit to their respective target extraocular muscles.
22. Examine the cut surface of the optic nerve and try to identify the **central artery of the retina**, which may be seen as a dark spot on the cut surface.
23. Refer to FIGURE 7.59.
24. If the removed eyeball is in dissectible condition, use a new scalpel blade to cut it in half in the coronal plane.
25. Observe that the **lens** separates the anterior and posterior chambers of the eye. *Note that the lens may be replaced by a prosthetic implant in some cadavers.*
26. Remove the **vitreous body** from the posteriorly located **vitreous chamber**.
27. Observe that the eye is composed of three layers or tunics. Identify the **fibrous (outer) layer** composed of the **sclera** (posterior five-sixths) and **cornea** (anterior one-sixth).
28. Identify the **choroid**, **ciliary body**, and **iris** comprising the **vascular (middle) layer**.
29. Use a probe to gently move the partially detached **retina**, which forms the **nervous (inner) layer**.
30. Observe that the retina is attached posteriorly near the **optic disc (blind spot)** where the optic nerve and retinal vessels enter or leave.
31. In well-preserved specimens, along the posterior aspect of the retina, it may be possible to identify the **macula**, the highest center for visual acuity in humans.
32. When you have finished your study of the explanted eye, place it in the tissue container.

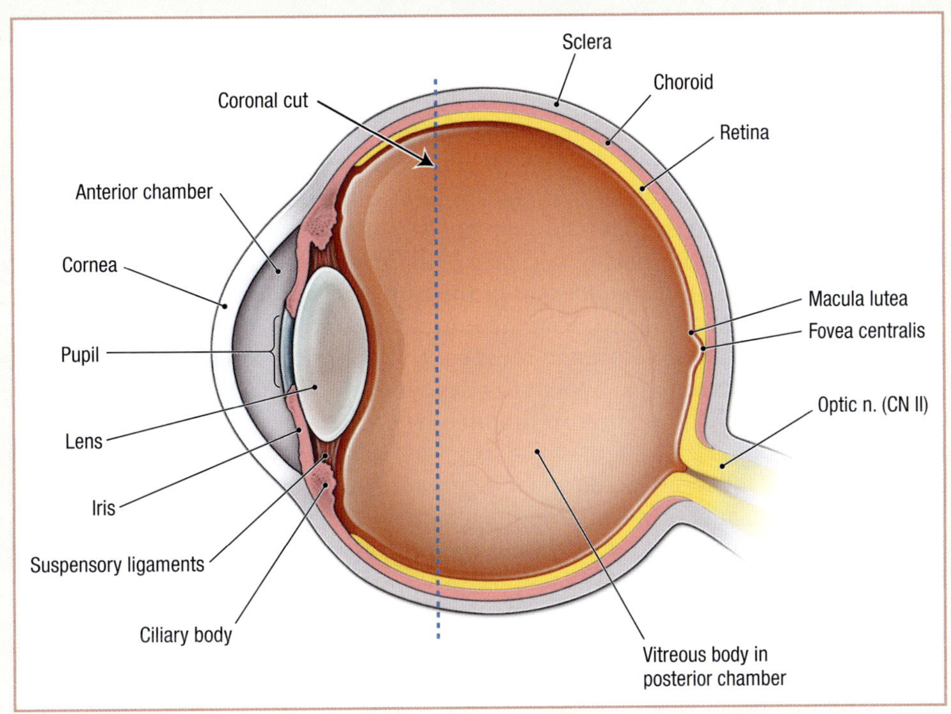

FIGURE 7.59 Transverse section through right eye. Superior view.

Dissection Follow-up

1. Use a skull to review the bones forming the margin, walls, and openings of the orbit.
2. Examine the middle cranial fossa and review the structures passing through the optic canal and superior orbital fissure.
3. Review the path of the nerves innervating the extraocular muscles within the cavernous sinus and their relationship to the common tendinous ring as they pass through the superior orbital fissure to reach the apex of the orbit.
4. Review the origin and course of the central artery of the retina and ophthalmic artery.
5. Review the attachments, actions, and innervations of the six extraocular muscles and levator palpebrae superioris in **TABLE 7.6**.
6. Review the location of the ciliary ganglion and describe the origin of its presynaptic parasympathetic axons, the course of its postsynaptic axons to the eyeball, and the functions of the two smooth muscles it innervates.
7. Return the reflected portions of the tissue back to their anatomical position.

TABLE 7.6 **Extraocular Muscles**

Muscle	*Anterior Attachments*	*Posterior Attachments*	*Actions*	*Innervation*
Levator palpebrae superioris	Tarsal plate of upper eyelid	Sphenoid bone	Elevation and retraction of upper eyelid	Superior division of oculomotor n. (CN III)
Superior rectus	Sclera (anterior, superior surface)	Common tendinous ring	Elevation and adduction of eye	
Superior oblique	Sclera (posterior, lateral, superior surface)	Sphenoid bone	Depression, intorsion, and abduction of eye	Trochlear n. (CN IV)
Lateral rectus	Sclera (anterior, lateral surface)	Common tendinous ring	Abduction of eye	Abducens n. (CN VI)
Medial rectus	Sclera (anterior, medial surface)		Adduction of eye	Inferior division of oculomotor n. (CN III)
Inferior rectus	Sclera (posterior, lateral, inferior surface)		Depression and adduction of eye	
Inferior oblique	Sclera (anterior, inferior surface)	Maxilla	Elevation, extorsion, and abduction of eye	

Note that the above actions are referenced from a neutral position of the eye.
Abbreviations: CN, cranial nerve; n., nerve.

DISARTICULATION OF HEAD

Dissection Overview

It is not possible to fully study the anatomical structures and relationships of the pharynx or nasal cavity without proper exposure through either bisection or disarticulation. As these techniques may feel particularly invasive to the donor, a moment of consideration for how to maintain proper care and respect, as well as thanking the donor, is once again suggested. It is also recommended that prior to beginning the disarticulation or bisection of the head, time be taken to discuss with your instructor and dissection team the appropriateness or necessity of these techniques for your course of study.

The cervical viscera are located within the anterior part of the neck and surrounded by pretracheal fascia. The retropharyngeal space separates the buccopharyngeal fascia, the posterior aspect of pretracheal fascia, from the prevertebral fascia surrounding the vertebral column and associated muscles. The alar fascia subdivides the retropharyngeal space to create a potential space for spread of infection known as the danger space. To study the cervical viscera from a posterior approach and clearly see the muscles and structures surrounded by prevertebral fascia, the head must be disarticulated or detached from the vertebral column.

The order of dissection will be as follows: The retropharyngeal space will be opened from the base of the skull superiorly to the superior thoracic aperture inferiorly. A wedge-shaped cut will be made in the occipital bone to facilitate disarticulation. The anterior aspect of the head will be reflected anteriorly off the vertebral column while remaining attached to the cervical viscera.

Skeletal Anatomy

Suboccipital Region

ATLAS 1.7A, 1.9, 1.11C, 8.5

Refer to an articulated skeleton and identify the following.

1. Refer to FIGURE 7.60.
2. Observe that the **atlas** (C1) does not have a body but that the **axis** (C2) has the **dens (odontoid process)**, the remnant of the body of C1 that fused to C2 during development.
3. On the atlas, identify the **anterior arch** and **anterior tubercle** at its midpoint anteriorly. *Note that the transverse ligament of the atlas holds the dens to the anterior arch of the atlas to provide stability.*
4. On the atlas, identify the **posterior arch** and **posterior tubercle** at its midpoint posteriorly, observing that the atlas does not have a spinous process.
5. On the superior aspect of the atlas bilaterally, identify the horizontally orientated **superior articular facets**.
6. On an articulated skeleton, observe that the articulation between the superior articular surface of the atlas and the **occipital condyles** at the base of the skull creates the **atlantooccipital joint**, which allows nodding movement or the "yes" type of motion, between the head and neck.
7. On the superior aspect of the axis bilaterally, identify the **superior articular facets**, which articulate with the **atlas**.
8. On an articulated skeleton, observe that the articulation between the atlas and axis creates the **atlantoaxial joint**, which allows rotational movement or the "no" type of motion, between the head and neck.
9. Refer to FIGURE 7.61.
10. From an inferior view, identify the **basilar part of the occipital bone** and the small, roughened area of the **pharyngeal tubercle** anterior to the **foramen magnum**. Recall that the foramen magnum allowed

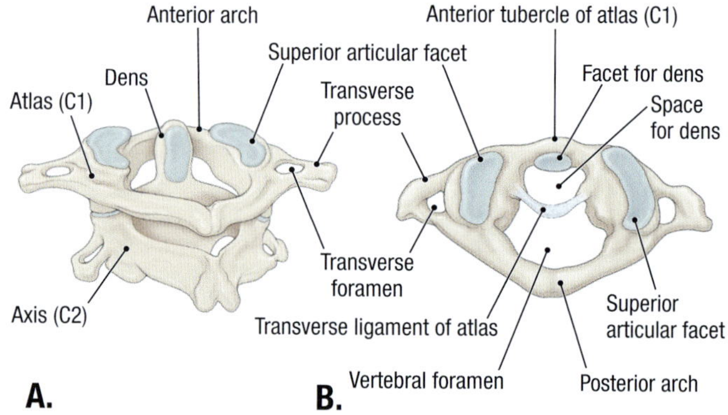

FIGURE 7.60 ● Skeleton and ligaments of atlantoaxial joint. **A.** Posterolateral view. **B.** Superior view.

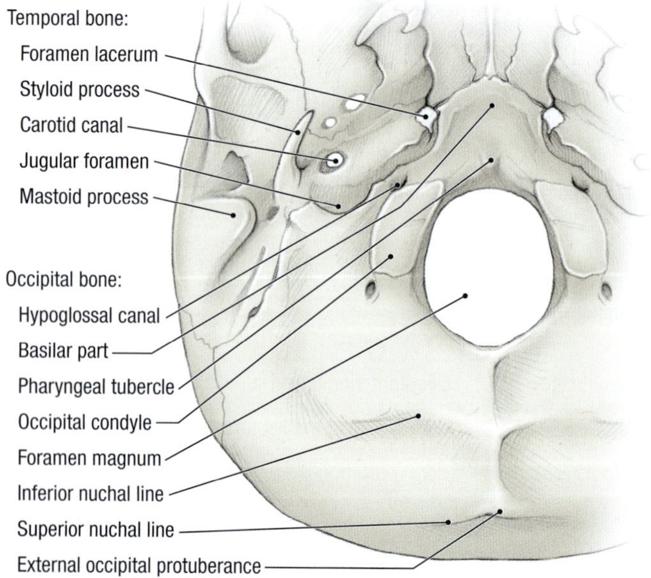

FIGURE 7.61 ● Temporal and occipital bones. Inferior view.

passage of the spinal cord, vertebral arteries (left and right), and cervical roots of the accessory nerves (left and right).

11. Identify the **hypoglossal canal** in the wall of foramen magnum and observe that the canal courses in the occipital bone superior to the **occipital condyle**.
12. Identify the **external occipital protuberance** in the posterior aspect of the skull as well as the horizontally oriented **superior** and **inferior nuchal lines**.
13. Identify the **jugular foramen** and observe that it is partially formed by the more anteriorly located temporal bone and more posteriorly located occipital bone. Recall that the glossopharyngeal nerve (CN IX), vagus nerve (CN X), accessory nerve (CN XI), and the internal jugular vein pass through the jugular foramen.
14. Identify the opening of the **carotid canal** medial to the **styloid process** and anterior to the jugular foramen.
15. Identify the **foramen lacerum** at the medial aspect of the carotid canal and recall that this opening is covered with cartilage in the living individual.
16. Identify the **mastoid process** and recall that this large prominence is the superior attachment of the SCM and posterior belly of digastric.

Dissection Instructions

Retropharyngeal Space

ATLAS 7.2, 7.21; VIDEO 7.14.1

1. Refer to FIGURE 7.62.
2. Place the body in a supine position.
3. Return to the cervical region and bilaterally gather the ends of the cutaneous branches of the cervical plexus (transverse cervical, great auricular, lesser occipital) and reflect them posteriorly so they remain attached to the cervical anterior rami near the vertebral column.
4. If not done previously, clean the anterior and posterior borders of the SCM to its superior attachment at the mastoid process bilaterally.
5. Reflect each SCM superiorly, taking care to preserve the accessory nerve on its deep surface.
6. Use blunt dissection to create a gap posterior to the contents of the right and left **carotid sheaths** to enter the **retropharyngeal (retrovisceral) space,** staying posterior to the **alar fascia** in the subdivision of the **danger space**.
7. Push your fingers medially through the newly created gap anterior to the scalenes and prevertebral muscles until they touch in the midline.
8. Use blunt dissection to enlarge the separation between the viscera and pretracheal fascia anteriorly and the vertebral column and prevertebral fascia posteriorly.
9. Place a probe in the retropharyngeal space posterior to the contents of the carotid sheaths so it passes

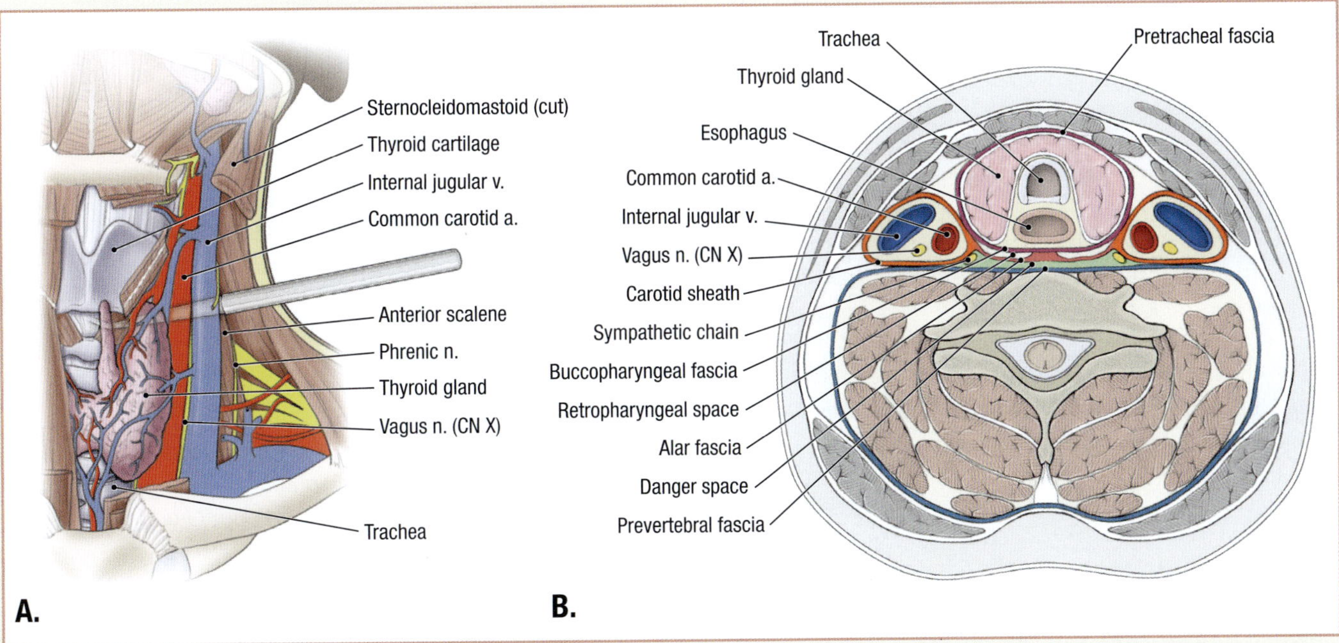

FIGURE 7.62 ● **A.** Insertion of probe into retropharyngeal space. Anterior view. **B.** Transverse section through retropharyngeal space. Inferior view.

completely across the neck within the retropharyngeal space.

10. Leave the probe traversing the neck and use your fingers or another blunt instrument to confirm that the retropharyngeal space extends superiorly all the way up to the base of the skull.
11. Use your fingers or another blunt instrument to confirm that the retropharyngeal space extends inferiorly into the mediastinum of the thorax. *Note that an infection may spread from the head to the thorax within the danger space.*

Disarticulation of Head

ATLAS 7.23, 7.28, 8.6A; VIDEO 7.14.2

Dissection Note: The head will be separated from the vertebral column at the atlantooccipital joint after making a wedge-shaped cut in the occipital bone.

1. Refer to FIGURE 7.63.
2. With the cadaver in the supine position, rotate the head until you can identify the accessory nerve and structures that exit the jugular foramina at the base of the skull bilaterally as you will keep them attached to the head during reflection.
3. Use a saw to make two oblique cuts through the occipital bone in the posterior cranial fossa parallel to the petrous ridge on each side (**Cut 1** and **Cut 2**). Internally, the saw cuts should be posterior to the jugular foramina, in order to preserve the structures passing through it, and posterior to the hypoglossal canals at the foramen magnum. Externally, the saw cuts should pass posterior to the mastoid process of the temporal bone so the attachments of the SCMs remain intact.

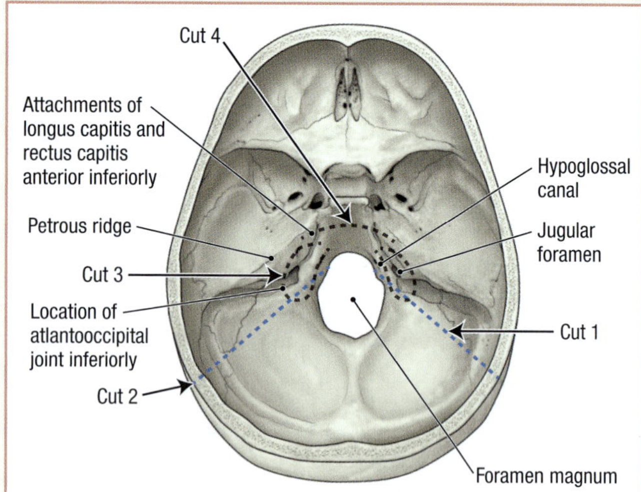

FIGURE 7.63 ● Cuts for head disarticulation. Superior view.

4. Slide a thin chisel from lateral to medial along the base of the skull adjacent to the atlantooccipital joint to widen the space at the base of the skull.
5. Use a scalpel to cut through the atlantooccipital joint capsules bilaterally (**Cut 3**).
6. Use the chisel to separate the articular surfaces of the atlantooccipital joints. *Note that if the joint is difficult to access from the supine position, the cadaver may be rotated to the prone position.*
7. Push the head anteriorly and insert a scalpel into the most superior part of the retropharyngeal space to cut the adhered soft tissues of the longus capitis, rectus capitis anterior, and anterior atlanto-occipital membrane to free the head for reflection (**Cut 4**).
8. Gently continue to force the head forward until it is freed from C1. *Note that if performed correctly, the head remains attached to the pharynx.*
9. With the head fully detached, but not yet reflected, identify the **sympathetic trunk** and **superior cervical sympathetic ganglion** on the anterior surface of the cervical vertebral column.
10. Reflect the right sympathetic trunk and superior cervical ganglion with the head, cervical viscera, and associated neurovascular structures anteriorly until the chin rests on the thorax.
11. On the left side, leave the left sympathetic trunk and associated cervical ganglion with the vertebral column and associated muscles structures posteriorly.
12. Inspect the reflected base of the skull from the posterior perspective and look for the structures associated with the jugular foramen and hypoglossal canal.

Prevertebral and Lateral Vertebral Regions

ATLAS 7.23, 7.24; VIDEO 7.14.3

1. Refer to FIGURE 7.64.
2. Identify the **prevertebral fascia** on the anterior surface of the cervical vertebral column.
3. Observe that prevertebral fascia covers the prevertebral (**longus colli** and **longus capitis**) and lateral vertebral (**anterior, middle,** and **posterior scalenes**) groups of muscles.
4. On the left side of the cervical vertebral column, identify the **superior, middle,** and **inferior cervical sympathetic ganglia** of the **sympathetic trunk.** *Note that frequently, the inferior cervical ganglion is connected with the first thoracic ganglion as the cervicothoracic (stellate) ganglion.*
5. Identify the **gray rami communicantes** connecting the sympathetic ganglia with the anterior rami of the cervical spinal nerves.

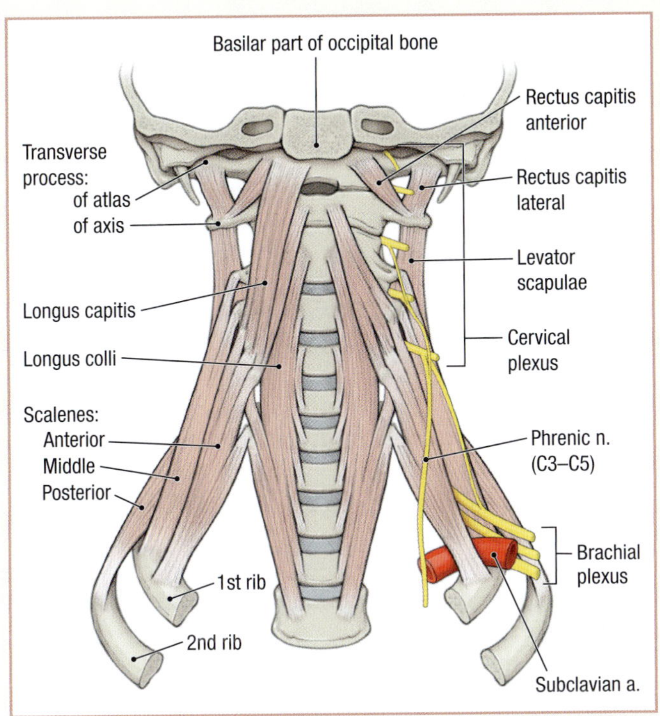

FIGURE 7.64 ● Prevertebral muscles. Anterior view.

6. Identify the roots of the brachial plexus made by the anterior rami of spinal nerves C5–T1, emerging between the anterior and middle scalenes.
7. At the base of the neck, follow the right and left vertebral arteries into the transverse foramina of vertebra C6, observing that as the vertebral artery ascends within the neck, it is well protected within the transverse foramina.
8. Superiorly, at the cut edge of the C1 vertebra, identify where the vertebral artery emerges from the transverse foramen of the atlas (C1). Recall that the right and left vertebral arteries ascend into the skull through foramen magnum prior to forming the basilar artery.
9. At the base of the skull, make an effort to identify the **rectus capitis anterior** and **lateralis**. *Note that during the disarticulation of the head, the rectus capitis anterior and lateralis may have been damaged.*

Dissection Follow-up

1. Use a skull to review the anatomy of the occipital bone.
2. Review the structures that pass through the foramen magnum, hypoglossal canal, and jugular foramen.
3. Review the course of the sympathetic trunk from the upper thorax to the base of the skull.
4. Review the origin and relationships of the roots of the brachial plexus to the scalenes.
5. Return the disarticulated head and attached structures of the neck back to their anatomical position.

PHARYNX

Dissection Overview

The pharynx extends from the base of the skull to the inferior border of the cricoid cartilage (vertebral level C6) where it is continuous with the esophagus. The pharynx can be subdivided from superior to inferior as the nasopharynx, oropharynx, and laryngopharynx. The nasopharynx communicates with the nasal cavity and serves as the primary pathway for air during respiration. The oropharynx receives air from the nasopharynx and food, liquids, and air from the oral cavity playing a key role in swallowing. The laryngopharynx is the point of separation for ingested food and liquids into the posteriorly located esophagus and air into the larynx anteriorly.

The pharyngeal wall consists of three layers. The outermost layer is composed of buccopharyngeal fascia, the adventitia of the pharynx, which is continuous with the connective tissue covering the buccinator. The middle layer is a muscular layer composed of an outer circular part and an inner longitudinal part. The innermost layer is composed of a mucous membrane with a thick submucosa that contributes to the pharyngobasilar fascia.

The order of dissection will be as follows: The external surface of the pharynx will be dissected from the posterior direction. The pharyngeal plexus of nerves will be identified, and the borders of the pharyngeal constrictors defined. The stylopharyngeus and glossopharyngeal nerve will be identified. The contents of the carotid sheath will be examined, and CN IX, CN X, CN XI, and CN XII will be followed from the base of the skull to their respective regions of distribution. The sympathetic trunk will be studied.

Dissection Instructions

Muscles of Pharyngeal Wall

ATLAS 7.27, 7.28, 7.29; VIDEO 7.15.1

Dissection Note: For the following dissection sequence, preserve the surrounding neurovascular structures and simply identify the muscles at this time.

1. Refer to FIGURE 7.65.
2. With the cadaver in the supine position, reflect the disarticulated head anteriorly and place the chin on the thorax to expose the pharynx along its posterior surface.
3. Palpate the tip of the **greater horn of the hyoid bone** and **posterior aspect of the thyroid cartilage**.
4. On the posterior aspect of the muscular pharynx, identify the **buccopharyngeal fascia**. As each muscle is identified in the following dissection steps, remove the **buccopharyngeal fascia** from the posterior surface of the muscle, sparing the neurovascular structures in the region.
5. In the midline of the posterior pharynx, identify the **pharyngeal raphe**, the posterior attachment of the three pharyngeal constrictors to their respective pair.
6. Beginning inferiorly on the posterior aspect of the pharynx at the height of the thyroid cartilage, identify the **inferior pharyngeal constrictor**.
7. The inferior pharyngeal constrictor can be subdivided into the more superiorly located **thyropharyngeus** and the more inferiorly located **cricopharyngeus** based on the anterior attachments of the fibers.
8. Observe that the fibers of the **cricopharyngeus** are continuous with the circular muscle fibers of the esophagus.
9. Identify the **middle pharyngeal constrictor** at the height of the greater horn of the hyoid bone and observe that it lies deep to the inferior pharyngeal constrictor.
10. Superior to the middle pharyngeal constrictor, identify the **superior pharyngeal constrictor.**
11. Observe that the inferior part of the superior pharyngeal constrictor lies deep to the middle pharyngeal constrictor.
12. Clear the buccopharyngeal fascia from the posterior surface of the pharyngeal constrictors near the midline.
13. Review the attachments and actions of the pharyngeal constrictors (see **TABLE 7.7**).
14. Use blunt dissection to define the superior border of the superior pharyngeal constrictor and identify the **pharyngobasilar fascia**, the dense connective tissue membrane attaching the superior edge of the superior constrictor to the base of the skull.

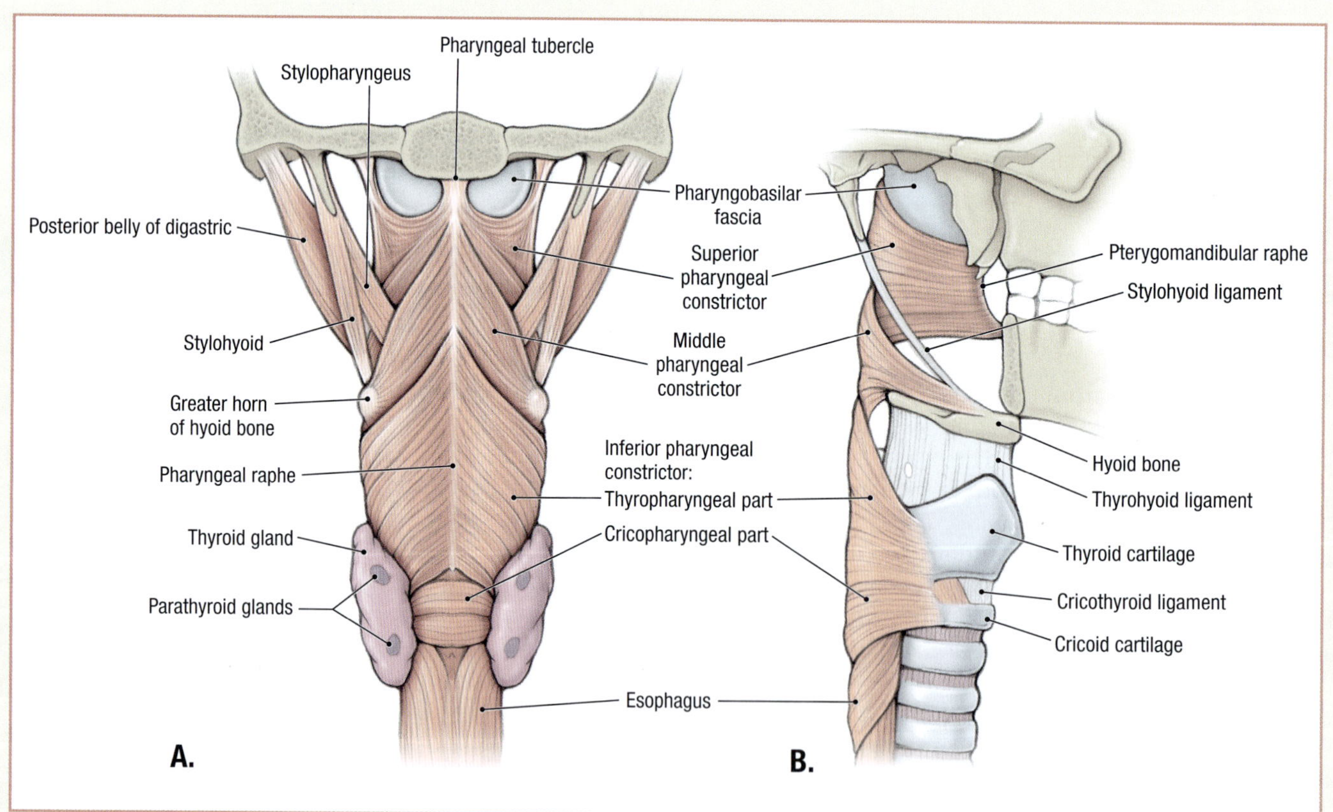

FIGURE 7.65 ● Muscles of pharynx. **A.** Posterior view. **B.** Right lateral view.

15. Identify the **stylopharyngeus** on the lateral aspects of the pharynx approximately one finger's width above the greater horn of the hyoid bone.
16. Follow the stylopharyngeus superiorly and palpate its attachment to the medial surface of the styloid process and inferiorly to the point where it pierces the pharynx. Observe that the stylopharyngeus enters the pharyngeal wall by passing between the superior and middle pharyngeal constrictors.
17. Review the attachments and actions the stylopharyngeus (see **TABLE 7.7**).

Nerves of Pharynx

ATLAS 7.27, 7.28, 7.29B, 7.31A; VIDEO 7.15.2

1. Refer to FIGURE 7.66.
2. Use blunt dissection to clean the posterior and lateral surfaces of the stylopharyngeus and identify the **glossopharyngeal nerve (CN IX)**. Observe that the glossopharyngeal nerve crosses the posterior and lateral surfaces of the stylopharyngeus to enter the pharynx.
3. Identify the **pharyngeal plexus of nerves** on the posterolateral aspect of the pharynx. *Note that the pharyngeal plexus receives branches from the glossopharyngeal nerve (sensory to the pharyngeal mucosa), vagus nerve (motor to the pharyngeal constrictors), and superior cervical sympathetic ganglion (vasomotor).*
4. Identify the **contents of the carotid sheath** from the posterior view.
5. Follow the internal carotid artery superiorly as far as possible and observe that it lies medial to the internal jugular vein.
6. Identify the glossopharyngeal nerve (CN IX), vagus nerve (CN X), and accessory nerve (CN XI) where they exit the jugular foramen medial to the internal jugular vein.
7. Follow the **glossopharyngeal nerve (CN IX)** inferiorly and observe that it passes between the internal and external carotid arteries as it approaches the stylopharyngeus.
8. Follow the **vagus nerve (CN X)** inferiorly to the thorax and observe that it lies posterior to the internal carotid artery and internal jugular vein in the carotid sheath.
9. Identify the **superior laryngeal nerve** arising from the vagus nerve about 2.5 cm inferior to the base of the skull. Trace the branches of the superior laryngeal nerve to the larynx.

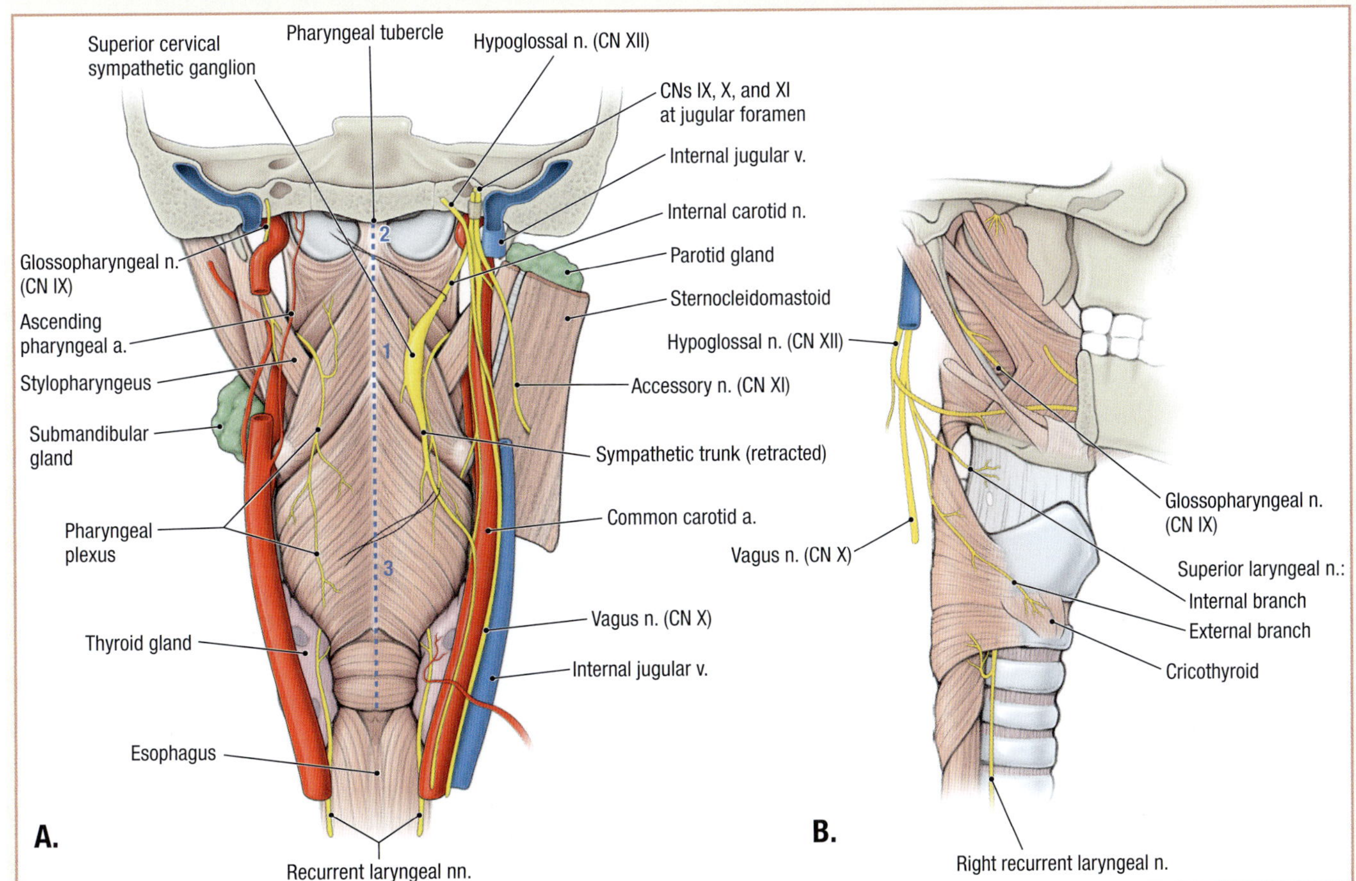

FIGURE 7.66 ■ Nerves and vessels of pharyngeal wall. **A.** Posterior view. **B.** Right lateral view.

10. Identify the **pharyngeal branch of the vagus nerve** arising near the base of the skull and follow it to the pharyngeal plexus.
11. Identify the **accessory nerve (CN XI)**, which usually passes between the internal jugular vein and internal carotid artery to reach the deep surface of the SCM.
12. Identify the **hypoglossal nerve (CN XII)** in the submandibular triangle and follow it posteriorly and superiorly as far as the base of the skull. Observe that the hypoglossal nerve passes lateral to the internal and external carotid arteries but medial to the internal jugular vein.
13. On the right side of the cadaver, verify that the **superior cervical sympathetic ganglion** and **sympathetic trunk** are posterior and medial to the carotid sheath.
14. Use a scalpel to make a small incision through the posterior wall of the pharynx in the midline at the approximate level of the oral cavity (**Cut 1**).
15. Use scissors to extend the incision superiorly through the pharyngeal raphe up to the pharyngeal tubercle at the base of the skull (**Cut 2**) and inferiorly through the inferior pharyngeal constrictor to a point just superior to the esophagus (**Cut 3**).

Opening of Pharynx

ATLAS 7.29; VIDEO 7.15.3

1. Refer to FIGURE 7.67.
2. Spread the cut edges of the pharynx and observe that the lumen of the pharynx communicates anteriorly with three cavities: nasal cavity, oral cavity, and larynx.
3. Identify the parts of the pharynx: **nasopharynx**, **oropharynx**, and **laryngopharynx**.
4. In the nasopharynx, identify the **posterior nasal apertures** on either side of the **nasal septum** superior to the **soft palate.**
5. In the oropharynx, identify the **uvula**, **base of the tongue**, **epiglottic valleculae**, and **epiglottis.**
6. In the laryngopharynx, identify the **laryngeal inlet.**

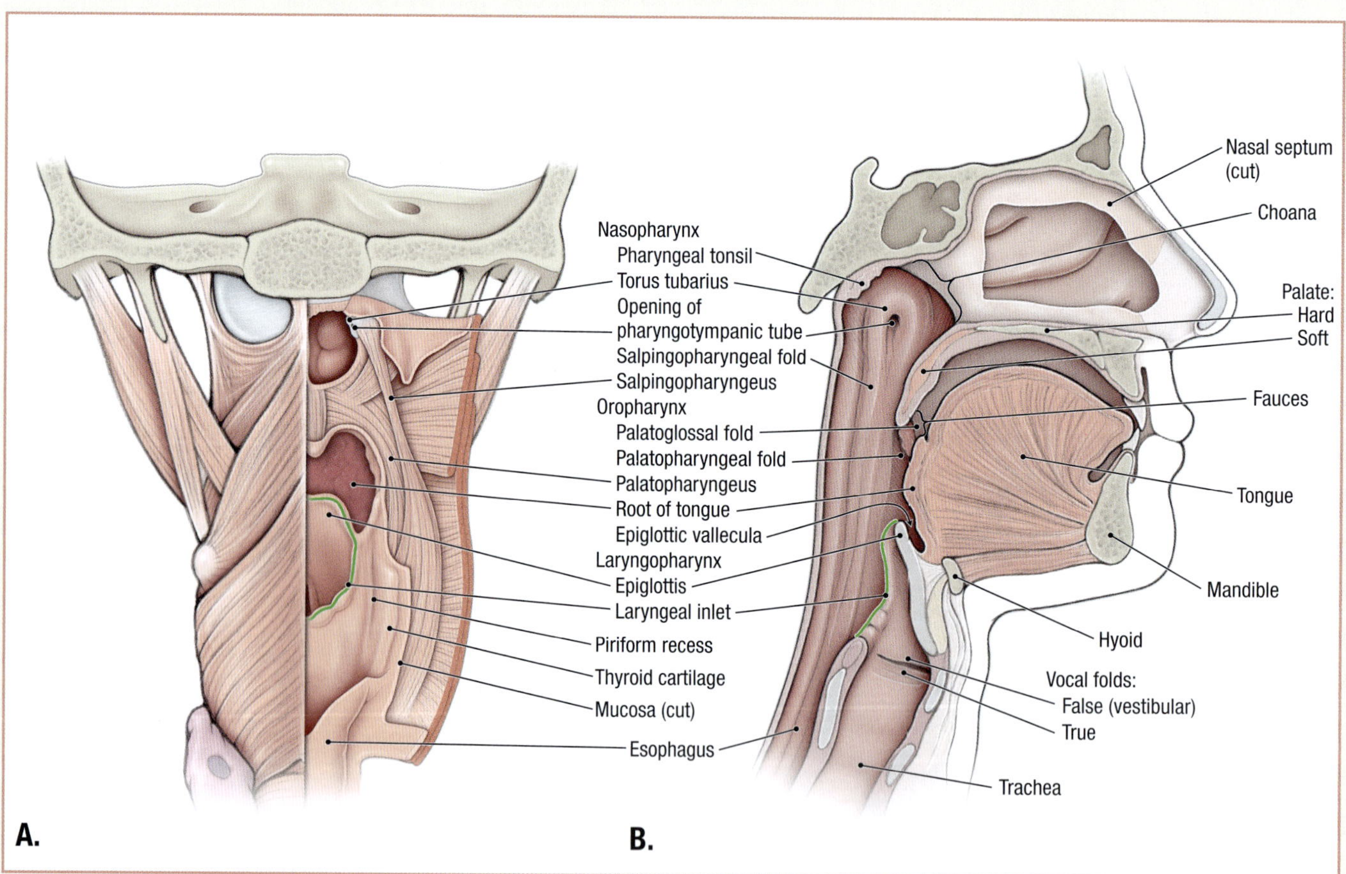

FIGURE 7.67 ■ **A.** Muscles of pharynx with right side opened. Posterior view. **B.** Midsagittal section of pharynx. Medial view.

Bisection of Head

ATLAS 7.2A, 8.24A, 8.77; VIDEO 7.15.4

Dissection Note: To view the nasal cavity, a sagittal cut must be made through the skull close to the median plane. The objective during the head bisection is to keep the nasal septum intact while cutting as close to the midline as possible.

1. Refer to FIGURE 7.68.
2. Begin the bisection of the head on the posterior aspect of the pharynx by using a scalpel to divide the uvula and soft palate along the median plane.
3. Turn the head and use a scalpel to cut through the upper lip and cartilages of the external nose on one side of the nasal septum, just off the midline (**Cut 1**).
4. Align a saw just lateral to the crista galli in line with your intended cut lateral to the septum so that as you cut through the skull from superior to inferior, you preserve the crista galli.
5. Cut inferiorly through the frontal and nasal bones until you reach the ethmoid bone in the floor of the anterior cranial fossa (**Cut 2**).
6. Once past the nasal septum, aim to cut through the midline of structures as much as possible.
7. Continue the midline cut through the sphenoid bone in the middle cranial fossa and into the basilar part of the occipital bone in the posterior cranial fossa (**Cut 3**).

Dissection Note: Take a moment to study the oral cavity of the cadaver to look for partial or full dentures as some of the cadavers may have false teeth, which may make cuts through the palate difficult if not removed.

8. Cut through the hard palate, stopping when the saw is free of the bone and rests in the oral cavity. Do not cut the tongue or mandible at this time.
9. The two superior halves of the head should separate from each other and expose the superior aspect of the tongue.

Internal Aspect of Pharynx

ATLAS 7.29, 8.67; VIDEO 7.15.5

1. Refer back to FIGURE 7.67.
2. In the bisected head, observe that the **nasopharynx** lies posterior to the nasal cavity and superior to the soft palate.
3. Identify the **posterior nasal aperture (choana, internal naris)**, the boundary between the nasal cavity and nasopharynx. Observe that the left and right choanae are separated by the posterior aspect of the nasal septum.
4. On the lateral wall of the nasopharynx, identify the **opening of the pharyngotympanic tube (auditory tube, eustachian tube)**.
5. Superior to the opening of the pharyngotympanic tube, identify the **torus tubarius**, the "horseshoe"-shaped cartilage of the pharyngotympanic tube covered by mucosa.
6. Extending posteroinferiorly from the torus tubarius, identify the **salpingopharyngeal fold**. *Note that the salpingopharyngeal fold is the mucosal fold overlying the salpingopharyngeus.*

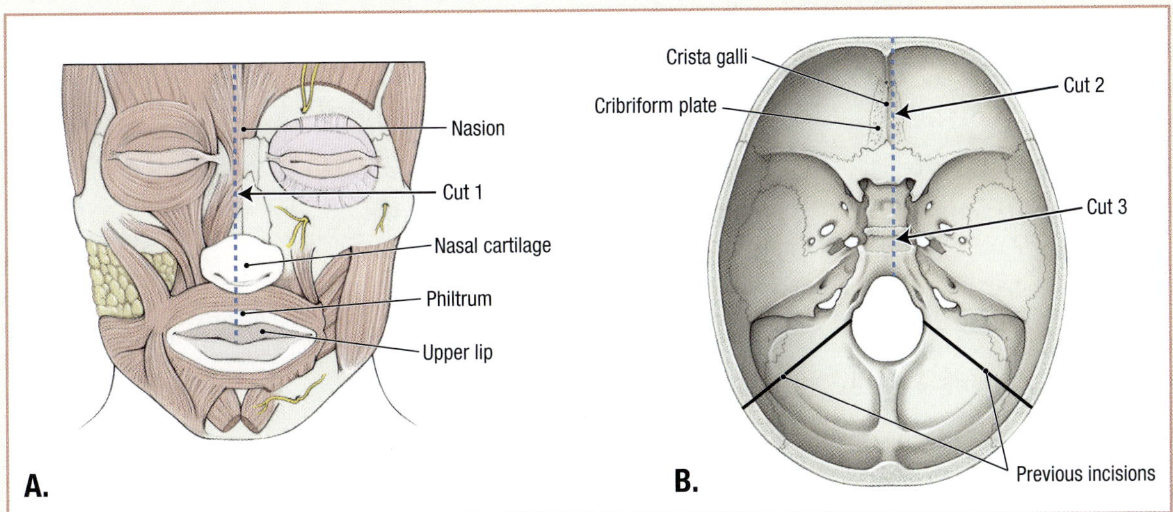

FIGURE 7.68 ■ **A.** Cuts through face for head bisection. Anterior view. **B.** Skeletal cuts for head bisection. Superior view.

7. Superior and posterior to the torus tubarius, identify the **pharyngeal recess**. Observe that the **pharyngeal tonsil (adenoid)** is located in the mucous membrane of the pharyngeal recess (see **Clinical Correlation 7.15**).

CLINICAL CORRELATION 7.15

Tonsillectomy and Adenoids

ATLAS 8.65, 8.66, 8.67

The tonsils are collections of lymphatic tissue around the oral and nasal cavities which assist the immune system. As the majority of lymphatic growth occurs prior to puberty, in young children, palatine tonsils appear large as compared to the adult. Inflammation of the tonsils (tonsillitis) caused by strep throat or other infections, as well as sleep apnea, may require removal of the tonsil (tonsillectomy). Typically, when "tonsils" are removed, it is in reference to the palatine tonsils, although it may also be necessary to remove the pharyngeal tonsils, and care must be taken to avoid damage to the glossopharyngeal nerve (CN IX) and internal carotid artery. Adenoids are enlarged pharyngeal tonsils and may obstruct the flow of air from the nose through the nasopharynx, making mouth breathing necessary thus compounding sleep apnea and snoring.

8. Observe that the **oropharynx** lies posterior to the oral cavity and is bounded superiorly by the soft palate and inferiorly by the epiglottis.
9. Inferior to the palate, identify the **palatoglossal fold (anterior pillar)** forming a dividing line between the oral cavity and oropharynx at the gap known as the **fauces**.
10. Identify the **palatopharyngeal fold (posterior pillar)** posterior to the palatoglossal fold descending along the lateral wall of the oropharynx.
11. Identify the location of the **palatine tonsil** between the palatoglossal and palatopharyngeal folds.
12. Identify the **laryngopharynx** posterior to the larynx extending from the hyoid bone to the lower border of the cricoid cartilage.
13. In the midline of the laryngopharynx, identify the cut edge of the **epiglottis** superior to the **laryngeal inlet (aditus)**. Observe that the margins of the laryngeal inlet are formed laterally by the **aryepiglottic folds**, which arch posteroinferiorly from the epiglottis.
14. Gently press the tip of a probe inferolateral to the aryepiglottic fold along the path of the **piriform recess**, the space bordered medially by the **larynx**, laterally by the **thyroid cartilage**, and posteriorly by the **inferior pharyngeal constrictor**.

Dissection Follow-up

1. Review the attachments, innervation, and actions of the pharyngeal constrictors in **TABLE 7.7**.
2. Review the nerves contributing to the pharyngeal plexus.
3. Trace the glossopharyngeal (CN IX), vagus (CN X), accessory (CN XI), and hypoglossal (CN XII) nerves from the posterior cranial fossa to their respective areas of distribution.
4. Review the relationships of the contents of the carotid sheath.
5. Review the boundaries and contents of each part of the pharynx.
6. Return the bisected head to its anatomical position.

TABLE 7.7 Muscles of Pharynx

Muscle	*Anterior Attachments*	*Posterior Attachments*	*Actions*	*Innervation*
Superior pharyngeal constrictor	Pterygoid hamulus and pterygomandibular raphe	Pharyngeal tubercle and pharyngeal raphe	Constrict wall of pharynx during swallowing	Vagus n. (CN X) via pharyngeal plexus
Middle pharyngeal constrictor	Greater horn of hyoid bone and inferior portion of the stylohyoid ligament	Pharyngeal raphe		
Inferior pharyngeal constrictor	Oblique line of thyroid cartilage and lateral surface of the cricoid cartilage			External branch of superior laryngeal n.
Stylopharyngeus	Styloid process (superior attachment)	Posterior and superior borders of thyroid cartilage with palatopharyngeus (inferior attachment)	Elevate pharynx and larynx during swallowing and speaking	Glossopharyngeal n. (CN IX)
Salpingopharyngeus	Cartilaginous part of pharyngotympanic tube	Posterior border of thyroid cartilage and side of pharynx and esophagus with palatopharyngeus		Vagus n. (CN X) via pharyngeal plexus

Abbreviations: CN, cranial nerve; n., nerve.

NOSE AND NASAL CAVITY

Dissection Overview

The right and left nasal cavities are separated by the nasal septum. The nostril (external naris) is the anterior entrance to the nasal cavity from the external environment. Posteriorly, each nasal cavity opens into the nasopharynx through a choana (internal naris). The nasal cavity is lined by mucosa directly attached to the bones and cartilages of the region, which give the walls of the nasal cavity their characteristic contours. The superior one-third of the nasal mucosa is olfactory in nature, and the lower two-thirds is respiratory in nature, although both are highly vascular and capable of engorgement.

The order of dissection will be as follows: The skeleton of the nasal cavity and nasal cartilages will be studied. The nasal septum will be examined. The features of the lateral nasal wall will be studied. The openings of the paranasal sinuses will be identified. The maxillary sinus will be examined.

Skeletal Anatomy

Nasal Cavity

ATLAS 8.2, 8.73E

Refer to a skeleton or disarticulated skull to identify the following skeletal features from an anterior view.

1. Refer to FIGURE 7.69.
2. Identify the **anterior nasal aperture** and observe that it is roughly heart shaped, with the apex of the "heart" directed superiorly toward the **nasal bones** on the bridge of the nose, and the broader aspect of the "heart" centered around the **anterior nasal spine** inferiorly.
3. Follow the margin of the nasal aperture superiorly and identify the **frontal process of the maxilla** between the **nasal** and **lacrimal bones**.
4. Identify the bony part of the **nasal septum** approximately in the midline of the skull creating a division between the right and left **nasal cavities**.
5. On the lateral wall of the nasal cavity, identify the **inferior nasal concha** curving away from the lateral wall.
6. Superior to the inferior nasal concha, identify the **middle nasal concha.** *Note that the middle nasal concha is part of the ethmoid bone, whereas the inferior nasal concha is an independent bone.*

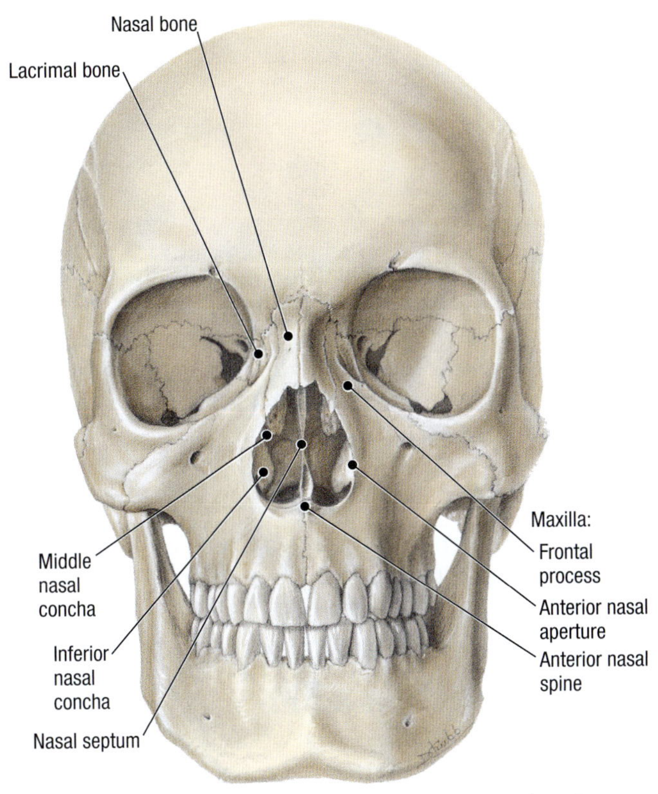

FIGURE 7.69 ■ Skeleton of nasal cavity. Anterior view.

Lateral Nasal Wall

ATLAS 8.74, 8.78B

Refer to a hemisected skull to identify the following skeletal features from a medial view.

1. Refer to FIGURE 7.70.
2. Identify the **cribriform plate of the ethmoid bone** and observe that it forms part of the floor of the anterior cranial fossa and roof of the nasal cavities. Recall that the small apertures of the cribriform plate contain branches of the olfactory nerve (CN I).
3. Identify the **perpendicular plate of the ethmoid bone** forming part of the bony nasal septum in the midline or medial wall of the nasal cavity.
4. Identify the **superior nasal concha** and **middle nasal concha**, which form part of the lateral wall of each nasal cavity.
5. Observe that the remainder of the lateral wall of the nasal cavity consists of portions of the **maxilla, lacrimal bone, inferior nasal concha**, and **perpendicular plate of the palatine bone**.
6. Observe that the perpendicular plate of the palatine bone lies anterior to the **medial pterygoid plate of the sphenoid bone**.
7. Pass a wire or the tip of a probe gently through the **sphenopalatine foramen** and observe that this opening connects the nasal cavity with the pterygopalatine fossa.

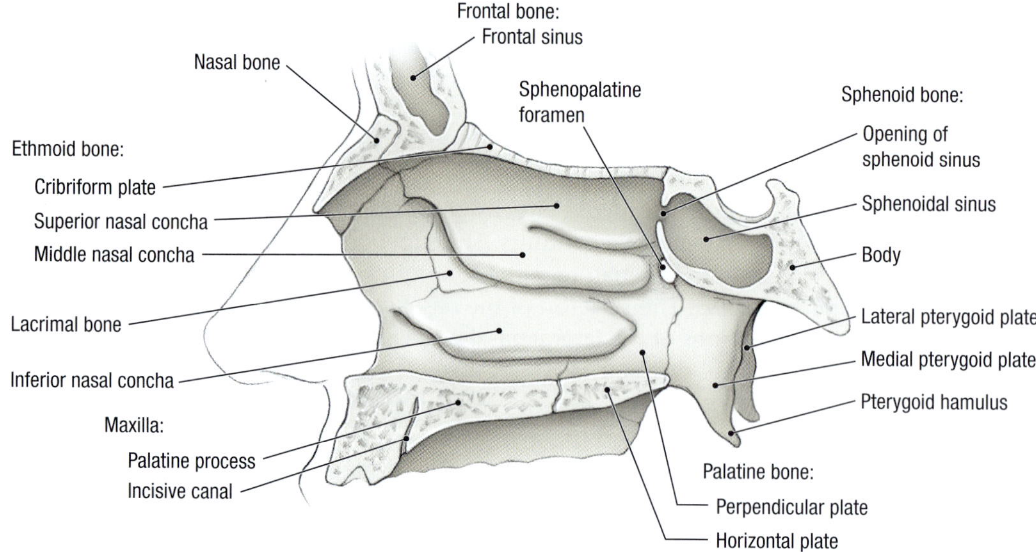

FIGURE 7.70 ■ Skeleton of lateral wall of right nasal cavity. Medial view.

8. Identify the **sphenoidal sinus** in the **body of the sphenoid** and observe that it is connected to the nasal cavity via the **opening of the sphenoidal sinus.**
9. Identify the **incisive canal** within the **palatine process of the maxilla.**
10. Observe that the **palatine process of the maxilla** forms the anterior aspect of the floor of the nasal cavity and hard palate, whereas the **horizontal plate of the palatine bone** forms the posterior aspect of the floor of the nasal cavity and hard palate.

Surface Anatomy

The surface anatomy of the external nose may be studied on a living subject or on a cadaver. On the cadaver, note that fixation of tissue during embalming may make it difficult to distinguish bone from well-preserved soft tissues in some specimens.

Nose

ATLAS 8.73A, 8.73B; VIDEO 7.16.1

1. Refer to FIGURE 7.71.
2. Identify the **root** of the nose overlying the nasal bones superiorly.
3. Follow the **bridge** of the nose inferiorly toward the **apex** of the nose, or tip.
4. Observe that the apex is in the midline superior to the **nasal septum** and **philtrum**, the slight depression between the nose and lips.
5. Lateral to the nasal septum to either side, identify a **nostril (naris)**, the aperture connecting the external environment with the nasal cavity.
6. Observe that the nostrils are bound laterally by the curve of tissue delineated by the **nasolabial groove**.
7. Palpate the **nasal bones** and **lateral nasal cartilages**. Observe that the lateral nasal cartilages give shape to the bridge of the nose.

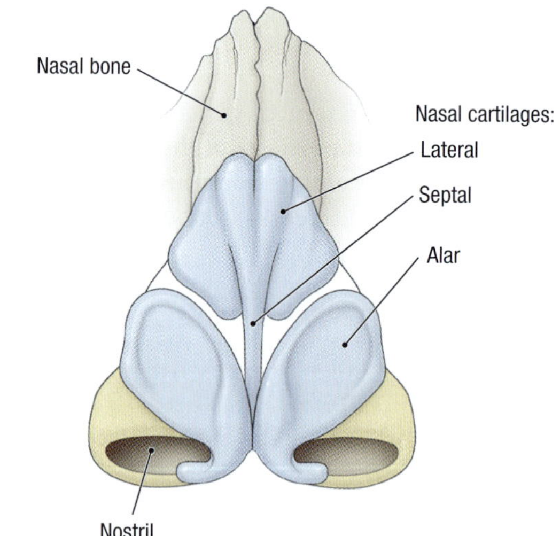

FIGURE 7.71 ■ Surface anatomy and cartilages of external nose. Anterior view.

8. Identify the **septal cartilage** on the anterior part of the nasal septum separating the right and left nasal cavities anteriorly. *Note that the lateral nasal cartilages are an extension of the septal cartilage.*
9. Lateral to the septal cartilage, palpate the **alar cartilages** that give shape to the medial side of the **nostril (naris)**.
10. On the cadaver, observe that the bones and cartilages of the nasal cavity are obscured by the mucosa covering them. *Note that the vessels and nerves of the nasal cavity are contained within this mucosa.*

Dissection Instructions

Nasal Septum

ATLAS 8.74B, 8.75B, 8.76B; VIDEO 7.16.2

1. Refer to FIGURE 7.72.
2. On the cadaver, examine the half of the head containing the intact **nasal septum**.
3. Use blunt dissection to peel away the mucosa on the nasal septum and identify the **sphenopalatine artery** and **nasopalatine nerve**, a branch of CN V_2.
4. Observe that the sphenopalatine artery and nasopalatine nerve pass diagonally down the nasal septum from the sphenopalatine foramen to the incisive canal. *Note that in addition to the nasal septum, the nasopalatine nerve and sphenopalatine artery supply a portion of the oral mucosa covering the hard palate.*
5. Make a brief effort to identify **internal nasal branches** arising from the **anterior ethmoidal nerve**, a branch of CN V_1.
6. Identify the **olfactory area**, the mucosa near the cribriform plate in the roof and superior aspect of the lateral wall of the nasal cavity.
7. Refer to FIGURE 7.73.
8. Strip the mucosa off the visible side of the nasal septum and identify the **perpendicular plate of the ethmoid bone** extending inferiorly from the ethmoid bone in line with the crista galli.
9. Identify the **vomer** in the posterior inferior aspect of the nasal septum subdividing the right and left **choanae** posteriorly.
10. Identify the **septal cartilage** anterior to the vomer and perpendicular plate of the ethmoid subdividing the **nostrils** anteriorly.

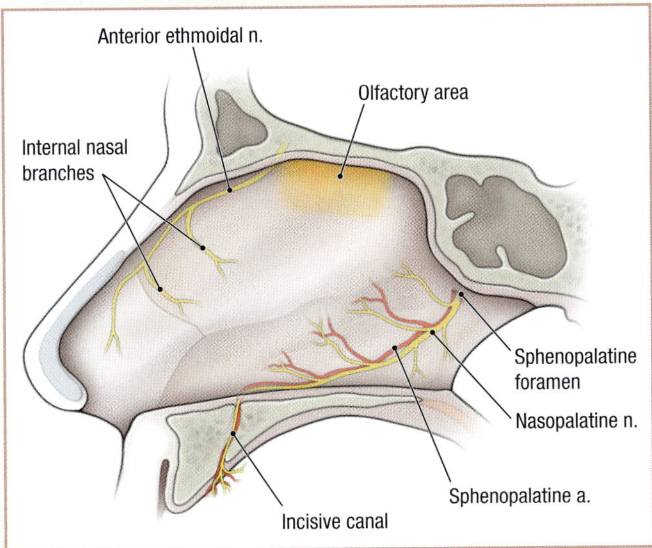

FIGURE 7.72 ● Innervation and arterial supply to mucosa of nasal septum. Lateral view.

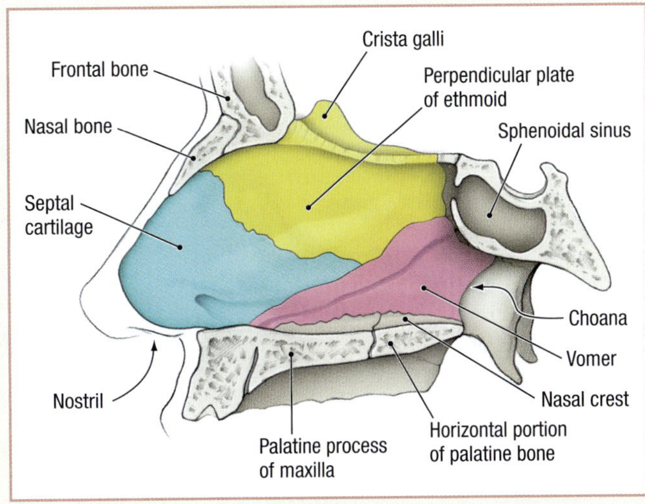

FIGURE 7.73 ● Nasal septum. Left lateral view.

11. Identify the **nasal crest** in the midline along the superior surface of the **palatine process of the maxilla** and at the junction of the right and left **horizontal plates of the palatine bones**.

Lateral Wall of Nasal Cavity

ATLAS 8.75A, 8.76A, 8.77, 8.78, 8.79A; VIDEO 7.16.3

1. Refer to FIGURE 7.74.
2. On the cadaver, examine the half of the head that does not contain the **nasal septum**.
3. Inspect the lateral wall of the nasal cavity and identify the **superior nasal concha**.

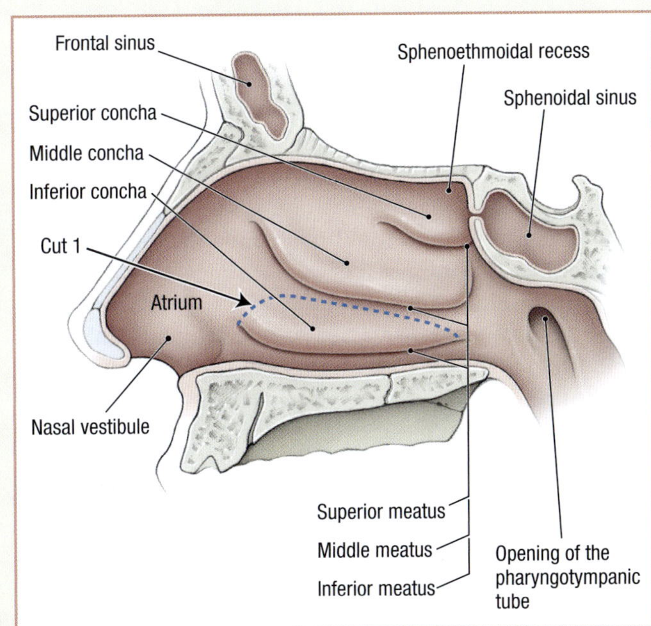

FIGURE 7.74 ● Nasal conchae and meatuses of right nasal cavity. Medial view.

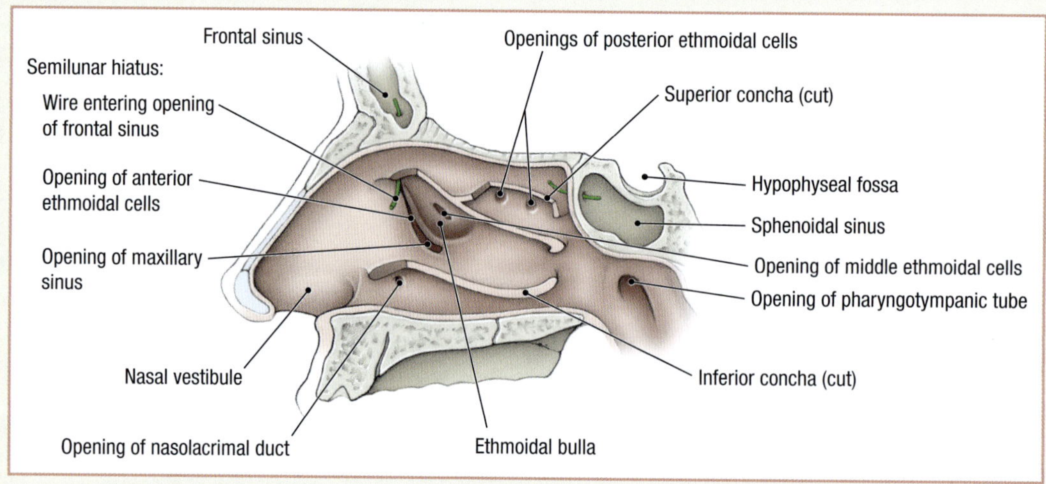

FIGURE 7.75 ● Openings in lateral wall of right nasal cavity. Medial view.

4. Superior and posterior to the superior nasal concha, identify the **sphenoethmoidal recess.** Inferior to the superior nasal concha, place the tip of the probe into the space of the **superior meatus.**
5. Identify the **middle concha** curving superior to the **middle meatus** and the **inferior concha** curving superior to the **inferior meatus.**
6. Identify the **vestibule,** the area superior to the nostril and anterior to the inferior meatus, and the **atrium,** the area superior to the vestibule and anterior to the middle meatus.
7. Use scissors to remove the **inferior concha** (**Cut 1**).
8. Refer to FIGURE 7.75.
9. Inferior to the cut edge of the inferior concha, identify the opening of the **nasolacrimal duct.**
10. Elevate the **middle concha** until you hear the bone break, and the concha can be reflected superiorly along a "hinge" of mucosa.
11. In the middle meatus, identify the curved slit of the **semilunar hiatus (hiatus semilunaris).**
12. Posterior to the curvature of the semilunar hiatus, identify the **ethmoidal bulla (bulla ethmoidalis)** bulging into the nasal cavity.
13. Within the semilunar hiatus, identify three openings from anterior to posterior of the **frontal sinus, anterior ethmoidal cells,** and **maxillary sinus.**

Dissection Note: A piece of wire may be passed through the openings to verify the orientation and continuity of each space with the nasal cavity.

14. On the summit of the ethmoidal bulla, identify the **opening of the middle ethmoidal cells.**
15. Identify the **opening of the posterior ethmoidal cells** in the superior meatus.
16. Identify the **opening of the sphenoidal sinus** in the sphenoethmoidal recess.
17. Examine the **sphenoid sinus.** Observe that the sphenoid sinus is lined by mucosa that is continuous with the mucosa of the nasal cavity (see **Clinical Correlation 7.16**).

CLINICAL CORRELATION 7.16

Pituitary Tumor Removal

ATLAS 8.30C, 8.77

The pituitary gland is often referred to as the "master gland" due to the high number of hormones it releases. Pituitary tumors may lead to large hormonal imbalances in the body, vision problems, headaches, or a variety of other symptoms. Depending on the size and severity of the tumor, it may be treated by medications or radiation, or it may need to be surgically removed. As the sphenoidal sinus lies directly inferior to the hypophyseal fossa containing the pituitary gland, relatively easy surgical access is available in a transsphenoidal approach. Transsphenoidal surgery may be done through the nostrils and nasopharynx, an endonasal approach, or by passing through the upper lip to open a path between the hard palate and nasal cavity in a sublabial approach.

18. Refer to FIGURE 7.76.
19. From a superior perspective, observe that the **ethmoidal cells** are located between the nasal cavity and orbit.
20. Observe that the ethmoidal cells consist of an **anterior** pair near the **frontal sinus,** a **middle** pair, and a **posterior** pair near the location of the **sphenoid sinus.** *Note that variation is common, and the individual air cells may be split or appear as clusters of smaller mucosal lined cavities.*
21. Refer back to FIGURE 7.47.

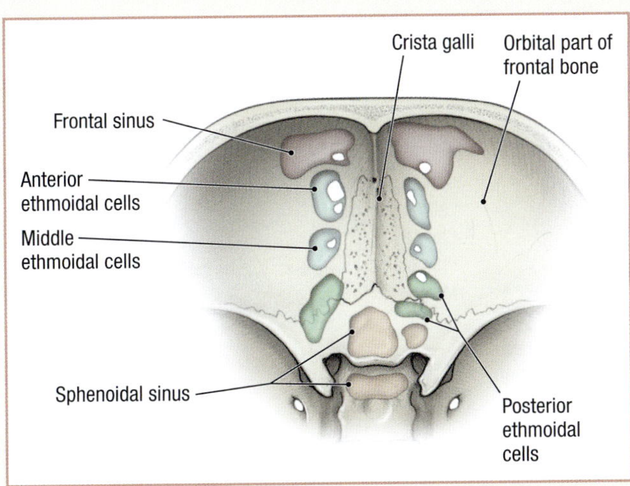

FIGURE 7.76 ● Paranasal sinuses. Superior view.

22. In a coronal cut of the head, observe that the **maxillary sinus** is approximately shaped like a three-sided pyramid.
23. Observe that the **floor of the orbit** forms the roof of the maxillary sinus and that the **opening of the maxillary sinus** is near its roof; thus, the maxillary sinus drains superiorly (see **Clinical Correlation 7.17**).

CLINICAL CORRELATION 7.17

Maxillary Sinus Infection

ATLAS 8.79A, 8.80, 8.83

When the head is in the upright position, the maxillary sinus cannot properly drain, leading to an increased likelihood of infection or inflammation (sinusitis). If infections of the maxillary sinus persist, an opening may be surgically created through the inferior meatus near the floor of the maxillary sinus to promote drainage.

If the roots of maxillary teeth project into the maxillary sinus, they are covered only by mucosa. During extraction of a maxillary molar or premolar tooth, the mucosa superior to the projecting root may be torn. As a result, a fistula may form between the oral cavity and maxillary sinus.

24. Observe that the floor of the maxillary sinus is the alveolar process of the maxilla and that the roots of the maxillary teeth may project into the maxillary sinus. *Note that the mucosa of the maxillary sinus is innervated by the infraorbital and posterior superior alveolar nerves.*

Dissection Follow-up

1. Review the features of the lateral wall of the nasal cavity.
2. Review the relationship of the paranasal sinuses to the orbit, anterior cranial fossa, and nasal cavity.
3. Review the drainage point of each paranasal sinus.
4. Return any reflected tissue and the bisected head to their anatomical position.

PALATE AND PTERYGOPALATINE FOSSA

Dissection Overview

The palate forms the floor of the nasal cavity and roof of the oral cavity; thus, it is covered by nasal mucosa on its superior surface and oral mucosa on its inferior surface. The palate consists of two portions: the hard palate, the anterior two-thirds surrounded by the upper dentition; and the soft palate, the posterior one-third extending into the pharynx. Numerous mucous glands (palatine glands) are present on the oral surface of the palate.

Many of the neurovascular structures supplying the hard and soft palate originate in the face and take a long intraosseous route to reach their target. As such, the neurovascular structures pass from the infratemporal fossa through the bones of the skull to enter the pterygopalatine fossa deep within the cheek to continue medially to the lateral aspect of the nasal cavity. From the lateral wall of the nasal cavity, the neurovascular path will either arch to the midline along the nasal septum or descend within the bone to reach their target destinations of the hard or soft palate.

The order of dissection will be as follows: The mucosal folds of the inner pharyngeal wall will be studied. The mucosa will be stripped from the inner surface of the pharynx and the muscles constituting the inner longitudinal layer examined. Muscles that move the soft palate will then be studied. The nerves and blood vessels of the palate will be identified. The palatine canal and pterygopalatine fossa will be dissected from the medial aspect. The pterygopalatine ganglion will be identified, and the nerves and vessels of the nasal cavity and palate summarized.

Skeletal Anatomy

Refer to a disarticulated skull to identify the following skeletal features from an inferior view.

Dentition

ATLAS 8.68, 8.69, 8.70, 8.71, 8.72

1. Refer to FIGURE 7.77.
2. The teeth can be subdivided into an **upper dentition (maxillary teeth)** and a **lower dentition (mandibular teeth)**.
3. Examine the upper dentition on the inferior aspect of the **maxilla**.
4. Observe that each tooth has an individual socket demarcated by an **alveolar process** extending inferiorly from the maxillary bone.
5. Identify the two **central incisors** to either side of the midsagittal plane anteriorly and the two **lateral incisors** immediately lateral to the central incisors on each side.
6. Continuing laterally, identify the two **canines (cuspids)**, noting the distinct difference in shape from the incisors.
7. Identify the four **premolars (bicuspids)** posterolateral to the canines, two on each side.
8. Identify the six **molars** posterior to the premolars, three on each side and numbered from 1 to 3 as they progress posteriorly from the premolars with the 3rd being the "wisdom tooth." *Note that often the wisdom teeth are removed to prevent overcrowding of the oral cavity.*
9. Observe that in the adult, there are 16 teeth on each dentition, making a total of 32 teeth.
10. Identify the corresponding numbers for the 16 maxillary teeth beginning with the right upper 3rd molar as number 1 and ending with the left upper 3rd molar as number 16, with the central incisors as numbers 8 and 9.
11. On a disarticulated mandible, identify the central and lateral incisors, canines, premolars, and molars.
12. Identify the corresponding numbers for the 16 mandibular teeth beginning with the left lower 3rd molar as number 17 and ending with the right lower 3rd molar as number 32, with the central incisors as numbers 24 and 25.
13. Alternatively, the teeth may be subdivided into quadrants as upper right, lower right, upper left, and lower left. With the quadrant numbering system, the teeth in each quadrant are numbered from 1 to 8 beginning with the central incisor of the quadrant being number 1 and the 3rd molar of the quadrant being number 8.
14. Observe that each tooth has five surfaces named for their respective orientations. Identify the facial surface, the aspect closest to the face, which can be subdivided into labial for the incisors and canines and buccal for the premolars and molars.
15. Opposite the facial surface, identify the lingual surface of each tooth, the aspect closest to the tongue.
16. Observe that each tooth has a mesial surface, the side of the tooth closest to the midsagittal plane; and a distal surface, the side furthest from the midsagittal plane as the teeth progress laterally and posteriorly.
17. Lastly, identify the incisal surface, the cutting edge of the anterior teeth; and the occlusal surface, the chewing surface for the posterior teeth.

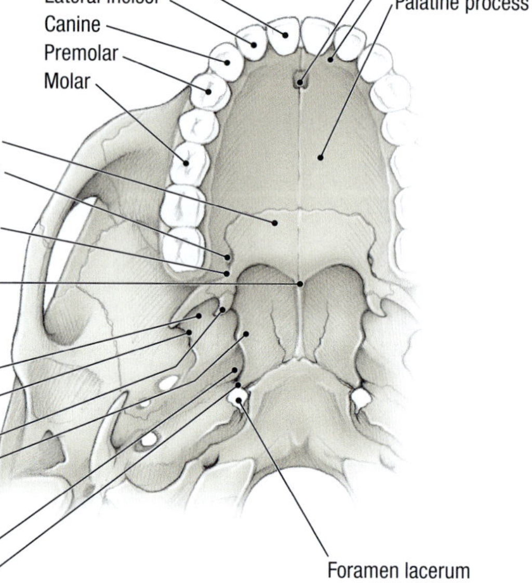

FIGURE 7.77 ■ Skeleton of palate. Inferior view.

Hard Palate

ATLAS 8.63A, 8.71B

1. Refer to FIGURE 7.77.
2. Identify the **hard palate** and observe that it is composed of the **palatine process of the maxilla** anteriorly and the **horizontal plate of the palatine bone** posteriorly.
3. Posterior to the incisors, identify the **incisive foramen** between the palatine processes of the fused maxillae.
4. Between the maxilla and palatine bone, identify the larger, more anteriorly located **greater palatine foramen**, and the slightly smaller, more posteriorly located **lesser palatine foramen**.
5. In the midline of the palatine bones on the posterior margin of the hard palate, identify the **posterior nasal spine** inferior to the nasal septum.

6. Identify the hook-like process of the **pterygoid hamulus** on the inferior aspect of the **medial pterygoid plate** of the sphenoid bone.
7. Observe that the medial pterygoid plate is separated inferiorly from the **lateral pterygoid plate** by the depression of the **pterygoid fossa**.
8. Identify the smaller, more superiorly located **scaphoid fossa** along the superior extent of the medial pterygoid plate near the base of the skull.

Pterygopalatine Fossa

ATLAS 8.9B, 8.50B

1. Refer to FIGURE 7.78.
2. Identify the **inferior orbital fissure** between the maxilla and greater wing of the sphenoid.
3. Identify the **pterygomaxillary fissure** between the lateral pterygoid plate and maxilla.
4. Pass a wire through the pterygomaxillary fissure and into the small cavity of the **pterygopalatine fossa**.
5. On the medial wall of the pterygopalatine fossa, identify the small opening of the **sphenopalatine foramen**.
6. Pass a wire through the sphenopalatine foramen and confirm that this opening connects the nasal cavity with the pterygopalatine fossa.
7. From an inferior view, identify the small opening of the **pterygoid canal** in the anterior margin of the **foramen lacerum**. Pass a thin wire through the pterygoid canal and observe that it connects to the pterygopalatine fossa.

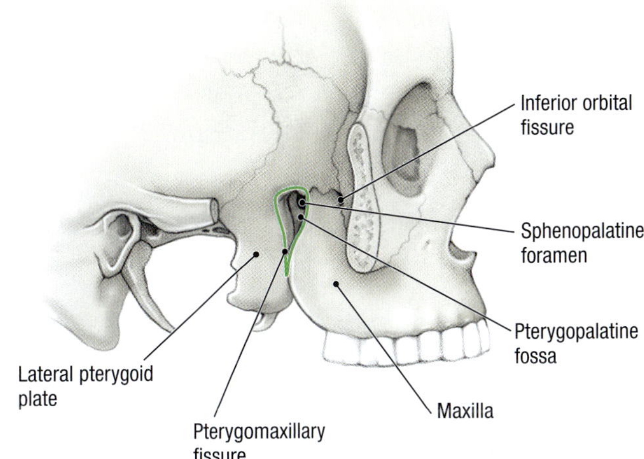

FIGURE 7.78 ● Right pterygopalatine and infratemporal fossae. Lateral view.

Dissection Instructions

Soft Palate

ATLAS 8.63B, 8.63C, 8.64; VIDEO 7.17.1

1. Refer to FIGURE 7.79.
2. Examine the edge of the **soft palate** where it is cut in the sagittal plane and observe that muscles attach to its posterior two-thirds provide the associated mobility of the structure.
3. Observe that the thickness of the soft palate is partly due to the presence of palatine glands and that the strength of the soft palate is primarily due to the **palatine aponeurosis**.
4. On the inner pharyngeal wall, identify the **opening of the pharyngotympanic tube** inferior to the mucous membrane–lined cartilage of the **torus tubarius**.
5. Observe that the **pharyngotympanic (auditory, eustachian) tube** connects the nasopharynx to the tympanic cavity. *Note that the part of the pharyngotympanic tube that is closest to the pharynx is cartilaginous (approximately two-thirds of its length) and the part that is closest to the middle ear passes through the temporal bone.*
6. Within the opening of the pharyngotympanic tube, identify the **torus levatorius**, the "bump" of mucosa overlying the **levator veli palatini** on the floor of the **pharyngotympanic tube**.
7. Identify the **salpingopalatine fold** arising from the anterior aspect of the torus tubarius and coursing to the soft palate.

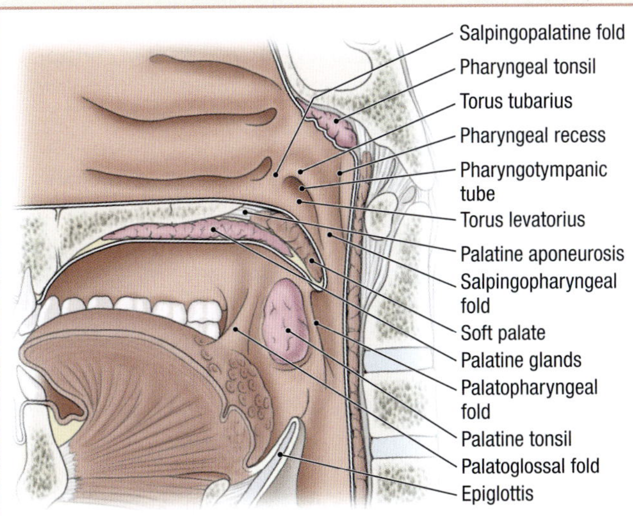

FIGURE 7.79 ● Mucosal folds in right pharynx. Medial view.

Dissection Note: Many of the pharyngeal and palatal mucosal folds have similar names to the underlying muscles of the region, with the fold name ending in "-al" and the muscle name ending in "-us."

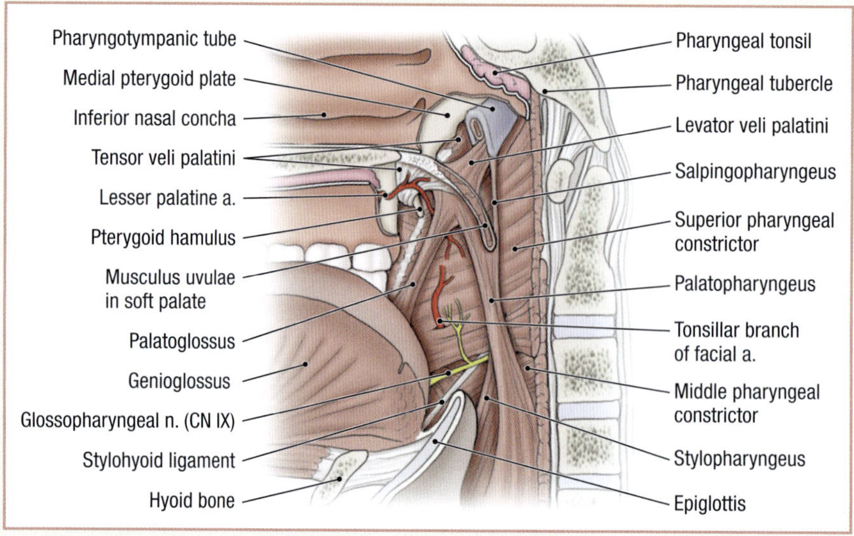

FIGURE 7.80 ● Muscles of right pharyngeal wall. Medial view.

8. Identify the **salpingopharyngeal fold** arising from the posterior aspect of the torus tubarius and coursing inferiorly into the pharynx.
9. Identify the **palatoglossal fold (anterior fauces)**, arching from the palate to the tongue, and the **palatopharyngeal fold (posterior fauces)**, arching from the palate to the pharynx.
10. Refer to FIGURE 7.80.
11. Use blunt dissection to remove the mucosa from the palatoglossal fold and identify the **palatoglossus**, which lies within the fold.
12. Remove the mucosa from the palatopharyngeal fold and identify the **palatopharyngeus**, which lies within the fold.
13. Remove the mucosa from the salpingopharyngeal fold and identify the **salpingopharyngeus**, which lies within the fold. *Note that the palatopharyngeus and salpingopharyngeus blend and contribute to the inner longitudinal muscle layer of the pharynx.*
14. Review the attachments, actions, and innervations of the palatoglossus, palatopharyngeus, and salpingopharyngeus (see **TABLE 7.8**).
15. Remove the remaining mucosa from the inner surface of the nasopharynx and oropharynx.
16. Identify the **stylopharyngeus**, which enters the pharynx between the **superior** and **middle pharyngeal constrictors**.
17. Observe that the stylopharyngeus lies anterior and parallel to the palatopharyngeus and salpingopharyngeus and that all three muscles blend near their inferior ends.
18. Review the attachments and actions of the stylopharyngeus (see **TABLE 7.7**).
19. Observe that the **pharyngobasilar fascia** closes the gap between the superior border of the superior pharyngeal constrictor and base of the skull. *Note that the pharyngotympanic tube and levator veli palatini pass through a gap in the pharyngobasilar fascia.*
20. Remove the mucosa from the torus levatorius and identify the **levator veli palatini** coursing along the floor of the auditory tube.
21. Remove the mucosa from the medial aspect of the **medial pterygoid plate**.
22. Carefully use bone cutters to chip away portions of the medial pterygoid plate and identify the **tensor veli palatini**. *Note that the belly of the tensor veli palatini is located between the medial and lateral plates of the pterygoid process.*
23. Palpate the **hamulus of the medial pterygoid plate** and find the tendon of the tensor veli palatini, which turns medially around the hamulus and attaches to the **palatine aponeurosis**.
24. Along the cut edge of the uvula, identify the **musculus uvulae**, which arise from the posterior nasal spine to elevate and retract the uvula. *Note that as the musculus uvulae and levator veli palatini contract, the soft palate thickens centrally and closes the pharynx between the nasopharynx and oropharynx.*
25. Review the attachments and actions of the levator veli palatini, tensor veli palatini, and musculus uvulae (see **TABLE 7.8**).
26. Refer to **TABLE 7.8** and note that five muscles of the soft palate and pharynx are innervated by the vagus nerve (CN X) via the pharyngeal plexus: salpingopharyngeus, levator veli palatini, palatoglossus, palatopharyngeus, and musculus uvulae. *Note that the tensor veli palatini is innervated by the mandibular division of the trigeminal nerve (CN V_3), not the vagus nerve.*
27. Use a probe to raise the mucosa on the inferior surface of the hard palate where it was cut during head bisection, and grasp it with forceps or a hemostat, and peel it from medial to lateral. *Note that the mucosa lining the palate is firmly attached and may require sharp dissection.*

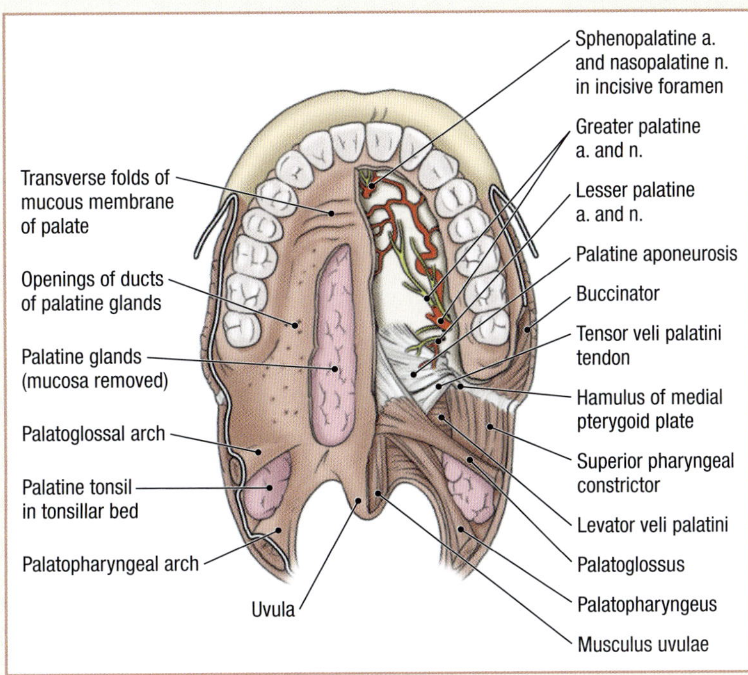

FIGURE 7.81 ■ Mucosa and glands (*right*) and underlying muscles, nerves, and vessels (*left*) of palate. Inferior view.

28. Detach the mucosa along the medial side of the alveolar process of the maxilla.
29. Refer to FIGURE 7.81.
30. Identify the **greater palatine artery** and **nerve** where they emerge from the **greater palatine foramen**.
31. Use blunt dissection to follow the greater palatine artery and nerve anteriorly. *Note that the distal end of the sphenopalatine artery and nasopalatine nerve supply the mucosa covering the anterior part of the hard palate.*
32. Posterior to the greater palatine nerve, identify the **lesser palatine artery** and **nerve**.
33. Use blunt dissection to follow the lesser palatine artery and nerve to the soft palate, which they supply.

Tonsillar Bed

ATLAS 8.65, 8.66, 8.67; VIDEO 7.17.2

1. Refer to FIGURE 7.81.
2. Identify the **palatine tonsil** in the **tonsillar bed (fossa)**. *Note that in older individuals, the palatine tonsil may be inconspicuous or may have been surgically removed.*
3. Identify the **anterior boundary** of the tonsillar bed formed by the **palatoglossal fold** and the **posterior boundary** of the tonsillar bed formed by the **palatopharyngeal fold**.
4. Observe that the **lateral boundary** of the tonsillar bed is formed by the **superior pharyngeal constrictor**.
5. If the cadaver has a palatine tonsil, use blunt dissection to remove it. Section the tonsil and observe the **crypts** that extend into its surface.
6. Remove the mucosa from the tonsillar bed and identify the **glossopharyngeal nerve (CN IX)**.
7. Observe that the glossopharyngeal nerve passes between the superior and middle pharyngeal constrictors to enter the tonsillar bed. *Note that the glossopharyngeal nerve innervates the mucosa of the posterior one-third of the tongue and posterior wall of the pharynx.*

Palatine Canal and Pterygopalatine Fossa

ATLAS 8.50B, 8.63C, 8.79A; VIDEO 7.17.3

Dissection Note: Dissection of the lateral nasal wall is quite difficult because the mucosa is firmly attached to the bone and the underlying nerve vessels are easily torn.

1. Refer to FIGURE 7.82.
2. Remove the mucosa from the posterior part of the lateral nasal wall.
3. Use a probe to locate the **sphenopalatine foramen** near the posterior end of the middle nasal concha.
4. Insert a probe into the sphenopalatine foramen and direct it inferiorly toward the greater palatine foramen of the hard palate. Pull the probe medially to break the medial wall of the palatine canal.
5. Identify the **greater palatine nerve** more anteriorly and the **lesser palatine nerve** more posteriorly within the palatine canal, which supply the hard and soft palates, respectively.
6. Identify the **descending palatine artery** in the palatine canal lateral to the greater and lesser palatine nerves. Recall that the descending palatine artery is one of the terminal branches of the maxillary artery.

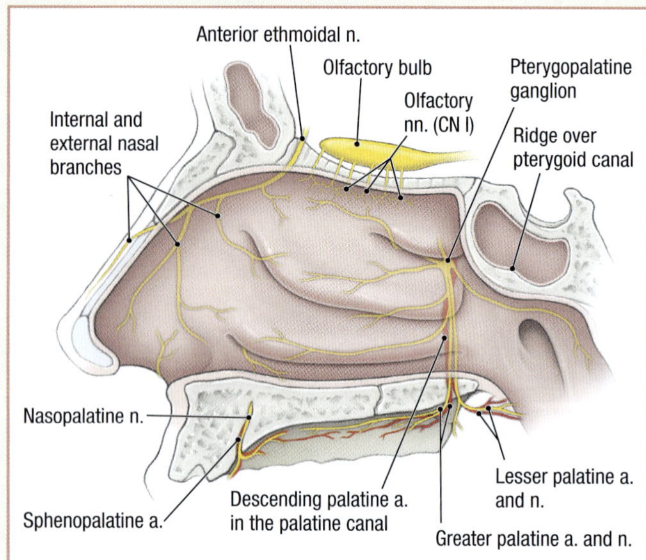

FIGURE 7.82 ● Arterial supply and innervation to mucosa of lateral wall of right nasal cavity. Medial view.

7. At the inferior end of the greater palatine canal, use a fine probe or needle to separate the nerves and vessels. Observe that the descending palatine artery divides into the **greater palatine artery** and **lesser palatine artery,** which supply the hard and soft palates, respectively.
8. Place a fine probe between the greater palatine nerve and the lesser palatine nerve and slide it superiorly until it meets resistance at the inferior border of the **pterygopalatine ganglion.** *Note that the pterygopalatine ganglion stimulates secretion from the mucosa of the nasal cavity, paranasal sinuses, nasopharynx, roof of the mouth, soft palate, and lacrimal gland.*
9. Remove the mucosa from the floor of the sphenoid sinus and look for a ridge marking the location of the pterygoid canal.
10. Use a probe to break open the ridge of bone and identify the **nerve of the pterygoid canal,** which enters the pterygopalatine fossa posteriorly.
11. Confirm that the nerve of the pterygoid canal ends anteriorly in the pterygopalatine ganglion. *Note that the nerve of the pterygoid canal contains presynaptic parasympathetic axons from the greater petrosal nerve and postsynaptic sympathetic axons from the deep petrosal nerve.*
12. Refer to FIGURE 7.83.
13. Turn the cadaver's head to perform the following dissection sequence from the lateral approach.
14. Deep in the **infratemporal fossa,** identify the **maxillary artery** where it courses deeply toward the pterygomaxillary fissure.
15. Near the pterygomaxillary fissure, observe that the maxillary artery gives rise to the **sphenopalatine artery,** which passes through the **pterygopalatine fossa** and then through the sphenopalatine foramen to enter the nasal cavity.
16. Branching from the maxillary artery, identify the **descending palatine artery,** which descends to enter the greater palatine canal, now visible from where it was dissected from the medial side.
17. Identify the **infraorbital artery,** which passes through the inferior orbital fissure to enter the infraorbital canal and emerge on the face through the infraorbital foramen.
18. Identify the **maxillary division of the trigeminal nerve (CN V_2)** where it courses from the foramen rotundum to the inferior orbital fissure. Observe that the maxillary division passes through the pterygopalatine fossa and gives pterygopalatine branches that will form the greater and lesser palatine nerves.

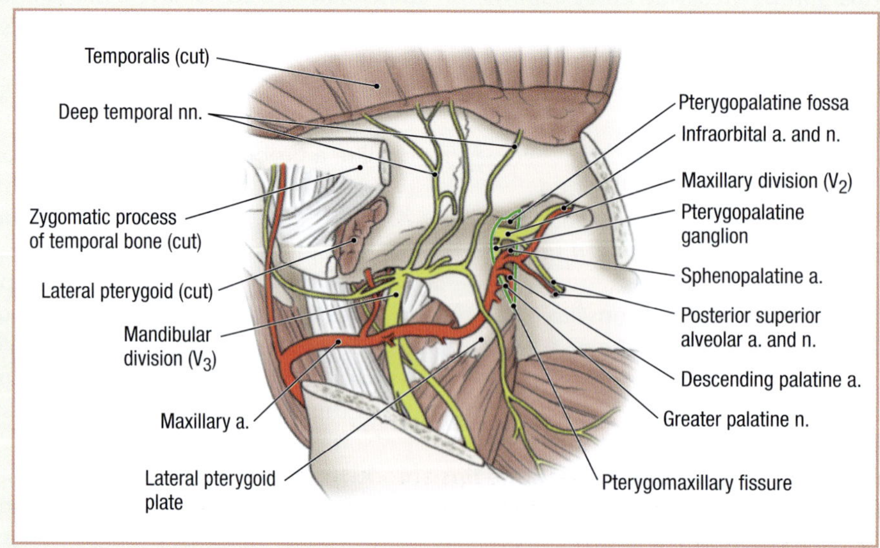

FIGURE 7.83 ● Arteries and nerves of pterygopalatine fossa. Lateral view.

Dissection Follow-up

1. Review the branching pattern of the maxillary division of the trigeminal nerve and use a skull to follow its course through the associated foramina.
2. Review the distribution of the following branches of the maxillary division of the trigeminal nerve: greater palatine, lesser palatine, nasopalatine, and infraorbital nerves.
3. Review the origin of the maxillary artery, its course through the infratemporal fossa, and the course of its branches.
4. Review the attachments, actions, and innervations of the muscles that move the soft palate in **TABLE 7.8**.
5. Review the attachments, actions, and innervations of the pharyngeal muscles in **TABLE 7.8**.
6. Review the pharyngeal plexus on the posterior surface of the pharynx and recall its role in innervation of the pharyngeal mucosa and muscles of the pharynx and soft palate.
7. Review the course of the glossopharyngeal nerve from the jugular foramen to the posterior one-third of the tongue.
8. Replace any reflected tissue back to its anatomical position.

TABLE 7.8 Muscles of Palate and Pharynx

<table>
<tr><th>Muscle</th><th>Superior Attachments</th><th>Inferior Attachments</th><th>Actions</th><th>Innervation</th></tr>
<tr><td>Palatoglossus</td><td>Palatine aponeurosis</td><td>Lateral aspect of tongue</td><td>Elevates tongue and depresses soft palate</td><td rowspan="5">Vagus n. (CN X) via pharyngeal plexus</td></tr>
<tr><td>Palatopharyngeus</td><td>Hard palate and palatine aponeurosis</td><td rowspan="2">Thyroid cartilage and pharyngeal wall</td><td rowspan="2">Elevate larynx during swallowing and speaking</td></tr>
<tr><td>Salpingopharyngeus</td><td>Cartilage of pharyngotympanic tube</td></tr>
<tr><td>Musculus uvulae</td><td>Posterior nasal spine (anterior attachment) and mucosa of uvula (posterior attachment)</td><td rowspan="3">Palatine aponeurosis</td><td rowspan="2">Elevates and retracts uvula</td></tr>
<tr><td>Levator veli palatini</td><td>Cartilage of pharyngotympanic tube and petrous part of temporal bone</td></tr>
<tr><td>Tensor veli palatini</td><td>Scaphoid fossa and spine of sphenoid bone</td><td>Tenses soft palate</td><td>Mandibular division of trigeminal n. (CN V_3)</td></tr>
</table>

Abbreviations: CN, cranial nerve; n., nerve.

ORAL REGION

Dissection Overview

The oral region includes the oral cavity and its contents (teeth, gums, and tongue), the palate, and the part of the oropharynx containing the palatine tonsils. The oral cavity can be subdivided into the oral vestibule, the area bounded by the lips and cheeks externally and the teeth and gums internally, and the oral cavity proper, the area between the alveolar arches and teeth. The largest content of the oral cavity proper is the tongue.

The order of dissection will be as follows: The superficial features of the oral region will be examined. The tongue will be inspected and bisected in the midline with the mandible. The intrinsic muscles of the tongue will be examined. The sublingual region will be studied, and dissection of the deep part of the submandibular gland completed. The extrinsic muscles of the tongue will be studied.

Surface Anatomy

Palpate the following structures in the oral cavity on the cadaver or use a mirror and a clean finger to examine your mouth.

Oral Vestibule

ATLAS 8.60B, 8.69E, 8.98A

1. Refer to FIGURE 7.84.
2. Identify the region of the **oral vestibule** between the **lips** anteriorly and the **teeth** posteriorly.
3. On the **maxilla**, identify the **alveolar processes** and **anterior surface**, the surface of the bone superior to the alveolar processes.
4. Elevate the **upper (superior) lip** and identify the **superior labial frenulum** in the midline attaching from the **gingivae (gums)** to the inner surface of the lip.

5. On the **mandible**, identify the **alveolar processes**.
6. Depress the **lower (inferior) lip** and identify the **inferior labial frenulum** in the midline attaching from the **gingivae (gums)** to the inner surface of the lip.

Oral Cavity Proper

ATLAS 8.64B, 8.65, 8.98A

1. Refer to FIGURE 7.84.
2. Observe that the anterior and lateral borders of the **oral cavity proper** are the teeth and gingivae (gums) of the upper and lower dentition.
3. The superior border (roof) of the oral cavity is the **hard palate** anteriorly and **soft palate** posteriorly, whereas the inferior border (floor) is the mucosa covering the **tongue** and sublingual area.
4. The posterior border of the oral cavity is defined by the **fauces**, the opening to the **oropharynx** bounded by the soft palate superiorly, base of the tongue inferiorly, and right and left **palatoglossal folds (arches)** and **palatopharyngeal folds (arches)** laterally.
5. Observe that the palatoglossal folds are anterior to the palatopharyngeal folds and more visible from the anterior perspective. *Note that the paired palatoglossal and palatopharyngeal folds are often referred to as the anterior and posterior pillars of fauces, respectively.*

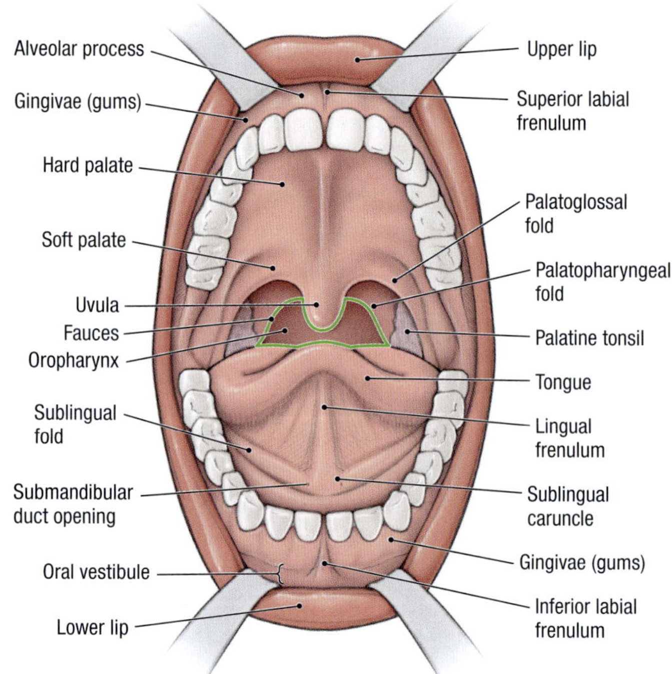

FIGURE 7.84 ● Oral cavity. Anterior view.

6. If present, identify the **palatine tonsil** between the palatoglossal and palatopharyngeal folds.
7. Observe that superiorly, the palatoglossal folds converge medially toward the **uvula**, the midline extension of soft tissue descending from the **soft palate**. *Note that if the head bisection has been completed, the uvula will have been cut in the midline.*
8. Elevate the **tongue** and examine the **sublingual area** to identify the **frenulum of the tongue**, the mucosal fold connecting the inferior aspect of the tongue to the floor of the mouth in the midline.
9. To either side of the frenulum of the tongue, identify a **sublingual fold (plica sublingualis)** overlying the path of the submandibular duct.
10. Observe that the sublingual folds terminate medially at the associated bump of the **sublingual caruncle**.
11. On the surface of the sublingual caruncle, identify the **opening of submandibular duct**. *Note that in a living individual, deep lingual veins are often visible beneath the mucosa on either side of the frenulum of the tongue, which may not be visible in the cadaver.*
12. Examine the inner surface of the cheek and observe that it is continuous with the lips, is lined by mucosa on the inner aspect, and contains the buccinator.
13. Make an effort to identify the opening of the parotid duct lateral to the 2nd maxillary molar on the inner aspect of the cheek.

Dissection Instructions

Tongue

ATLAS 8.57B, 8.58A; VIDEO 7.18.1

1. Refer to FIGURE 7.85.
2. Examine the **tongue** and identify its **apex**, **body** (anterior two-thirds), and **root** (posterior one-third). Observe that the body and root of the tongue are delineated by the **terminal sulcus (sulcus terminalis)**. *Note that the tongue is a muscular organ that can assume a variety of shapes and positions to accommodate speech and swallowing and assist in mastication, taste, and oral cleansing.*
3. Observe that the **lingual tonsils** lie posterior to the terminal sulcus on the root of the tongue.
4. On the **dorsum** of the tongue, follow the **median sulcus** posteriorly to the terminal sulcus and identify the **foramen cecum** in the midline.
5. Examine the surface of the dorsum of the tongue and identify the **lingual papillae** on its mucosal surface anteriorly. *Note that there are four types of lingual papillae: vallate, fungiform, foliate (containing taste buds), and filiform (containing nerve endings for touch).*
6. Observe that the **body of the tongue** lies horizontally in the oral cavity and the **root of the tongue** lies more vertically. *Note that the root of the tongue constitutes the*

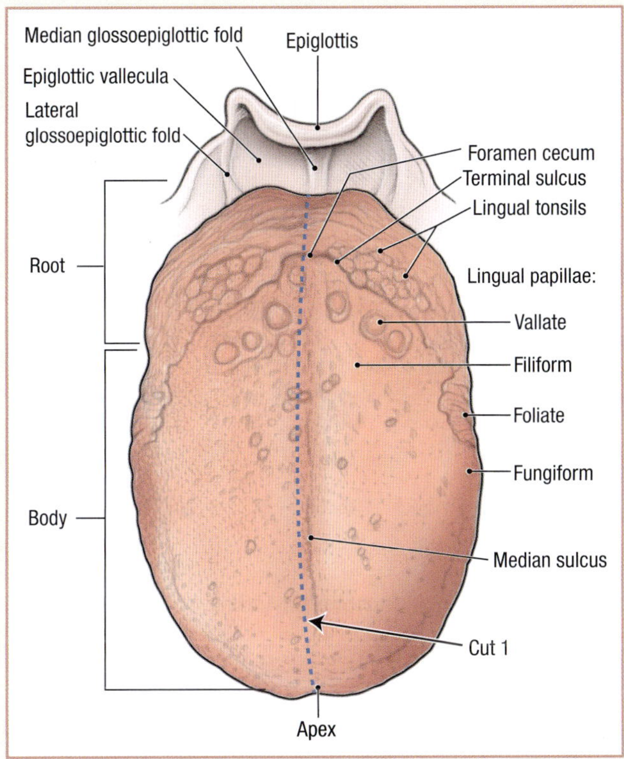

FIGURE 7.85 Dorsum of tongue and incision for tongue bisection. Superior view.

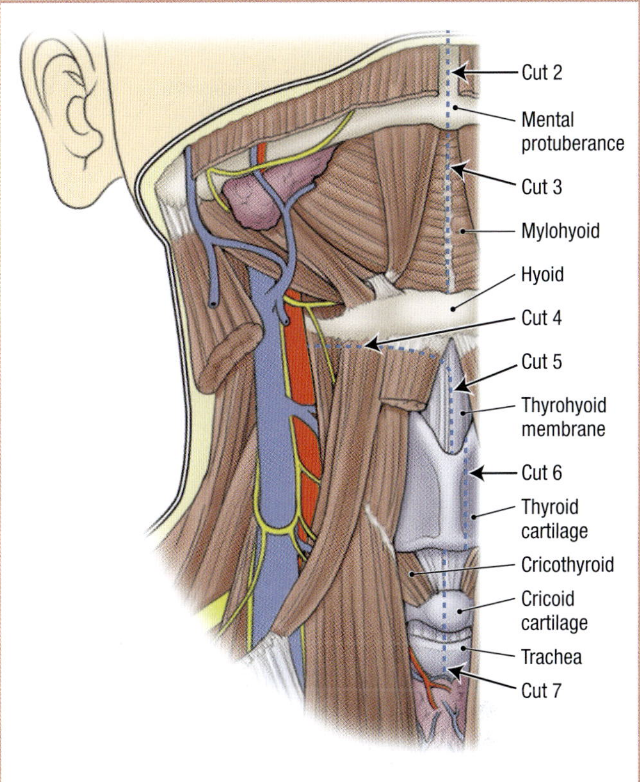

FIGURE 7.86 Incision and cut lines for bisection of mandible, floor of mouth, and larynx. Anterior view.

lower part of the anterior boundary of the oropharynx and contains more lymphatics than taste receptors.

7. At the root of the tongue, identify the **median glossoepiglottic fold**, a midline fold of mucosa between the dorsum of the tongue and **epiglottis**.
8. Lateral to the median glossoepiglottic fold, identify the **lateral glossoepiglottic fold** between the dorsum of the tongue and lateral border of the epiglottis.
9. Identify the **epiglottic valleculae**, the depressions between the median and right and left lateral glossoepiglottic folds.

Bisection of Tongue and Mandible

ATLAS 8.57A, 8.59B, 8.61A; VIDEO 7.18.2

1. Refer to FIGURE 7.85.
2. Use a scalpel to bisect the tongue in the median plane, beginning at the apex and proceeding toward the epiglottis (**Cut 1**), but do not yet cut through the epiglottis. Make the incision through the midline of the tongue through the bulk of the intrinsic muscles, stopping at the level of the floor of the mouth.
3. Refer to FIGURE 7.86.
4. Turn the head to expose the submental triangle.
5. Use a saw to cut through the mandible in the median plane (**Cut 2**).

Dissection Note: Do not allow the saw to pass between the genioglossus on the deep side of the mandible and do not bisect the epiglottis, hyoid bone, or larynx at this time.

6. Use a scalpel to cut the **mylohyoid** along the median raphe (**Cut 3**).
7. Use blunt dissection to separate the mylohyoid from deeper structures.

Sublingual Region

ATLAS 8.58C, 8.62A; VIDEO 7.18.3

Dissection Note: Perform the following dissection sequence on only one side of the head.

1. Refer back to FIGURE 7.80 and to FIGURE 7.87.
2. Identify the cut edge of the **mylohyoid** in the sagittal view of the head.
3. Deep to the mylohyoid, use blunt dissection to identify the **geniohyoid**.
4. On the sectioned surface of the tongue, identify the **genioglossus**.
5. Review the attachments, actions, and innervations of the geniohyoid and genioglossus (see **TABLE 7.9**).
6. Carefully use a scalpel to incise the **sublingual mucosa** along the medial surface of the mandible beginning at the frenulum of the tongue and stopping near the 2nd mandibular molar.
7. Use forceps and blunt dissection to peel the cut edge of mucosa medially and remove it from the dissection field.
8. Identify the **sublingual gland** immediately deep to the mucosa and observe that the sublingual gland

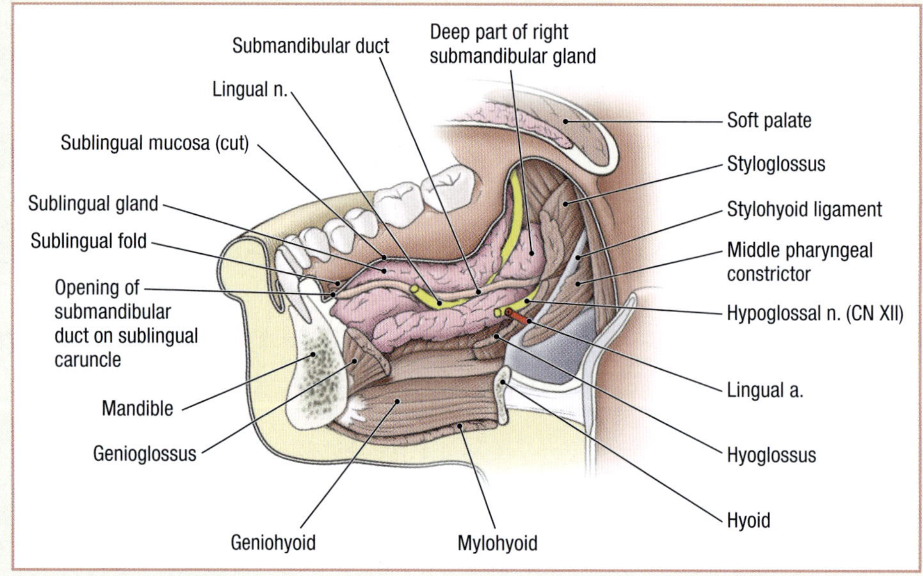

FIGURE 7.87 ● Dissection of right sublingual region with tongue removed. Medial view.

rests on the mylohyoid. *Note that the sublingual gland has about 12 short ducts that drain along the summit of the sublingual fold.*

9. Identify the **submandibular duct** along the medial side of the sublingual gland.
10. Use blunt dissection to follow the submandibular duct anteriorly to its **opening on the sublingual caruncle**.
11. Use blunt dissection to follow the submandibular duct posteriorly to the **deep part of the submandibular gland**. *Note that the deep part of the submandibular gland is located on the superior surface of the mylohyoid.*
12. Turn the cadaver to find the **lingual nerve** in the infratemporal fossa and trace it into the sublingual region.
13. Observe that the lingual nerve first passes lateral, then inferior, and then medial to the submandibular duct. *Note that the lingual nerve has several branches that supply the mucosa of the anterior two-thirds of the tongue with general sensation and taste and general sense to the mucosa on the floor of the mouth and lingual side of the alveolar ridge.*
14. Near the 3rd mandibular molar, identify the **submandibular ganglion** suspended from the lingual nerve. *Note that the submandibular ganglion contains the postsynaptic parasympathetic cell bodies associated with the facial nerve (CN VII) to the submandibular and sublingual glands as well as taste to the anterior two-thirds of the tongue. Recall that the presynaptic parasympathetic fibers from the chorda tympani, a branch of the facial nerve, joined the lingual nerve in the infratemporal fossa to reach the submandibular ganglion.*
15. Refer to FIGURE 7.88.
16. Turn the cadaver so the submandibular triangle is exposed.
17. Use blunt dissection to define the attachment of the **mylohyoid** to the hyoid bone.
18. Use scissors to detach the mylohyoid from the hyoid bone and reflect it superiorly.
19. Identify the **hyoglossus** attaching from the hyoid bone to the root of the tongue.
20. Find the **hypoglossal nerve (CN XII)** and use a probe to trace it into the sublingual region where it passes between the deep part of the submandibular gland and hyoglossus.
21. Observe that both the hypoglossal nerve and lingual nerve pass between the hyoglossus and mylohyoid to enter the sublingual region. *Note that the course of the hypoglossal nerve is inferior to the course of the lingual nerve.*

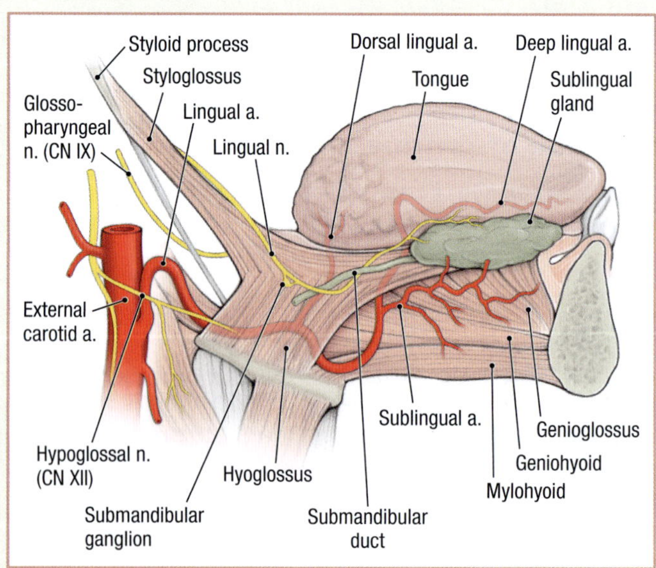

FIGURE 7.88 ● Extrinsic muscles and blood supply to tongue with right half of mandible removed. Right lateral view.

22. Near the superior end of the hyoglossus, identify the **styloglossus**.
23. Review the attachments, actions, and innervations of the hyoglossus and styloglossus (see **TABLE 7.9**).
24. Identify the **intrinsic muscles of the tongue** and observe that they consist of vertical, transverse, superior longitudinal, and inferior longitudinal groups of fibers (see **Clinical Correlation 7.18**). *Note that the intrinsic muscles and three extrinsic muscles of the tongue (styloglossus, genioglossus, and hyoglossus) are innervated by the hypoglossal nerve (CN XII). The palatoglossus, another extrinsic muscle of the tongue, is innervated by CN X via the pharyngeal plexus.*

CLINICAL CORRELATION 7.18

Carotid Endarterectomy and Hypoglossal Nerve Injury

ATLAS 7.14, 7.16, 9.22F

Carotid artery occlusion from atherosclerotic plaque buildup may lead to stenosis and thus require removal of the plaque surgically (carotid endarterectomy). As the hypoglossal nerve courses lateral to the carotid vessels, it is prone to damage during an open carotid endarterectomy. To test hypoglossal nerve function, a physician will ask the patient to protrude or "stick out" the tongue. As the genioglossus protrudes the tongue and is innervated by the hypoglossal nerve, the functional side of the tongue will protrude normally, whereas the dysfunctional side protrudes less or not at all. Therefore, in testing for hypoglossal nerve lesions, the protruded tongue deviates toward the side of the nerve lesion.

25. Return to the carotid triangle and locate the **lingual artery** where it arises from the external carotid artery.
26. Follow the lingual artery superiorly until it passes medial to the hyoglossus where it gives rise to the **dorsal lingual artery**.
27. Continue to follow the lingual artery to the point where the **sublingual artery** branches arise and the name changes to the **deep lingual artery**. *Note that the deep lingual artery is usually located within 5 mm of the inferior surface of the tongue.*

Dissection Follow-up

1. Review the surface features of the tongue.
2. Review the innervation of the lingual mucosa.
3. Review the path of the submandibular duct from the submandibular triangle to the sublingual caruncle.
4. Trace the lingual nerve from the infratemporal fossa to the tongue, noting its relationship to the submandibular duct, hyoglossus, and mylohyoid.
5. Review the location of the chorda tympani and the role it plays in sensory innervation of the tongue and parasympathetic innervation of the submandibular and sublingual glands.
6. Trace the hypoglossal nerve from the base of the skull to the tongue, noting its relationships to arteries and muscles.
7. Review the attachments, actions, and innervations of the extrinsic muscles of the tongue and oral cavity in **TABLE 7.9**.
8. Review the origin and course of the facial and lingual arteries.
9. Return any reflected tissue back to its anatomical position.

TABLE 7.9 Muscles of Tongue and Oral Cavity

Muscle	*Superior Attachments*	*Inferior Attachments*	*Actions*	*Innervation*
Geniohyoid	Inferior mental spine of mandible (anterior attachment)	Body of hyoid bone (posterior attachment)	Pulls hyoid bone anteriorly	C1 via hypoglossal n. (CN XII)
Genioglossus	Superior mental spine of mandible (anterior attachment)	Hyoid bone and tongue (posterior attachment)	Depresses and protrudes tongue	Hypoglossal n. (CN XII)
Hyoglossus	Side and inferior aspect of tongue	Body and greater horn of hyoid bone	Depresses and retracts tongue	
Styloglossus	Styloid process and stylohyoid ligament	Side and inferior aspect of tongue	Retracts tongue and draws it superiorly	

Abbreviations: C, cervical vertebrae; CN, cranial nerve; n., nerve.

LARYNX

Dissection Overview

The larynx is contained in the visceral compartment of the neck anterior to the pharynx and medial and posterior to the thyroid gland. In its neutral position, the larynx is located at vertebral levels C3–C6, although its height varies during speech and swallowing. The skeleton of the larynx is responsible for maintaining a patent airway and consists of a series of articulated cartilages united by thin membranes. The glottis, a valve-like opening in the larynx, serves the dual function of controlling the airway and producing sound during phonation. The *intrinsic* muscles of the larynx control the glottis. The *extrinsic* muscles of the larynx (infrahyoids, suprahyoids, and stylopharyngeus) control the position of the larynx in the neck.

The order of dissection will be as follows: The cartilages of the larynx will be studied. The mucosa of the posterior part of the larynx will be to expose two intrinsic muscles. The left lamina of the thyroid cartilage will be removed to expose the remaining intrinsic muscles. The larynx will be opened and the mucosal features studied. The nerves to the larynx will be reviewed.

Skeletal Anatomy

Skeleton of Larynx

ATLAS 7.30

Use a model of the larynx and the cadaver to study the laryngeal cartilages and membranes.

1. Refer to FIGURE 7.89.
2. Identify the unpaired **epiglottic cartilage** posterior to the tongue and hyoid bone.
3. Observe that the **stalk** of the epiglottic cartilage is attached to the inner surface of the angle formed by the thyroid laminae.
4. Inferior to the hyoid bone, identify the **thyroid cartilage** and palpate the **laryngeal prominence (Adam's apple)** where the two **laminae** join in the anterior midline.
5. Identify the **thyrohyoid membrane** between the superior border of the thyroid cartilage and the inferior border of the hyoid bone. *Note that when the suprahyoid and infrahyoid muscles move the hyoid bone, the larynx also moves because of the thyrohyoid membrane.*
6. Observe that the **superior horn** of the thyroid cartilage projects superiorly, whereas the **inferior horn** of the thyroid cartilage projects inferiorly and articulates with the **cricoid cartilage** at the small synovial **cricothyroid joints**.
7. Observe that the **cricoid cartilage** is shaped like a ring, its **lamina** is a broad flat area positioned posteriorly, and its **arch** is located anteriorly.

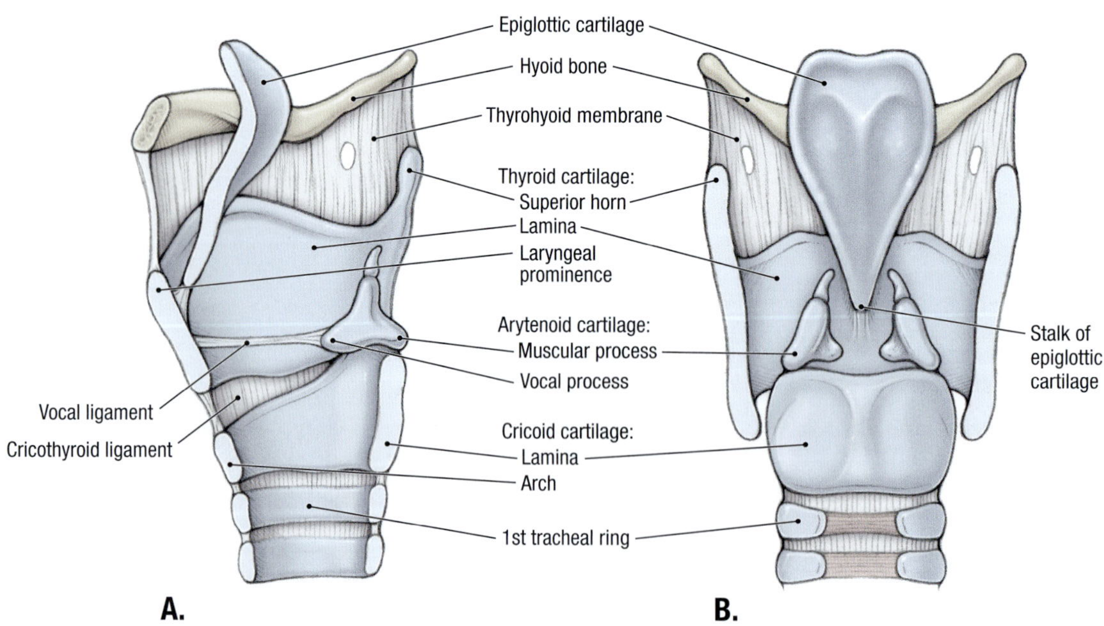

FIGURE 7.89 ● Laryngeal skeleton. **A.** Medial view in midsagittal section. **B.** Posterior view.

8. Identify the **arytenoid cartilages** on the posterior aspect of the superior border of the lamina of the cricoid cartilage.
9. Observe that each arytenoid cartilage is pyramid shaped and articulates with the cricoid cartilage through a synovial joint.
10. On the arytenoid cartilage, identify the **muscular process**, the attachment site for intrinsic laryngeal muscles, and the **vocal process**, the posterior attachment site of the **vocal ligament**.
11. Observe that the anterior end of each vocal ligament is attached to the inner surface of the thyroid cartilage at the angle formed by the laminae. *Note that each arytenoid cartilage can tilt anteriorly and posteriorly, rotate, slide toward the other side (adduction), and slide away from the other side (abduction).*

Dissection Instructions

Intrinsic Muscles of Larynx

ATLAS 7.31, 7.33; VIDEO 7.19.1

1. Refer back to FIGURE 7.86 and to FIGURE 7.90.
2. Identify the **cricothyroid** on the external surface of the larynx and recall that it was innervated by external branch of the superior laryngeal nerve while the internal branch pierced the **thyrohyoid membrane**.
3. To expose the posterior surface of the larynx, move the cadaver's head forward and allow the chin to rest on the thoracic wall.
4. Spread open the posterior wall of the pharynx to expose the posterior surface of the larynx and palpate the **lamina of the cricoid cartilage**.
5. Lateral to the lamina, identify the depression of the **piriform recess**.
6. Examine the vocal folds from a superior view and identify the **rima glottidis**, the interval between the vocal folds. *Note that the rima glottidis and the vocal folds collectively are called the glottis.*
7. Use blunt dissection to remove the mucosa from the piriform recess and identify the **internal branch of the superior laryngeal nerve** and **superior laryngeal artery**.
8. Observe that the **recurrent laryngeal nerve** enters the larynx by passing posterior to the **cricothyroid joint** where its name changes to **inferior laryngeal nerve**. *Note that physicians often refer to the entire length of the nerve as simply the recurrent laryngeal nerve.*
9. Use blunt dissection to strip the mucosa from the lamina of the cricoid cartilage and expose the **posterior cricoarytenoid**, the only muscle that opens the rima glottidis.

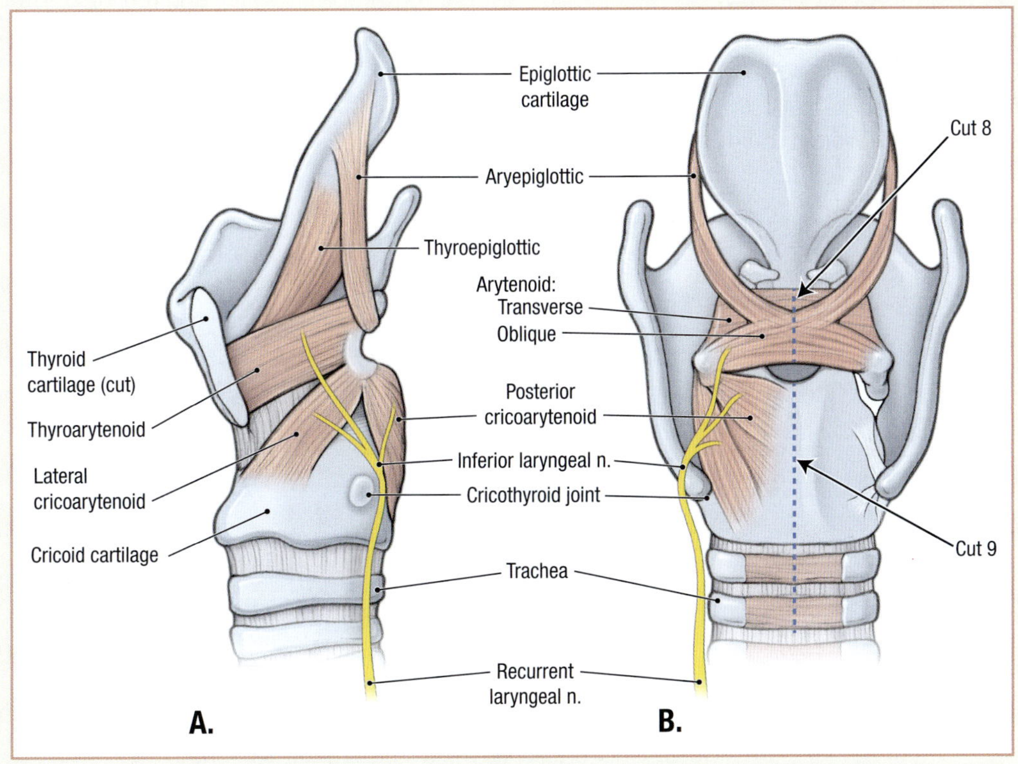

FIGURE 7.90 ● Intrinsic muscles of larynx. **A.** Lateral view. **B.** Posterior view.

10. Superior to the posterior cricoarytenoid, identify the **arytenoid** attaching to both arytenoid cartilages.
11. Observe that the arytenoid has **transverse** and **oblique fibers**. *Note that the arytenoid slides the arytenoid cartilages together (adduction of the vocal folds).*
12. On the left side only, use scissors to disarticulate the cricothyroid joint. *Note that the cricothyroid joint is a synovial joint that is reinforced by short ligaments.*
13. Return the head back to its anatomical position.
14. On the left side only, use scissors to make a horizontal incision through the thyrohyoid near its attachment to the hyoid (**Cut 4**) and reflect the muscle inferiorly. Similarly, if not already done previously, make horizontal incisions through the superior attachments of the sternohyoid and sternothyroid on the left side and reflect them inferiorly.
15. Make a horizontal incision through the **thyrohyoid membrane** near its attachment to the hyoid and a vertical incision through the midline of the membrane (**Cut 5**) while sparing the internal branch of the superior laryngeal nerve and superior laryngeal artery.
16. Make a vertical incision through the left lamina of the thyroid cartilage 5 mm to the left of the midline (**Cut 6**). Reflect the thyroid lamina inferiorly and detach it from the cricothyroid.
17. Medial to the thyroid lamina that was removed, identify the **lateral cricoarytenoid**.
18. Identify the **thyroarytenoid** superior to the lateral cricoarytenoid. *Note that the vocalis is formed by the medial fibers of the thyroarytenoid, although often difficult to distinguish in the cadaver. The vocalis is attached to the vocal ligament and modifies the tension in localized parts of the vocal fold, modulating pitch.*
19. Make an effort to identify the delicate muscles of the larynx superior to the thyroarytenoid, the **thyroepiglottic** and **aryepiglottic**.
20. Review the attachments, actions, and innervations of the muscles of the larynx (see **TABLE 7.10**).
21. Continue to cut inferiorly in the anterior midline through the cricothyroid ligament, cricoid cartilage, and 1st tracheal ring (**Cut 7**).

Interior of Larynx

ATLAS 7.32, 7.34B, 7.34D; VIDEO 7.19.2

1. Refer to FIGURE 7.90.
2. To expose the posterior surface of the larynx, move the cadaver's head forward and allow the chin to rest on the thoracic wall.
3. In the posterior midline, cut the transverse and oblique arytenoids (**Cut 8**).
4. Cut the cricoid cartilage and trachea in the midline posteriorly (**Cut 9**).
5. Refer to FIGURE 7.91.
6. Open the larynx and examine the **laryngeal cavity**.
7. Inspect the mucosa that lines the interior of the larynx and identify the **vestibular fold (false vocal fold)** superiorly, and the **vocal fold (true vocal fold)** inferiorly, which contains the **vocal ligament** (see **Clinical Correlation 7.19**).

CLINICAL CORRELATION 7.19

Laryngospasm

ATLAS 7.32, 7.35

Laryngospasm is a life-threatening spasmodic closure of the glottis, the opening between the vocal folds. Spasms of the intrinsic laryngeal muscles that close the glottis may be produced by irritating chemicals, severe allergic reactions, and sometimes as a side effect of medications.

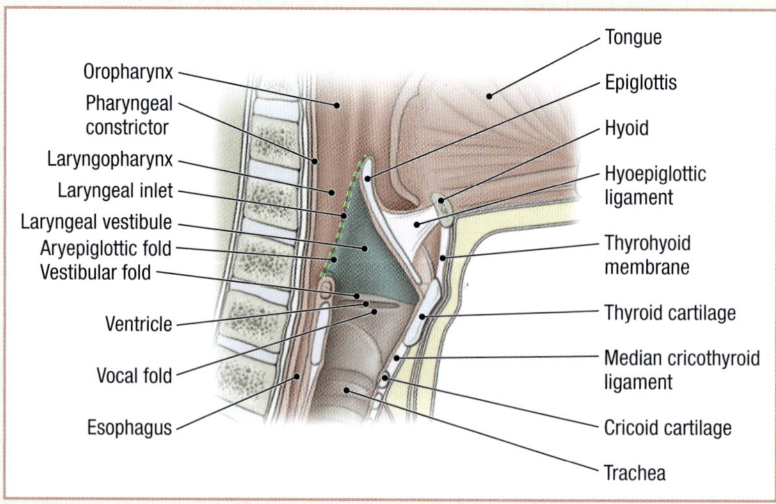

FIGURE 7.91 ● Mucosal features of larynx in midsagittal section. Medial view.

The vocal cords and larynx can be visualized using direct laryngoscopy (viewed with a direct line of sight by a rigid laryngoscope) or indirect laryngoscopy (viewed through a mirror or camera by a flexible laryngoscope). Persistent hoarseness is an indication for laryngoscopy and may be caused by changes of the vocal folds or may indicate that the recurrent laryngeal nerve is compromised in the thorax or neck.

8. Identify the **vestibule**, the space superior to the vestibular folds; the **ventricle**, the depression between the vestibular and vocal folds; and the **infraglottic cavity**, the region inferior to the vocal folds continuous with the trachea.
9. Examine the **epiglottis** and note that it moves inferiorly during swallowing to close the laryngeal inlet as the remainder of the larynx elevates.
10. Use a blunt probe to explore the space of the **ventricle** and, if present, the **saccule**, a small recess arising from the cavity of the ventricle.
11. Observe that the **internal branch of the superior laryngeal nerve** passes through the thyrohyoid membrane to provide sensory innervation to the mucosa of the vocal fold and mucosa superior to the vocal folds.
12. Observe that the **external branch of the superior laryngeal nerve** remains external to the larynx to innervate the cricothyroid and inferior pharyngeal constrictors.
13. Observe that the **inferior laryngeal branch of the recurrent laryngeal nerve** enters the larynx inferiorly to innervate the intrinsic muscles of the larynx, except the cricothyroid, and provides sensory innervation to the mucosa inferior to the vocal folds.

Dissection Follow-up

1. Use a cross-sectional drawing of the neck and the dissected specimen to review the relationship of the larynx to the vertebral column, carotid sheaths, and other cervical viscera.
2. Trace the right and left vagus nerves into the thorax and follow the recurrent laryngeal nerves from the thorax to the larynx, noting the differences.
3. Review the blood supply to the larynx beginning at the external carotid artery.
4. Review the pattern of sensory innervation to the larynx.
5. Review the attachments, actions, and innervations of the intrinsic laryngeal muscles in **TABLE 7.10**.
6. Replace the head and reflected laryngeal tissue in their correct anatomical positions.

TABLE 7.10 Muscles of Larynx

Muscle	*Superior Attachments*	*Inferior Attachments*	*Actions*	*Innervation*
Cricothyroid	Inferior margin and inferior horn of thyroid cartilage	Anterolateral surface of cricoid cartilage	Tilts thyroid cartilage anteriorly to lengthen (tense) vocal folds	External branch of superior laryngeal n. (CN X)
Posterior cricoarytenoid	Muscular process of arytenoid cartilage	Posterior surface of lamina of cricoid cartilage	Rotates arytenoid cartilage laterally to abduct vocal folds	Inferior laryngeal n. (continuation of recurrent laryngeal n.) (CN X)
Lateral cricoarytenoid		Arch of cricoid cartilage	Rotates arytenoid cartilage medially to adduct vocal folds	
Thyroarytenoid		Posterior surface of thyroid cartilage	Tilts arytenoid cartilage anteriorly to relax vocal folds	

Abbreviations: CN, cranial nerve; n., nerve.

EAR

Dissection Overview

The ear is composed of three parts: external, middle, and internal. The external ear consists of the auricle and external acoustic meatus. The middle ear (tympanic cavity) is enclosed within the temporal bone and contains the ossicles (bones of the middle ear). The internal ear (vestibulocochlear organ) is the neurologic part of the ear and is contained within the petrous part of the temporal bone.

The order of dissection will be as follows: The parts of the external ear will be examined. The facial nerve will be followed into the internal acoustic meatus, and the roof of the tympanic cavity will be removed. The auditory ossicles will be identified, and one ossicle will be removed. The temporal bone will be cut to reveal the medial and lateral walls of the tympanic cavity. The tympanic membrane will be studied. Features of the medial wall of the tympanic cavity will be examined.

Skeletal Anatomy

Skeleton of Ear

On a skull with the calvaria removed, review the following skeletal features.

Temporal Bone

ATLAS 8.3A, 8.10, 8.82A, 8.94A

1. Refer to FIGURE 7.92.
2. On the floor of the middle cranial fossa, identify the **tegmen tympani**, the portion of temporal bone forming the roof of the tympanic cavity.
3. Identify the **groove for the greater petrosal nerve** coursing medially near the roof of the carotid canal.
4. On the posterior surface of the petrous part of the temporal bone within the posterior cranial fossa, identify the **internal acoustic meatus**.
5. From a lateral view, identify the **external acoustic meatus** anterior to the **mastoid process**.
6. From an inferior view, identify the **stylomastoid foramen** between the mastoid process and **styloid process**.
7. Medial to the stylomastoid foramen, identify the **jugular fossa**, the depression immediately anterior to the jugular foramen. Observe the proximity of the jugular fossa and **opening of the carotid canal**.
8. Anterior to the round opening of the **carotid canal**, identify the irregular borders leading to the bony portion of the **pharyngotympanic tube**.

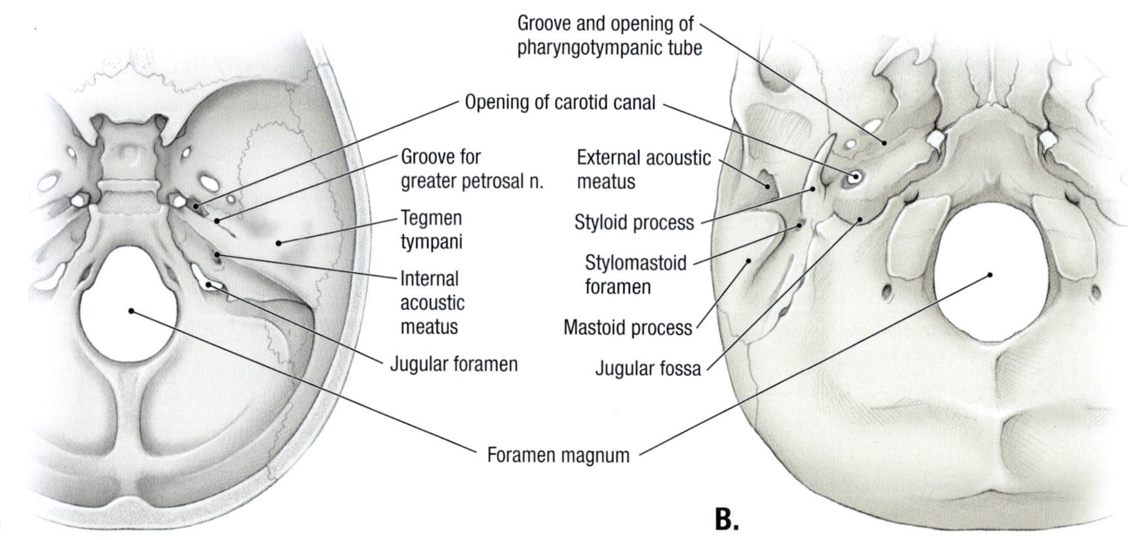

FIGURE 7.92 ● Temporal bone. **A.** Superior view. **B.** Inferior view.

Surface Anatomy

External Ear

ATLAS 8.85

1. Refer to FIGURE 7.93.
2. On the cadaver, examine the **auricle (pinna)**, the visible portion of the external ear.
3. Identify the **helix**, the rim of the auricle paralleled by a more anteriorly located, rounded prominence of auricular cartilage, the **antihelix**.

4. Follow the helix superiorly and anteriorly until it curves around the antihelix and leads to the **concha**, the deepest part of the auricle.
5. Anterior to the opening of the **external acoustic meatus**, identify the **tragus** and observe that it is directed posteriorly toward the **antitragus**.
6. On the inferior aspect of the auricle, identify the **lobule of the auricle (earlobe)**. Observe that **auricular cartilage** gives the auricle its shape. *Note that there is no cartilage in the lobule.*
7. Palpate the auricular cartilage and verify that it is continuous with the cartilage of the external acoustic meatus. *Note that the external acoustic meatus begins at the deepest part of the concha and ends at the tympanic membrane (a distance of about 2.5 cm in adults). The wall of the outer one-third of the external acoustic meatus is cartilaginous and the inner two-thirds is bony.*

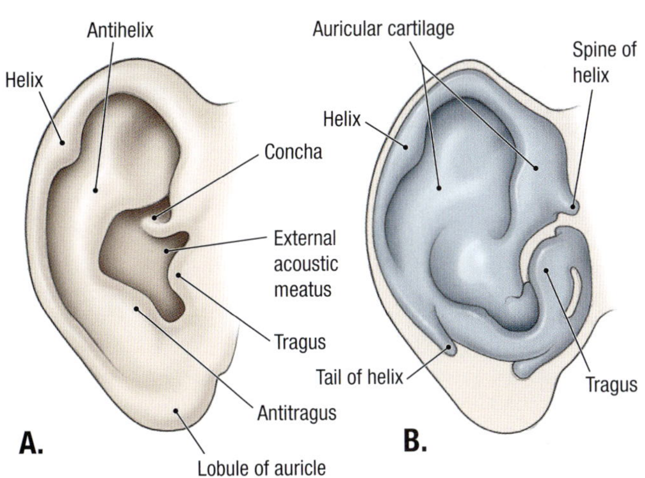

FIGURE 7.93 ● **A.** Surface anatomy of external ear. **B.** Auricular cartilage. Lateral views.

Dissection Instructions

Tympanic Cavity from Superior Approach

ATLAS 8.86, 8.91, 8.94; VIDEO 7.20.1

Dissection Note: The tympanic cavity (middle ear) will be approached by removing the tegmen tympani portion of the floor of the middle cranial fossa on only one side of the head. Remember to wear eye protection when cutting bone.

1. Refer to FIGURE 7.94.
2. If the dura mater is still present in the middle cranial fossa of the cadaver, peel it off the superior surface of the temporal bone beginning at the superior border of the petrous part of the temporal bone in an anterior direction.
3. Look for the **greater petrosal nerve** in the groove for the greater petrosal nerve. *Note that the greater petrosal nerve lies between the dura mater and bone.*
4. In the posterior cranial fossa, identify the **facial nerve (CN VII)** and **vestibulocochlear nerve (CN VIII)** as they enter the internal acoustic meatus.
5. Use a hammer and the tip of a probe or small chisel to gently break through the roof of the internal acoustic meatus. Follow the **facial** and **vestibulocochlear nerves** laterally as they pass through the internal acoustic meatus, remaining superior to the nerves when cutting the roof of the internal acoustic meatus.
6. Remove the small portions of the broken tegmen tympani and follow the facial nerve laterally until it makes a sharp bend in the posterior direction and identify the **geniculate ganglion**. *Note that the geniculate ganglion contains cell bodies of sensory neurons.*
7. Make an effort to identify the origin of the greater petrosal nerve from the geniculate ganglion within the bone. *The greater petrosal nerve carries presynaptic parasympathetic fibers to the pterygopalatine ganglion for innervation of the mucous membranes of the nasal and upper oral cavities and lacrimal gland.*
8. Follow the greater petrosal nerve and observe that it passes inferiorly and medially in the **groove for the greater petrosal nerve** on the surface of the temporal bone.
9. Observe that the greater petrosal nerve joins the deep petrosal nerve to form the **nerve of the pterygoid canal** on the surface of the internal carotid artery after it emerges from the carotid canal near the opening of the foramen lacerum. *Note that the nerve of the pterygoid canal carries the presynaptic fibers of the greater petrosal nerve to the pterygopalatine ganglion.*
10. Observe that at the geniculate ganglion, the facial nerve travels a short distance in a posterolateral direction and then turns inferiorly to exit the skull at the stylomastoid foramen via the facial canal. Do not attempt to follow the facial nerve deeply through the temporal bone.
11. Identify the location of the **cochlea** anterior to the internal acoustic meatus in the angle formed by the facial nerve, geniculate ganglion, and greater petrosal nerve.
12. Remove a portion of the tegmen tympani anterior to the facial nerve to identify the **modiolus of the cochlea**, the central axis. *Note that the visibility of the modiolus in the cadaver largely depends on the plane of the cut.*
13. In the dissected cadaver, remove a portion of the tegmen tympani posterior to the facial nerve and identify the **semicircular canals**, which appear as a series of tiny holes in the bone posterior to the internal acoustic meatus.

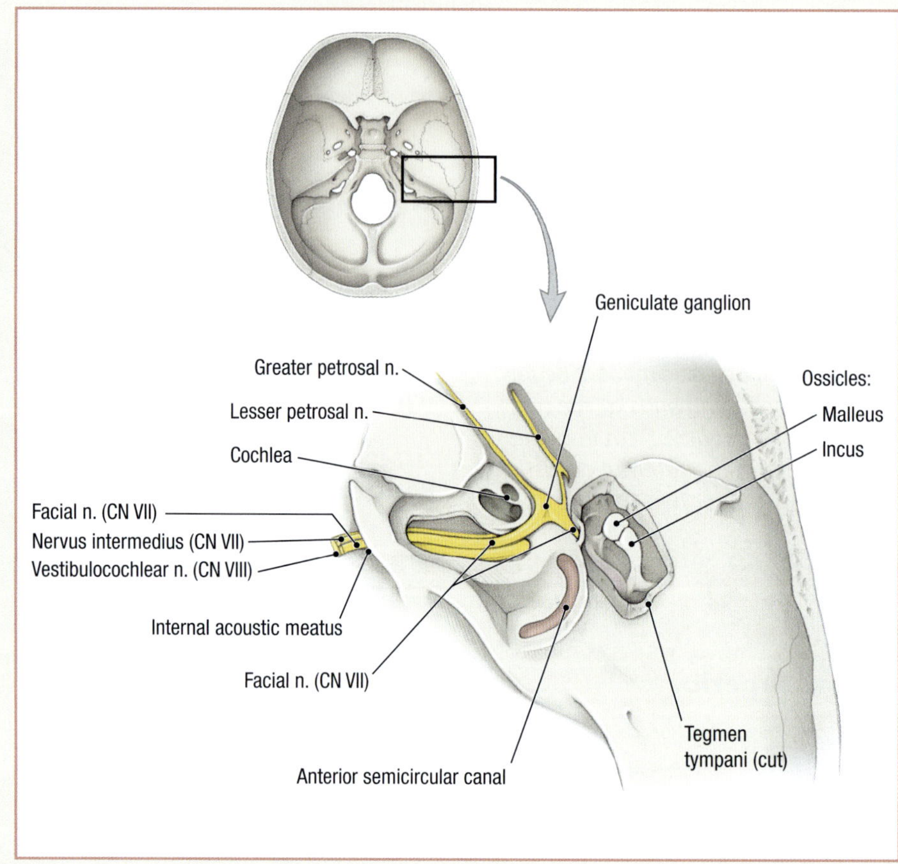

FIGURE 7.94 ● Right middle ear after removal of tegmen tympani. Superior view.

14. Expand the opening in the roof of the **tympanic cavity** by removing additional portions of the **tegmen tympani** laterally and confirm it is an air-filled space within the temporal bone.
15. Within the tympanic cavity, identify the **auditory ossicles**.
16. Observe that the **malleus** is attached to the tympanic membrane, the **incus** occupies an intermediate position, and the **stapes** is the most medial of the auditory ossicles. *Note that the malleus and incus should easily be seen from the superior view but that the stapes is located more inferiorly and may be harder to see.*
17. Use fine forceps to disarticulate and remove the incus leaving the malleus attached to the tympanic membrane.
18. Looking down from above, identify the **tympanic membrane** on the lateral wall of the tympanic cavity. Attempt to identify the tendon of the tensor tympani, a thin strand of tissue spanning from the medial wall of the tympanic cavity to the handle of the malleus.

Sectioning of Tympanic Cavity

ATLAS 8.87, 8.92

Dissection Note: The following dissection approach is intended for use on a decalcified temporal bone. If a decalcified temporal bone is not available, you may skip the following dissection protocol and proceed to the middle ear sequence.

1. Refer to FIGURE 7.95.
2. With the blade angled parallel to the internal surface of the tympanic membrane, insert a scalpel blade into the opening created after removal of the incus. Make a

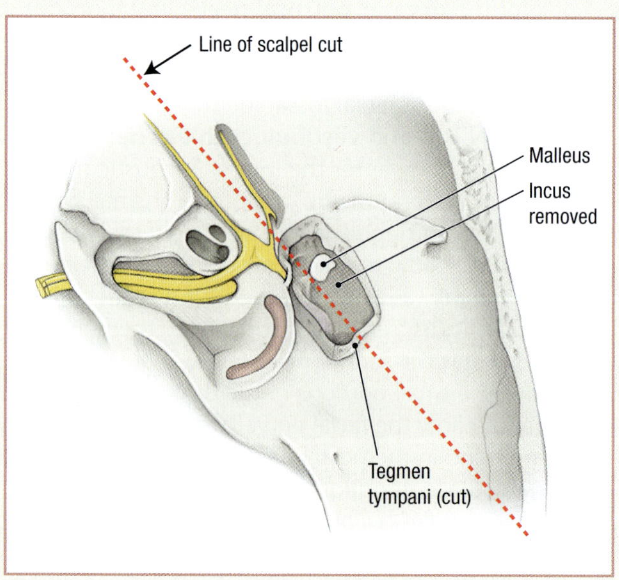

FIGURE 7.95 ● Angle of cut to separate medial and lateral walls of tympanic cavity. Superior view.

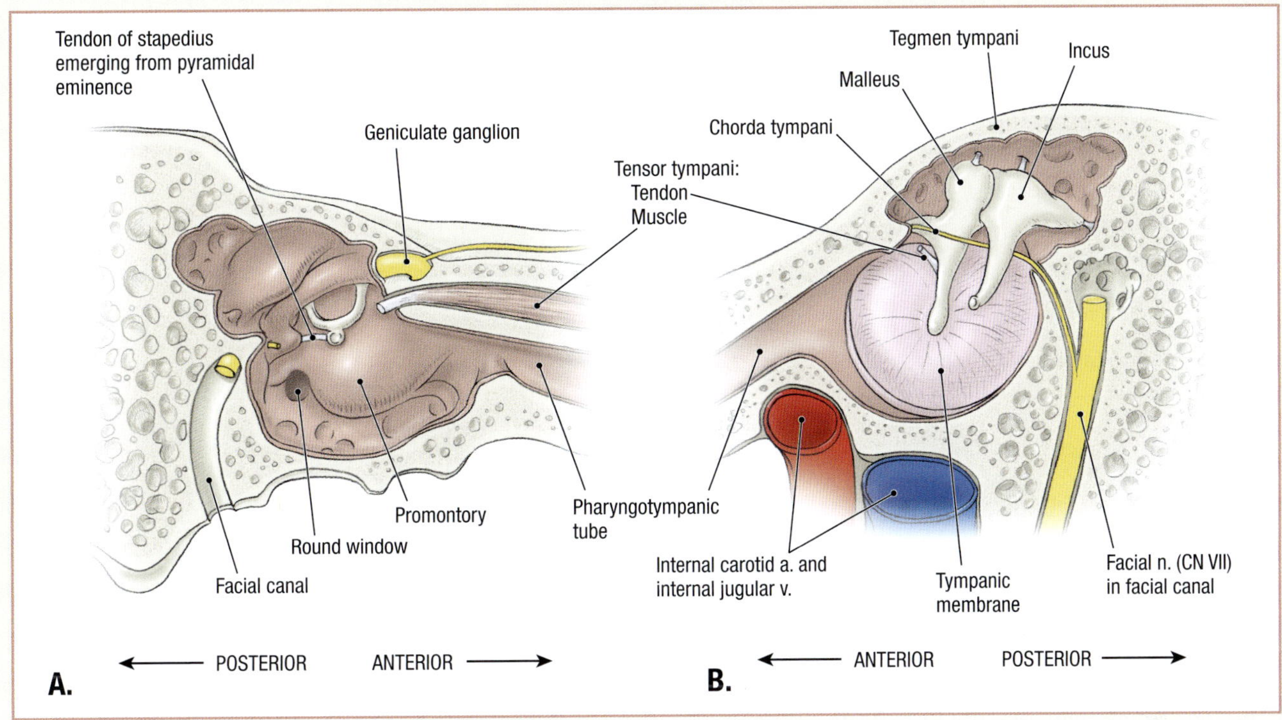

FIGURE 7.96 ■ Walls of right tympanic cavity opened like a book. **A.** Medial wall. **B.** Lateral wall.

cut extending anteriorly down the pharyngotympanic tube that divides the middle ear into medial and lateral walls. *Note that the cut through the pharyngotympanic tube should course parallel to the superior border of the petrous part of the temporal bone.*

3. Refer to FIGURE 7.96.
4. On the lateral wall of the tympanic cavity, examine the tympanic membrane and identify the **chorda tympani**. Observe that the chorda tympani courses between the malleus and incus.
5. On the medial wall of the tympanic cavity, identify the elevation of the **promontory**.
6. Superior to the promontory, identify the **stapes** still attached to the **oval window (fenestra vestibuli)**. Look for the **stapedius tendon**, about 1 mm long, passing from the pyramidal eminence to the stapes. *Note that the stapedius is innervated by the facial nerve (CN VII).*
7. Inferior to the stapes, identify the **round window (fenestra cochleae)** posteroinferior to the promontory.
8. Identify the **tensor tympani** attaching to the pharyngotympanic tube and sphenoid bone medially and the manubrium (handle) of the malleus laterally. *Note that the tensor tympani is innervated by the mandibular division of the trigeminal nerve (CN V_3).*
9. Observe that the tendon of the tensor tympani crosses the tympanic cavity.
10. Observe that the tympanic cavity and its associated recesses and air cells are covered with mucous membrane. *Note that the tympanic branch of the glossopharyngeal nerve (CN IX) innervates the mucous membrane of the tympanic cavity and forms the tympanic plexus under the mucosa covering the promontory.*

Walls of Tympanic Cavity

ATLAS 8.90, 8.92, 8.93D, 8.93E

1. Refer to FIGURE 7.97 to familiarize yourself with the features of the tympanic cavity.
2. Observe that the tympanic cavity is separated from the external acoustic meatus by the **tympanic membrane** and from the middle cranial fossa by the **tegmen tympani**.
3. Identify the **lateral wall** of the tympanic cavity formed by the tympanic membrane (see **Clinical Correlation 7.20**).

CLINICAL CORRELATION 7.20

Otitis Media

ATLAS 8.87, 8.88, 8.90

An "ear infection" is typically caused by inflammation of the middle ear cavity (otitis media), which may occur rapidly with ear pain, difficulty sleeping, loss of appetite, and fever, or may be painless with effusion (fluid accumulation) over time. A burst "ear drum" or perforation of the tympanic membrane may result from otitis media, foreign bodies entering the external acoustic meatus, trauma, or increased pressure.

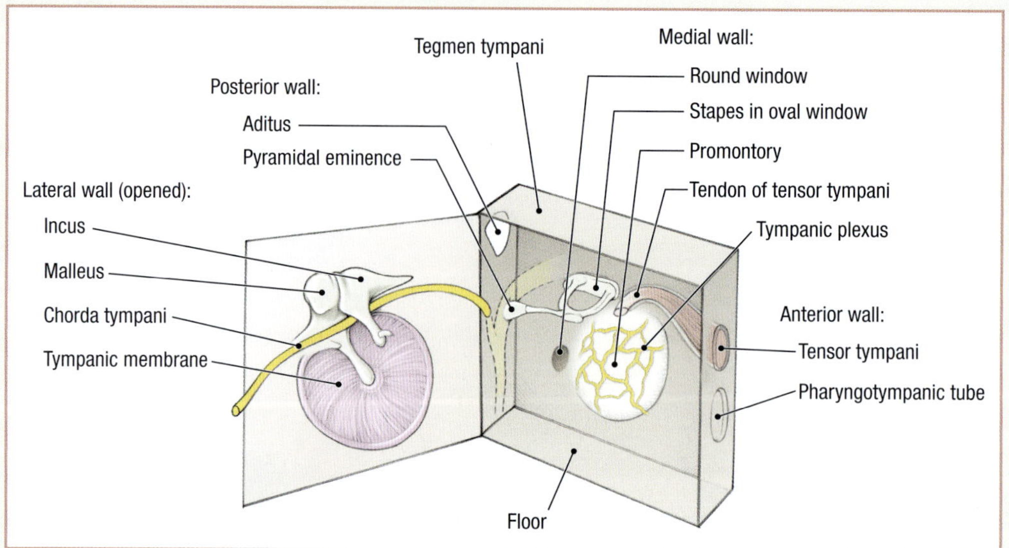

FIGURE 7.97 ■ Schematic of walls of right tympanic cavity with lateral wall opened. Anterolateral view.

4. Along the superior aspect of the **posterior wall** of the tympanic cavity, identify the **aditus**, an opening into the **mastoid air cells** within the mastoid process.
5. Identify the **medial wall** of the tympanic cavity containing the rounded **promontory** and **oval window (fenestra vestibuli)** occupied by the base (footplate) of the **stapes**.
6. Observe that the **anterior wall** of the tympanic cavity contains the opening of the **pharyngotympanic tube**.
7. Identify the **superior wall (roof)** of the tympanic cavity formed by the tegmen tympani of the temporal bone.
8. Observe that the **inferior wall (floor)** of the tympanic cavity is closely related to the **jugular fossa** and **jugular bulb**.

Dissection Follow-up

1. Review the external appearance of the tympanic membrane.
2. Relate the tympanic membrane to the handle of the malleus and chorda tympani.
3. Review the course of the facial nerve from the internal acoustic meatus to the muscles of facial expression.
4. Review the course of the greater petrosal nerve from the geniculate ganglion to the pterygopalatine ganglion and summarize the distribution of the postsynaptic axons that arise in the pterygopalatine ganglion.
5. Review the location of the cell bodies for the sensory axons of special sense related to the chorda tympani.
6. Review all branches of the glossopharyngeal nerve, including those that give rise to the lesser petrosal nerve.
7. Return all reflected tissue to its anatomical position.

Index

NOTE: Page numbers followed by the letter *b* refer to boxes; those followed by letter *f* refer to figures; and those followed by the letter *t* refer to tables.

B

C

G

H

I

J

M

N

Q

R

S

T